Manual for Pharmacy Technicians

Second Edition

 American Society of Health-System Pharmacists®

Any correspondence regarding this publication should be sent to the publisher, American Society of Health-System Pharmacists, 7272 Wisconsin Avenue, Bethesda, MD 20814.

The information presented herein reflects the opinions of the contributors and reviewers. It should not be interpreted as an official policy of ASHP or as an endorsement of any product.

Drug information is constantly evolving because of ongoing research and clinical experience, and it is often subject to interpretation and the uniqueness of the clinical situation. ASHP has made every effort to ensure the accuracy and completeness of the information presented in this book. However, the reader is advised that the publisher, contributors, and reviewers cannot be responsible for the continued currency of the information, for any errors or omissions, or for any consequences arising therefrom.

Produced by the American Society of Health-System Pharmacists' Product Development Office.

Cover and Page Design: Hector L. Coronado

ISBN: 1-879907-79-8

Preface

This second edition of the *Manual for Pharmacy Technicians* was published by the American Society of Health-System Pharmacists in cooperation with the Illinois Council of Health-System Pharmacists (ICHP). The purpose of the second edition is to provide a comprehensive text that addresses topics and subjects relevant to pharmacy technicians in all practice settings. With this in mind, ICHP conscientiously selected a mix of technicians and pharmacists from various practice settings to contribute to the publication.

The focus of the second edition was broadened to include new chapters on the home care and ambulatory care practice settings, drug classifications and pharmacologic actions, and drug information resources that are commonly used in pharmacy practice. The chapters from the first edition were updated and revised to focus on ambulatory care, home care, and institutional pharmacy practice. In addition, the usefulness of the book as a learning tool was enhanced by the addition of a glossary, and learning objectives and self assessment questions to each chapter. The objectives and questions allow the reader to evaluate his/her learning before progressing to the next chapter.

The book is intended to apply to pharmacy technicians and pharmacists in all practice settings. Furthermore, the book is intended to be:

- a tool to supplement instruction in a classroom-type setting or on the job,
- a resource for people with varying ranges of experience—from people who have been pharmacy technicians for years to those who have never worked in a pharmacy,
- one of several tools used by employers to develop a technician training program, and
- one of several tools used by pharmacy technicians to prepare for the pharmacy technician certification exam.

Readers may want to use this edition in conjunction with other texts that cover topics of primary interest to them. In fact, several chapters contain lists of publications that readers may also find useful. Educators may find ASHP's *Model Curriculum for Pharmacy Technician Training* useful. The curriculum includes a guide and instructions for adapting the model to the needs of individual technician programs.

Listed on the next page are organizations that pharmacy technicians may be able to use as resources in their practice.

PHARMACY ORGANIZATIONS

American Council on Pharmaceutical Education
311 W. Superior Street, Suite 512
Chicago, IL 60610
(312) 664-3575; FAX (312) 664-4652

American Pharmaceutical Association
2215 Constitution Avenue, NW
Washington, DC 20037-2985
(800) 237-AphA; (202) 628-4410
FAX (202) 783-2351

American Society for Pharmacy Law
P.O. Box 7163
Auburn, CA 95604-7163
(916) 801-5865; FAX (916) 823-5259

American Society of Health-System Pharmacists
7272 Wisconsin Avenue
Bethesda, MD 20814
(301) 657-3000; FAX (301) 657-8817

Joint Commission on Accreditation of Health Care Organizations
One Renaissance Boulevard
Oakbrook Terrace, IL 60181
(630) 792-5000; FAX (630) 792-5005

National Association of Chain Drug Stores
P.O. Box 1417-D49, 413 N. Lee Street
Alexandria, VA 22313-1480
(703) 549-3001; FAX (703) 836-4869

National Community Pharmacists Association (formerly NARD)
205 Daingerfield Road
Alexandria, VA 22314
(703) 683-8200; FAX (703) 683-3619
www.ncpanet.org

National Council for Prescription Drug Programs, Inc.
4201 N. 24th Street, Suite 365
Phoenix, AZ 85016-6268
(602) 957-9105; FAX (602) 955-0749

TECHNICIAN ORGANIZATIONS

American Association of Pharmacy Technicians
P.O. Box 1447, 620 S. Elm
Greensboro, NC 27402
(910) 275-1700; FAX (910) 275-7222

Pharmacy Technician Certification Board
2215 Constitution Avenue, NW
Washington, DC 20037-2985
(202) 429-7576; FAX (202) 429-7596

Pharmacy Technician Educators Council
1426 Prince Street
Alexandria, VA 22314
(703) 683-9493; FAX (703) 836-8982

GOVERNMENT AGENCIES

Food and Drug Administration, general information
(301) 827-4420

Food and Drug Administration's MEDWATCH Program
(800) FDA-1088; FAX (800) FDA-0178

Acknowledgments

Acknowledgments are meant to recognize the efforts of those behind the scenes. ASHP gratefully acknowledge ICHP and Linda Fred for their assistance in producing the second edition of the *Manual for Pharmacy Technicians*.

—ASHP Product Development Team

As I looked back through my documents used to produce this book, I realize it has taken more time than anyone thought it would. However, I would not trade the experience I've gained over the course of this project. I crossed paths with many committed and extremely capable and helpful people who shared in this challenging yet worthy project. I would like to thank ICHP for its faith in me and willingness to allow me to participate in such an important undertaking; Amy Zannikos and Ben Dickinson, ASHP pharmacist editors, for their guidance and efforts toward completing this book; the authors for all their hard work and enduring patience; the reviewers who added their perspective to each chapter along the way; and Allen Kent, Jack Lemanowicz, Sandra Carroll, and John Snyder who have each been my supervisor at some stage of the project and have willingly supported me throughout the project. Finally, I'd especially like to thank Mike and Ellen for evenings and weekends I spent with a good book when I might have been spending time with them.

—Linda Y. Fred, R.Ph.
January 1998

Contributors

Stephen J. Allen, M.S., FASHP, Director of Pharmacy, Suburban Hospital, Bethesda, MD

Gail Bernstein, Pharm.D., BCPS, Elmhurst Memorial Hospital Pharmacy, Elmhurst, IL

Karen E. Bertch, Pharm.D., Clinical Pharmacist, Coram Healthcare, Mt. Prospect, IL; Clinical Pharmacy Specialist, Veteran's Administration Central Office, Pharmacy Benefits Management, Hines, IL; and Clinical Associate Professor, University of Illinois, College of Pharmacy, Chicago, IL

Edward Donnelly, R.Ph., MBA, FASHP, Owen Healthcare Inc., Director of Pharmacy, Edward Hospital, Naperville, IL

Linda Y. Fred, R.Ph., Director of Inpatient Pharmacy Services, Carle Foundation Hospital, Urbana, IL

Dennis Fruin, R.Ph., General Manager, Apothecare Inc., Chicago, IL

Melissa Hogan, Pharm.D., Assistant Professor, Midwestern University, Chicago College of Pharmacy, Chicago, IL

Charmaine Hunt, Pharm.D., Drug Information Clinical Pharmacist, Lutheran General Hospital, Park Ridge, IL

Kristin Y. Izenstark, M.S., R.Ph., Pharmacy Manager, Lutheran General Hospital-Advocate, Park Ridge, IL

Rebecca S. Kentzel, C.Ph.T., Saint Francis Medical Center, Peoria, IL

Jacqueline Z. Kessler, M.S., R.Ph., Lutheran General Hospital, Park Ridge, IL

Mary Ann Kliethermes, B.S., Pharm.D., Vice-President, Clinical Services, Clinical Pharmacy Systems, Inc., Elmhurst, IL

Connie Larson, Pharm.D., Assistant Director, Hospital Pharmacy, University of Illinois at Chicago Medical Center, Chicago, IL

Richard K. Lewis, Pharm.D., MBA, Director of Pharmacy, Ambulatory Care Pharmacy Services, University of Illinois HMO, and Clinical Assistant Professor, University of Illinois at Chicago, College of Pharmacy, Department of Pharmacy Practice, Chicago, IL

Steven C. Lundquist, Pharm.D., System Clinical Manager, Owen Healthcare, Inc., Columbia Chicago Division, Chicago, IL

Douglas J. Scheckelhoff, M.S., FASHP, Director of Pharmacy, Childrens National Medical Center, Washington, DC

Michele F. Shepherd, Pharm.D., BCPS, Abbott Northwestern Hospital, Minneapolis, MN

Gerald A. Storm, R.Ph., Saint Francis Medical Center, Peoria, IL

Reviewers

ASHP and ICHP gratefully acknowledge the following individuals who donated their time and expertise in reviewing the chapters for this book.

Angela Barnes

Robert Beagley

Jan Begando

Sue Bevill

Alice Blatner

Susan Boswell

Maria F. Brackney

Bill Brooks

Toby Clark

Mark David

Jayne Gayman

Daniel H. Good

Christopher Hatwig

Joseph P. Hickman

Holly Houghton

Mihyun Kim

David Lourwood

Phil Ludwig

Nan Lundquist

Mary Lynn Moody

Diane Nitzki-George

Mike Novario

Delores Novy

Fred Ottolino

Henry A. Palmer

Marjorie F. Parker

Louise Petroka

Lisa Reitmaier

Annie Rubino

Bonnie Senst

Phillip Schneider

Glen Schumock

Joan Stachnik

Todd Thompson

Elaine K. Tompary

Henry F. Wedemeyer

Table of Contents

1 Introduction to Pharmacy

Michele F. Shepherd, Pharm.D., BCPS

The primary responsibility of any employee in the profession of pharmacy is to ensure that patients receive the proper drug therapy for their specific medical conditions. To achieve this goal, pharmacy personnel in hospitals, community pharmacies, and other health care settings perform a variety of duties designed to deliver the correct drug in the correct amount to all patients at all times in a timely manner. These duties range from ordering medications from suppliers, to distributing drugs to patients, to monitoring patients. Pharmacists are assisted by pharmacy technicians in several capacities to fulfill these obligations.

The pharmacy profession has ancient roots dating back thousands of years and is based in the sciences of mathematics, chemistry, and medicine. Knowledge from these sciences is applied to the development of drugs and the study of how drugs affect the human body. Pharmacists must be honest and ethical, and protect the rights and privacy of patients. To establish and maintain a profession consistent with these credences, state boards of pharmacy enforce pharmacy laws and regulations and require practicing pharmacists to meet minimum education and experience standards.

This chapter emphasizes the differences between the duties and responsibilities of pharmacy technicians and pharmacists and introduces technician competency expectations. Various pharmacy practice settings are outlined, with an emphasis on hospitals.

LEARNING OBJECTIVES

After completing the chapter the reader will be able to

1. Outline the differences in responsibilities of pharmacy technicians and licensed pharmacists.
2. List four settings in which pharmacy is practiced.
3. Define pharmaceutical care.
4. State the purpose of a policy and procedure manual.
5. Define differences between licensing and certification.
6. List five functions that pharmacy technicians perform in various pharmacy settings.
7. Explain why the use of outpatient pharmacy and medical services is increasing.

1

PHARMACY TRAINING AND EDUCATION

A profession is an occupation or vocation that requires advanced training in a liberal art or science. Technicians are persons skilled in the practical or mechanical aspects of a profession. Technicians assist professionals in routine, day-to-day functions that do not require professional judgment. Although technicians may be capable of functioning efficiently and safely without supervision, professionals are ultimately responsible for the technicians' activities and performance. Legally, professionals, such as pharmacists, are held liable for the performance of technicians, which necessitates the technicians' work be approved by professionals.

Pharmacy Technicians

Pharmacy technicians assist licensed pharmacists by completing tasks that do not require the professional judgment of a pharmacist and can be reviewed by a licensed pharmacist to ensure accuracy. The assistance of technicians is essential because it allows pharmacists to spend more time engaged in activities that require their professional judgment, such as patient care.

Pharmacy technician training prerequisites vary from employer to employer, but most employers require pharmacy technicians to have earned at least a high school diploma. As the degree of technician responsibility increases, so too does the amount of required training or previous experience. Many employers have established criteria to classify technicians based on the amount of training or experience they have had. For instance, a pharmacy technician 1 (PT-1) may be a newly hired technician who is responsible only for filling hospital unit-dose medication carts. A pharmacy technician 2 (PT-2) in that same hospital may have 5 years of job experience and be able to fill unit-dose medication carts, charge and credit patient accounts, compound intravenous (IV) solutions, and inventory narcotics. Technicians may be trained on-the-job or by completing a formal program, such as an associate degree program or course work at a community or technical college.

On-the-job Training: This type of training is often offered to technicians by employers. Technicians are trained to perform tasks specific to the particular job or position for which they were hired. Usually, technicians are taught only those skills they need to perform the particular job. For example, a technician may be trained on-the-job to fill unit-dose medication carts, compound IV solutions, or enter patient information into a computer database. When this type of training is very informal, the trainee is instructed by another technician who is familiar with the job; when it is more structured the trainee participates in a training course developed for the position by the employer. Some hospitals offer training courses that consist of classroom teaching combined with hands-on experience that last from 1 week to 6 months. In addition to covering general pharmacy topics such as aseptic technique, pharmaceutical calculations, technician responsibilities, and pharmacy rules and regulations, these courses cover job-related issues such as organizational policies and procedures and employee responsibilities.

Formal Programs: Community and technical college programs are broader in scope. These programs may be completed in 6 to 24 months and are more rigorous than on-the-job training. They cover all of the technical duties related to pharmacy plus topics such as medical terminology, pharmaceutical calculations, drug distribution systems, IV admixture procedures, and medication packaging techniques. In these programs, student technicians gain skills, knowledge, and experience by attending classes and completing clerkships at local hospitals or community pharmacies. Most programs offer full-time, part-time, and night classes plus financial assistance to those who qualify.

Pharmacists

Pharmacists are professionals who have had advanced training in the pharmaceutical sciences. In all states, pharmacists must be licensed by the state's board of pharmacy before they can practice pharmacy and must continue to follow the board of pharmacy regulations as they practice. In all states, the activities of technicians are supervised by licensed pharmacists who are held accountable for the technicians' performance.

Pharmacists must earn a college or university degree in pharmacy to become eligible to take the licensing examination offered by the state boards of pharmacy. This education teaches them how to use medical information to evaluate health care–related situations in a safe and effective manner. Often, there are no black and white answers, so pharmacists must rely on their education and professional judgment to make the best decision. There are two types of entry level degrees, two main types of postgraduate degrees, and a number of postgraduate training opportunities for pharmacists.

To be eligible for enrollment into an entry level pharmacy degree program, students must have completed a minimum of 2 years of college course work. The first professional college degree that pharmacists usually earn is a bachelor of science (B.S.) in pharmacy or a doctor of pharmacy (Pharm.D.). Pharmacists with B.S. degrees have completed 5 years of college, including 2 years of general college courses followed by 3 years of pharmacy courses.

In the past, a pharmacist would have earned a Pharm.D. degree by attending 6 years of pharmacy school or by completing a 5-year B.S. program followed by an additional 2-year program. Currently, most schools of pharmacy are, or will be, offering only a 6-year Pharm.D. degree.

After earning an entry level degree, many pharmacists elect to pursue postgraduate degrees such as a master's in science (M.S.) that emphasizes the pharmaceutical sciences, or a master's in business administration (M.B.A.) that stresses the business aspects of pharmacy. Generally, a master's degree (M.S. or M.B.A.) requires 2 years of full-time study and production of a thesis. By completing two additional years of course work and another thesis, pharmacists with a master's degree can also earn a doctor of philosophy (Ph.D.) degree in the pharmaceutical sciences or social and administrative pharmacy. In some cases, pharmacists combine their pharmacy degree with other degrees such as law (J.D.) or medicine (M.D.).

Many pharmacists have also completed a 1- or 2-year postgraduate training program, called a residency. Residencies provide the opportunity to gain clinical experience, usually in a hospital setting, after earning a degree. Fellowships, usually 2 or 3 years in length, also provide postgraduate training, but focus on pharmacy research experience rather than clinical pharmacy practice experience.

Before filling prescriptions or orders prescribed by physicians, pharmacists must rely on their education and professional judgment to determine if the prescription is appropriate for each patient. They must verify that the medication dosage is correct, that the patient is not allergic to the drug, and that the prescribed medication will not interact with other medications the patient is taking. They must also counsel and educate the patient on how to properly take the medication and alert the patient to possible side effects of the drug. These functions are performed by pharmacists every time that a prescription or order is filled.

Policies and Procedures

Technicians must observe the policies and procedures (P&P) established by their practice site and the pharmacy department. Guidance concerning the employer's expectations of the employees is provided in P&P documents. P&P documents provide guidance and are compiled in a readily available manual as a reference for all employees. Many accrediting organizations, such as the Joint Commission on Accreditation of Healthcare Organizations (JCAHO), require that pharmacy departments develop P&P manuals.

Policy and procedure manuals cover broad areas, such as hiring requirements and employee benefits, which makes the P&P manual relevant to all employees working for the organization. Departmental P&P are developed by individual departments in the organization and give direction on issues specific to that department. However, there may be some P&P applicable to more than one department. For example, the pharmacy and laboratory may share the same policy on disposal of used needles.

Policy and procedure manuals provide a guide for consistent orientation, training, and evaluation of personnel. The manuals set expectations for all employees ahead of time so that employees know how they should perform their jobs and how their job performance will be evaluated. Managers who evaluate employees use these written standards and expectations to measure employee performance so that they can detect personnel who are not performing up to the standard as well as recognize those employees who are surpassing job expectations. Managers can evaluate the performance of the pharmacy department as a whole by comparing the performance to the criteria set forth by the P&P.

Policies and procedures help coordinate the activities of the many departments in a hospital or other organization. When each department knows what it can expect from the others, use of resources is more efficient, duplication of services may be reduced, and patient care is improved.

Pharmacy department P&P address issues concerning the delivery of efficient, quality drug therapy. Such issues include

- Correct aseptic (sterile) technique when compounding IV admixtures
- The monitoring of patients for drug allergies
- Proper handling of cancer chemotherapeutic agents
- Distribution and control of all drugs used in the organization
- Procedures for ensuring that patients receive the correct drugs
- Use of investigational (experimental) drugs
- Management of toxic or dangerous drugs
- Provision for pharmacy services in the event of a disaster
- Identification of medications brought into the organization by patients
- Management of drug expenditures and the pharmacy budget

Pharmacy department P&P are developed by the director of pharmacy with input from pharmacists, appropriate physicians, and other health care professionals. After the P&P are written, they are reviewed by a committee before they are implemented. P&P are usually revised and updated annually. Most often, pharmacy P&P are reviewed by the Pharmacy and Therapeutics Committee, but other committees may also review the P&P that are pertinent to them. For example, the Infection Control Committee may review the pharmacy P&P on disposal of needles used to compound IV solutions, or the Oncology Committee may review the P&P on cleaning up spilled chemotherapy drugs. Figures 1-1 and 1-2 show examples of a preface to a pharmacy P&P manual and a table of contents, respectively.

Position Descriptions

Position, or job, descriptions are included in the P&P manual. Position descriptions define the functions and tasks for which employees are responsible. They outline the authority of the positions, that is, who reports to the employee and to whom the employee reports. Other expectations such as dress code, work schedule, and the physical requirements of the position may be included. Every position in the pharmacy, from director to pharmacy technician to staff pharmacist, has a written position description. Two example pharmacy technician position descriptions are shown in Figures 1-3 and 1-4. As can be seen by the examples, position descriptions vary from organization to organization and

may even vary within an organization. A pharmacy department often has several different technician position descriptions, each with its own set of duties and expectations.

A pharmacy technician (PT-1) may be hired as a unit-dose technician and be responsible for the duties as outlined in that position description such as entering medication orders into the pharmacy computer system, filling medication orders or prescriptions, stocking medication storage shelves, and maintaining automated unit-dose dispensing systems. As the PT-1 gains more experience and demonstrates competence in that position, he or she may move into a PT-2 position, which requires more responsibility and/or skill. An example of a PT-2 position is an IV admixture technician position. This position requires the technician to be comfortable with mathematical calculations, have manual dexterity, and be able to follow sterile (aseptic) technique. Often IV medications are costly or may pose some risk to the technician if not handled and prepared properly, so it is very important that the technician be well trained for such a position. Technicians should be familiar with the position description for the position or positions they fill in a pharmacy since they are often able and expected to perform in a number of positions, each with its own set of required skills and duties.

LICENSURE AND CERTIFICATION

The American Society for Health-System Pharmacists (ASHP) Task Force on Technical Personnel in Pharmacy has compiled definitions of the following terms:

- Credentialing—The general process of formally recognizing professional or technical competence.[1]
- Accreditation—The process of granting recognition or vouching for conformance with a standard (usually refers to recognition of an *institution*).
- Certification—The process by which a nongovernmental agency or association grants recognition to an *individual* who has met certain predetermined qualifications specified by that agency or association.
- Licensure—The process by which an agency of government grants permission to an individual to engage in a given occupation upon finding that the individual applicant has attained the minimal degree of competency necessary to ensure that the

I. PURPOSE

The purpose of a policy and procedure manual is to provide an authoritative source of official organizational policies, procedures, and practices, as well as to define operational responsibilities and the line of authority in the various areas within a department. The departmental *Policy and Procedure Manual* will serve:
A. As a means of standardizing and coordinating procedures
B. As a reference and guide for daily operations
C. As a means of orientation for new pharmacy personnel
D. As a central record of the departmental policies

II. MATERIALS INCLUDED IN THE MANUAL

The *Policy and Procedure Manual* is divided into five main areas:
- DIVISION 01 General
- DIVISION 02 Drug Distribution Division
- DIVISION 03 Administration and Technology Division
- DIVISION 04 Drug Information Division
- DIVISION 05 Clinical Services, Education, and Research Division

The divisions are subdivided into various chapters as listed in the table of contents to cover the topics included in each division.

III. AUTHORITY OF THIS MANUAL

A. The instructions contained in this manual are official and shall be relied upon as the basis for the performance of work. It is the responsibility of each employee to be thoroughly familiar with each policy and procedure covered in the manual that affects the scope of responsibility of that employee. Questions about any specific policy or procedure should be referred to the employee's supervisor for clarification. Since all conceivable work situations cannot be anticipated by an instruction, the policies and procedures set forth in this manual shall be regarded as guides to performance under related or analogous conditions.
B. Situations may arise where conformance with the instructions in this manual may not be possible. This may be because the original instructions may not have anticipated additional factors that may be present in a given situation. Whenever such a situation arises, the supervisor is expected to exercise judgment as to whether the instruction shall be suspended pending review by the director of pharmacy or in emergency situations whether other action is required, provided there is no violation of law or fixed hospital policy. This does not mean that the supervisor may, at will, suspend the effect of instruction with which he or she may not be in agreement. This shall be regarded as an emergency authority only, and in every case of the exercise of this authority, a full written report shall be made to the director of pharmacy. This report shall justify why emergency exception to the rules was taken without prior authorization.

IV. OTHER GENERAL PUBLISHED INSTRUCTIONS

A. Other general published instructions of the Department of Pharmacy shall be within the framework of the policies and procedures of this manual or shall be supplementary to it. In the event of conflict between other published instructions and this manual, the manual shall take precedence, unless otherwise specified.
B. Occasionally, it may be necessary to issue temporary instructions that will take precedence over materials in the manual. When this is done, the temporary instruction shall clearly state the exceptions and shall include a time limit for the temporary instructions.
C. If a supervisor should issue oral or written instructions in conflict with this manual, such superseding instructions shall be followed, but it is the responsibility of the person receiving them to point out the conflict with the manual. This shall be regarded as an emergency authority only, and in every case of the exercise of this authority, a full report shall be made to the director of pharmacy. This report shall justify why emergency exception to the rules was taken without prior authorization.

V. HOW TO FIND MATERIAL

The material covered by this manual has been organized into divisions, chapters, sections, parts, and subparts. All subdivisions are numbered with Arabic numerals. A typical section designation, therefore, would be 01-20-15:
- DIVISION 01 General
- CHAPTER 20 Policy and Procedure Manual
- SECTION 15 Distribution

When more than one page is required for a particular part or subpart, a dash and the letter "A" shall follow the first page number. The second page would be "B" and so on, as necessary. Through reference to the table of contents, one may ordinarily find all related material together. Sample forms will appear at the end of each division and will be numbered consecutively within each division.

VI. NEW MATERIAL AND REVISIONS

Chapters, sections, parts, and subparts are numbered so that additional information may be inserted without altering the numbering system; that is, originally every fifth digit was used. In most cases, a draft of proposed new material will be sent to all concerned individuals so that suggestions and recommendations can be made. All new material, as well as revisions of old material, will be placed in each volume of the manual by the secretarial staff, at which time a copy, under cover of a transmittal memorandum, where necessary, will be sent to each employee concerned, stating that the attached policy and procedure has been placed in the manuals. A copy of the *Policy and Procedure Manual* will be located in each area of the Department of Pharmacy and will be available to any departmental employee.

Figure 1-1. Preface to pharmacy policy and procedure manual.

Source: Hethcox JM. The policy and procedure manual. In: Brown TR, editor. *Handbook of Institutional Pharmacy Practice*, 3rd ed. Bethesda, MD: American Society of Hospital Pharmacists; 1992. p. 60.

public health, safety, and welfare will be reasonably well protected.
- Registration—The process of making a list or being enrolled in an existing list. (In an occupational setting, it may or may not be illegal to carry out a particular function without being registered.)

Technicians

Some professional organizations, such as ASHP, the American Pharmaceutical Association (APhA), the American Association of Colleges of Pharmacy (AACP), and the National Association of Boards of Pharmacy (NABP),

DIVISION 01 General

CHAPTER	05	Introduction	
SECTION	05	Anytown Hospital	
PART	05	General Statement	
	10	Statement of Mission and Goals	
	15	Maps	
SECTION	10	Department of Pharmaceutical Services	
PART	05	General Statement	
	10	Statement of Mission and Goals	
	15	Division Purposes	
	20	Objectives for the Current Year	
	25	Floor Plan and Location Guide	
	30	Departmental Appearance	
CHAPTER	10	Department of Pharmaceutical Services Organization	
SECTION	05	Organization Chart	
	10	Acting Authority	
	15	Position Descriptions	
PART	05	Drug Distribution Division	
SUBPART	05	Assistant Director	
	10	Inpatient Supervisor	
	15	Outpatient Supervisor	
	20	Staff Pharmacist	
	25	Senior Data Entry Operator	
	30	Pharmacy Technician	
	35	Pharmacy Intern	
SECTION	20	Committees	
CHAPTER	15	Standards	
SECTION	05	American Pharmaceutical Association Code of Ethics	
	10	Joint Commission on Accreditation of Healthcare Organizations—Pharmaceutical Services	
	15	American Society of Hospital Pharmacists—Minimum Standard for Pharmacies in Institutions	
	20	State Board of Health—Pharmacy Standards	
	25	American Society of Hospital Pharmacists—Accreditation Standard for Hospital Pharmacy Residency Training with Guide to Interpretation	
	30	Minimum Expectations of a Pharmacist	
	35	Hospital Code of Ethics	
	40	Patient's Bill of Rights	

CHAPTER	20	Policy and Procedure Manual	
SECTION	05	Format	
	10	Writing Style	
	15	Distribution	
	20	Responsibility	
	25	Revisions and Additions	
	30	Review	
CHAPTER	25	Personnel Policies	
	30	Staffing and Scheduling	
	35	Security	
	40	Interdepartmental Relationships	
	45	Communications	
	50	Safety Program—Accident Prevention	
	55	Fire Emergency Plan	
	60	Disaster Plan	
	65	Bomb Threat	
	70	Public Relations	

DIVISION 02 Drug Distribution

CHAPTER	05	General
	10	Central Inpatient Pharmacy Service
	15	Outpatient Pharmacy Service
	20	Satellite Pharmacies

DIVISION 03 Administration and Technology

CHAPTER	05	Administration
	10	Purchasing and Inventory
	15	Quality Assurance
	20	Technology
	25	Transportation

DIVISION 04 Drug Information

CHAPTER	05	Drug Information Requests
	10	Pharmacy and Therapeutics Committee
	15	Publications
	20	Investigational Drugs
	25	Library
	30	Adverse Drug Reaction Reporting Program
	35	Drug Allergy Reporting Program
	40	Drug Interaction Reporting Program

DIVISION 05 Clinical Services, Education, and Research

CHAPTER	05	Clinical Services
	10	Education
	15	Research

Figure 1-2. Portion of a table of contents of a pharmacy department policy and procedure manual, illustrating content organization based on departmental management responsibilities.

Source: Ginnow WK, King CM Jr. Revision and reorganization of a hospital pharmacy policies and procedures manual. *Am J Hosp Pharm.* 1978;35:698–704.

became jointly involved with the Scope of Pharmacy Practice Project. The objective of the project was to perform a validated task analysis of the functions, responsibilities, and tasks of pharmacists and technicians. This analysis documented what pharmacy technicians do and what knowledge is necessary for them to have in order to effectively perform those activities.

Participants in the Scope of Pharmacy Practice Project recognized the need for a national technician certification program for credentialing, accrediting, certifying, licensing, or registering technicians, rather than the various state programs that now exist. In 1995, APhA, ASHP, the Illinois Council of Hospital Pharmacists (ICHP), and the Michigan Pharmacists Association (MPA) established the Pharmacy Technician Certification Board (PTCB). The PTCB was created to develop a voluntary national pharmacy technician certification program.[1] Prior to the PTCB, the pharmacy profession had not established standardized technician training programs or licensing procedures to the extent it had for pharmacists. Now, the PTCB's duties include the

---

POSITION DESCRIPTION OF A PHARMACY TECHNICIAN

DIVISION	01	General
CHAPTER	10	Department of Pharmaceutical Services
SECTION	15	Position Description
PART	05	Drug Distribution
SUBPART	30	Pharmacy Technician

Immediate Superior: Appropriate Section Supervisor or Pharmacist on duty during Supervisor's absence
Immediate Subordinate: None
Authority: Proceed within the expressed limits of established policies and procedures securing approval from the Supervisor or Pharmacist on duty for deviations from same.

Responsibilities

1. Be familiar with, understand, and comply with all policies and procedures affecting the scope of responsibility as compiled in the Department of Pharmaceutical Services Policy and Procedure Manual.
2. Respond to the Hospitals' Disaster Call at any time of day or night.
3. Work cooperatively with all Hospitals and Health Science Center employees and promote and maintain good interpersonal and interdepartmental relationships.
4. Maintain good relationships with the public in behalf of the Department of Pharmaceutical Services and the University of Minnesota Hospitals.
5. Advise Supervisor of malfunctioning equipment and unsafe equipment.
6. Make recommendation to the Supervisor as to how methods and procedures can be improved.
7. Observe and report to the Supervisor any unusual situations, occurrences, conditions, or complaints including those related to drugs, drug requests, drug usage, or security within the Pharmacy or the Hospitals.
8. Perform other related duties as assigned by authorized personnel or as may be required to meet emergency situations.
9. Keep work area in a clean and orderly manner.
10. Perform oral and/or written requests given by the Supervisor or other Pharmacists. Conflicting instructions should be resolved by the Supervisor or in his (or her) absence, the Administrative Pharmacy Officer.
11. Be accountable for the time period in which scheduled to work in dispensing area to the Supervisor or to the Pharmacist in charge. Notify the Supervisor or Pharmacist in charge when leaving the area assigned for breaks or meals.
12. Have all work checked by a Pharmacist.
13. When assigned to Inpatient area, perform duties according to Policy and Procedure on Inpatient Responsibility of Personnel (02-10-10-20). The ratio of technicians to pharmacists in this area shall not exceed 1 to 1.
14. When assigned to unit dose activities in the pharmacy satellites, perform duties according to Policy and Procedure on Technician Daily Procedures (02-20-10). The ratio of technicians to pharmacists in this area shall not exceed 3 to 1.

   a. Maintain adequate supplies of controlled substances on all nursing areas served by the satellite.
   b. Change unit dose medication cassettes.
   c. Periodically inventory the area and reorder additional supplies of drugs from Central Pharmacy as needed.
   d. Restock shelves in the dispensing areas upon receipt of stock replacement.
   e. Fill unit dose medication drawers.
   f. Prepare IV admixture solutions as required.
   g. Prepare extemporaneous package injectable and oral dosage forms.
   h. Fill new medication orders.
   i. Enter new medication orders into the computer.
   j. Type accurate and legible labels for IV admixtures, packaged doses, and pass/self meds.

15. When assigned to the Outpatient area, perform duties according to Policy and Procedure on Outpatient Responsibilities to Personnel (02-15-10).
16. When assigned to the IV Admixture Sterile Prep Packaging Service:
   a. Prepare IV Admixtures, Total Parenteral Nutrition Solutions (TPN), Antilymphocytic Globulin Solutions (ALG, ATG, IGG), skin test antigens, antibiotic piggybacks and syringes, and other sterile products as requested.
   b. Perform all clerical work associated with the IV Admixture Service such as calculations, computer processing, typing, coordinating, and workload statistics.
   c. Monitor credits returned, reissuing appropriate preparations and discarding expired ones.
   d. The ratio of technicians to pharmacists in this area shall not exceed 3 to 1.
17. When assigned as the Controlled Substance Courier, maintain adequate supplies of controlled substances on all nursing areas' maintained controlled substance floorstock.
18. Answer the telephone in assigned areas as per Departmental Policy and Procedures on Telephone Communications (01-45-05).

Figure 1-3. Example of a position description for a pharmacy technician.

Source: Ploetz PA, Woller TW. Pharmacy technicians. In: Brown TR, editor. *Handbook of Institutional Pharmacy Practice*, 3rd ed. Bethesda, MD: American Society of Hospital Pharmacists; 1992. p. 401.

development and implementation of policies related to such a voluntary certification process.

Technicians who wish to become certified may take the National Pharmacy Technician Certification Examination offered by the PTCB. The first such examination was held in 1995. To take the examination, candidates must have a high school diploma or a graduate equivalency diploma (GED) and submit the appropriate application form, fees, and supporting docu-

JOB DESCRIPTION: SUPPORTIVE PERSONNEL

REPORTS TO: Director of pharmacy and staff pharmacist(s)

SUPERVISES: N/A

EDUCATION/ TRAINING: High school diploma or equivalent preferred; typing skills required

EXPERIENCE: Institutional pharmacy experience preferred

WORK SCHEDULE: May be required to work rotating shifts, including weekends and holidays

PHYSICAL REQUIREMENTS: May require standing for long periods; may require lifting of heavy boxes

OCCUPATIONAL HAZARDS: May be exposed to potentially hazardous and toxic substances

APPEARANCE: Neat, professional appearance required

ATTITUDE: Courteous, cooperative attitude required

Responsibilities and Duties

Responsibilities of pharmacy supportive personnel include compliance with all applicable policies, procedures, codes, and standards of the facility. Supportive personnel work under the direct supervision of a licensed pharmacist and do not perform duties that can legally be performed only by a licensed pharmacist.

The following duties are *representative* of the position. Additional duties and projects may be assigned.

- Assist pharmacists in providing effective, appropriate, and safe pharmacy services.
- Participate in pharmacy orientation programs, training programs for pharmacy supportive personnel, pharmacy staff meetings, and inservice educational programs.
- Assist in maintaining the cleanliness and orderliness of the pharmacy.
- Maintain records.
- Issue supplies to other departments.
- Assist in stock control (inventorying, stocking, pricing, and monitoring usage).
- Pick up and deliver drug orders.
- Participate in activities that resolve unsafe and unsanitary practices.
- Attend and participate in other programs, committees, meetings, and functions required by the facility or the pharmacy.

Reviewed and accepted:

_____   _____
Supportive Staff Member   Date

_____   _____
Supervisor   Date

Figure 1-4. Example of a position description for a pharmacy technician.

Source: Coe CP. *Elements of Quality in Pharmaceutical Care,* Bethesda, MD: American Society of Hospital Pharmacists; 1992. p. 219.

ments. This closed-book examination consists of 125 multiple choice questions. There are four possible answers to choose from, with only one being the correct or best answer. The final score is based on the total number of correctly answered questions.

The questions are written to assess the candidates' knowledge and skills that are deemed necessary to perform the activities encountered in the work of pharmacy technicians. As outlined in the guide for the certification examination, the exam divides these activities into three broad functions:

I. *Assisting the pharmacist in serving patients*, including activities related to dispensing prescriptions, distributing medications, and collecting and organizing information,

II. *Medication distribution and inventory control systems*, pertaining to those activities related to purchasing medications and supplies, controlling inventory, and preparing and distributing medications according to policies and procedures, and

III. *Operations*, including administrative activities that deal with issues such as operations, human resources, facilities and equipment, and information systems.

Fifty percent of the examination tests the candidate on topics in function I, 35% in function II, and the remaining 15% in function III.

There are several references available to assist candidates to prepare for the examination. More information about the certification exam can be obtained from the Professional Examination Service, c/o PTCB (701) Testing Office, 475 Riverside Drive, New York, NY 10115-0089.

Currently, ASHP accredits hospital pharmacy technician training programs. Accreditation serves to standardize the formal training that hospital pharmacy technicians receive; it also provides hospitals that offer a technician training program with guidelines on how to adequately train competent pharmacy technicians. Pharmacy technician training programs must meet the minimum criteria set by ASHP before the program can earn accreditation.

The ASHP Technical Assistance Bulletin (TAB) on Outcome Competencies and Training Guidelines for Institutional Pharmacy Technician Training Programs (appendix 1) was developed to ensure that technicians who master the competency standards set forth in the TAB can function capably in most pharmacy environments. This manual provides the information pharmacy technicians need to meet the objectives and expectations of TAB.

Pharmacists

After earning a B.S. degree or Pharm.D. degree, degree holders must pass an examination administered by their state's board of pharmacy. Members of a board of pharmacy include pharmacists and public members who have been appointed to the board by the governor of their state. The members of a state board of pharmacy are responsible for protecting the citizens of their state. The board does so by passing pharmacy rules and regulations to be followed in addition to the laws enacted by that state's legislature.[2] Once degree holders have successfully passed their state's board of pharmacy examination, they become registered pharmacists (R.Ph.) and are allowed to practice pharmacy in that state.

Some pharmacists choose to become certified as pharmacotherapy specialists. After passing a day-long certification examination, they earn the title of Board Certified Pharmacy Specialist, and may attach the initials BCPS to their credentials. These pharmacists must still comply with the requirements of their state's board of pharmacy. There are also certification examinations in nutrition, nuclear pharmacy, and oncology. Other specialty certification examinations are in development.

PHARMACY PRACTICE SETTINGS

Pharmacy is practiced in many environments, which are commonly divided into ambulatory care and institutional settings. Ambulatory care settings are those such as community, home care, and mail order that serve the patients who live in their own homes or similar situations. Institutional settings are those where patients receive long- or short-term care by health professionals. The two primary settings are the community pharmacies and institutions. Other settings include managed care, hospice care, research facilities, educational centers, and pharmaceutical industry.

Although the specific pharmacy activities of practice settings may vary, the primary goal of each remains the same, to ensure that patients receive the proper drug therapy for their medical conditions.

Community Pharmacy

The community pharmacy is the corner drug store or the local retail or grocery store pharmacy; the average person is probably most familiar with this practice site. Community pharmacies can be members of a chain of pharmacies or can be independently owned. Usually patients are customers who are being treated by doctors as outpatients and come into the store with prescriptions. They are not admitted to a hospital or cared for by professionals in a health care facility. Generally, these patients live in their own homes under their own care.

Technicians in community settings often prepare prescription labels to be checked by a pharmacist, order and maintain drug inventory, process insurance claims, and operate a cash register.

Mail Order Pharmacy

Pharmacists and technicians also work in mail order facilities where patients may have their prescriptions filled and refilled through the mail. A major difference between mail order pharmacies and community pharmacies is that there is no face-to-face contact with the patients. However, mail order pharmacists must use the same degree of professional judgment that is used in community or institutional settings. Technician duties in a mail order pharmacy are similar to those in the community setting.

Managed Care

A managed care program is simply a type of health insurance program where patients pay a blanket fee for their health care services rather than the traditional fee-for-service. Managed care programs attempt to improve the quality of health care delivery and patient outcomes. One definition of a managed care prescription program is "the application of management principles to achieve maximum health outcomes at the lowest cost."[3] Pharmacists who work in managed care environments usually do not have direct patient contact but instead manage drug therapy on a global basis. They collect information from the patients' computerized medication profiles and pool it into a large database. Prescription drug use and physician prescribing patterns are analyzed for trends that indicate optimal or sub-optimal medication therapy. Pharmacists then try to minimize drug costs and improve patient outcomes or results through the development of drug formularies and disease-specific drug therapy guidelines.

Technicians in a managed care setting may collect data, research information, or assist pharmacists in writing reports.

Hospital Pharmacy

Patients are admitted to hospitals for short-term supervised medical care by health care professionals in a structured, formal manner. Pharmacists are directly involved with patient care and have daily interactions with physicians, nurses, and other health care givers. They develop plans of pharmaceutical care and, with the other caregivers, monitor the patients' drug therapy. Depending on the size of the hospital, some pharmacists provide specialized services in areas such as pediatrics, oncology, infectious diseases, nutrition support, and drug information. In addition to the provision of direct patient care, among other things, pharmacists also evaluate trends in medication use and physician prescribing, develop guidelines for medication use, educate patients and health care professionals, and implement and maintain drug distribution systems. They also work together with nurses, physicians, and other members of hospital committees and work groups, both within the pharmacy department and outside of the department.

Technicians who work in hospitals work with pharmacists to accomplish many of the pharmacy's goals. Generally, technicians spend time entering physician medication orders into a computer, preparing intravenous drug admixtures, repackaging and labeling unit-dose medications, delivering medications, and completing paperwork for quality assurance or billing purposes.

Long-term Care

Long-term facilities are those where patients stay for extended periods of time. They include settings such as nursing homes, mental or psychiatric institutions, intermediate-care facilities for mentally retarded patients, and skilled nursing facilities. Patients in these settings require professional care but not to the same degree that hospitalized patients do. Pharmacists and technicians in long-term care practices perform many of the same activities as those in hospital settings.

Home Health Care

Home health care is defined as physician ordered services provided to patients at their residences, be it their own homes or any other setting in which the patients live.[4] Such services may include personal care, respite care, shopping assistance, drug and infusion therapy, or speech, physical, or occupational therapy.[4,5] Home care pharmacists assess the patient for the appropriateness of home medication administration, and if so, go on to assess and develop a pharmaceutical care plan to monitor and educate the patient. Medications administered in the home setting may be as simple as oral tablets or capsules, or as complex as drug therapy administered intravenously.

Technician duties in a home care setting may include preparing intravenous and sterile products, maintaining computerized patient profiles and accompanying a pharmacist to a patient's home.

Expansion of Technician Responsibilities

Table 1-1 lists some of the functions that pharmacy technicians perform in pharmacy settings around the country. Some of the functions listed are not routinely performed by technicians in most inpatient or outpatient pharmacies, but are viewed by some pharmacists as appropriate for the future if appropriate training is provided and current limitations are removed.[6]

TRENDS IN PHARMACY PRACTICE

Focus on Providing Pharmaceutical Care

The concept of pharmaceutical care was introduced in the early 1990s. Pharmaceutical care is defined as "the direct, responsible provision of medication-related care for the purpose of achieving definite outcomes that improve a patient's quality of life."[7]

Pharmaceutical care involves cooperation between a pharmacist, patient, and other health care professionals in designing, implementing, and monitoring a therapeutic medication plan. This involves three major functions: (1) identification of potential and actual drug-related problems, (2) resolution of actual drug-related problems, and (3) prevention of potential drug-related problems. Pharmaceutical care makes the pharmacist directly responsible to the patient for the quality of that care. The basic goals,

processes, and relationships of pharmaceutical care exist regardless of practice setting.[7]

Increasing Impact of Technology

Technical advances are changing the practice of pharmacy. New technical machines and systems have been developed to help dispense medications and monitor medication use in a more accurate, timely, and cost efficient manner. Since advanced computer systems collect and store patient information, it is more accurate and easier to access. Checks and balances (e.g., checks for drug interactions, patient allergies, and duplicate therapy) are built into computer systems and fewer errors may be committed. Automation of these checks and balances and other traditional functions allows pharmacists to do more activities that require their professional judgment and expertise. In turn, pharmacists are relying more than ever on technicians to operate and maintain these new systems.

Increasing Use of Outpatient Services

More and more, patients are cared for and treated as outpatients. This is a result of the increased need to contain the skyrocketing costs of health care. In the past, patients who would have been admitted to a hospital 2 or 3 days before surgery, now are admitted on the day of the procedure and discharged earlier than in the past. Many hospitals have outpatient surgery centers established where patients come to the center for surgery and are released a few hours later. For many diagnostic tests, patients are no longer admitted to a hospital, but are seen as outpatients and allowed to go home shortly after the tests.

The practice of pharmacy is changing to meet this new environment. Some clinics and outpatient centers have pharmacists and pharmacies available on site. In these settings, pharmacists have a shorter length of time to gather patient information and perform pharmaceutical care.

SUMMARY

Pharmacy technicians now commonly review and fill medication orders or prescriptions that are checked by a pharmacist at a later time. Most of the IV admixture and sterile compounding is done by technicians. More and more of the computer-entry functions, such as patient billing and order entry, are also the responsibility of technicians. In

Table 1–1[6, 12-14]

Functions of Pharmacy Technicians

Information Management
- Assist with drug use evaluations
- Collect data for drug therapy monitoring activities
- Collect data for pharmacokinetic activities
- Enter orders into a computer or patient profile
- Maintain patient medication profiles
- Provide drug information to patients, nurses, and physicians

Medication Preparation
- Compound and reconstitute medications
- Perform mathematical calculations
- Prepare parenteral nutrient solutions and antineoplastic agents
- Prepare IV fluids and medications
- Repackage and label unit dose drugs

Medication Dispensing
- Certify the complete drug order/prescription
- Check the work of other technicians:
    - Check medication orders/prescriptions filled by other technicians
    - Check IV admixtures made by other technicians
    - Check order entries made by other technicians
- Contact physicians for clarification of prescriptions/orders
- Deliver medications and controlled substances to patient care areas
- Fill and price outpatient prescriptions
- Fill orders for floor stock drugs
- Fill patient medication carts/cabinets
- Inspect and maintain emergency medication carts
- Inspect drug storage and patient care areas
- Provide drugs for medical emergency responses
- Receive oral requests from a nurse or oral orders/prescriptions from a physician
- Review patient profiles for appropriateness of therapy
- Verify the appropriateness (drug, strength, and regimen) of a physician's order/prescription

Medication Inventory Management
- Audit controlled substances
- Control pharmacy purchases and inventory
- Initiate purchase orders
- Obtain drugs for decentralized pharmacists

Training
- Train other technicians

some hospitals technicians may check each other's work,[8] dispense medications from a pre-approved list,[9] or even administer medications.[10,11]

Given the changes occurring in the pharmacy profession, the roles of pharmacy technicians are expanding and more is expected from technicians than in the past. Increasingly, technicians have become primarily responsible for the mechanical, and routine aspects of pharmacy practice in order to allow pharmacists to expand their practices.

RECOMMENDED READING

American Society of Hospital Pharmacists. ASHP statement on pharmaceutical care. *Am J Hosp Pharm.* 1993;50:1720–3.

Blake KM. How to achieve teamwork between pharmacists and technicians: a technician's perspective. *Am J Hosp Pharm.* 1992;49:2133, 2137.

Knapp DA. Pharmacy practice in 2040. *Am J Hosp Pharm.* 1992;49:2457–361.

McFarland HM. How to achieve teamwork between pharmacists and technicians: a pharmacist's perspective. *Am J Hosp Pharm.* 1992;49:1665–6.

Smith JE. The national voluntary certification program for pharmacy technicians. *Am J Health-Syst Pharm.* 1995;52:2026–9.

Whitney HAK Jr. Pharmacy's version of "The Wizard of Oz." *Ann Pharmacother.* 1992;26:996–8.

REFERENCES

1. Zellmer WA. Pharmacy technicians, part 1: national certification. *Am J Health-Syst Pharm.* 1995;52:918. Editorial.
2. Vandel JH. A board of pharmacy member's viewpoints on the technician issue. *Am J Hosp Pharm.* 1989;46:545–7.
3. Schafermeyer KW. Overview of pharmacy in managed health care. In: *A Pharmacist's Guide to Principles and Practices of Managed Care Pharmacy.* Alexandria, VA: Foundation for Managed Care Pharmacy; 1995. p. 15–26.
4. Catania PN. Introduction to home health care. In: *Home Health Care Practice,* 2nd ed. Palo Alto, CA: The Pocket Press; 1994. p. 1–11.
5. American Society of Hospital Pharmacists. ASHP guidelines on the pharmacist's role in home care. *Am J Hosp Pharm.* 1993;50:1940–4.
6. Govern VL, Birdwell SW, Sherrin TP. Attitudes of Ohio pharmacists toward pharmacy technicians. *Am J Hosp Pharm.* 1991;48:1228–33.
7. Hepler CD, Strand LM. Opportunities and responsibilities in pharmaceutical care. *Am J Hosp Pharm.* 1990;47:533–43.
8. Woller TW, Stuart J, Vrabel R, *et al.* Checking of unit dose cassettes by pharmacy technicians at three Minnesota hospitals. *Am J Hosp Pharm.* 1991;48:1952–6.
9. Kalman MK, Witkowski DE, Ogawa GS. Increasing pharmacy productivity by expanding the role of pharmacy technicians. *Am J Hosp Pharm.* 1992;49:84–9
10. Scala SM, Schneider PJ, Smith GL Jr, *et al.* Activity analysis of pharmacy-directed drug administration technicians. *Am J Hosp Pharm.* 1986;43:1702–6.
11. Fillmore AD, Schneider PJ, Bourret JA, *et al.* Costs of training drug-administration technicians. *Am J Hosp Pharm.* 1986;43:1706–9.
12. Raehl CL, Pitterle ME, Bond CA. Legal status and functions of hospital-based pharmacy technicians and their relationship to clinical pharmacy services. *Am J Hosp Pharm.* 1992;49:2179–87.
13. Hogan GF. ASHP survey of use of pharmacy technicians—1985. *Am J Hosp Pharm.* 1985;42:2720–1.
14. Phillips CS, Ryan MR, Roberts KB. Current and future delegation of pharmacy activities to technicians in Tennessee. *Am J Hosp Pharm.* 1988; 45:577–83.

SELF-ASSESSMENT QUESTIONS

1. What is the primary responsibility of anyone who works in the field of pharmacy?

2. Define pharmaceutical care.

3. A _____ provides guidance in areas such as personnel orientation, training and evaluation, correct aseptic (sterile) technique, and administration of medications by personnel other than registered nurses.

4. Match the following terms with their correct definitions:
   ___ Certification
   ___ Accreditation
   ___ Licensure
   ___ Registration

   a. The process of granting recognition or vouching for conformance with a standard
   b. The process by which a nongovernmental agency or association grants recognition to an individual who has met certain predetermined qualifications specified by that agency or association
   c. The general process of formally recognizing professional or technical competence
   d. The process of making a list or being enrolled in an existing list
   e. The process where a government agency grants permission to an individual to engage in a given occupation

5. A _____ setting of pharmacy practice is one where pharmacists care for patients in their own places of residence.

6. Pharmaceutical care implies the establishment of a relationship and commitment between the _____ and the _____.

7. True or False: Pharmacists in community settings are not able to practice pharmaceutical care.

8. True or False: Pharmacy technicians must pass the National Pharmacy Technician Certification Examination before they may be hired to work in a hospital.

9. List four activities that pharmacy technicians perform that free time for the pharmacists so

that they can better practice pharmaceutical care.

ANSWERS TO SELF-ASSESSMENT

1. The primary responsibility of any employee in the profession of pharmacy is to ensure that patients receive the proper drug therapy for their specific medical conditions. Pharmacy personnel in hospitals, community pharmacies, and other health care settings perform a variety of duties designed to deliver the correct drug in the correct amount to all patients at all times.

2. According to Hepler and Strand, pharmaceutical care is the part of pharmacy practice that involves direct interaction of the pharmacist with the patient about that patient's drug-related needs.

3. Policy and Procedure Manual

4. ___ Certification (b)
   ___ Accreditation (a)
   ___ Licensure (e)
   ___ Registration (d)

5. Home care

6. Pharmacist, patient. A key element of pharmaceutical care is the ongoing relationship between the pharmacist and patient.

7. False. Pharmaceutical care is a responsibility of any pharmacist practicing in any pharmacy setting.

8. False. The National Pharmacy Technician Certification Examination is, at this time, a voluntary certification process.

9. Information Management, Medication Preparation, Medication Dispensing, Medication Inventory Management Training (see Table 1-1).

APPENDIX 1

ASHP Technical Assistance Bulletin on Outcome Competencies and Training Guidelines for Institutional Pharmacy Technician Training Programs

Preamble

Definitions. The term "supportive personnel" has been recommended as standard nomenclature to be used in referring collectively to all nonprofessional hospital pharmacy personnel. This document describes the training outcome competencies for those supportive personnel designated "pharmacy technicians." A technician may be defined as a person skilled in the technique of a particular art (technique being the mechanical ability required to perform an activity).

For purposes of this document, a pharmacy technician shall be defined as someone who, under the supervision of a licensed pharmacist, assists in the various activities of the pharmacy department not requiring the professional judgment of the pharmacist. Such duties include, but need not be limited to: maintaining patient records; setting up, packaging, and labeling medication doses; filling and dispensing routine orders for stock supplies of patient-care areas; maintaining inventories of drug supplies; and mixing drugs with parenteral fluids. Technicians function in strict accordance with standard, written procedures and guidelines, any deviation from which must be approved by the supervising pharmacist.

Supportive personnel primarily engaged in duties not associated with the techniques of preparing and dispensing medications (e.g., secretaries, clerks, typists, and delivery personnel) are not considered "pharmacy technicians" and their competencies are not covered in this document. Likewise, competencies of supportive personnel who administer medication ("medication technicians") are also excluded. This document addresses the training of a "generalist" technician, one who can function appropriately in most hospitals, both small and large, in the kinds of activities for which there is generally the greatest need for supportive personnel manpower.

Application of the Outcome Competencies. The competencies described in this document are representative ones, and no attempt has been made to develop an exhaustive listing. It is believed that any technician who can demonstrate attainment of these competencies should be able to perform satisfactorily in any organized health-care setting after a reasonable period of orientation. It is not expected, however, that all institutional pharmacy technicians will, in fact, possess these competencies.

The competencies are described in behavioral terms; thus, it should be possible to evaluate the trainee's attainment of each competency in the manner described in each statement. In some instances, this can be by paper and pencil tests; in other instances, it can be by oral statement; and in yet other cases, it can be by actually performing the activity or function under the observation of the evaluator. In the latter instances, it is extremely important that the evaluator judges the trainee's performance strictly on the basis of the objectives previously established for the respective training activity relating to the competency.

Omitted from most of the competency statements are references to time or error limits. Obviously, they must be taken into account in the evaluation process. It is suggested that reasonable time and error limits be imposed where indicated, based on the evaluator's experience.

The training guidelines following the list of competencies for each objective statement consist of suggested topics to be covered in the didactic portion of the training program. Again, these are not exhaustive lists; every training institution is expected to add or delete topics as it deems necessary.

The training guidelines do not include training activities necessary for the development of manipulative skills. These are clearly implied in the statements listed under the competencies for each of the 11 objectives.

The qualifications of applicants to be admitted to the training program are discussed in Appendix A.

Objective I

The technician should demonstrate appropriate knowledge and understanding of the health-care institution and its pharmacy department.

Competencies. The technician should be able to

1. Interpret the institution's organizational chart in terms of the name and title of the administrative person to whom the director of pharmacy reports and the administrative and professional relationship of the pharmacy department to any other departments in the institution.
2. Describe the general responsibilities and job status of personnel in other institutional departments with whom the technician will have contact in carrying out assigned duties and activities.
3. Interpret the organizational chart for the pharmacy department in terms of names and general responsibilities of all departmental supervisory and administrative personnel.
4. Describe the location of the major hospital departments and service units, and escort another person to any department or unit.
5. State at least three reasons why information about patients must be kept confidential.
6. State at least five reasons for initiation of a disciplinary action in the institution (e.g., absenteeism, incompetency, and dishonesty).

Source: American Society of Hospital Pharmacists. *Am J Hosp Pharm.* 1982;39:317–20.

Training Guidelines. Suggested topics include

1. Organization, functions, and responsibilities of the hospital.
2. Organization, functions, and responsibilities of the pharmacy.
3. Hospital and departmental policies and procedures.

Objective II

The technician should demonstrate a thorough knowledge and understanding of the duties and responsibilities of his/her position, including standards of ethics governing pharmacy practice.

Competencies. The technician should be able to

1. State all of the technician's primary job responsibilities, the duties falling under each, and how they differ from the primary responsibilities of the pharmacist.
2. State the institutional and departmental policies applicable to each of the primary job responsibilities, and describe the procedures for each.
3. Define what is meant by "a decision requiring a pharmacist's judgment," and cite at least 10 examples.
4. Demonstrate the use of correct telephone communication technique and protocol, both in receiving and in initiating calls.
5. Demonstrate the use of correct written communication by drafting a memorandum to the supervisor requesting a change in work assignment schedule to take care of personal business.
6. State the general requirements of any local, state, or federal laws that specifically affect any of the technician's responsibilities.

Training Guidelines. Suggested topics include

1. Orientation to technician duties (job description).
2. Relationship of technicians to pharmacists, hospital staff, and patients.
3. Communication principles and techniques.
4. Legal aspects of technician functions such as:
   a. Accountability.
   b. Pharmacy regulations.
   c. Use and storage of controlled substances.

Objective III

The technician should have a working knowledge of the pharmaceutical–medical terms, abbreviations, and symbols commonly used in the prescribing, dispensing, and charting of medications in the institution.

Competencies. The technician should be able to

1. Transcribe without error any 12 inpatient medication orders selected at random from at least four different patient units in the institution.
2. Define in lay terms the meaning of names of all

clinical, diagnostic, and treatment units and services in the institution.

Training Guidelines. Suggested topics include

1. Pharmaceutical–medical terminology.
2. Pharmaceutical–medical abbreviations and symbols.
3. Drug classification systems and drug nomenclature.

Objective IV

The technician should have a working knowledge of the general chemical and physical properties of all drugs handled in manufacturing and packaging operations in the pharmacy department.

Competencies. The technician should be able to

1. Designate from a list of 50 drug names those that are light sensitive and those that must be refrigerated.
2. State what precautions and procedures must be used in handling caustic, poisonous, and flammable substances.
3. List the titles of at least four reference books where stability information on drug compounds can be found.

Training Guidelines. Suggested topics include

1. Pharmaceutical solutes, solvents, and basic solution theory.
2. Basic principles of stability (effects of heat, cold, light, and moisture on drugs and chemicals).
3. Storage requirements for drugs and chemicals.
4. Safety considerations regarding:
   a. Toxic and caustic substances.
   b. Flammable chemicals and drugs.
   c. Operating pharmacy equipment.
   d. Control of microbiological contamination.
   e. Cleaning and housekeeping.
   f. Control records.

Objective V

The technician should demonstrate an ability to carry out the calculations required for the usual dosage determinations and solutions preparation, using weight and volume equivalents in both the metric and apothecary systems.

Competencies. The technician should be able to

1. List without error the metric equivalents for the apothecary doses and for household doses written in 12 randomly selected medication orders.
2. Convert without error all metric or apothecary weights and volumes to the other system in at least four manufacturing formulas.
3. Perform the calculations necessary to prepare weight-in-volume and volume-in-volume solutions.

Training Guidelines. Suggested topics include

1. Weights and measures (apothecary and metric systems,

household measures, potency units and strengths, equivalents, and conversions).
2. Review of fractions, decimals, ratios, and percentages.
3. Dosage calculations and preparation of solutions.

Objective VI

The technician should demonstrate the ability to perform the essential functions relating to drug purchasing and inventory control.

Competencies. The technician should be able to

1. Prepare a written report of a physical inventory of a representative stock of pharmacy drugs and supplies using prepared forms and records.
2. Determine from existing reorder levels which inventoried items should be ordered and in what quantity.
3. Demonstrate an ability to check in a drug shipment by using the packing list or invoice and purchase order, completing the receiving report, and adding the items to the inventory.
4. Demonstrate the ability to retrieve from the drug storeroom at least 10 randomly designated drug items.
5. Describe the procedure for returning outdated drugs to the manufacturer.

Training Guidelines. Suggested topics include

1. Inventory and purchasing procedures and records.
2. Maintaining controlled substances records.
3. Inspection of nursing unit drug supplies.
4. Use of computer terminals.

Objective VII

The technician should demonstrate a working knowledge of drug dosages, routes of administration, and dosage forms.

Competencies. The technician should be able to

1. List at least:
   a. Six routes of drug administration.
   b. Ten dosage forms of drugs and their respective routes.
2. State the lumen size, length, and primary use for each of five different needles.
3. Identify, by name and use, each of five different syringes.

Training Guidelines. Suggested topics include

1. Sources of drugs.
2. Rationales for drug use (preventive, curative and restorative, and limiting disease processes).
3. Dose–response relationships.
4. Absorption, biotransformation, and excretion of drugs.
5. Risk–benefit ratios.
6. Patient variables and drug therapy (age, weight, pathological conditions, and genetic factors).
7. Local administration (to skin and mucuous membranes, to ears and eyes, and irrigations).
8. Systemic administration (oral, sublingual–buccal, inhalation, rectal, and parenteral).
9. Dosage forms (tablets, capsules, solutions, suspensions, ointments, suppositories, powders, and injectables).

Objective VIII

The technician should have a working knowledge of the procedures and operations relating to the manufacturing, packaging, and labeling of drug products.

Competencies. The technician should be able to

1. Repackage and label 25 unit doses from a bulk supply of drugs and correctly complete all necessary control records.
2. Demonstrate for each of five randomly selected formulation and packaging requests:
   a. Correct selection of necessary equipment.
   b. Proper assembly and use of the equipment.
   c. Proper cleaning and storing of the equipment.
   d. Proper selection of each ingredient.
   e. Accurate calculation and measurement of each ingredient.
   f. Proper completion of worksheet record of weights and volumes, manufacturers' lot numbers, and other required information.
   g. Correct procedure for mixing and preparing product.
   h. Proper selection and preparation of packages/containers and closures.
   i. Proper packaging technique.
   j. Correct selection and preparation of labels.
   k. Proper quarantine procedure.
3. Identify from a list of 10 different steps in manufacturing and packaging operations those functions that must be performed by a pharmacist only.

Training Guidelines. Suggested topics include

1. Measurements of quantity (weights, volumes, and numbers).
2. Use, assembly, and maintenance of equipment and apparatus.
3. Control and recordkeeping procedures (formula mastersheets, worksheets and batch records, labeling and label control, quarantine, and product testing and monitoring).
4. Packaging considerations (drug containers and closures).
5. Storage and inventory control.
6. Lot numbers and expiration dates and times.
7. Types of drug packages and containers (multiple dose, single dose, treatment size, large-volume parenteral containers, small-volume parenteral containers, aerosols and sprays, tubes, droppers, etc.).
8. Labeling of drug containers and packages.

Objective IX

The technician should have a working knowledge of the procedures and techniques relating to aseptic compounding and parenteral admixture operations.

Competencies. The technician should be able to

1. List five different possibilities for contamination of an injectable solution during its preparation and for each possibility a precaution that would prevent the contamination.
2. Demonstrate the proper technique for using a syringe and needle for aseptic withdrawal of the contents of:
   a. A rubber-capped vial.
   b. A glass ampul.
3. Demonstrate the proper technique for aseptic reconstitution of an antibiotic injection.
4. Describe the occasions when hand washing is required, and demonstrate the proper technique.
5. Demonstrate the correct techniques and procedures for preparing at least three parenteral admixtures, including the proper preparation of the label and completion of the control records.
6. Identify the major components of a laminar-flow hood, and state their functions.
7. Define or describe:
   a. Microbial growth and transmission.
   b. Origin, pharmacologic effect, and prevention of pyrogens.
   c. Sterility.
   d. Heat sterilization.
   e. "Cold" sterilization.
8. Designate from a list of 10 different sterile preparations those that may be safely heat sterilized.
9. Demonstrate the proper technique for visual inspection of parenteral solutions.

Training Guidelines. Suggested topics include

1. Parenteral routes of administration (rationale, precautions, and problems; routes; and methods of parenteral administration).
2. Equipment and systems used in parenteral administration (needles and syringes, administration sets, fluid containers, filters, and pumps).
3. Equipment used to prepare parenteral admixtures (laminar-flow hoods, filters, pumps and vacuum sets, drug additive systems and packages, Cornwall pipetters, etc.).
4. Aseptic compounding techniques (specific to the fluid system in use and including the prefilling of syringes, preparing ophthalmic solutions, etc.).
5. Labeling and recordkeeping (bottle labels, fluid orders and profiles, and compounding records).
6. Incompatibilities (visual and chemical incompatibilities, pH and concentration effects, and reference sources).
7. Quality control (particulate matter inspection and monitoring of contamination).

Objective X

The technician should demonstrate the ability to perform the usual technician functions associated with an institutional drug distribution system.

Competencies. The technician should be able to

1. Prepare the drug profile for five newly admitted patients.
2. Pick all doses for one patient unit, and complete the necessary dispensing records.
3. Describe the special dispensing and recordkeeping procedures that apply to the dispensing of:
   a. Controlled drugs.
   b. Investigational drugs.
   c. Nonformulary drugs.
4. List for each of 30 commonly prescribed tradename drugs:
   a. The generic name.
   b. The usual dose.

Training Guidelines. Suggested topics include

1. Physicians' order sheets and patient medication profiles.
2. Setting up doses for patients.
3. Checking doses.
4. Delivery and exchange of medications.

Objective XI

The technician should demonstrate the ability to perform manipulative and recordkeeping functions associated with the dispensing of prescriptions for ambulatory patients.

Competencies. The technician should be able to

1. Carry out the following functions for any 10 randomly selected ambulatory patient prescriptions:
   a. Correctly type the label.
   b. Select the proper drug from the dispensing stock.
   c. Accurately count or measure the product, and place it in the proper container.
   d. Complete the necessary records and documents.
   e. Calculate the charge for the prescription.
2. Describe the special procedures and documentation required in dispensing ambulatory patient prescriptions for:
   a. Controlled drugs.
   b. Investigational drugs.
   c. Nonprescription drugs.
3. Designate from a list of 10 steps involved in ambulatory patient prescription dispensing those functions that only a pharmacist may carry out.

Training Guidelines. Suggested topics include

1. Prescriptions and patient profiles.
2. Preparing prescription labels.
3. Counting and measuring drugs.

Appendix A: Qualifications for Training Program Applicants

Applicants to the technician training program should have certain demonstrated abilities as evidenced by successful completion of relevant high school courses or other appropriate educational programs or by acceptable grades on a written entrance examination. These abilities and knowledge include general basic chemistry, arithmetic, basic algebra, reading, and writing. Other requirements are: adequate command of the English language; ability to acquire skill in the use of pharmaceutical apparatus, instruments, and equipment; ability to work with sustained attention and care on routine repetitive tasks; ability to follow oral and written instructions with accuracy, precision, and dependability; and ability to distinguish routine functions from those requiring a pharmacist's judgment. These requirements should be clearly understood by applicants to the program.

2 | Medication Dosage Forms, Routes of Administration, and Abbreviations

Michele F. Shepherd, Pharm.D., BCPS

When most people think of taking a medication, they think of swallowing a tablet or capsule. Although this is the most common way people take medications, other forms of administration are used to introduce medications into the body by routes other than the mouth. Solutions, suspensions, suppositories, and sprays may be used to deliver medications into body areas such as the ear, nose, eye, rectum, or bloodstream.

This chapter describes common dosage forms and routes of administration. It is not intended to be all inclusive; other references are available that are more extensive and detailed. Included in this chapter is a list of frequently used abbreviations; it is not meant to be all inclusive.

LEARNING OBJECTIVES

After completing the chapter the reader will be able to

Medication Dosage Forms

1. List three advantages of liquid medication dosage forms over other dosage forms.
2. List three disadvantages of solid medication dosage forms.
3. Outline characteristics of each of the following categories of liquid dosage forms: solutions, emulsions, and suspensions.
4. Describe two situations in which an ointment may be preferred over a cream.
5. Explain the differences between various solid dosage forms such as tablets, capsules, lozenges, powders, and granules.

Routes of Administration

6. List six routes of administration by which drugs may enter or be applied to the body.
7. Identify special considerations for each route of administration.
8. List five parenteral routes of administration.
9. Explain the difference between the topical and transdermal routes.

10. Distinguish between the sublingual and buccal routes.

Abbreviations
11. Give the abbreviations for right eye, left eye, and both eyes.
12. Interpret the abbreviations qd, qam, and qod.
13. Define the abbreviations ASAP, APAP, and ASA.
14. List the abbreviations for the oral, rectal, intravenous, intramuscular, and subcutaneous routes of medication administration.

MEDICATION DOSAGE FORMS

Liquid Medication Dosage Forms

Liquid medication dosage forms are those that deliver medication in a fluid medium. The fluid serves as a carrier, or delivery system, for the medication and is referred to as the vehicle. Common vehicles are water, alcohol, and mineral oil. The medication may be dissolved in the vehicle or may be present as very fine solid particles suspended, or floating, in the vehicle. Liquid dosage forms may pour freely as water or have the thick consistency of syrup. They may be intended for oral consumption or for use in, or on, other parts of the body.

Liquid medication dosage forms have some advantages over other medication dosage forms:

- Oral liquid dosage forms usually are faster acting than solid dosage forms. Medications are absorbed into the bloodstream in a dissolved state. The medication in a liquid dosage form is already dissolved or is present in small particles so it can readily be absorbed. In contrast, tablets must dissolve before they can be absorbed so it takes more time for the medication to be absorbed.
- For patients who have difficulty swallowing, oral liquid medications may be easier to take than an oral solid dosage form.
- There is more flexibility in liquid doses than some other dosage forms because liquid medications are usually dispensed in bulk containers rather than distinct dosage units. For example, a liquid medication may contain 500 milligrams (mg) of a drug in 10 milliliters (ml) of liquid. The same medication is also available in 500 mg tablets. To take a 600 mg dose of the liquid medication, a patient would simply need to measure out

12 ml of liquid. However, to take a 600 mg dose of the tablet the patient would need to take 1.2 tablets, which would be difficult.
- Liquid medications may be used where solid dosage forms are not practical to administer. For example, medications that need to be placed directly into the ear or eye may be more practically administered as a liquid rather than a solid.

Liquid dosage forms also have some disadvantages:

- Often they have a shorter time to expiration than other dosage forms.
- Most drugs have a bad taste as the drug dissolves or is chewed into small particles. Drug particles present in the oral liquid medications come in contact with the taste receptors on the tongue and leave a bad taste. Sweeteners and flavoring agents are necessary to make these liquid medications more palatable. Tablets, on the other hand, are often coated and swallowed quickly to avoid contact with the taste receptors.
- Patients do not always find liquid medications convenient to take because they may be spilled, require careful measuring before administration, or have special storage or handling requirements such as refrigeration or shaking before use.

Liquid medication dosage forms are categorized based on several characteristics: the type of liquid medium (e.g., water or alcohol) in which the medication is delivered, whether the medication is dissolved or suspended as particles in the liquid, and the intended use of the medication. Other characteristics are further explained in the following paragraphs. Table 2-1 gives examples of liquid dosage forms.

Solutions

Solutions are evenly distributed, homogeneous mixtures of dissolved medication in a liquid vehicle. Molecules of a solid, liquid, or gaseous medication are equally distributed among the molecules of the liquid vehicle. Because the medication is already dissolved in the solution, it is absorbed from the stomach, skin, or other site of administration more quickly than other medication dosage forms.

Solutions may be subdivided based on characteristics of the vehicle:

- *Aqueous* and *viscous aqueous* solutions use purified water as the vehicle. Aqueous solutions may be ingested orally, applied topi-

Table 2–1

Examples of Liquid Medication Dosage Forms

Solutions
- Aqueous (water) solutions
  - Douches
  - Irrigations
  - Enemas
  - Gargles
  - Washes
  - Sprays
- Viscous (thick) aqueous solutions
  - Syrups
  - Jellies
  - Mucilages
- Nonaqueous solutions
  - Hydroalcoholic
    - Elixirs
    - Spirits
  - Alcoholic
    - Collodions
    - Spirits
  - Glycerites
  - Miscellaneous
    - Inhalants
    - Liniments

Emulsions
- Oil-in-water
- Water-in-oil

Suspensions
- Lotions
- Magmas and milks
- Gels

Extractives
- Tinctures
- Fluidextracts
- Extracts

cally, or injected into the bloodstream. Viscous aqueous solutions are sticky, thick, sweet solutions that are either liquid or semisolid.

- *Nonaqueous* solutions are those that utilize solvents, or dissolving liquids, in addition to or instead of water. Commonly used nonaqueous solvents include alcohol (ethyl alcohol or ethanol), glycerin, and propylene glycol. Nonaqueous solutions that employ alcohol as their solvent are called *alcoholic* solutions.
- *Hydroalcoholic* solutions are nonaqueous solutions that contain a mixture of alcohol and water. Nonaqueous solutions that contain alcohol but no water are called *alcoholic* solutions. A *glycerite*, which uses glycerin as a solvent, vehicle, or both, is another nonaqueous solution.
- *Inhalants* and *liniments* do not fit neatly into any category and are classified as miscellaneous solutions.

Aqueous Solutions

Douches are solutions that are directed into a body cavity or against a part of the body to clean or disinfect. Douches are used to remove debris from the eyes, or to cleanse the nose, throat, or vagina. Examples of commercially available vaginal douche products are Massengill (Smith-Kline Beecham) and Summer's Eve (Fleet).

Irrigating solutions are used to wash or cleanse part of the body such as the eyes, urinary bladder, open wounds, or abraded skin. They often contain medications such as antibiotics or other antimicrobial agents. Irrigating solutions may be used in surgical procedures to clear the surgical field of blood and surgical debris. While similar to douches, irrigating solutions usually are used in larger volumes and over larger areas of the body for a more general cleansing than douches.

Enemas are solutions that are introduced into the rectum to empty the bowel or to treat diseases of the lower gastrointestinal tract. Enemas, such as Fleet enemas (Fleet), are often given to relieve serious constipation or to cleanse the bowel before surgery.

Gargles are solutions that treat conditions of the throat. The gargle is held in the throat as the patient gurgles air through the solution. Although gargles are admitted into the mouth, they should not be swallowed. A familiar example of a gargle is Chloraseptic mouth rinse and gargle.

A *wash* is a solution that cleanses or bathes a body part, such as the eyes or mouth. A *mouthwash* is a solution used to deodorize, refresh, or disinfect the mouth, primarily for cosmetic reasons. Although many people use mouthwashes as gargles, technically they are in different classes of solutions; gargles are used to treat throat conditions such as a sore throat, while mouthwashes are used to freshen the mouth. Like gargles, mouthwashes should not be swallowed. Common mouthwashes include Scope and Listerine.

Frequently Used Abbreviations

acetaminophen	apap; APAP	eye, right	OD
after	p; P	left	OS
after meals	pc; PC	both	OU
after meals and at bedtime	pchs; PC&HS	Fahrenheit	F; °F
aluminum hydroxide	Al(OH)3; Al(OH)$_3$	ferrous gluconate	FeGluc
around the clock	atc; ATC	ferrous sulfate	FeSO4; FeSO$_4$
as desired	ad lib	fluid ounce	$f\!\!\!З$; fl oz
as directed	u.d.; U.D.	fluid dram	$f\!\!\!З$
as much as suffices	q.s.	four times daily	qid
as needed	prn; PRN	give of such doses	d.t.d.
aspirin (acetylsalicyclic acid)	ASA	grain	gr.
as soon as possible	ASAP	gram	G; gm; GM; g
bedtime	hs	headache	HA; H/A
before meals	ac; AC	heart rate	HR
before meals and at bedtime	achs; AC&HS	history	Hx
belladonna and opium	B&O	hour	h; hr; °
blood pressure	BP	hydrochlorothiazide	HCTZ
blood sugar	BS	hydrogen peroxide	H2O2; H$_2$O$_2$
bowel movement	BM	immediately, now	stat
by	per; p	increase	↑; incr
by mouth, orally	po; PO	intradermal	ID
calcium	Ca; C^{++}	intramuscular	IM
capsule	cap	intravenous	IV
Celsius	C; °C	intravenous piggyback	IVPB
chlorine/chloride	Cl/Cl$^-$	intravenous push	IVP
cubic centimeters (same as ml)	cc	iron	Fe; Fe^{++}
decrease	↓; decr	isoniazid	INH
dextrose		keep vein open	KVO
5% in water	D5W; D5	kilogram	kg
5% in Ringer's injection, lactated	D5RL; D5LR	label (let it be labeled)	sig.
		laxative of choice	LOC
5% in sodium chloride 0.9%	D5NS; D5/NS	leave of absence	LOA
		liquid	liq
5% in sodium chloride 0.45%	D5 1/2 NS; D5/0.45NS	liter	L
		magnesium	Mg; Mg^{++}
5% in sodium chloride 0.225%	D5 1/4 NS; D5/0.2NS	magnesium oxide	MgO; MagOx
		magnesium sulfate	MgSO4; MgSO$_4$
10% in water	D10W; D10	may repeat (time 1 dose, 2 doses)	MR; (MR × 1); (MR × 2)
diagnosis	Dx		
discharge	D/C	metered dose inhaler	MDI
discontinue	D/C	microgram	mcg; ug; μg
dispense	disp	milk of magnesia	MOM
dispense as written	DAW	milligram	mg
dram	З	milliequivalent	mEq
drop	gtt	milliliter (same as cc)	mL; ml
each, of each	aa	minims	♏
ear, right	AD	morphine sulfate	MS; MSO$_4$
left	AS	multiple vitamin	MV; MVI
both	AU	nausea and vomiting	N&V; N/V
every	q	nitroglycerine	NTG
day	qd	no known allergies	NKA
evening	qpm	no known drug allergies	NKDA
morning	qam	nothing by mouth	NPO
other day	qod	ointment	oint; ung
___hours	q__h; q__hr; q___°	on call (to surgery, lab, etc.)	on-call

Frequently Used Abbreviations (*Continued*)

one	†	sterile water (for injection)	SW; (SWFI)
one-half	ss.; s̄s̄	subcutaneous	SC; SQ; subQ
one-time dose	once; × 1	sublingual	SL
operating room	OR	suppository	supp
ophthalmic	OP; opth	tablespoon	tbsp; TBS
ounce (apothecary)	oz; (℥)	tablet	tab
over the counter	OTC	take (take thou, prescription)	Rx
oxygen	O; O₂	teaspoon	tsp
penicillin	PCN	telephone order	T.O.
potassium	K; K⁺	temperature	T
potassium chloride	KCl	tetracycline	TCN
pound	lb; #	three	ⅲ
pulse	P	three times daily	tid
recovery room	RR	tincture	tinct.
rectally (per rectum)	PR	tissue plasminogen activator	TPA
respiration	R	total parenteral nutrition	TPN
Ringer's injection	R	treatment	Tx
lactated	LR; RL	twice daily	bid
scruples	℈	two	ii
sodium	Na; Na⁺	units *	units; u; U
sodium bicarbonate	NaHCO3; NaHCO₃	vaginally (per vagina)	PV
sodium chloride	NaCl	verbal order	V.O.
sodium chloride solution		water	H2O; H₂O
0.9% (normal saline)	NS; NSS	with	c; c̄
0.45 (1/2 normal saline)	1/2 NS; 1/2 NSS; 0.45 NS	without	s; x̄
0.225% (1/4 normal saline)	1/4 NS; 1/4 NSS; 0.2NS	write (let it be written)	sig.
		while awake (when awake)	WA; W/A
solution	sol'n; sol		

* should always be spelled out

Sprays are solutions that are delivered as a mist against the mucous membranes of the nose and throat. Nasal decongestants (e.g., Afrin and Neo-Synephrine) and antiseptic throat solutions (e.g., Cheracol Sore Throat) are common spray formulations.

Viscous Aqueous Solutions

A *syrup* is a concentrated mixture of sugar and purified water. The high sugar content distinguishes syrups from other types of solutions. Syrups may or may not contain medication or added flavoring agents. Syrups without a medication, but with a flavoring agent, are called nonmedicated or flavored syrups. Flavored syrups are often used as vehicles for unpleasant tasting medications; the result is a medicated syrup. The high amount of sugar present in syrups predisposes them to bacterial contamination, so they often contain a preservative.

The advantage of a syrup is its ability to disguise the bad taste of medications. Syrups are thicker than aqueous solutions, therefore only a portion of the medication dissolved in the syrup comes in contact with the taste buds. The remainder of the medication is held above the tongue by the thick syrup so it is not tasted as it is swallowed. The high sugar content of syrups gives them a sweet taste that helps conceal the bad taste of the medicine. This is why syrups are commonly used for pediatric medications.

The thick character of syrups also has a soothing effect on irritated tissues of the throat, so syrups are often used for cough formulations. Robitussin and Triaminic Syrup are examples of two well-known cough and cold syrups.

Jellies are semisolid solutions that contain a high proportion of water. Jellies are used as lubricants for surgical gloves and rectal thermometers. K-Y Jelly is an example of a commonly used biological lubricant. It may be used to aid in the insertion of rectal thermometers or other diagnostic probes into orifices, as a sexual lubricant, or to reduce surface friction during ultrasound procedures. Jellies are also used as vehicles for vaginal contraceptive agents.

Mucilages are thick, viscous, adhesive liquids. They are solutions of water containing the sticky, pulpy components of vegetable matter. Mucilages are useful dosage forms that prevent insoluble solid medication particles from settling to the bottom of liquids. Bulk-producing laxative/psyllium products such as Metamucil form a mucilage when the powder is added to water or juice.

Hydroalcoholic Solutions

Hydroalcoholic solutions are nonaqueous and differ from aqueous solutions in that they contain alcohol in addition to water. Elixirs and spirits are examples of hydroalcoholic solutions.

Elixirs are clear, sweet, flavored water-and-alcohol mixtures intended for oral ingestion. The alcohol content in various elixirs varies greatly depending on the ability of the other ingredients in the elixir to dissolve in water. Many drugs do not dissolve easily in pure water but do so in a water-and-alcohol mixture. The alcohol in an elixir helps to dissolve these drugs. Some elixirs may have as little as 3% alcohol while others may contain almost 25% alcohol. The advantage of an elixir, its alcohol content, may also be a disadvantage or a contraindication in patients who should not or cannot ingest alcohol. In addition, alcohol can have undesired interactions with other medications the patients may be taking. Pediatric, elderly, and alcoholic patients should be made aware of the alcohol content of elixirs, because these patients may be especially sensitive to even a small amount of alcohol. Phenobarbital elixir and digoxin pediatric elixir are two widely prescribed medicated elixirs.

Aromatic and licorice elixirs are used as flavoring agents. An aromatic elixir is an unmedicated elixir commonly used as a vehicle for other medications. "Simple elixir," which contains orange, lemon, coriander, and anise oils in syrup, water, and alcohol, is such an example.

Spirits, or essences, are alcoholic or hydroalcoholic solutions that contain volatile, or easily evaporated, substances. Because the volatile substances dissolve more readily in alcohol, spirits can contain a greater concentration of these materials than water. Perhaps the most familiar spirits administered internally are the alcoholic beverages brandy (Spiritus Vini Vitis) and whiskey (Spiritus Frumenti). Other spirits may be inhaled (e.g., aromatic ammonia spirits, popularly known as smelling salts), while still others, such as peppermint spirits, are used as flavoring agents.

Alcoholic Solutions

Alcoholic solutions are nonaqueous solutions that contain alcohol but no water.

A *collodion* is a liquid preparation of pyroxylin (found in cotton fibers) dissolved in ethyl ether and ethanol. After application to the skin, the ether and ethanol evaporate and leave a pyroxylin film. Collodions that contain medication are useful in the treatment of corns and warts. Unmedicated collodions, such as liquid adhesive bandages (New-Skin), may be applied to the skin to protect and seal small wounds.

Spirits, as mentioned above, may be either alcoholic or hydroalcoholic solutions.

Glycerite Solutions

Glycerites are nonaqueous solutions of medication dissolved in glycerin, a sweet oily fluid made from fats and oils. Glycerin can be used alone as a vehicle, in combination with water, alcohol, or both. Because glycerin easily mixes with water and alcohol, it can be used as a solvent for medications that do not dissolve in either alone. After dissolving a medication in glycerin, the medication/glycerin mixture can then be easily added to a water and/or alcohol vehicle. Most glycerite solutions are very viscous, some to the point of being jelly-like. Glycerites are not commonly used today.

Miscellaneous Solutions

Inhalants are fine powders or solutions of drugs delivered as a mist through the mouth into the respiratory tract. Many drugs used to treat asthma are formulated as inhalants. The over-the-counter product Primatene Mist and the prescription drug Proventil are two examples.

A *liniment* is a medication dosage form that is applied to the skin with friction and rubbing. Liniments may be solutions, emulsions, or suspensions. Some liniments contain agents that produce a mild irritation or reddening of the skin. This irritation produces a counterirritation, or mild inflammation, of the skin that relieves inflammation of deeper structures such as muscles. Ben-Gay Original Ointment is a liniment widely used to relieve minor aches and pains of muscles.

Emulsions

Emulsions are mixtures of two liquids that normally do not mix. In an emulsion, one liquid is broken into small particles and evenly scattered throughout the other. The liquid present in small particles is referred to as the internal phase; the other liquid is called the external, or continuous, phase. To keep the two liquids from separating, an emulsifying agent is added to the formulation. The emulsifying agent prevents the small particles of the internal phase from fusing together and eventually separating out from the external phase to form two distinct layers. Oil-and-vinegar salad dressing is a common household emulsion that is formed by shaking the two liquids together. Because no emulsifying agent is added, the oil and vinegar separate within seconds after shaking and the emulsion is broken.

In most emulsions, the two liquids are oil and water. An *oil-in-water* (O/W) emulsion consists of small oil globules dispersed throughout water; a *water-in-oil* (W/O) emulsion is the reverse: water droplets are distributed throughout the oil. Most emulsions intended for oral use are of the O/W type; those to be applied to the skin may be of either type.

Oil-in-Water Emulsions

The O/W emulsions are desirable for oral use for several reasons. Unpalatable oily medications are broken into small particles and dispersed throughout a sweetened, flavored aqueous vehicle. These small particles are then carried past the taste buds and swallowed without the patient tasting the oily medication. The small particle size increases medication absorption from the stomach into the bloodstream. Mineral oil and castor oil are available as emulsions that make them taste better.

Water-in-Oil Emulsions

Water-in-oil emulsions are often used on unbroken skin. They spread more evenly than O/W emulsions since the natural oils on the skin readily mix with the external oil phase of the emulsion. They also soften the skin better because they retain moisture and are not readily washed off with water. However, they stain clothing and have a heavy, greasy feel. On the other hand, O/W emulsions may be more desirable in some cases since they are water washable and do not stain clothing. They feel lighter and non-greasy and are particularly advantageous when the emulsion is to be applied to a hairy part of the body such as the scalp.

The choice of O/W or W/O emulsion for preparations applied to the skin depends on several factors. Medications that are irritating to the skin are better tolerated if they are applied to the skin as small particles present in the internal phase. The external phase keeps them from directly contacting and irritating the skin. Therefore, medications that dissolve more readily in oil are applied to the skin as O/W emulsions, in which the oil is the internal phase, while those that dissolve in water are applied as W/O emulsions, in which the water is the internal phase.

Some emulsions may also be injected into the bloodstream. Intravenous fat emulsion (Intralipid and Liposyn) is an example of a O/W emulsion that is infused into the bloodstream through a vein. Oil-in-water and water-in-oil emulsions are compared in Table 2-2.

Suspensions

Suspensions are mixtures of fine particles of an undissolved solid distributed through a gas, liquid, or solid. Most suspensions are solids dispersed in liquids. The difference between a solution and a suspension is that in a solution the particles are dissolved where in a suspension they are not. Suspensions are useful for administering a large amount of solid medication that would be inconvenient to take as a tablet or capsule. The fine particles dissolve more quickly in the stomach and thus are absorbed into the bloodstream more quickly than the medication of a solid tablet or capsule. Usually suspensions need to be shaken before use to redistribute particles that may have settled to the bottom or risen to the top of the container during storage.

Most suspensions are intended for oral use, but some may be administered by other routes such as the rectal, otic, ophthalmic, or parenteral routes. Orally administered suspensions usually use water as the vehicle; some given by parenteral routes, such as the intramuscular route, use an oil as the vehicle.

Lotions are suspensions intended for external application. They contain finely powdered medications, and they cool, soothe, dry, or protect the skin. Lotions are usually applied without rubbing and work easily into large areas of the skin without leaving a greasy or oily feeling. Calamine lotion is a commonplace example of a protective lotion.

Magmas and *milks* are thick, viscous suspensions of undissolved drugs in water. Milk of magnesia may be the most familiar example of a magma. Magmas and milks are usually intended for oral administration and should be shaken well before each use.

Table 2–2

Comparison of O/W and W/O Emulsions

Oil-in-Water (O/W)

Advantages
- Improve taste of oral medications
- Better absorption of oral medications into the bloodstream
- Light, non-greasy feel
- Water washable

Disadvantages
- May easily wash off with water, or if patient sweats
- Does not spread easily on the skin

Water-in-Oil (W/O)

Advantages
- Spread more evenly on skin
- Soften skin
- Not easily washed off (may also be a disadvantage)

Disadvantages
- May stain clothing
- Heavy, greasy feel

Gels are similar to magmas and milks except that the suspended particle size in gels is smaller. Gels, too, are often intended for oral administration. Many commercially available antacids are gels.

Extractives

Extractives are concentrated preparations of active components obtained from plant or animal tissue. The crude drug is extracted, or withdrawn, from the dried plant or animal tissue by soaking it in a solvent. The solvent is then evaporated, leaving the active component behind. Tinctures, fluidextracts, and extracts are examples of formulations prepared in this manner. They differ only in their potency.

Tinctures are alcoholic or hydroalcoholic solutions whose potency is adjusted so that each milliliter of tincture contains the equivalent potency of 100 mg of crude drug. Iodine tincture and paregoric tincture are common examples.

Fluidextracts are more potent than tinctures; each milliliter of fluidextract contains the equivalent of 1000 mg of crude drug. Cascara sagrada fluidextract and senna fluidextract are commonly used to clear the bowels.

Extracts are prepared in the same manner as tinctures and fluidextracts but are two to six times as potent as the crude drug. Vanilla, almond, and peppermint extracts are examples of extracts.

Solid Medication Dosage Forms

Medications are commonly formulated in a solid form. Examples of solid medication dosage forms include tablets, capsules, suppositories, and lozenges. Solid medication dosage forms are used to deliver medications orally, rectally, or vaginally. It is important to remember that, like some liquid medication dosage forms, some solid medication dosage forms may be used by more than one route. For example, tablets are used for oral medications, but they may also be used to deliver medications into the vagina. Suppositories are usually given rectally (e.g., glycerin rectal suppositories) but may also be used to deliver medications into the vagina (e.g., Monistat 3 vaginal suppositories) or, very rarely, into the urethra. Table 2-3 summarizes the solid medication dosage forms that are discussed in this chapter.

Solid medication dosage forms have several advantages over other dosage forms:
- They often have longer shelf lives and are easier to package, store, and transport.
- Patients receive accurate medication doses since solid medications are formulated in distinct units.
- Techniques have been developed to create dosage forms of solid medications, in which the medication is released from the solid over a long period of time, these are sustained-release dosage forms. Patients need not take the medication as often as they would if they would have to take a non-sustained-release form.
- Patients find solid dosage forms more convenient to self-administer.
- Often, the oral solid medication dosage forms have little or no taste.

Oral solid dosage forms also have disadvantages:
- Some oral solid dosage forms are large enough to present a problem for patients unable to swallow larger tablets or capsules.
- Unconscious patients are not able to take oral solid medications. This is especially a problem if the desired medication is not

available in a form that can be administered by another route.

- Solid dosage forms must be dissolved—in the stomach or rectum for instance—before they are absorbed into the bloodstream. This results in a time delay before the drug can begin to act. Delay is not desirable for situations such as a heart attack or severe asthma episode, in which immediate drug action is necessary.

Tablets

Tablets are compacted solid medication dosage forms; they may be further classified on the basis of their method of manufacture. *Molded tablets* are made from wet materials placed in molds. *Compressed tablets* are formed by die punch compression of powdered, crystalline, or granular substances.

Other ingredients that have no medicinal activity may be included in a compressed tablet. These inactive, or inert, ingredients (e.g., binders, lubricants, diluents, colorants) are necessary for the manufacturing process or to make the tablet more effective (e.g., disintegrators). Binders help keep the compressed tablet from crumbling and hold it together. Diluents are fillers that are added to the active medication to make the tablet a practical size, and lubricants ease removal of the tablet from the die. Colorants add color to the product, and disintegrators are included to help the tablet dissolve in the stomach or elsewhere in the body.

Compressed tablets may have a sugar, film, or enteric coating on the outside. Sugar coating or film coating may be used to mask noxious-tasting or -smelling drugs, to add color to the tablet, or to protect the drug from exposure to the air and humidity. A film coating also coats the tablet with a hard shell to make it more durable and easier to swallow.

Enteric-coated oral tablets have a coating that protects the tablet from stomach acid and protects the lining of the gastrointestinal tract from irritation by the drug. Enteric-coating is also a technique used in making sustained-release tablets.

Tablets may also be described by a number of other terms. *Sublingual* and *buccal* tablets are useful solid dosage forms that are absorbed through the lining under the tongue or lining of the cheek directly into the bloodstream. Medications that are destroyed by stomach acid or are poorly

Table 2–3

Examples of Solid Medication Dosage Forms

Tablets
- Sublingual
- Buccal
- Effervescent
- Chewable
- Vaginal

Capsules

Lozenges

Extended-Release

Miscellaneous
- Powders
- Granules
- Aerosols
- Ointments
  Oleaginous
  Anhydrous
  Emulsion; O/W, W/O
  Water soluble
- Creams
  O/W
  W/O

absorbed into the bloodstream may be formulated as either of these types of tablets.

Effervescent tablets contain ingredients that bubble and release the active drug when placed in a liquid. The advantage to effervescent tablets is that they quickly disintegrate and dissolve before administration; therefore, the drug can be absorbed quickly. Original Alka-Seltzer Effervescent Tablets is an example.

Chewable tablets are those that do not need to be swallowed whole and may or should be chewed. They are pleasantly flavored and are especially useful for pediatric medications (e.g., chewable baby aspirin). Some adult tablets are also chewable. Antacid tablets (e.g., Rolaids Tablets and Tums) may be chewed before swallowing.

Vaginal tablets are inserted into the vagina. The tablet dissolves and the medication is absorbed through the vaginal mucous lining. Gyne-Lotrimin vaginal tablets is one such commercially available medication.

Capsules

Capsules are solid medication dosage forms in which the drug, with or without inactive or inert ingredients, is contained within a gelatin shell. Gelatin shells are made of protein derived from animals.

Hard gelatin capsules are two-piece oblong casings filled with powdered ingredients. Most often, these are intended for oral use and are swallowed whole. However, in some instances the capsule may be or should be opened and the powdered ingredients sprinkled on food or in water before administration (e.g., Theo-Dur Sprinkle capsules). Other capsules contain powders that are meant to be inhaled through the mouth into the lungs where the drug takes effect. These capsules are inserted into a mechanical device that punctures the capsule and releases the powder. Patients then inhale the powder into their lungs through the mouthpiece on the mechanical device. Ventolin Rotacaps is a medication administered in this fashion to treat asthma.

Soft gelatin capsules have ingredients added to the gelatin to give it soft, squeezable elastic consistency. The two halves of the capsule are sealed shut and, unlike hard gelatin capsules, cannot be opened. Soft gelatin capsules may be round, elliptical, or oblong in shape and are filled with liquid, pasty, or powdered medications. Vitamin A and vitamin D preparations are often available in a soft gelatin capsule. Colace, a stool softener, is also a soft gelatin capsule.

Lozenges

Lozenges, also known as *troches* or *pastilles*, are hard disk-shaped solid medication dosage forms that contain medication in a sugar base. Lozenges are used to deliver antiseptic, local anesthetic, antibiotic, analgesic, antitussive, astringent, or decongestant drugs to the mouth or throat. The lozenge is held in the mouth and sucked. As it dissolves, the lozenge releases the medication. Sucrets Sore Throat and Cēpacol Throat lozenges contain local anesthetic, antiseptic, and other ingredients useful for treating minor sore throats. Mycelex troches contain a fungicide and are used to treat oral fungal infections.

Extended-Release Dosage Forms

In some instances, it is desirable to have a medication dosage form that slowly and consistently releases the drug over an extended period of time—instead of all at once. These medication dosage forms are called extended-release, sustained-release, long-acting, or controlled-release. While the exact meaning of these terms differs in some respects, each of these terms implies a gradual release of medication over a longer period of time than standard dosage forms. Table 2-4 lists common abbreviations for extended-release. Oral tablets and capsules are the most common dosage forms that are formulated as extended-release. There are other dosage forms, such as implants and some intramuscular injections, that are also extended-release and they will be discussed later.

Extended-release dosage forms may be advantageous in several ways:

- They deliver medication in a slow, controlled, and consistent manner so that the patient is absorbing the same amount of medication throughout the given time period.
- The risk of drug side effects is reduced because the medication is delivered over an extended period of time.
- The patient may need to take the medication less frequently during the day, often only once or twice.
- Patients are more likely to take their medications properly if they have to take them less often and are less likely to experience side effects.
- The daily medication cost to the patient may be decreased. While extended-release products may be more expensive on a per-dose basis, the total daily cost may be less since the patient may need to take only one or two doses a day rather than three or four.

Several technologies are available to give medication dosage forms extended-release properties. Many small beads of medication in varying sizes may have varying thicknesses of a coating material. These beads are then put in a hard gelatin capsule. In the stomach, the gelatin capsule quickly dissolves and releases the small beads, which then dissolve and release medication at varying rates over a long period of time. The cold product Contac 12-Hour Capsules is formulated in this manner.

Other extended-release products use a slowly eroding matrix to provide the extended-release characteristic. In this situation, a portion of the medication is treated and made into special granules. These granules are then combined with untreated portion of the medication granules and made into a tablet or capsule. The

Table 2–4

Common Abbreviations for Extended-Release

CD	Controlled-diffusion
CR	Controlled-release, continuous-release
CRT	Controlled-release tablet
LA	Long-acting
SA	Sustained-action
SR	Sustained-release, slow-release
TD	Time delay
TR	Time-release
XL	Extra-long
XR	Extended-release

untreated drug granules immediately release the drug in the stomach while the treated ones slowly erode to provide the prolonged effect. Slow-K potassium tablets are such a product.

Some extended-release products are formulated in two or more layers. One layer immediately dissolves to produce an immediate effect while the remaining layers dissolve and release the drug gradually.

Other products, such as Procanbid, embed drug in an inert plastic or wax matrix. The drug is then released into the body as it slowly leaches from the matrix. The matrix does not dissolve and is passed through the gastrointestinal tract and excreted in the feces.

A very sophisticated extended-release system uses an osmotic pump to slowly deliver medication over time. This system utilizes the principle of osmosis, which states that fluids tend to flow from areas with a low concentration of a substance to areas with a high concentration. The pump system is composed of a special membrane surrounding a core of medication. As fluid in the stomach passes through the membrane, the drug core inside swells and forces medication out of a small hole drilled in the membrane. Procardia XL is one product that uses an osmotic pump system.

Miscellaneous Dosage Forms

A number of medication dosage forms do not fit neatly into a specific category. They may be either unique in and of themselves, or may be a combination of medication dosage forms.

Powders

Powders, as a medication dosage form, can be used externally or internally. External powders, or dusting powders, are finely ground mixtures of dry drugs and inactive ingredients that are sprinkled or dusted on the area to be medicated. An example is Mycostatin powder, which is often used to treat fungal infections of the skin. Internal powders are meant to be dissolved in a liquid prior to ingestion. Many potassium products are available as powders intended to be dissolved in water or juice. Some powders, such as powdered toothpaste, are mixed with water and used in the wetted state.

Powders are packaged in bulk containers or, when the amount delivered must be accurate, in powder papers. Powder papers are envelopes of folded paper that contain enough powder for one dose or application. BC Powder and Arthritis Strength BC Powder are analgesic powders packaged in powder papers.

Granules

When powders are wetted, allowed to dry, and ground into coarse pieces, the resulting medication dosage form is called a granule.

Granules differ from powders in that the particle size is larger and usually more stable. Many antibiotics are formulated as granules. The pharmacist or technician adds water to form a solution or suspension at the time of dispensing. Senokot Granules, a common laxative, is added to water before administration.

Aerosols

Aerosols are suspensions of very fine liquid or solid particles distributed in a gas and packaged under pressure. Medication is released from the container in a spray (e.g., Bactine Antiseptic Anesthetic), foam (e.g., ProctoFoam-HC), or solid (e.g., Tinactin). Aerosols are conveniently packaged and easy to use.

Aerosols may be used to deliver medications to internal and external sites. Aerosols inhaled internally, such as Proventil and Ventolin, are used to treat conditions such as asthma. The aerosol delivers the drug directly to the lungs, where it begins acting immediately. The drug does not first have to be dissolved in the stomach and absorbed into the bloodstream as it would if it were formulated as a tablet or capsule. External aerosols, such as Tinactin and Bactine Antiseptic Anesthetic sprays, may also be applied topically (externally) for skin conditions. An external aerosol can deliver medication to a hard-to-reach area of the skin and can be applied to inflamed or irritated skin with little or no further irritation.

Ointments

Ointments are semisolid medication dosage forms intended to be applied to the skin or mucous membranes. They are used to lubricate and soften or as a base (a vehicle that contains a drug) for drug delivery. However, ointments do not always contain a drug. Ointments are categorized on the basis of their characteristics. The primary types are oleaginous, anhydrous, emulsion, and water soluble.

Oleaginous, or *hydrocarbon*, *bases* are emollients that soothe the skin or mucous membrane. They are occlusive and protect the skin or mucous membrane from the air. They are hydrophobic, or repel water, and therefore do not wash off with water. They feel greasy to the touch. Oleaginous bases are used primarily for their lubricating effect because they do not allow moisture to escape from the skin, do not dry out, and remain on the skin for a long time. Vaseline petroleum jelly is an example of an oleaginous base.

Anhydrous, or *absorption*, *bases* contain no water and are similar to oleaginous bases but differ, in that instead of repelling water, they absorb it. They also soften skin but not to the same degree as the oleaginous bases. Anhydrous bases are used to absorb an aqueous, or water-based, drug into an ointment base. They do not contain water as part of their formula but as they absorb water, a water-in-oil (W/O) emulsion is formed. Anhydrous lanolin and cold cream are widely used anhydrous bases.

Emulsion bases may be W/O or O/W. The W/O types are also emollient, occlusive, and greasy. They contain water and some may be able to absorb additional water. Lanolin, mentioned above as an anhydrous base, and cold cream are considered to be W/O emulsions when water is added to them.

Emulsion bases of the O/W type, or water-washable bases, are quite different. They are non-greasy and readily wash off with water. They are non-occlusive and may be diluted, or thinned with the addition of water. They are often used to absorb watery discharge in certain skin conditions or may be used to help the skin absorb certain medications. Hydrophilic Ointment is an O/W ointment base.

Water-soluble bases are non-greasy, non-occlusive, and water-washable. They do not contain

any fats and usually do not contain any water. Nonaqueous or solid medications are added to this type of ointment base. Polyethylene glycol ointment is one such base.

Ointment bases are chosen primarily on the basis of the characteristics described above. A W/O emulsion base may be used if a liquid medication is to be added to the ointment. Some medications may be more stable or more readily absorbed by the skin when delivered in some types of ointment bases over others. However, the softening or drying characteristics of the ointment base may also influence the choice of a base. For instance, a non-greasy ointment base may be chosen if the ointment is to be applied to the face since a greasy base may leave an unpleasant feeling.

remember O/W : OFF w/ water

Creams

Creams are semisolid O/W or W/O emulsions that may or may not contain medication. They are easily worked into the skin and feel lighter than ointments. They too serve to soften the skin. Creams may be preferred over ointments because they are easier to spread, have a cooling effect on the skin, and (in the case of O/W creams) are easier to wash off with water. Many products are available as creams or ointments to cater to the preferences of patients and physicians. Creams are also widely used in many cosmetic products.

remember: W/O WITHOUT water

ROUTES OF ADMINISTRATION

Drugs can be administered by several different routes. Although the oral route is most common, it may not always be the most convenient or practical. Drugs may be administered via any body orifice, through the skin, or an artificially made opening.

Oral

Medications taken by the oral route are introduced into the body through the mouth. The oral route is abbreviated PO, which is from the Latin *per os* (by mouth). Tablets, capsules, solutions, suspensions, and emulsions are some of the medication dosage forms that may be taken orally.

The oral route has many advantages. It is safe and convenient, and medications taken orally are generally less expensive than those administered by other routes. Oral dosage forms may be modified to deliver drugs in an extended-release fashion.

There are disadvantages to the oral route. It cannot be used to administer medications to unconscious patients or those who have trouble swallowing. Because an oral medication must be dissolved in the stomach before entering the bloodstream, there is a lag time between ingestion and the time the drug begins to act. This time lag is a problem if an immediate action is desired. Food, other drugs, acid, or lack of acid in the stomach may interfere with the dissolution or absorption of the drug.

There may be times when a patient cannot swallow a medication orally (e.g., the patient is mechanically ventilated with an endotracheal tube in the throat). In these situations, medications may be given through a tube inserted through the nose, throat, or even the abdomen. Although these tubes are usually inserted for other reasons, they may offer alternatives to the usual oral route.

Sublingual and Buccal

The terms *sublingual* (under the tongue) and *buccal* (inside the cheek) not only refer to types of tablets but also to routes of oral medication administration.

To administer a drug sublingually, a *sublingual* tablet is placed under the tongue where the medication dissolves and is absorbed into the bloodstream through the underlining of the tongue. Nitroglycerin sublingual tablets are administered under the tongue. Sublingual tablets are used when a rapid drug effect is desired, such as the use of nitroglycerin to treat chest pain.

To administer a drug bucally, *buccal* tablets are used. They are placed inside the pouch of the cheek, where the medication dissolves and is absorbed through the cheek lining into the bloodstream over time. Metandren Linguets, a male sex hormone product, are administered via the buccal route.

Parenteral

Parenteral routes of administration are those that bypass the gastrointestinal tract. Medications administered parenterally are most commonly introduced into the body intravenously, intramuscularly, or subcutaneously. They may be injected over a short period of time (seconds to minutes) with a needle and syringe or infused into the body at a constant rate over hours or days. Drugs that are given parenterally are most commonly formulated as solutions (e.g., potassium chloride, dextrose, many antibiotics, regular insulin). Less often, suspensions (e.g., Sus-Phrine, penicillin G benzathine) and emulsions (e.g., intravenous fat emulsion) are administered parenterally.

Parenterally administered drugs are given to patients who are unable to take oral medications, when faster drug action is desired, or when a drug is not available in a form that can be administered by another route. A disadvantage of parenteral routes is that they are often invasive, that is, a needle penetrates the skin to enter into veins, arteries, and other areas of the body. This penetration maybe painful for the patient and could introduce bacteria or other contaminants into the body resulting in an infection.

Intravenous (IV) medications are introduced into the body through a needle placed directly in a vein. These drugs are usually given as solutions that must be sterile and free of particulate matter. Drugs given by the IV route are immediately available to act in the body. Because IV drugs act quickly, one must be careful giving IV medications. If too high a dose is given or if the patient experiences an adverse reaction, it is difficult to reverse the drug's effects.

Intravenously administered drugs may be given as a *bolus* or by *continuous infusion*. A bolus drug dose is injected into the body over a relatively short period of time—seconds to minutes. The term *IV push* also refers to this administration technique; the drug is pushed into the body by means of a syringe. Lidocaine, a drug used to treat abnormal heart rhythms, may be given as a bolus. In contrast, some medications may be infused into veins over hours to days using a constant infusion or drip, which provides a constant supply of drug to the body. Bolus doses and continuous infusions are often used together. For example, after lidocaine is given as an IV push, a lidocaine drip is often started to maintain a certain level of lidocaine in the blood.

Intramuscular (IM) administration involves direct injection of medication into a large muscle mass such as the upper arm, thigh, or buttock. The drug is then absorbed from the muscle tissue into the bloodstream. IM drugs may be given as solutions or suspensions. Drugs given by the IM route act more quickly than orally administered drugs but not as quickly as IV drugs. Some drugs may be formulated in extended-release forms that slowly release drug from the muscle tissue into the bloodstream over hours, days, or even months. Some types of penicillin are formulated in this manner. Disadvantages to the IM route are that it is difficult to reverse the drug's effects once the injection has been given, the injection is painful to receive and may cause bruising, and drug absorption from the muscle into the bloodstream may be erratic and incomplete.

Solutions or suspensions injected *subcutaneously* (SC, subQ, SQ) are deposited in the tissue immediately under the skin and are sometimes referred to as hypodermic injections. Drugs given by the SC route are absorbed to a lesser extent and act slower than those given by the IV or IM routes. Patients can easily be taught to administer SC injections to themselves. Many diabetic patients give themselves daily SC injections of insulin.

A limitation of both the SC and IM routes is the volume of drug that can be injected under the skin or into the muscle. It may be undesirable to use the SC route in patients with frail skin or the IM route in patients with decreased muscle mass or bleeding problems.

Caution must be exercised when interpreting abbreviations that refer to the route of medication administration. The abbreviation IV usually refers to the intravenous route, but it could also refer to the *intravitreous* (into the eye) or *intraventricular* (into the brain) routes, or could be interpreted as the roman numeral four. Like extended-release abbreviations, abbreviations for drug administration routes must be carefully interpreted in the context of each medication order.

The IV, IM, and SC routes of medication administration are the most commonly used parenteral routes. However, drugs can be injected into almost any body space. Several other parenteral medication dosage routes are used for specialized purposes or to limit drug delivery to the immediate area of the injection. These routes include intradermal, intraarterial, intraarticular, intracardiac, intraperitoneal, intrapleural, intraventricular, intravesicular, intravitreous, and intrathecal.

The *intradermal* (ID) route involves drug being injected into the top layers of the skin. ID injections are not injected as deep as those given subcutaneously. The ID route is used to administer drugs for skin testing of patients to see if they are allergic to drugs or other substances such as dust, pet dander, or pollen. It can also be used to administer diagnostic skin tests to check if patients have been exposed to certain microorganisms such as those that cause mumps or tuberculosis.

Intraarterial (IA) injections involve administering an agent directly into arteries. It has the advantage of delivering drugs, such as cancer chemotherapy agents, directly to the desired location and thus may decrease some of the side effects caused when the drug acts in other parts of the body. This more direct route involves greater risk than the IV route and may be more toxic if the drug was not originally intended for arterial administration.

The *intraarticular* route involves injecting a drug into a joint, such as a knee or elbow. These drugs act to treat diseases in the joint. For example, steroid drugs are injected intraarticularly to treat the inflammation caused by arthritis.

The *intracardiac* route, injection directly into the heart muscle, is used in life-threatening emergencies. This route is not often used because it entails the risk of rupturing the heart.

Intraperitoneal injections are given into the peritoneal, or abdominal, cavity. This route is used to administer antibiotics to treat infections in the peritoneal cavity. One method of dialysis, peritoneal dialysis, uses the intraperitoneal route to remove waste products from the blood of patients with kidney failure.

Intrapleural describes the injection of drugs into the sac surrounding the lungs, or the pleura. Drugs are injected intrapleurally to stimulate inflammation and scarring of the pleural tissues so that excessive and bothersome fluid can no longer accumulate in the pleural sac.

The *intraventricular* route is used to administer drugs into the ventricles, or cavities, of the brain to treat infections or cancerous tumors of brain.

The *intravesicular* route delivers drugs directly into the urinary bladder. This route is used to treat bladder infections or bladder cancer.

Intravitreous administration is direct injection into the eye. Many drugs do not enter the eye from the bloodstream, and often the only way to deliver medications inside the eye is to inject them intravitreously. Antibiotics to treat sight-threatening eye infections are administered via this route.

Intrathecal is the route by which drugs are injected into the space around the spinal cord. This route may be used to deliver agents that treat infections or cancerous tumors of the central nervous system.

An *implant* is a medication pump or device inserted semi-permanently or permanently into the body. Medication is released from the implant and delivered in a controlled fashion. Implants are often used to treat chronic, or long-term, conditions or diseases. Some diabetic patients have a small pump that delivers insulin implanted in their bodies. Certain types of cancers may be treated with chemotherapeutic agents that are delivered into the arteries that enter the cancerous organ. A small pump filled with the drug is implanted into the body and infuses the chemotherapy drug into the artery. A form of contraception, Norplant (Wyeth-Ayerst), has been developed in which an implant is inserted under the skin of a woman's arm and slowly releases birth control medication for up to 5 years.

Topical

The topical route of administrating medication refers to the application of medications to the surface of the skin or mucous membranes. Medications administered topically include antibiotics, antiseptics, astringents, emollients, and corticosteroids. Topical medication dosage forms include creams, ointments, lotions, sprays, and aerosols. In most cases, the skin or mucous membrane acts as a barrier to prevent the medication from entering the bloodstream. As a result, drugs used for treating diseases of the skin and mucous membranes can be applied in higher concentrations than drugs administered internally.

Some ointments and creams (e.g., topical corticosteroid ointments) are formulated to deliver a drug into the skin to treat a condition of the deeper skin layers. Sometimes creams or ointments may be designed so that the drug diffuses through the skin into the bloodstream. The drug is then available to the whole body. This is called systemic absorption. Nitroglycerin ointment used to treat chest pain is an example.

In some cases, systemic absorption is not desired and may result in unwanted side effects. For example, when topical corticosteroids are absorbed systemically over prolonged periods of time, the patient may develop cataracts or glaucoma. Penetration of topical medications into the bloodstream is more likely when the skin is not intact (e.g., when it is inflamed or burned).

Other Routes of Administration

Transdermal

The *transdermal,* or *percutaneous,* route of medication administration delivers drugs across the skin. The topical route is used for medications not intended to enter the body and bloodstream, but the transdermal route is meant to deliver medications to the bloodstream and consequently, the rest of the body. Medications are continuously absorbed into the bloodstream when the transdermal route is used. Transdermal medications are applied to the skin, released from a vehicle, and absorbed into the bloodstream. Adhesive patches, similar to plastic bandages, contain drugs in a small reservoir and are commonly used to deliver medications transdermally. Patches are convenient to use. Depending on the patch, they may be applied to the skin from once a day to once a week.

Transdermal patches are formulated in one of two ways. One type of patch is formulated so that the patch itself controls the rate of delivery of drug to the skin. A special membrane in the patch is in contact with the skin. The membrane controls the amount of drug delivered from a drug reservoir contained in the patch, through the membrane and skin, and into the bloodstream. The second type of transdermal patch is designed so that the skin itself controls the rate of drug delivery. The drug moves from an area of high concentration (the drug reservoir) into an area of low concentration (the skin and bloodstream). The disadvantage to this type of patch is that the release of drug is less controlled and a large amount of drug could suddenly be released from the patch into the blood.

Medications that are available in a patch formulation include a narcotic analgesic (Duragesic), female hormones (Estraderm), and drugs to treat high blood pressure (Catapres-TTS), chronic chest pain (Nitro-Dur, Nitrodisc, Transderm-Nitro, and others), and motion sickness (Transderm Scōp), and to help patients quit smoking (Habitrol, Pro-Step, Nicoderm, and Nicotrol).

Ointments are sometimes used to deliver drugs percutaneously. Nitroglycerin ointment for chronic chest pain was often used in the past. Its use has been widely replaced by the nitroglycerin transdermal patches although the ointment may still be used to transition, or wean, patients from continuous nitroglycerin IV infusions to oral nitroglycerin medications.

Rectal

Drugs inserted through the anus into the rectum are delivered by the rectal route. Rectally administered drugs may be formulated as solids (suppositories), liquids or suspensions (enemas), and aerosol foams. Once the drug reaches the rectum, its activity may be limited to the lower gastrointestinal tract, or the drug may be absorbed into the bloodstream and delivered to its site of action elsewhere in the body. The rectal route is often used for children and patients who are unable to take oral medications.

Vaginal

Drugs may also be inserted into the vagina. Drugs delivered by the vaginal route may be in the form of a vaginal suppository (e.g., AVC vaginal suppositories), tablet (e.g., Mycostatin vaginal tablets), cream (e.g., Terazol), ointment (Vagistat-1), gel (e.g., Ortho-Gynol Contraceptive), or solution (e.g., Massengill Douche).

The drug's activity may be limited to the vagina—as it is when vaginal medications are used to treat vaginal infections—or the drug may be absorbed into the bloodstream and delivered to a remote site where the drug takes effect. Prostaglandin suppositories used for premenstrual syndrome are an example of a drug administered vaginally to produce effects in other parts of the body (systemic).

Otic

The otic route is used to deliver drugs into the ear canal. Otic drugs may be formulated as solutions or suspensions. Local conditions of the ear, such as ear infections or excessive ear wax, may be treated with otically administered drugs.

Ophthalmic

Drugs that are administered into the eye are given via the ophthalmic route. Ophthalmic medications are formulated as solutions, suspensions, gels, or ointments. Special medicated inserts (e.g., Ocusert Pilo) intended to be placed in the pouch of the lower eyelid can also be used to deliver medications to the eye. The ophthalmic route is advantageous in that conditions of the eye, such as glaucoma and infections of the conjunctiva, may be treated without administering the drug systemically. As a result, medication can reach the intended site without exposing the patient to unnecessary side effects in other parts of the body.

Nasal

Drugs are administered into the nostrils by the nasal route. Solutions may be nasally administered as sprays or drops. This route is advantageous because conditions of the nose, such as nasal congestion or allergic rhinitis, may be treated without administering the drug systemically. Often drugs given nasally act more quickly than if they were administered by a route, such as the mouth or vein, that introduces medication into the whole body. In other instances, drugs may be nasally administered to treat conditions not involving the nose (e.g., Stadol NS nasal spray for the relief of migraine headaches).

Inhalation

Drugs may be inhaled through the mouth into the lungs. This route is used when a rapid drug effect is desired to treat lung conditions. The inhalation route is most often used to deliver medications for the treatment of asthma. Examples, such as the over-the-counter product Primatene Mist and the prescription drug Proventil, have been previously discussed.

DOSAGE FORM VERSUS ROUTE OF ADMINISTRATION

A particular medication dosage form often implies a specific administration route; and a particular route often implies a specific dosage form. For instance, the tablet dosage form is most often administered orally, but it is also used to administer drugs intravaginally. When the rectal route is used, the suppository is the dosage form commonly considered. However, suppositories are not necessarily the only dosage form used for the rectal route since many medications are formulated as rectal foams or enemas. Finally, as discussed previously, a term may be used to describe both a route and a dosage form, for example, the terms *sublingual* and *buccal*.

Many drugs are available in a number of dosage forms and may be delivered via a number of administration routes. In some instances, a condition may be treated using two or more routes. For example, meningitis, an infection of the brain, may be treated with antibiotics administered intravenously and intraventricularly. Glaucoma, a condition of the eye, may be treated locally with ophthalmic drops or systemically with oral capsules. Physicians and pharmacists select the most appropriate dosage form and route based on the patient's condition, the need for immediate drug action, or the availability of a drug in a particular dosage form or administration route.

RECOMMENDED READING

Ansel HC. *Introduction to Pharmaceutical Dosage Forms.* 6th ed. Philadelphia, PA: Lea & Febiger; 1995.

Davis NM. *Medical Abbreviations: 7000 Conveniences at the Expense of Communications and Safety,* 7th ed. Huntingdon Valley, PA: Neil M. Davis Associates; 1995.

Gennaro AR, editor. *Remington's Pharmaceutical Sciences,* 19th ed. Easton, PA: Mack Publishing Company; 1995.

Stanaszek WF, Stanaszek MJ, Holt RJ, *et al. Understanding Medical Terms: A Guide for Pharmacy Practice.* Lancaster, PA: Technomic Publishing Company, Inc.; 1992.

SELF-ASSESSMENT QUESTIONS

1. Common vehicles for liquid medication forms are _____, _____, and _____.

2. For the following situations, would a liquid or solid medication dosage form be a better choice?
   a. The patient has just had throat surgery and cannot easily swallow.
   b. A patient is very sensitive to unpleasant tastes and refuses to take "bad" tasting medicine.
   c. A traveling salesman needs to take a medication on a regular basis.
   d. A patient has an ear infection.

3. Define "internal phase."

4. The IV route of administration may be advantageous over the IM route because _____.

5. Intraventricular medication administration means that the medication is injected directly into the _____.

6. A parenteral route of medication administration is one that bypasses the _____.

7. A patient must apply a topical medication to her scalp. Would an O/W or W/O emulsion be more appropriate?

8. Match the term with the route of administration.
   a. sublingual
   b. intrapleural
   c. intraarticular
   d. intravenous
   e. intravitreous
   f. subcutaneous
   ___ injection into the eye
   ___ injection into the pleura of the lungs
   ___ injection beneath the skin
   ___ injection directly into a vein
   ___ administration and absorption of drug from under the tongue
   ___ injection of a drug into a joint, such as the knee or elbow

9. List three types of nonaqueous solutions.

10. Lozenges are also known as _____ or _____.

ANSWERS TO SELF-ASSESSMENT

1. water, alcohol, mineral oil

2. a. Liquid, since liquids are usually easier to swallow.
   b. Solid, since they often have little or no taste especially when compared to a liquid medication.
   c. Solid, since solid medications are more convenient to package and transport and do not need to be measured.
   d. Liquid, since it is not practical to administer solid medication forms into the ear.

3. In an emulsion, one liquid is broken into small particles and is evenly scattered throughout the other. The liquid present in small particles is referred to as the internal phase.

4. IV medications are injected into the bloodstream and do not need to be absorbed through the muscle into the blood before they can act.

5. ventricles of the brain (Be careful not to think that this means the ventricles of the heart.)

6. gastrointestinal tract

7. O/W emulsions may be more desirable since they are easily water washable, feel lighter,

and are particularly advantageous when the emulsion is to be applied to a hairy part of the body.

8. _e_ injection into the eye
   _b_ injection into the pleura of the lungs
   _f_ injection beneath the skin
   _d_ injection directly into a vein

_a_ administration and absorption of drug from under the tongue

_c_ injection of a drug into a joint, such as the knee or elbow

9. hydroalcoholic (elixirs, spirits), alcoholic (collodions, spirits), glycerites

10. troches, pastilles

3 Pharmacy Calculations

Gerald A. Storm, R.Ph.
Rebecca S. Kentzel, C.Ph.T.

Most calculations pharmacy technicians and pharmacists use involve basic math. However, basic math is easily forgotten when it is not used routinely. This chapter reviews the fundamentals of calculations and how those calculations are applied in pharmacy.

LEARNING OBJECTIVES

After completing this chapter the reader will be able to
1. Calculate conversions between different numbering and measuring systems.
2. Calculate medication doses from various medication dilutions.
3. Calculate and define osmolarity, isotonicity, body surface area, and flow rates.

REVIEW OF BASIC MATHEMATICS

Numerals

A numeral is a word or a sign, or a group of words or signs, that express a number.

Kinds of Numerals

Arabic

Examples: 0, 1, 2, 3, 4, 5, 6, 7, 8, 9, etc.

Roman

In pharmacy practice, these numerals are only used to denote quantities on prescriptions.

ss or $\overline{ss}$ = 1/2	L or l = 50
I or i = 1	C or c = 100
V or v = 5	D or d = 500
X or x = 10	M or m = 1000

This chapter was adapted with permission from the Johns Hopkins Hospital Technician Training Course 1991. p. 106–38.

It is important to note that when a smaller Roman numeral (e.g.,"I") is placed before a larger Roman numeral (e.g., "V"), the smaller Roman numeral is subtracted from the larger Roman numeral.

Example: I = 1 and V = 5; therefore, IV = 4 because 5 − 1 = 4.

Problem Set #1:

Convert the following roman numerals to arabic numerals:

a. ii = _____   b. DCV = _____   c. xx = _____
d. iii = _____   e. vii = _____   f. iv = _____
g. IX = _____   h. xv = _____   i. xi = _____
j. MXXL = _____ k. xiv = _____   l. xvi = _____

Numbers

A number is a total quantity or amount that is made of one or more numerals.

Kinds of numbers

Whole Numbers

Examples: 10, 220, 5, 19

Fractions

Fractions are parts of whole numbers.

Examples: 1/4, 2/7, 11/13, 3/8

Always try to express a fraction in its simplest form.

Examples: 2/4 = 1/2, 10/12 = 5/6, 8/12 = 2/3

The whole number above the fraction line is called the numerator, and the whole number below the fraction line is called the denominator.

Mixed Numbers

These numbers contain both whole numbers and fractions.

Examples: 1 1/2, 13 3/4, 20 7/8, 2 1/2

Decimal Numbers

Decimal numbers are actually another means of writing fractions and mixed numbers.

Examples: 1/2 = 0.5, 1 3/4 = 1.75

Note: Decimal numbers can be identified by the period appearing somewhere in the number. The period in a decimal number is called the decimal point.

The following two points about zeros in decimal numbers are VERY important:

1. Do NOT write a whole number in decimal form.

   In other words, when writing a whole number, avoid placing a period followed by a zero (e.g., 5.0).

   Why? Periods are sometimes hard to see, and errors may result from misreading the number. For example, the period in 1.0 may be overlooked, and the number could appear to be 10 instead. This could cause a 10-fold dosing error, which could kill someone.

2. On the contrary, when writing a fraction in its decimal form, always precede the period with a zero.

   Why? Once again, periods are sometimes difficult to see, and .5 may be misread as 5. However, if the period in 0.5 was illegible, the zero would alert the reader that a period is supposed to be there.

WORKING WITH FRACTIONS AND DECIMALS

Please note that this section is meant only to be a basic overview. These are fundamental skills that a practicing pharmacy technician should already possess. The problems and examples found in this section should serve as basic building blocks for all calculations reviewed later in this chapter. If you do not know how to do these basic functions, you need to seek further assistance.

Review of Basic Mathematical Functions Involving Fractions

When adding, subtracting, multiplying, and/or dividing fractions, all units (or terms) must be alike. Also, when working with fractions, be sure that the smallest reduced fraction is the way that you express your answer (i.e., if your answer is 6/8, be sure to reduce it to 3/4).

Addition

Add the following: 3/4 g + 7/8 g + 1/4 kg

First, convert all terms to common units:
   1000 g/kg × 1/4 kg = 250 g

Convert all fractions to common denominators:
   3/4 g × 2/2 = 6/8 g

Now, add: 6/8 g + 7/8 g + 250 g = 250 13/8 g

Reduce to the smallest fraction:
250 13/8 g = 251 5/8 g

Subtraction

Subtract the following: 7/8 g – 1/4 g

All terms are already in common units, so you can proceed to converting the fractions to common denominators:
1/4 g × 2/2 = 2/8 g

Now, subtract: 7/8 g – 2/8 g = 5/8 g

Multiplication

Multiply the following: 1/6 m × 2/3

When multiplying and dividing fractions, you do NOT have to convert to common denominators.

First, multiply the numerators: 1 × 2 = 2

Next, multiply the denominators: 6 × 3 = 18

Express your answer as a fraction: 2/18 m

Be sure to reduce your fraction: 2/18 m = 1/9 m

Division

Divide the following: 1/2 m ÷ 1/4

Once again, you do NOT have to convert to common denominators.

To divide two fractions, the first fraction must be multiplied by the inverse (or reciprocal) of the second fraction.

Let's go back to our example:

1/2 m ÷ 1/4 is the same as 1/2 m × 4/1

Now, multiply: 1/2 m × 4/1 = 4/2 m

Reduce to lowest fraction: 4/2 m = 2 m

Review of Basic Mathematical Functions Involving Decimals

As with fractions, when adding, subtracting, multiplying, and/or dividing decimals, all units (or terms) must be alike.

Addition

Note: It is important to remember to line up decimal points when adding and/or subtracting decimal numbers (as shown in the next column).

Add the following: 0.1 mg + 0.1247 g

First, convert to common units:
0.1247 g × 1000 mg/g = 124.7 mg

Add the terms by lining up the decimal points:

```
   0.1 mg
+124.7 mg
─────────
 124.8 mg
```

Subtraction

Subtract the following: 2.1 g – 20.5 mg

Subtraction is treated the same as addition. We must first convert to common units:
2.1 g × 1000 mg/g = 2100 mg

Now, subtract. Don't forget to line up decimal points:

```
 2100.0 mg
 – 20.5 mg
──────────
 2079.5 mg
```

Multiplication

Note: When multiplying decimal numbers, the number of decimal places in the product must equal the total number of decimal places in the numbers multiplied, as shown below.

Multiply the following: 0.6 L × 24

In our example, there is a total of one digit to the right of the decimal point in the numbers being multiplied, so our answer will have one digit to the right of the decimal point.

Answer: 0.6 L × 24 = 14.4 L

Division

Note: When dividing decimal numbers, move the divisor's decimal point to the right to form a whole number. Remember to move the dividend's decimal point the same number of places to the right. When using long division, place the decimal point in the answer immediately above the dividend's decimal point.

Divide the following: 60.75 ml ÷ 4.5

Move the decimal points: 607.5 ml ÷ 45

Answer: 607.5 ml ÷ 45 = 13.5 ml

Converting Fractions to Decimal Numbers

Simply divide the numerator by the denominator.

For example, 1/2 = one divided by two = 0.5

Converting Mixed Numbers to Decimal Numbers

This process involves the following two steps:

Step 1. Write the mixed number as a fraction.

Method: Multiply the whole number and the denominator of the fraction. Add the product (result) to the numerator of the fraction, keeping the same denominator.

Example: 2 3/4 = two times four plus three over four = 11/4

Step 2. Divide the numerator by the denominator.

Example: 11/4 = eleven divided by four = 2.75

Or use this alternate method

The alternate method involves the following three steps:

Step 1. Separate the whole number and the fraction.

Example: 2 3/4 = 2 and 3/4

Step 2. Convert the fraction to its decimal counterpart.

Example: 3/4 = three divided by four = 0.75

Step 3. Add the whole number to the decimal fraction.

Example: 2 plus 0.75 = 2.75

Converting Decimal Numbers to Mixed Numbers or Fractions

Step 1: Write the decimal number over one, dividing it by one. (Remember that dividing any number by one does not change the number.)

Example: 3.5 = 3.5/1

Step 2: Move the decimal point in both the numerator and denominator an equal number of places to the right. The number of places the decimal point needs to be moved is determined by the number of digits following the decimal point in the numerator.

Example: Since there is only one digit following the decimal point in 3.5, move the decimal point one place to the right in both the numerator and the denominator: 3.5/1 = 35/10.

Remember that the number will remain the same as long as you do exactly the same things to the numerator and the denominator. You also have to remember that the decimal point of a whole number always follows the last digit.

Step 3: Simplify the fraction.

Example: 35/10 = 7/2 = 3 1/2

Problem Set #2:

Convert the following fractions to decimal numbers:

a. 1/2   b. 3/4   c. 1   d. 2/5
e. 1/3   f. 5/8   g. 50/100   h. 12/48
i. 1 1/2   j. 2 2/3   k. 5 1/4   l. 3 4/5

Convert the following decimal numbers to fractions or mixed numbers:

m. 0.25   n. 0.4   o. 0.75   p. 0.35
q. 2.5   r. 1.6   s. 3.25   t. 0.33

PERCENTAGES

Percentage (%) means "by the hundred" or "in a hundred." Percents are just fractions, but fractions with a set denominator. The denominator is always one hundred (100).

Example: "50%" means "50 in a hundred" or "50/100" or "1/2"

Converting Percentages to Fractions

Write the number preceding the percent sign over 100 and simplify the resulting fraction.

Example: 25% = 25/100 = 1/4

Converting Fractions to Percentages

Convert the fraction to one in which the denominator is a hundred. This is easiest when the fraction is in the form of a decimal.

Step 1: Write the fraction in its decimal form.

Example: 3/4 = three divided by four = 0.75

Step 2: Write the decimal over one.

Example: 0.75/1

Step 3: To obtain 100 as the denominator, move the decimal point two places to the right. To avoid changing the number, move the decimal point two places to the right in the numerator as well.

Example: 0.75/1 = 75/100

Step 4: Since we already know that "out of a hundred" or "divided by a hundred" is the same as percent, we can write 75/100 as 75%.

Concentration Expressed as a Percentage

Percent weight-in-weight (w/w) is the grams of a drug in 100 grams of the product.

Percent weight-in-volume (w/v) is the grams of a drug in 100 ml of the product.

Percent volume-in-volume (v/v) is the milliliters of drug in 100 ml of the product.

The above concentration percentages will be discussed in further detail a little later in this chapter.

Problem Set #3

Convert the following percentages to fractions (remember to simplify the fractions):

a. 23%	b. 67%	c. 12.5%	d. 50%
e. 66.7%	f. 75%	g. 66%	h. 40%
i. 100%	j. 15%		

Convert the following fractions to percentages:

k. 1/2	l. 1/4	m. 2/5	n. 6/25
o. 4/100	p. 0.5	q. 0.35	r. 0.44
s. 0.57	t. 0.99		

UNITS OF MEASURE

Metric System

The metric system is based on the decimal system, in which everything is measured in multiples or fractions of ten. Appendix 3 lists the conversion charts reviewed on the following pages.

Standard Measures

The standard measure for length is the meter, the standard measure for weight is the gram, and the standard measure for volume is the liter.

Prefixes

The prefixes below are used to describe multiples or fractions of the standard measures for length, weight, and volume.

Latin prefixes

micro- (μ):	1/1,000,000	= 0.000001
milli- (m):	1/1000	= 0.001
centi- (c) :	1/100	= 0.01
deci- (d) :	1/10	= 0.1

Note that Latin prefixes denote fractions.

Greek prefixes

deca- (da): 10
hecto- (h): 100
kilo- (k): 1000
mega- (M): 1,000,000

Note that Greek prefixes denote multiples.

Prefixes with Standard Measures

Length

Standard measure is the meter (m).

1 kilometer (km)	= 1000 meters (m)
0.001 kilometer (km)	= 1 meter (m)
1 millimeter (mm)	= 0.001 meter (m)
1000 millimeters (mm)	= 1 meter (m)
1 centimeter (cm)	= 0.01 meter (m)
100 centimeters (cm)	= 1 meter (m)

Volume

Standard measure is the liter (L).

1 milliliter (ml)	= 0.001 liter (L)
1000 milliliters (ml)	= 1 liter (L)
1 microliter (μl)	= 0.000001 liter (L)
1,000,000 microliters (μl)	= 1 liter (L)
1 deciliter (dl)	= 0.1 liter (L)
10 deciliters (dl)	= 1 liter (L)

Weight

Standard measure is the gram (g).

1 kilogram (kg)	= 1000 grams (g)
0.001 kilogram (kg)	= 1 gram (g)
1 milligram (mg)	= 0.001 gram (g)
1000 milligrams (mg)	= 1 gram (g)
1 microgram (μg)	= 0.000001 gram (g)
1,000,000 micrograms (μg)	= 1 gram (g)

Apothecary System

The apothecary system is sometimes used in prescription writing.

Weight

The standard measure for weight is the grain (gr).

Pound (lb.)	Ounces (3)	Drams (3)	Scruples (Ə)	Grains (gr)
1 =	12 =	96 =	288 =	5760
	1 =	8 =	24 =	480
		1 =	3 =	60
			1 =	20

Volume

The standard measure for volume is the minim.

Gallons (gal)	Pints (pt)	Fluid ounces (f3 or fl oz)	Fluid drams (f3)	Minims (ℳ)
1 =	8 =	128	= 1024 =	61,440
	1 =	16	= 128 =	7,680
		1	= 8 =	480
			1 =	60

Avoirdupois System

This system is mainly used in measuring the bulk medications encountered in manufacturing. Be sure to note that the pounds-to-ounces equivalent is different in the apothecary and avoirdupois systems. The avoirdupois system is most commonly used to measure weight, and the apothecary system is most commonly used to measure volume. Be sure to take note of the difference in symbols used for the two systems. Also, note that fluid ounces, which measures volume, is often mistakenly shortened to "ounces," which is actually a measure of weight. Since ounces measure weight, pay close attention to the measure you are working with and convert accordingly.

Weight

The standard measure for weight is the grain (gr).

Pound (lb)	Ounces (oz)	Grains (gr)
1 =	16	= 7000
	1	= 437.5

Household System

The household system is the most commonly used system of measuring liquids in outpatient settings. The measuring equipment usually consists of commonly used home utensils (i.e., teaspoons, tablespoons, etc.).

1 teaspoonful (tsp) = 5 ml
1 dessertspoonful = 10 ml

1 tablespoonful (TBS) = 15 ml = 0.5 fluid ounces (fl oz)
1 wineglassful = 60 ml = 2 fl oz
1 teacupful = 120 ml = 4 fl oz
1 glassful/cupful = 240 ml = 8 fl oz
3 tsp = 1 TBS
2 TBS = 1 fl oz
8 fl oz = 1 cup
2 cups = 1 pint (pt)
2 pt = 1 quart (qt)
4 qt = 1 gallon (gal)

Note: The term drop is commonly used; however, caution should be used when working with this measure, especially with potent medications. The volume of a drop depends not only on the nature of the liquid but also on the size, shape, and position of the dropper used. To accurately measure small amounts of liquid, use a 1-ml syringe (with milliliter markings) instead of a dropper. Eye drops are an exception to this rule; they are packaged in a manner to deliver a correctly sized droplet.

Problem Set #4:

Fill in the blanks:

  a. 1 liter (L) = _____ ml
  b. 1000 g = _____ kg
  c. 1 g = _____ mg
  d. 1000 μg = _____ mg
  e. 1 TBS = _____ tsp
  f. 1 TBS = _____ ml
  g. 240 ml = _____ cupfuls
  h. 1 cup = _____ ml
  i. 15 ml = _____ TBS
  j. 1 tsp = _____ ml
  k. 240 ml = _____ TBS
  l. 1 pt = _____ ml
  m. 1 fl oz = _____ TBS
  n. 1 qt = _____ pt

Equivalencies Between Systems

The systems lack a close relationship among their units. For this reason, the preferred system of measuring is the metric system. The table of weights and measures below gives the approximate equivalencies used in practice.

Length Measures

1 meter (m) = 39.37 (39.4) inches (in)
1 inch (in) = 2.54 centimeters (cm)
1 micron (μ) = 0.000001 meter (m)

Volume Measures

1 milliliter (ml) = 16.23 minims (℞)
1 fluid ounce (fl oz) = 29.57 (30) milliliters (ml)
1 liter (L) = 33.8 fluid ounces (fl oz)
1 pint (pt) = 473.167 (480) milliliters (ml)
1 gallon (cong) = 3785.332 (3785) milliliters (ml)

Weight Measures

1 kilogram (kg) = 2.2 pounds (lb)
1 pound (avoir) (lb) = 453.59 (454) grams (g)
1 ounce (avoir) (oz) = 28.35 (28) grams (g)
1 ounce (apoth) (oz) = 31.1 (31) grams (g)
1 gram (g) = 15.432 (15) grains (gr)
1 grain (gr) = 65 milligrams (mg)
1 ounce (avoir) (oz) = 437.5 grains (gr)
1 ounce (apoth) = 480 grains (gr)

Temperature Conversion

Temperature is always measured in the number of degrees centigrade (°C), also known as degrees Celsius, or the number of degrees Fahrenheit (°F). The following equation shows the relationship between degrees centigrade, and degrees Fahrenheit: $[9(X°C)] = [5(X°F)] - 160°$

Example: Convert 110°F to °C.
$$[9(X°C)] = [5(110°)] - 160°$$
$$X°C = (550 - 160)/9$$
$$°C = 43.3°$$

Example: Convert 15°C to °F
$$[9(15°)] = [5(X°F)] - 160°$$
$$(135 + 160)/5 = X °F$$
$$59° = °F$$

Conversion Between Systems

Example question: How many kilograms are in 44 lbs?

Step 1: Write down the statement of equivalency between the two units of measure and make sure that the unit corresponding with the unknown in the question is on the right.
2.2 lbs = 1 kg

Step 2: Write down the problem with the unknown underneath the equivalency.
Equivalency: 2.2 lbs = 1 kg
Problem: 44 lbs = ? kg

Step 3: Cross multiply and divide.
1 times 44 divided by 2.2 = $[(1 \times 44) / 2.2]$ = 20 kg

Determining Body Surface Area

The Square Meter Surface Area (Body Surface Area) is a measurement that is used instead of kilograms to estimate the amount of medication a patient should receive. Body Surface Area (BSA) takes into account the patient's weight and height. BSA is always expressed in meters squared (m^2). When using the equation listed below, units of weight (W) should be kilograms (kg) and height (H) should be centimeters. The following equation is used to determine BSA:

$$BSA = (W^{0.5378}) \times (H^{0.3964}) \times (0.24265)$$

Now, using the formula, calculate the BSA of a patient who weighs 150 pounds and is 5 feet 8 inches tall.

Step 1. Convert weight to kilograms.

$$\frac{150 \text{ lb}}{2.2 \text{ lb/kg}} = 68.2 \text{ kg}$$

Step 2. Convert height to centimeters.

5 feet × 12 inches/foot = 60 inches
+ 8 inches = 68 inches
68 inches × 2.54 cm/inch = 172.7 cm

Step 3. Insert the converted numbers into the formula.

$$BSA = (W^{0.5378}) \times (H^{0.3964}) \times 0.024265$$
$$BSA = (68.2^{0.5378}) \times (172.7^{0.3964}) \times 0.024265$$
$$BSA = (9.69) \times (7.71) \times 0.024265$$
$$BSA = 1.81 \text{ m}^2$$

Problem Set #5:

Convert the following:

a. 30 ml = _____ fluid ounces
b. 500 mg = _____ g
c. 3 teaspoons = _____ fluid ounces
d. 20 ml = _____ teaspoons
e. 3.5 kg = _____ g
f. 0.25 mg = _____ g
g. 1500 ml = _____ L
h. 48 pints = _____ gallons
i. 6 gr = _____ mg
j. 120 lb = _____ kg
k. 3 fluid ounces = _____ ml
l. 72 kg = _____ pounds
m. 946 ml = _____ pints
n. 800 g = _____ lb
o. 3 tsp = _____ milliliters
p. 2 TBS = _____ fluid ounces
q. 2 TBS = _____ ml
r. 2.5 cups = _____ fl oz
s. 0.5 gr = _____ mg
t. 0.5 L = _____ ml

u. 325 mg = _____ gr

v. 2 fl oz = _____ TBS

w. 60 ml = _____ fl oz

x. 144 lb = _____ kg

y. 1 fl oz = _____ tsp

z. 4 tsp = _____ ml

aa. 83°F = _____ °C

bb. –8°F = _____ °C

cc. 5°C = _____ °F

dd. 32°C = _____ °F

ee. What is the BSA of a patient who weighs 210 pounds and has a height of 5 feet 1 inch?

RATIO AND PROPORTION

A ratio states a relationship between two quantities.

> Example: 5 g of dextrose in 100 ml of water (this solution is often abbreviated "D5W").

A proportion is two equal ratios.

> Example: 5 g of dextrose in 100 ml of a D5W solution equals 50 g of dextrose in 1000 ml of a D5W solution.

> or

$$\frac{5 \text{ g}}{100 \text{ ml}} = \frac{50 \text{ g}}{1000 \text{ ml}}$$

A proportion consists of two unit (or term) types (e.g., kilograms and liters, or milligrams and milliliters). If three of the four terms are known, the fourth term can be calculated.

Problem Solving by the Ratio and Proportion Method

The ratio and proportion method is an accurate and simple way to solve some problems. In order to use this method, you should learn how to arrange the terms correctly, and you must know how to multiply and divide.

There is more than one way to write a proportion. The most common is the following:

$$\frac{\text{Term \#1}}{\text{Term \#2}} = \frac{\text{Term \#3}}{\text{Term \#4}}$$

This expression is read: Term #1 is to Term #2 as Term #3 is to Term #4.

By cross multiplying, the proportion can now be written as:

(Term #1) × (Term #4) = (Term #2) × (Term #3)

Example 1: How many grams of dextrose are in 10 ml of a solution containing 50 g of dextrose in 100 ml of water (D50W)?

Step 1: Determine which is the known ratio and which is the unknown ratio. In this example, the known ratio is "50 g of dextrose in 100 ml of solution." The unknown ratio is "X g of dextrose in 10 ml of solution."

Step 2: Write the unknown ratio (Terms #1 and #2) on the left side of the proportion. Be sure that the unknown term is on the top.

$$\frac{X \text{ g}}{10 \text{ ml}} = \frac{\text{Term \#3}}{\text{Term \#4}}$$

Step 3: Write the known ratio (Terms #3 and #4) on the right side of the proportion. The units of both ratios must be the same—the units in the numerators and the units in the denominators must match. In this case, that means grams in the numerator and milliliters in the denominator. If units of the numerators or the denominators differ, then a conversion to the same units must be completed.

$$\frac{X \text{ g}}{10 \text{ ml}} = \frac{50 \text{ g}}{100 \text{ ml}}$$

Step 4: Cross multiply.

$$X \text{ g} \times 100 \text{ ml} = 50 \text{ g} \times 10 \text{ ml}$$

Step 5: Divide each side of the equation by the known number on the left side of the equation. This will leave only the unknown value on the left side of the equation:

$$X \text{ g} = \frac{50 \text{ g} \times 10 \text{ ml}}{100 \text{ ml}}$$

Step 6: Simplify the right side of the equation to solve for X grams:

Answer: X g = 5 g

Example 2: You need to prepare a 500-mg chloramphenicol dose in a syringe. The concentration of chloramphenicol solution is 250 mg/ml. How many milliliters should you draw up into the syringe?

Step 1: Determine the known and unknown ratios.

$$\text{Known: } \frac{1 \text{ ml}}{250 \text{ mg}}$$

$$\text{Unknown: } \frac{X \text{ ml}}{500 \text{ mg}}$$

Step 2: Write the proportion.

$$\frac{X \text{ ml}}{500 \text{ mg}} = \frac{1 \text{ ml}}{250 \text{ mg}}$$

Step 3: Cross multiply.

$$X \text{ ml} \times 250 \text{ mg} = 1 \text{ ml} \times 500 \text{ mg}$$

Step 4: Divide.

$$X \text{ ml} = \frac{1 \text{ ml} \times 500 \text{ mg}}{250 \text{ mg}}$$

Step 5: Simplify.

$$X \text{ ml} = 2 \text{ ml}$$

Answer: Draw up 2 ml in the syringe to prepare a 500-mg dose of chloramphenicol.

Problem Set #6:

a. How many milligrams of magnesium sulfate are in 10 ml of a 100 mg/ml magnesium sulfate solution?
b. A potassium chloride (KCl) solution has a concentration of 2 mEq/ml.
   1. How many milliliters contain 22 mEq?
   2. How many milliequivalents (mEq) in 15 ml?
c. Ampicillin is reconstituted to 250 mg/ml. How many milliliters are needed for a 1-g dose?

CONCENTRATION AND DILUTION

Terminology

1. 5% dextrose in water is the same as D5W
2. 0.9% sodium chloride (NaCl) is the same as normal saline (NS).
3. Saline is NOT the same as NS.
4. Half-normal saline is half the strength of normal saline (0.9% NaCl), or 0.45% NaCl. This may also be referred to as 0.5 NS or 1/2 NS.

Concentration Expressed as a Percentage

The concentration of one substance in another may be expressed as a percentage or as a ratio strength.

As stated earlier in this chapter, concentrations expressed as percentages are determined using one of the following formulas:

1. Percent weight-in-weight (w/w) is the grams of a drug in 100 grams of the product.

2. Percent weight-in-volume (w/v) is the grams of a drug in 100 ml of the product.
3. Percent volume-in-volume (v/v) is the milliliters of drug in 100 ml of the product.

Example 1:

0.9% sodium chloride (w/v) = 0.9 g of sodium chloride in 100 ml of solution.

Example 2:

5% dextrose in water (w/v) = 5 g of dextrose in 100 ml of solution.

Example 3:

How many grams of dextrose are in 1 L of D5W?

Use the ratio and proportion method to solve this problem:

Known ratio: D5W means $\dfrac{5 \text{ g}}{100 \text{ ml}}$

Unknown ratio: $\dfrac{X \text{ g}}{1 \text{ L}}$

Write the proportion:

$$\frac{X \text{ g}}{1 \text{ L}} = \frac{5 \text{ g}}{100 \text{ ml}}$$

Are you ready to cross multiply? No. Remember, you must first convert the denominator of either term so that both are the same. Since we know that 1 L = 1000 ml, we can convert the unlike terms in the following manner:

$$\frac{X \text{ g}}{1000 \text{ ml}} = \frac{5 \text{ g}}{100 \text{ ml}}$$

Now that the units are both placed in the same order and the units across from each other are the same, you can cross multiply.

$$X \text{ g} \times 100 \text{ ml} = 5 \text{ g} \times 1000 \text{ ml}$$

Divide:

$$X \text{ g} = \frac{5 \text{ g} \times 1000 \text{ ml}}{100 \text{ ml}}$$

Simplify:

$$X \text{ g} = 50 \text{ g}$$

Answer:

There are 50 g of dextrose in 1 L of D5W.

Before attempting problem sets #7 and #8, here are a few suggestions for solving concentration and dilution problems:

1. Calculate the number of grams in 100 ml of solution first. That is your "known" side of the ratio.

2. Then calculate the number of grams in the volume requested in the problem by setting up a ratio.
3. Check to make sure your units are in the same order in the ratio.
4. Make sure the units that are across from each other in the ratio are the same.
5. After you have arrived at the answer, convert your answer to the requested units.

Problem Set #7:

a. In 100 ml of a D5W/0.45 NaCl solution:

    1. How many grams of NaCl are there?
    2. How many grams of dextrose are there?

b. How many grams of dextrose are in 1 L of a 10% dextrose solution?
c. How many grams of NaCl are in 1 L of 1/2 NS?
d. How many milligrams of neomycin are in 50 ml of a 1% neomycin solution?
e. How many grams of amino acids are in 250 ml of a 10% amino acid solution?

Problem Set #8:

a. An order calls for 5 million units (MU) of aqueous penicillin. How many milliliters are needed if the concentration is 500,000 units/ml?
b. How many milliliters are needed for a 15-MU aqueous penicillin dose if the concentration of the solution is 1 MU/ml?
c. Pediatric chloramphenicol comes in a 100 mg/ml concentration. How many milligrams are present in 5 ml of the solution?
d. How many milliliters of a 250 mg/ml chloramphenicol solution are needed for a 4-g dose?
e. Oxacillin comes in a 500 mg/1.5 ml solution. How many milliliters will be required for a dose of 1.5 g?
f. How many grams of ampicillin are in 6 ml of a 500 mg/1.5 ml solution?
g. How many milliliters contain 3 g of cephalothin if the concentration of the solution is 1 g/4.5 ml?
h. Use the following concentrations to solve these problems:

Hydrocortisone 250 mg/2 ml
Tetracycline 250 mg/5 ml
Potassium chloride (KCl) 2 mEq/ml
Thiamine 100 mg/ml
Mannitol 12.5 g/50 ml
Heparin 10,000 units/ml
Heparin 1000 units/ml

1. 10 mEq KCl = _____ ml
2. 50 mg thiamine = _____ ml
3. 750 mg hydrocortisone = _____ ml
4. 1 g tetracycline = _____ ml
5. 25 g mannitol = _____ ml
6. 20,000 units heparin = _____ ml OR _____ ml
7. 35 mEq KCl = _____ ml
8. 6000 units heparin = _____ ml OR _____ ml
9. 40 mEq KCl = _____ ml
10. 600 mg hydrocortisone = _____ ml
11. _____ mg hydrocortisone = 4 ml
12. _____ mg tetracycline = 15 ml
13. _____ mEq KCl = 15 ml
14. _____ g mannitol = 75 ml
15. _____ units or _____ units heparin = 2 ml
16. _____ mEq KCl = 7 ml
17. _____ g tetracycline = 12.5 ml
18. _____ units or _____ units heparin = 10 ml
19. _____ mEq KCl = 45 ml
20. _____ g thiamine = 3 ml

i. How many grams of magnesium sulfate are in 2 ml of a 50% magnesium sulfate solution?
j. How many grams of dextrose are in 750 ml of a D10W solution?
k. How many milliliters of a D5W solution contain 7.5 grams of dextrose?
l. How many grams of NaCl are in 100 ml of a NS solution?
m. How many grams of NaCl are in 100 ml of a 1/2 NS solution?
n. How many grams of NaCl are in 100 ml of a 1/4 NS solution?
o. How many grams of NaCl are in 1 L of a 0.45% NaCl solution?
p. How many grams of NaCl are in 1 L of a 0.225% NaCl solution?
q. How many grams of dextrose are in 100 ml of a D5W/0.45% NaCl solution?
r. How many milliliters of a 70% dextrose solution are needed to equal 100 g of dextrose?
s. How many milliliters of a 50% dextrose solution are needed for a 10-g dextrose dose?
t. How many grams of dextrose are in a 50 ml NS solution?

Concentration Expressed as a Ratio Strength

Concentrations of weak solutions are frequently expressed as ratio strength.

Example: Epinephrine is available in three concentrations: 1:1000 (read one to one thousand); 1:10,000; and 1:200.

A concentration of 1:1000 means that there is 1 g of epinephrine in 1000 ml of solution.

What does a 1:200 concentration of epinephrine mean?

It means 1 g of epinephrine in 200 ml of solution.

What does a 1:10,000 concentration of epinephrine mean?

It means 1 g of epinephrine in 10,000 ml of solution.

Now you can use this definition of ratio strength to set up the ratios needed to solve problems.

Problem Set #9:

a. How many grams of potassium permanganate should be used in preparing 500 ml of a 1:2500 solution?

b. How many milligrams of mercury bichloride are needed to make 200 ml of a 1:500 solution?

c. How many milligrams of atropine sulfate are needed to compound the following prescription?

 ℞

Atropine sulfate	1:200
Dist. water qs ad	30 ml

d. How many milliliters of a 1:100 solution of epinephrine will contain 300 mg of epinephrine?

e. How much cocaine is needed to compound the following prescription?

 ℞

Cocaine	1:100
Mineral oil qs ad	15 ml

f. How much zinc sulfate and boric acid are needed for the following prescription?

 ℞

Zinc sulfate	1%
Boric acid	2:100
Distilled water qs ad	50 ml

Dilutions Made from Stock Solutions

Stock solutions are concentrated solutions used to prepare various dilutions of the original stock solution. To prepare a solution of a desired concentration, you must calculate the quantity of stock solution that must be mixed with diluent to prepare the final product.

Calculating Dilutions

Example 1: You have a 10% NaCl stock solution available. You need to prepare 200 ml of a 0.5% NaCl solution. How many milliliters of the stock solution do you need to make this preparation? How much more water do you need to add to produce the final product?

Step 1: How many grams of NaCl are in the requested final product?

$$\frac{X \text{ g NaCl}}{200 \text{ ml soln}} = \frac{0.5 \text{ g NaCl}}{100 \text{ ml soln}}$$

Therefore, 200 ml of 0.5% NaCl solution contains 1 g of NaCl.

Step 2: How many milliliters of the stock solution will contain the amount calculated in Step 1 (i.e., 1 g)?

Remember, 10% means the solution contains 10 g/100 ml.

$$\frac{X \text{ ml}}{1 \text{ g}} = \frac{100 \text{ ml}}{10 \text{ g}}$$

$$X \text{ ml} = 10 \text{ ml}$$

The first part of the answer is 10 ml of stock solution.

Step 3: How much water will you need to finish preparing your solution?

Keep in mind the following formula:

(final volume) – (stock solution volume) = (volume of water)

Therefore, for our problem,

200 ml – 10 ml = 190 ml of water

The second part of the answer is 190 ml of water.

Example 2: You have to prepare 500 ml of a 0.45% NaCl solution from a 10% NaCl stock solution. How much stock solution and water do you need?

Step 1: How many grams of NaCl are in the requested volume? In other words, 500 ml of a 0.45% NaCl solution contains how much NaCl?

$$\frac{X \text{ g NaCl}}{500 \text{ ml}} = \frac{0.45 \text{ g}}{100 \text{ ml}}$$

$$X \text{ g} \times 100 \text{ ml} = 0.45 \text{ g} \times 500 \text{ ml}$$

$$X \text{ g} = \frac{0.45 \text{ g} \times 500 \text{ ml}}{100 \text{ ml}}$$

$$X \text{ g} = 2.25 \text{ g}$$

Step 2: How many milliliters of stock solution will contain the amount in Step 1 (i.e., 2.25 g)?

$$\frac{X \text{ ml}}{2.25 \text{ g}} = \frac{100 \text{ ml}}{10 \text{ g}}$$

$$X \text{ ml} \times 10 \text{ g} = 2.25 \text{ g} \times 100 \text{ ml}$$

$$X \text{ ml} = \frac{2.25 \text{ g} \times 100 \text{ ml}}{10 \text{ g}}$$

$$X \text{ ml} = 22.5 \text{ ml}$$

You will need 22.5 ml of stock solution.

Step 3: How much water will you need?

(Final volume) – (stock solution volume) = volume of water

500 ml – 22.5 ml = 477.5 ml water

Answer: You will need 22.5 ml of stock solution and 477.5 ml of water to make the final product.

Problem Set #10:

a. You need to prepare 1000 ml of a 1% neomycin solution for a bladder irrigation. You only have a 10% neomycin stock solution available in the pharmacy.

   1. How many milliliters of the stock solution do you need to make this preparation?
   2. How many milliliters of sterile water do you need to add to complete the product?

b. Sorbitol is available in a 70% stock solution. You need to prepare 140 ml of a 30% solution.

   1. How many milliliters of the stock solution are needed to formulate this order?
   2. How much sterile water still needs to be added to complete this product?

c. You need to make 1 L THAS/CAS solution containing a 35% dextrose.

   1. How many milliliters of the D70W do you use?
   2. How much sterile water for injection still has to be added?

d. You have a 10% amino acid solution. You need to make 500 ml of a 6% amino acid solution.

   1. How many milliliters of the stock solution are needed to prepare this solution?
   2. How many milliliters of sterile water for injection need to be added?

e. You receive the following prescription:

   ℞

Boric acid	300 mg
Dist. water qsad	15 ml

   1. How many milliliters of a 5% boric acid solution are needed to prepare this prescription?
   2. How many milliliters of distilled water do you need to add?

f. You need to prepare 180 ml of a 1:200 solution of potassium permanganate ($KMnO_4$). A 5% stock solution of $KMnO_4$ is available.

   1. How much stock solution is needed?
   2. How much water is needed?

g. How many milliliters of a 1:400 stock solution should be used to make 4 L of a 1:2000 solution?

h. You receive the following prescription:

   ℞

Atropine sulfate	0.05%
Dist. water qsad	10 ml

You have a 1:50 stock solution of atropine sulfate available.

   1. How many milliliters of stock solution are needed?
   2. How many milliliters of water are needed to compound this prescription?

DOSAGE AND FLOW RATE CALCULATIONS

Dosage Calculations

Basic Principles

1. Always look for what is being asked:
   - Number of doses
   - Total amount of drug
   - Size of a dose

   If you are given any two of the above, you can solve for the third.
2. Number of doses, total amount of drug, and size of dose are related in the following way:

$$\text{Number of doses} = \frac{\text{Total amount of drug}}{\text{Size of dose}}$$

This proportion can also be rearranged to:

Total amount of drug = (number of doses) × (size of dose)

OR

$$\text{Size of dose} = \frac{\text{Total amount of drug}}{\text{Number of doses}}$$

Calculating Number of Doses

Problem Set #11:

a. How many 10-mg doses are in 1 g?

b. How many 5-ml doses can be made out of 2 fl oz?

(Remember: Terms across from each other must be in the same units.)

Calculating Total Amount of Drug

Problem Set #12:

a. How many milliliters of ampicillin do you have to dispense if the patient needs to take 2 teaspoonfuls four times a day for 7 days?

Note: First, calculate the total number of doses the patient needs to receive, then multiply this number by the dose.

b. How many milligrams of theophylline does a patient receive per day if the prescription indicates 300 mg tid?

c. How many fluid ounces of antacid do you have to dispense if the patient is to receive 1 TBS with meals and qhs for 5 days?

Calculating Dose Size

Problem Set #13:

a. If a patient is to receive a total of 160 mg of propranolol each day, and the patient takes one dose every 6 hours, how many milligrams are in each dose?

b. If a daily diphenhydramine dose of 300 mg is divided into six equal doses, how much do you have to dispense for every dose?

Calculating the Correct Dose

Dosage calculations can be based on weight, body surface area, or age.

Calculating Dose Based on Weight

Dose (in mg) = [Dose per unit of weight (in mg/kg)] × [Weight of patient (in kg)]

Dose/day (in mg/day) = [Dose/kg per day (in mg/kg per day)] × [Weight of patient (in kg)]

To find the size of each dose, divide the total dose per day by the number of doses per day as illustrated in the following formula:

$$\text{Size of Dose} = \frac{\text{Total amount of drug}}{\text{Number of doses}}$$

Problem Set #14:

a. A patient who weighs 50 kg receives 400 mg of acyclovir q8h. The recommended dose is 5 mg/kg every 8 h.

   1. Calculate the recommended dose for this patient.
   2. Is the dose this patient is receiving greater than, less than, or equal to the recommended dose?

b. The test dose of amphotericin is 0.1 mg/kg. What dose should be prepared for a patient weighing 220 lbs? (Remember, terms must be in the same units before beginning calculations.)

c. A 20-kg child receives erythromycin 25 mg q6h. The stated dosage range is 30–100 mg/kg per day divided into four doses.

   1. What is the dosage range (in mg/day) this child should receive?
   2. Is the dose this child is being given within the dosage range that you have just calculated?

Calculating Dose Based on Body Surface Area

As noted previously in this chapter, body surface area (BSA) is expressed as meters squared (abbreviated m^2).

Problem Set #15:

a. An adult with a BSA of 1.5 m^2 receives acyclovir. The dose is 750 mg/m^2 per day given in three equal doses.

   1. Calculate the daily dose for this patient.
   2. Calculate the size of each dose for this patient.

Note: These problems are done exactly like the weight problems; however, meters squared should be substituted everywhere kilograms appeared before.

Calculating Dose Based on Age

The following is an example of information that might be found on the label of an over-the-counter children's medication:

St. Joseph's Cough Syrup for Children
Pediatric Antitussive Syrup

Active ingredient: Dextromethorphan hydro-bromide 7.5 mg per 5 ml
Indications: For relief of coughing associated with colds and flu for up to 8 hours
Actions: Antitussive
Warnings: Should not be administered to children for persistent or chronic cough such as occurs with asthma or emphysema, or when cough is accompanied by excessive secretions (except under physician's advice)
How supplied: Cherry-flavored syrup in plastic bottles of 2 and 4 fl oz
Dosage: (see table below)

Age	Weight	Dosage
Under 2 yr	below 27 lb	As directed by physician
2 to under 6 yr	27 to 45 lb	1 tsp every 6 to 8 h (not to exceed 4 tsp daily)
6 to under 12 yr	46 to 83 lb	2 tsp every 6 to 8 h (not to exceed 8 tsp daily)
12 yr and older	84 lb and greater	4 tsp every 6 to 8 hrs (not to exceed 16 tsp daily)

Problem Set #16:

a. Based on the preceding dosing table:
   1. What is the dose of St. Joseph's for a 5-year-old child?
   2. What should you dispense for a 12-year-old child weighing 30 kg?

b. The usual dose of ampicillin is 100 mg/kg per day. The prescription for a 38-kg child is written as 1 g q6h.
   1. Is this dose acceptable?
   2. If not, what should it be?

c. Propranolol is given as 0.5 mg/kg per day every 6 h.
   1. What should a 10-kg child receive per day?
   2. What is the size of every dose?

d. Aminophylline is given at a rate of 0.6 mg/kg per hr.
   1. What daily dose will a 50-kg patient receive?
   2. If an oral dose is given every 12 h, what will it be?

IV Flow Rate Calculations

Using flow rates, you can calculate the volume of fluid and/or the amount of drug a patient will be receiving over a certain time period. Prefilled IV bags are available in the following volumes: 50, 100, 250, 500, and 1000 ml.

Calculating Volume of Fluid

Daily volume of fluid (in ml/day) = [Flow rate (in ml/h)] × [24 h/day]

Problem Set #17:

a. D5W is running at 40 ml/hr.
   1. How many milliliters of D5W does the patient receive per day?
   2. Which size D5W container will you dispense?

b. D5W/NS is prescribed to run at 100 ml/h.
   1. How much IV fluid is needed in 24 h?
   2. How will you dispense this volume?

c. A patient has two IVs running: D5W/0.5NS at 10 ml/h and a hyperalimentation solution at 70 ml/h. How much fluid is the patient receiving from these IVs per day?

Calculating Amount of Drug

Problem Set #18:

a. An order is written as follows: 1 g of aminophylline in 1 L D5W/0.225% NaCl to run at 50 ml/h. How much aminophylline is the patient receiving per day?

b. The dose of aminophylline in a child is 1 mg/kg per hour.
   1. If the child weighs 40 kg, at what rate should the IV in question a be running?
   2. What should the daily dose be?

c. You add 2 g of aminophylline to 1 L of D5W. If this solution is to run at 10 ml/h, how much drug will the patient receive per day?

d. If the dose of aminophylline should be 0.6 mg/kg per hour, and the patient weighs 40 kg, what rate should the IV in question c be running?

Calculation of IV Flow (Drip) Rates

Calculation of IV flow (drip) rates is necessary to ensure that patients are getting the amount of medication the physician ordered. For example, if an order is written as: 25,000 units of heparin in 250 ml D5W to infuse at 1000 units/h, what is the correct rate of infusion (in ml/h)?

$$\text{Concentration of IV} = \frac{\text{Total amount of drug}}{\text{Total volume}}$$

$$\text{Concentration of IV} = \frac{25,000 \text{ units heparin}}{250 \text{ ml D5W}}$$

Concentration of IV = 100 units/ml of D5W

Now that you have calculated the concentration per milliliter, you can determine exactly what the rate should be by using the following formula:

$$\text{IV Rate} = \frac{\text{Dose desired}}{\text{Concentration of IV}}$$

$$\text{IV Rate} = \frac{(1,000 \text{ units/h})}{(100 \text{ units/ml})}$$

IV Rate = 10 ml/h

Problem Set #19

a. An order is written for 2 g of xylocaine in 250 ml of D5W to infuse at 120 mg/h. What is the correct rate of infusion (in ml/h)?
b. An order is written for 25,000 units of heparin in 250 ml of D5W. The doctor writes to infuse 17 ml/h. How many units of heparin will the patient receive in a 12-h period?

MOLES, EQUIVALENTS, OSMOLARITY, ISOTONICITY, AND PH

Moles and Equivalents

A mole is one way of expressing an amount of a chemical substance or a drug.

Examples: A mole of NaCl weighs 58.45 g.
A mole of KCl weighs 74.55 g.

An equivalent usually expresses the amount of a particle of a chemical substance or a drug.

Examples: One mole of NaCl contains one equivalent of Na^+ (which weighs 23 g).

One mole of NaCl also contains one equivalent of Cl^- (which weighs 35.45 g).

Remember: 1 equivalent (Eq) = 1000 milliequivalents (mEq)

Numbers to Remember

Note: If you should forget these numbers, these equivalents can be found on the labels of the large-volume sodium and dextrose solutions.

a. 0.9% NaCl contains 0.9 g NaCl in every 100 ml of solution,

or

0.9% NaCl contains 9 g NaCl in every liter of solution.

b. 0.9% NaCl contains 15.4 mEq Na^+ in every 100 ml of solution,

or

0.9% NaCl contains 154 mEq Na^+ in every liter of solution.

c. 0.45% NaCl (1/2 NS) contains 0.45 g NaCl in every 100 ml of solution, or 7.7 mEq of Na^+ in every 100 ml of solution

or

0.45% NaCl contains 4.5 g NaCl in every liter of solution or 77 mEq of Na^+ in every liter of solution.

d. The table below summarizes some of the data.

	grams of NaCl/ 100 ml	grams of NaCl/ liter	milli-equivalents of Na^+/liter
0.9 % NaCl (NS)	0.9	9	154
0.45% NaCl (1/2 NS)	0.45	4.5	77
0.225% NaCl (1/4 NS)	0.225	2.25	38.5

Problem Set #20:

a. You need to make 1 L of NS. You have 1 L of SWI (Sterile Water for Injection) and a vial of NaCl (4 mEq/ml). How will you prepare this solution?
b. An order calls for D10W/0.45% NaCl to run at 40 ml/h. You have 1 L of D10W and a vial of NaCl (4 mEq/ml) available. How would you prepare this bottle?
c. How would you prepare 500 ml of a D10W/0.225% NaCl solution if you have SWI, NaCl (4 mEq/ml), and a 50% dextrose solution available?
d. You have D10W and a vial of NaCl (4 mEq/ml). How would you prepare 250 ml of a D10W/NS solution?

Osmolarity and Isotonicity

Osmolarity expresses the number of particles (osmols) in a certain volume of fluid.

Remember: 1 osmol (Osm) = 1000 milliosmols (mOsm)

The osmolarity of human plasma is about 280 to 300 mOsm/L.

The osmolarity of NS is about 300 mOsm/L, and the osmolarity of D5W is about 280 mOsm/L.

Solutions of the same osmolarity are called isotonic.

Example: NS and plasma are isotonic.

If parenteral fluids are administered that are not isotonic, it could result in irritation of veins and swelling or shrinking of red blood cells.

Solutions having osmolarities higher than that of plasma are known as hypertonic solutions.

Examples: Hyperalimentation solutions and D5W/NS are hypertonic.

Solutions having osmolarities lower than that of plasma are called hypotonic solutions.

Example: 1/2 NS is hypotonic.

pH

pH refers to the acidity or basicity of a solution. The pH scale ranges from 1 to 14.

> pH = 7 is neutral
> pH < 7 is acidic
> pH > 7 is basic

Normal human plasma has a pH of approximately 7.4.

Parenteral solutions with pHs different from that of normal human plasma can be very irritating to tissue when injected. Examples are phenytoin and diazepam. Ophthalmalogic preparations are buffered to maintain a pH as close to 7.4 as possible.

Some drugs are not stable at a certain pH. One example is ampicillin, which is not very stable in acidic solutions. D5W solutions are slightly acidic, whereas NS solutions are more neutral. Therefore, ampicillin injection is dispensed in NS rather than D5W.

PRACTICE CALCULATIONS 1

1. What does $\overline{ss}$ mean:_____
2. Convert II to its arabic equivalent:
   _____
3. Write 2/5 as a decimal fraction:
   _____
4. The fraction form of 0.1 is:_____
5. 25% expressed as a fraction:_____

6. Write 0.88 as a percentage:_____
7. 1/4 expressed as a percentage:_____
8. The fraction form of 0.4 is:_____
9. xiv expressed in arabic numbers:_____
10. 1 1/2 in decimal form:_____
11. The standard metric system measure for weight is the _____
12. The standard metric system measure for length is the _____
13. The standard metric system measure for volume is the _____
14. 1 km = _____ m
15. 1 L = _____ ml
16. 1 kg = _____ g
17. 1 g = _____ mg
18. 1 µg = _____ g
19. 0.01 g = _____ mg
20. 1 ml = _____ L
21. 1 tsp = _____ TBS
22. 1 cup = _____ ml
23. 1 TBS = _____ fl oz
24. 15 ml = _____ TBS
25. 1 cup = _____ fl oz
26. 1000 ml = _____ L
27. 2 kg = _____ g
28. 1 gal = _____ qt
29. 1 pt = _____ cups
30. 1 mg = _____ g
31. 1 tsp = _____ ml
32. 5 gr = _____ g
33. 3 cups = _____ ml
34. 70 kg = _____ lb
35. 45 ml = _____ fl oz
36. 80 mg = _____ gr
37. 250 mg = _____ g
38. 3 TBS = _____ tsp
39. 2 fl oz = _____ TBS
40. 3 qt = _____ pt
41. 120 ml = _____ cups
42. 10 ml = _____ tsp
43. 45 ml = _____ TBS
44. 50 µg = _____ mg
45. 2 gal = _____ qt
46. 0.5 pt = _____ ml
47. 20 kg = _____ lb
48. 750 mg = _____ g
49. 25 ml = _____ tsp
50. 6 tsp = _____ TBS

PRACTICE CALCULATIONS 2

1. 6% (w/w) = _____
   10% (w/v) = _____
   0.5% (v/v) = _____

2. A patient needs a 300-mg dose of amikacin. How many milliliters do you need to draw from a vial containing 100 mg/2 ml of amikacin?
3. A suspension of naladixic acid contains 250 mg/5 ml. The syringe contains 15 ml. What is the dose (in milligrams) contained in the syringe?
4. How many milligrams of neomycin are in 200 ml of a 1% neomycin solution?
5. 1/2 NS = _____ g NaCl / _____ ml solution
6. How many grams of pumpkin are in 300 ml of a 30% pumpkin juice solution?
7. Express 4% hydrocortisone cream as a ratio. (Remember that solids, such as creams, are usually expressed as weight-in-weight).
8. You have a solution labeled D10W/NS.

   a) How many grams of NaCl are in 50 ml of this solution?
   b) How many milliliters of this solution contain 50 g dextrose?

9. A syringe is labeled "cat tails 5 mg/ml, 20 ml." How many milligrams of cat tails are in the syringe?
10. Boric acid 2:100 is written on a prescription. This is the same as _____ boric acid in _____ solution.
11. How much epinephrine do you need to prepare 20 ml of a 1:400 epinephrine solution?
12. Calculate the amounts of boric acid and zinc sulfate to fill the following prescription:

   ℞
Zinc sulfate	0.5%
Boric acid	1:50
Distilled water qs. ad	100 ml

13. Use the following concentrations to solve the problems:

Gentamicin	80 mg/ml
Magnesium sulfate	50%
Atropine	1:200

   a) 120 mg gentamicin = _____ ml
   b) 100 mg atropine = _____ ml
   c) _____ g magnesium sulfate = 150 ml

PRACTICE CALCULATIONS 3

1. You need to prepare 1 L of 0.25% acetic acid irrigation solution. The stock concentration of acetic acid is 25%.

   a. How many milliliters of stock solution do you need to use?
   b. How many milliliters of sterile water do you need to add?

2. A drug order requires 500 ml of a 2% neomycin solution.

   a. How much neomycin concentrate (1 g/2 ml) is needed to fill the order?
   b. How many milliliters of sterile water need to be added to the concentrate before dispensing the drug?

3. a. Calculate the amount of atropine stock solution (concentration 0.5%) needed to compound the following prescription:

   ℞
   | Atropine sulfate | 1:1500 |
   | Sterile water qs ad | 300 ml |

   b. How much sterile water do you have to add to complete the order?

4. How many tablets do you have to dispense for the following prescription?

   ℞
   Obecalp ii tablets tid for 10 days

5. How many 2-tsp doses can a patient take from a bottle containing 3 fl oz?
6. A patient is receiving a total daily dose of 2 g of acyclovir. How many milligrams of acyclovir is he receiving per dose if he takes the drug five times a day?
7. The recommended dose of erythromycin to treat an ear infection is 50 mg/kg per day given q6h. Answer the following questions regarding this drug:

   a. If a child weighs 20 kg, how much erythromycin should he receive per day?
   b. How much drug will he receive per dose?

8. The dose of prednisone for replacement therapy is 2 mg/m² per dose. The drug is administered twice daily. What is the daily prednisone dose for a 1.5-m² person?
9. An aminophylline drip is running at 1 mg/kg per hour in a 10-kg child. How much aminophylline is the child receiving per day?
10. A child with an opiate overdose needs naloxone. The recommended starting dose is 5–10 µg/kg. The doctor writes for 0.3 mg naloxone stat. Answer the following questions based on the child's weight of 40 kg:

a. What is the dosage range of the starting dose, based on the child's weight?

b. On the basis of the answer to "a," does 0.3 mg sound like a reasonable dose?

11. An IV fluid containing NS is running at 80 ml/h.

a. How much fluid is the patient receiving per day?

b. How many 1-L bags will be needed per day?

12. A patient has two IVs running: an aminophylline drip at 20 ml/h and saline at 30 ml/h. How much fluid is the patient receiving per day from his IVs?

13. a. You prepare a solution by adding 2 g of Bronkospaz to 1 L of NS. What is the concentration of Bronkospaz ?

b. If the solution of Bronkospaz you made in "a" runs at 30 ml/h, how much Bronkospaz is the patient receiving per day?

c. If a 60-kg patient should receive 1 mg/kg per hour, will the dose in "b" be appropriate?

ANSWERS TO PROBLEM SETS

Problem Set #1:

a. 2	b. 605	c. 20	d. 3
e. 7	f. 4	g. 9	h. 15
i. 11	j. 1030	k. 14	l. 16

Problem Set #2:

a. 0.5	b. 0.75	c. 1	d. 0.4
e. 0.33	f. 0.625	g. 0.5	h. 0.25
i. 1.5	j. 2.67	k. 5.25	l. 3.8
m. 1/4	n. 2/5	o. 3/4	p. 7/20
q. 2 1/2	r. 1 3/5	s. 3 1/4	t. 1/3

Problem Set #3:

a. 23/100	b. 67/100	c. 1/8	d. 1/2
e. 66.7/100	f. 3/4	g. 33/50	h. 2/5
i. 1	j. 3/20	k. 50%	l. 25%
m. 40%	n. 24%	o. 4%	p. 50%
q. 35%	r. 44%	s. 57%	t. 99%

Problem Set #4:

a. 1000 ml

b. 1 kg

c. 1000 mg

d. 1 mg

e. 3 tsp

f. 15 ml

g. 1 cup

h. 240 ml

i. 1 TBS

j. 5 ml

k. 16 TBS

l. 480 ml

m. 2 TBS

n. 2 pt

Problem Set #5:

a. 1 fl oz

b. 0.5 g

c. 0.5 fl oz

d. 4 tsp

e. 3500 g

f. 0.00025 g

g. 1.5 L

h. 6 gal

i. 390 mg

j. 54.5 kg

k. 90 ml

l. 158 lb

m. 1.97 pt

n. 1.76 lb

o. 15 ml

p. 1 fl oz

q. 30 ml

r. 20 fl oz

s. 32.5 mg

t. 500 ml

u. 5 gr

v. 4 TBS

w. 2 fl oz

x. 65.5 kg

y. 6 tsp

z. 20 ml

aa. 28.3°C

bb. −22.2°C

cc. 41°F

dd. 89.6°F

ee. 2.1 m²

Problem Set #6:

a. 1000 mg

b. 1. 11 ml
   2. 30 mEq

c. 4 ml

Problem Set #7:

a. 1. 0.45 g
   2. 5 g

b. 100 g

c. 4.5 g

d. 500 mg

e. 25 g

Problem Set #8:

a. 10 ml

b. 15 ml

c. 500 mg

d. 16 ml

e. 4.5 ml

f. 2 g

g. 13.5 ml

h. 1. 5 ml
   2. 0.5 ml
   3. 6 ml
   4. 20 ml
   5. 100 ml
   6. a. 2 ml of heparin 10,000 units/ml or
      b. 20 ml of heparin 1000 units/ml
   7. 17.5 ml
   8. a. 0.6 ml of heparin 10,000 units/ml or
      b. 6 ml of heparin 1000 units/ml
   9. 20 ml
   10. 4.8 ml
   11. 500 mg
   12. 750 mg
   13. 30 mEq
   14. 18.75 g
   15. 20,000 units or 2000 units
   16. 14 mEq
   17. 0.625 g
   18. 100,000 units or 10,000 units
   19. 90 mEq
   20. 0.3 g

i. 1 g

j. 75 g

k. 150 ml

l. 0.9 g

m. 0.45 g

n. 0.225 g

o. 4.5 g

p. 2.25 g

q. 5 g

r. 142.9 ml

s. 20 ml

t. 0

Problem Set #9:

a. 0.2 g

b. 400 mg

c. 150 mg

d. 30 ml

e. 150 mg

f. 500 mg of zinc sulfate and 1 g of boric acid

Problem Set #10:

a. 1. 100 ml of stock solution
   2. 900 ml of water

b. 1. 60 ml of stock solution
   2. 80 ml of water

c. 1. 500 ml of D70W
   2. 500 ml of sterile water

d. 1. 300 ml of stock solution
   2. 200 ml of sterile water

e. 1. 6 ml of 5% boric acid
   2. 9 ml of distilled water

f. 1. 18 ml of stock solution
   2. 162 ml of water

g. 800 ml of stock solution

h. 1. 0.25 ml of stock solution
   2. 9.75 ml of water

Problem Set #11:

a. 100 doses

b. 12 doses

Problem Set #12:

a. 280 ml of ampicillin

b. 900 mg of theophylline

c. 10 fl oz

Problem Set #13:

a. 40 mg of propranolol

b. 50 mg for every dose

Problem Set #14:

a. 1. 250 mg q8h
   2. greater than the recommended dose

b. 10 mg

c. 1. 600–2000 mg/day
   2. no

Problem Set #15:

a. 1. 1125 mg
   2. 375 mg

Problem Set #16:

a. 1. 1 tsp every 6 to 8 h not to exceed 4 tsp daily
   2. 2 tsp every 6 to 8 h not to exceed 8 tsp daily

b. 1. no
   2. 3800 mg/day

c. 1. 5 mg/day
   2. 1.25 mg per dose

d. 1. 720 mg
   2. 360 mg every 12 hours

Problem Set #17:

a. 1. 960 ml
   2. 1000 ml
b. 1. 2400 ml
   2. 3000 ml, three 1-L bags
c. 1920 ml of fluid

Problem Set #18:

a. 1.2 g
b. 1. 40 ml/h
   2. 960 mg/day
c. 480 mg/day
d. 12 ml/hr

Problem Set #19:

a. 15 ml/h
b. 20,400 units

Problem Set #20:

a. Add 38.5 ml NaCl to 1 L SWFI
b. Add 19.25 ml NaCl to 1 L D10W
c. 4.81 ml NaCl plus 100 ml D50W; qs with SWFI to 500 ml
d. 9.625 ml NaCl; qs with D10W to 250 ml

27. 2000
28. 4
29. 2
30. 0.001
31. 5
32. 0.325
33. 720
34. 154
35. 1.5
36. 1.23
37. 0.25
38. 9
39. 4
40. 6
41. 0.5
42. 2
43. 3
44. 0.05
45. 8
46. 240
47. 44
48. 0.75
49. 5
50. 2

ANSWERS TO PRACTICE CALCULATIONS 1

1. 1/2
2. 2
3. 0.4
4. 1/10
5. 1/4
6. 88%
7. 25%
8. 2/5
9. 14
10. 1.5
11. gram
12. meter
13. liter
14. 1000
15. 1000
16. 1000
17. 1000
18. 0.000001
19. 10
20. 0.001
21. 1/3
22. 240
23. 0.5
24. 1
25. 8
26. 1

ANSWERS TO PRACTICE CALCULATIONS 2

1. 6 g/100 g
   10 g/100 ml
   0.5 ml/100 ml
2. 6 ml
3. 750 mg
4. 2000 mg
5. 0.45 g/100 ml
6. 90 g
7. 4 g/100 g
8. a. 0.45 g
   b. 500 ml
9. 100 mg
10. 2 g in 100 ml
11. 0.05 g or 50 mg
12. 0.5 g zinc sulfate and 2 g boric acid
13. a. 1.5 ml
    b. 20 ml
    c. 75 g

ANSWERS TO PRACTICE CALCULATIONS 3

1. a. 2.5 g acetic acid = 10 ml stock solution
   b. 990 ml sterile water

2. a. 10 g neomycin = 20 ml stock solution
   b. 480 ml stock solution
3. a. 0.2 g atropine sulfate = 40 ml stock solution
   b. 260 ml sterile water
4. 60 tablets
5. 9 doses
6. 400 mg per dose
7. a. 1000 mg per day
   b. 250 mg per dose
8. 6 mg per day
9. 240 mg per day
10. a. Acceptable dosage range: 200–400 µg
    b. Yes, it falls within the accepted calculated range.
11. a. 1920 ml per day
    b. 2 1-L bags per day
12. 1200 ml per day
13. a. 2000 mg/1000 ml or 2 mg/ml or 2 g/1000 ml or 2 g/L or 2:1000
    b. 1440 mg/day
    c. Yes, dose is appropriate.

APPENDIX 3

Table #1

micro-(µ)	:	1/1,000,000	= 0.000001
milli-(m)	:	1/1000	= 0.001
centi-(c)	:	1/100	= 0.01
deci-(d)	:	1/10	= 0.1

Table #2

deca-(da) : 10
hecto-(h) : 100
kilo-(k) : 1000
mega-(M) : 1,000,000

Table #3

1 kilometer (km) = 1000 meters (m)
0.001 kilometer (km) = 1 meter (m)
1 millimeter (mm) = 0.001 meter (m)
1000 millimeters (mm) = 1 meter (m)
1 centimeter (cm) = 0.01 meter (m)
100 centimeters (cm) = 1 meter (m)

Table #4

1 milliliter (ml) = 0.001 liter (L)
1000 milliliters (ml) = 1 liter (L)
1 microliter (µl) = 0.000001 liter (L)
1,000,000 microliters (µl) = 1 liter (L)
1 deciliter (dl) = 0.1 liter (L)
10 deciliters (dl) = 1 liter (L)

Table #5

1 kilogram (kg) = 1000 grams (g)
0.001 kilogram (kg) = 1 gram (g)
1 milligram (mg) = 0.001 gram (g)
1000 milligrams (mg) = 1 gram (g)
1 microgram (µg) = 0.000001 gram (g)
1,000,000 micrograms (µg) = 1 gram (g)

Table #6

Pound (lb)		Ounces (ʒ)		Drams (ʒ)		Scruples (Ə)		Grains (gr)
1	=	12	=	96	=	288	=	5760
		1	=	8	=	24	=	480
				1	=	3	=	60
						1	=	20

Table #7

Gallons (gal)		Pints (pt)		Fluid ounces (fʒ)		Fluid drams (fʒ)		Minims (ℳ)
1	=	8	=	128	=	1024	=	61,440
		1	=	16	=	128	=	7,680
				1	=	8	=	480
						1	=	60

Table #8

Pound (lb)		Ounces (oz)		Grains (gr)
1	=	16	=	7000
		1	=	437.5

Table #9

1 meter (m) = 39.37 (39.4) inches (in)
1 inch (in) = 2.54 centimeters (cm)
1 micron (µ) = 0.000001 meter (m)

Table #10

1 milliliter (ml) = 16.23 minims (ℳ)
1 fluidounce (fl oz) = 29.57 (30) milliliters (ml)
1 liter (L) = 33.8 fluid ounces (fl oz)
1 pint (pt) = 473.167 (480) milliliters (ml)
1 gallon (cong) = 3785.332 (3785) milliliters (ml)

Table #11

1 kilogram (kg) = 2.2 pounds (lb)
1 pound avoir (lb) = 453.59 (454) grams (g)
1 ounce avoir (oz) = 28.35 (28) grams (g)
1 ounce apoth (oz) = 31.1 (31) grams (g)
1 gram (g) = 15.432 (15) grains (gr)
1 grain (gr) = 65 milligrams (mg)
1 ounce (avoir) (oz) = 437.5 grains (gr)
1 ounce (apoth) = 480 grains (gr)

Table #12

	grams of NaCl/ 100 ml	grams of NaCl/ liter	milli-equivalents of Na^+/liter
0.9% NaCl (NS)	0.9	9	154.5
0.45% NaCl (1/2 NS)	0.45	4.5	77
0.225% NaCl (1/4 NS)	0.225	2.25	38.5

4 | Pharmacy Law

Edward Donnelly, R.Ph., MBA, FASHP

This chapter provides an overview of pharmacy law and how it relates to the pharmacy technician. Some of the more influential laws regulating the practice of pharmacy will be discussed as well as the requirements for filling prescriptions and medication orders.

Federal law will be primarily covered since state laws regarding technicians and pharmacists tend to vary among states. Each state has its own laws pertaining to the manufacturing, distribution, and dispensing of drugs; the definition and requirements of a technician; the pharmacist to technician ratio required for practice; and the duties a technician is allowed to perform.

The laws are usually located in the state's pharmacy practice act. When federal and state laws differ, the stricter of the two laws applies. Therefore, it is important that technicians become familiar with state law and federal regulations.

Another source of information pertaining to pharmacy practice is the Code of Ethics for Pharmacists (appendix 4-A). This code provides the principles of professional conduct for pharmacists, but much of the information also pertains to technicians.

LEARNING OBJECTIVES

After reading the chapter the reader should be able to
1. Differentiate and describe the various drug classifications.
2. State the major intent of the Food, Drug, and Cosmetic Act and its two major amendments, the Durham-Humphrey Amendment and Kefauver-Harris Amendment.
3. Describe who may prescribe medications, including controlled substances, and list the prescription, prescription label, refill, and record requirements associated with these medications.
4. State the intent of the Controlled Substances Act (CSA) and differentiate the five schedules of medications that are regulated by the CSA.
5. Describe the requirements of the CSA, including ordering and record requirements.
6. State the intent of the Poison Prevention Packaging Act of 1970 as well as the exemptions and method of enforcement of the act.
7. State the history, counseling guidelines, documentation requirements, standards, and enforcement of the Omnibus Budget Reconciliation Act of 1990 (OBRA 90).

LIABILITY

Liability is a legal responsibility, either criminal or civil. It is the condition of being bound in law and justice to pay an indebtedness or discharge some obligation. Civil liability is a legally enforceable debt owed for a wrong committed against an individual. Criminal liability is a legally enforceable debt owed for a wrong (crime) committed against society (the State). It occurs when there has been a statute violation. A statute is law enacted by legislation. Criminal liability may result in fines, imprisonment, and loss of property depending on the severity and penalties outlined in the statute.[1]

Probably the most common source of civil liability for pharmacists is professional negligence or malpractice. Malpractice occurs when a practitioner fails to follow an established standard of care, thus causing injury or damages to another person. Standard of care is the type of care that would be rendered by a competent pharmacist under the same or similar conditions. Damages to the patient may be mental, physical, or financial. Damages to husband-wife or parent-child relationships may also be considered.[2]

It should be noted that pharmacists are liable for the actions of technicians under their supervision. As a result, technicians should not attempt to do more than what is allowed under state or federal regulations. State pharmacy practice acts are not consistent with regard to pharmacy technicians. Some states imply functions able to be performed by technicians by outlining the duties that pharmacists must perform, while other states specifically authorize functions for technicians.[3]

Other types of liability relevant to pharmacy practice include product and employer liability. Product liability is a legal method whereby a patient can make claims for injuries caused by drugs. The patient usually sues the drug manufacturer because the essence of this claim is that the drug product itself is defective. Employer liability holds an employer responsible for the negligent acts of an employee, even if the employer is otherwise without fault. The thought behind this rule is that an employer has the authority to manage the conduct of the employee, and therefore should be liable for the employee's negligent conduct.[4]

PRODUCT CLASSIFICATION

In order to better understand federal laws, it is necessary to be familiar with general terminology used to classify products. There are three classifications: non-prescription drugs, prescription drugs, and other.

Nonprescription Drugs

Nonprescription drugs, or over-the-counter (OTC) drugs, are recognized as safe and effective for use without a prescription. Nonprescription drugs must be properly labeled with directions for safe and effective consumer use.

Prescription Drugs

Prescription drugs, or legend drugs, may be obtained only with a prescription and are not considered safe for use without medical supervision. Prescription drugs are not intended for anyone other than the person for whom they are prescribed, and must be labeled by the manufacturer with the federal legend (hence the name legend drugs): "Caution: Federal law prohibits dispensing without a prescription."

Federal and some state laws may give certain controlled substances, such as codeine when used in a cough medicine, exempt status and allow pharmacists to dispense them without a prescription (see Controlled Substances section).

USP/NF Designation

The Federal Pure Food and Drugs Act of 1906 recognized *The United States Pharmacopeia (USP)* and *The National Formulary (NF)* as "official compendia," thereby giving official status to the drugs and the standards set forth in these volumes.

These reference texts list the therapeutic agents used in medical practice that are approved with respect to source, chemistry, physical properties, and purity, among other indicators. Although originally designed to help physicians choose a drug to prescribe, these compendia are now used primarily by the Food and Drug Administration (FDA) and pharmaceutical industry as the official standards for quality and purity of drugs. In addition, physicians know that the drugs listed in these references have met the standards set for quality and chemical uniformity.

Investigational Drugs

Investigational drugs are defined as those that are being considered but have not yet been approved by the FDA for human use. In addition, FDA approved drugs are considered investigational when they are being studied for new indications, new routes of administration, or new dosage forms.[5] Once an investigational drug receives FDA approval, it is considered a new drug.

Studies using investigational drugs can be performed on an inpatient or outpatient basis. These studies are classified into one of three types:

Phase I: The primary goal of a phase I study is to determine a maximally tolerated dose of the investigational drug. Generally, these studies use a small number of healthy adult volunteers.

Phase II: The primary goals of this type of study are to determine whether a new drug has clinical activity and to expand knowledge regarding the study dose and schedule, and toxicity of the drug. It is administered to a larger number of individuals who have the disease the drug is intended to treat.

Phase III: This type of study compares the investigational drug and/or new treatment to an existing standard treatment or placebo to gather further data on safety and efficacy. Information from these studies is used to determine if the new drug/treatment has a superior patient response and/or survival when compared to conventional therapy.[6]

Postmarketing surveillance occurs after the investigational drug has been approved by the FDA and is available for use in the general population. Information is collected on the use of the drug in a large number of patients. Adverse effects and other problems that were not evident in the smaller phase I–III trials may be uncovered at this time.

All studies in which investigational drugs are used must be approved by an institutional review board (IRB). Patients must sign an informed consent (a document explaining the study and its risks) before participating in studies involving investigational drugs. Participation in these studies is voluntary and the patient may withdraw from the study at any time. Likewise, the patient can be withdrawn from the study by the principal investigator if necessary.

Investigational drugs are usually stored in the pharmacy and dispensed by pharmacy personnel. The prescription labels for investigational drugs should distinguish them from non-investigational drugs (e.g., "caution: new drug limited by US Federal law to investigational use"). Accurate dispensing and inventory records must be maintained of all investigational drugs. As a general rule, records should be maintained for two years following the date of an approved new drug application (NDA) for the indication that is investigated or, if the application is not approved or no application is filed, for 2 years after the investigation is discontinued for an indication.[7]

New Drugs

A new drug is a chemical substance for medical use that is determined by the FDA to be safe and effective for use under the conditions for which it was studied. Usually, a new drug has not been used extensively or for a long period of time outside the studies investigating its safety and efficacy. However, an established agent may also be considered a new drug if it is offered in a new dosage form, with new medical claims, or in a new dosage.

Proprietary Drugs

A proprietary, or brand name drug, refers to a chemical entity that was the first to be approved by the FDA via the NDA process, (e.g., Procardia, Lasix, Valium). As soon as a chemical entity displays encouraging pharmacological activity, the pharmaceutical company files a patent application. After the patent is granted, the pharmaceutical company has exclusive rights to the agent for 17 years. A large portion or all of the patent time is usually spent researching and developing the agent. Once the patent has expired, generic versions may be manufactured by other companies. Pharmaceutical companies try to get products to the market while they are still under patent before a generic version is available in order to recover some or all of the money spent researching and developing the agent.

Generic Drugs

A generic drug is a medication that contains the same active component(s) as the brand name drug. Generic drugs became more prevalent after the passage of the Drug Price Competition and Patent Term Restoration Act in 1984. This act was meant to increase competition within the pharmaceutical industry by facilitating the generic drug marketing process.

Prior to this act, a complete NDA had to be submitted to the FDA to get approval for a generic version of a drug marketed after 1962.

Very few generic pharmaceutical companies had the resources to conduct the efficacy and safety studies required for a NDA, so generic drugs were not common. The 1984 act allowed generic versions of brand name drugs to be marketed after receiving approval of an abbreviated new drug application (ANDA). This is a much simpler process in which the generic company refers to the information supporting the brand name drug and proves that the generic version of the brand name drug is of sufficient equivalency to the proprietary drug (bioequivalency). For a generic oral dosage form, meeting bioequivalency standards is one of the most important tests.

BASIC PHARMACY LAW

The Food, Drug, and Cosmetic Act (FDCA), the Controlled Substances Act (CSA), and the Omnibus Budget Reconciliation Act of 1990 (OBRA 90) are three of the more influential Federal laws affecting the practice of pharmacy.

The FDCA, passed in 1938, requires product manufacturers to prove their product was safe and effective for use under conditions set forth on the label. This act also prohibits the introduction of misbranded or adulterated foods, drugs, and devices, including cosmetics and diagnostic aids. The FDA enforces and regulates this act and governs the quality, strength, purity, and labeling of drugs as defined by the FDCA.

In 1951, the Durham-Humphrey Amendment (DHA), also known as the prescription drug amendment, was enacted. It requires that drugs which cannot be used safely without medical supervision be labeled for sale and be dispensed only upon the prescription of an authorized prescriber. This includes a prescriber's oral prescription that is reduced promptly to writing and filled by a pharmacist, and refilling of any written or oral prescription, if refills are authorized by the prescriber. If these conditions are not met and a prescription drug is dispensed, the drug may be considered misbranded.

The Kefauver-Harris Amendment (KHA) of 1962 requires drug manufacturers prove to the FDA the effectiveness of their products before marketing them. The KHA applies to all drugs introduced after 1962 and to drugs for which NDAs had been approved from 1938 to 1962.

This amendment strengthened the FDA's authority over human drug testing. As a result, drug manufacturers conduct better-controlled and more appropriate clinical studies, which improved the likelihood that problems with the safety or efficacy of a drug will be detected before it reaches the market.

Food, Drug, and Cosmetic Act (FDCA)

Legal Prescribers

Each state may decide who is authorized to prescribe drugs and the scope of their prescribing authority. For instance, medical doctors would have wide latitude for prescribing medications. Other health care professionals allowed to prescribe within a limited scope in some states include dentists, nurses, podiatrists, optometrists, physician assistants, and pharmacists. However, the prescriptive authority for these groups is restricted by state law. For example, a dentist may be allowed to prescribe antibiotics for a tooth infection or analgesics for a painful procedure, but not blood pressure medications.

Legislation in an increasing number of states grants prescriptive authority to pharmacists based on specific guidelines or protocol. For example, in New Mexico, state law has created a special category of pharmacists called pharmacist clinicians. They are able to prescribe medications as long as they have received additional education training at least equivalent to that received by a physician's assistant. Pharmacist clinicians must have a written agreement that delegates prescriptive authority from a doctor or physician group in active practice in order to prescribe.[8]

Prescription Requirements

Prescription requirements are specified only for controlled substances (see Controlled Substances section), but many of these requirements are useful for noncontrolled substances. These include full name and address of the patient; name, strength, and quantity of medication; directions for use; date of issuance; and actual signature of prescriber.

Requirements for Prescription Label

Under the FDCA, the prescription label must have the following information:
- Name and address of the dispenser (pharmacy)
- Serial number of the prescription
- Date of the prescription or its date of filling or refilling
- Name of the prescriber

- Name of the patient, if stated on the prescription[9]
- Directions for use with precautions, if any, as indicated in the prescription

State law may further require
- Address of the patient
- Initials or name of the dispensing pharmacist
- Telephone number of the pharmacy
- Drug name, strength, and manufacturer's lot or control number
- Expiration date of the drug, if any, and the name of the manufacturer or distributor
- Amount of drug dispensed
- Refill information

In addition, all labelling for prescription drug products must include the statement, "Federal law prohibits dispensing without a prescription."

Requirements for Prescription Refills

A prescription can usually be refilled as many times as the prescriber indicates on the prescription, within a time period determined by the state. This time period is usually one year from the date the prescription was written. If the number of refills does not appear on the prescription it is assumed that refills are not authorized.

Although the number of refills should be written as a number, prescribers often write p.r.n. to indicate that the prescription may be refilled as needed. While p.r.n. is not really acknowledged by the FDA as a valid designation, a pharmacist may use professional judgment in determining whether to refill the prescription. Refills should be consistent with directions for use, and the prescriber should be contacted after a reasonable time period to ensure that the refills are consistent with what the prescriber intended.

When a prescription is refilled, state laws usually requires that a note be made on the back of the prescription indicating the quantity dispensed, the date dispensed, and the pharmacist's initials. Many states allow this information to be kept electronically.

Patients who do not have refills remaining may request that the pharmacist asks the prescriber to authorize refills. If the prescriber authorizes refills, the pharmacist may create a new prescription or add refills to the existing prescription.

An *emergency supply* of medication, usually not more than a 72-hour supply, may be dispensed to a patient if the pharmacist is unable to obtain refill authorization. The pharmacist must use professional judgment to determine whether the situation warrants dispensing an emergency supply.

Record Requirements

The Food, Drug, and Cosmetic Act describes the records that pharmacists are required to keep. One of the main reasons pharmacists are required to record the receipt, disposition, and accountability of drugs, is to ensure that the pharmacy can contact patients who received a drug that has been recalled.

Purchase invoices are records of drug receipt, prescriptions are records of drug disposition, and inventories provide a record of drugs in stock. Any sales, disposals, returns, destruction, or theft of drugs should be evidenced by some type of written document.

These records should be kept at least as long as the state or federal statute of limitations on crime. Most of the time this is usually 5 or 6 years from the date of the alleged felony offense. The reasoning for this is that the records provide evidence of the transactions involved. This proof may be a valid defense to an alleged drug law violation.

Controlled Substances

At the federal level, the Attorney General of the United States designates a drug as a controlled substance. The Secretary of Health and Human Services evaluates the substance against eight criteria and makes a recommendation to the Attorney General on whether or not to classify the substance as controlled. The eight criteria are
- The actual or relative potential for abuse
- The scientific evidence of its pharmacological effect, if known
- The state of current scientific knowledge about the drug or substance
- Its history and current pattern of abuse
- The scope, duration, and significance of the abuse
- The extent of risk to public health
- The liability for psychological or physiological dependence
- The chemical similarity to another controlled substance

State boards of pharmacy or legislatures also have the authority to classify a drug as a controlled substance.[10]

The Controlled Substances Act (CSA) is the main federal law regulating the manufacture, distribution, and dispensing of controlled substances. The CSA is enforced and regulated by the Drug Enforcement Administration (DEA), an agency of the Department of Justice. The FDA, however, retains authority to regulate some habit-forming drugs, and these drugs may be subject to regulation by both the FDA and the DEA. Laws dealing with controlled drugs are usually more stringent than those governing noncontrolled drugs.

Although the CSA is quite comprehensive, ASHP has produced a technical assistance bulletin on use of controlled substances in organized health-care settings (appendix 4-B). The bulletin addresses topics from the CSA that apply to institutional settings. Note that the third paragraph states, "The guidelines should be used in connection with the law and regulations. They are not intended as a substitute for knowledge of the law and regulations." Pertinent issues regarding the CSA not covered in appendix 4-B are discussed in this section.

Substances that fall under the CSA are generally divided into five schedules, schedule I through schedule V. The schedules, also known as classes, are sometimes called C-I through C-V, and are assigned this way to provide a rational basis for assigning penalties and for applying security and record-keeping controls. The penalties and controls are consistent with the abuse potential of each drug. Only schedule II through V drugs may be marketed for medical use in the United States; schedule I substances, with the highest abuse potential, may not be marketed in the United States.

Classification

- *Schedule I (C-I)*—Drugs with no accepted medical use in the United States, high potential for abuse, and lack of accepted safety for use under medical supervision. Examples are heroin, marijuana, and lysergic acid diethylamide (LSD).
- *Schedule II (C-II)*—Drugs with acceptable medical use but a high potential for abuse, including severe psychologic or physical dependence. Examples are amphetamines, cocaine, codeine, hydromorphone, meperidine, methadone, morphine, and opium.
- *Schedule III (C-III)*—Drugs with acceptable medical use and less potential for abuse than drugs in schedules I and II, plus high potential for psychologic and low to moderate potential for physical dependence. One example is Paregoric. Some of the

schedule II drugs are also classified as schedule III drugs when limited quantities of the drug are present in a product. One example is acetaminophen with codeine.
- *Schedule IV (C-IV)*—Drugs with acceptable medical use and less potential for abuse than drugs in schedule III, and a limited potential for psychologic and physical dependence. Examples are chloral hydrate, phenobarbital, and benzodiazepines.
- *Schedule V (C-V)*—Drugs with acceptable medical use and less potential for abuse than drugs in schedule IV, and a limited potential for psychologic and physical dependence. Some examples are Lomotil and cough medicines with codeine.

The DEA may place a nonscheduled drug into a scheduled, controlled status after consultation with the FDA. For example, in 1991 certain anabolic steroids were classified as schedule III drugs because of their abuse potential.

Schedule I drugs are not often dealt with in practice. Appendix 4-B and other sources often differentiate and group controlled drugs. Schedule II drugs have the most stringent requirements and are often handled specially as a group. Schedule III and IV drugs have many similar requirements and are often grouped together. Schedule V drugs have the least stringent requirements and may not require the same strict handling as other schedules, or they may be grouped with schedule III and IV drugs.

Generally, commercial containers of scheduled drugs are required to bear labels designating the schedule, with the appropriate C symbol in the upper right corner twice the size of the largest type or overprinted over at least half the label.

Some state laws permit certain controlled drugs to be dispensed without a prescription. These are limited to schedule V drugs, such as cough medicines with codeine; and

(1) sales must be made by a pharmacist;
(2) no more than 240 ml or 48 dosage units of opium-containing substances, or 120 ml or 24 dosage units of other controlled substances, may be sold in a period of 48 hours;
(3) the purchaser must be 18 years or older; and
(4) sales must be recorded in a bound book and include the name of the drug and quantity sold, name and address of purchaser, date of purchase, and pharmacist's initials.

Prescription Requirements

A prescription for a controlled substance may be issued only by individuals authorized to prescribe controlled substances by the jurisdiction in which they are licensed to practice the profession. A hospital's DEA registration will permit its employed physician interns, physician residents, and foreign physicians to dispense, administer, or prescribe controlled substances for hospital patients (see appendix 4-B for more detail).

Under the CSA, prescriptions for drugs in schedules II to V must be written in ink or indelible pencil or typed. They must be issued for legitimate medical purposes only. They must contain the following:

- Full name and address of the patient
- Name, strength, and quantity of medication
- Directions for use, if any
- Date of issuance. The prescription may not be predated or postdated by the prescriber.
- Actual signature of the prescriber. Prescriptions may be handwritten or typed by an agent of the prescriber, such as a nurse, but the signature must be handwritten by the prescriber as he or she would sign a legal document. A stamp bearing the prescriber's name may not be used. See appendix 4-B for requirements of oral prescriptions and refill information for controlled substances.
- Full name, address, and DEA number of the prescriber. The DEA number should be verified before the drug is dispensed. Valid DEA numbers have two letters and seven digits and will pass the following test. Add the second, fourth, and sixth digits and multiply the sum by two. Add the resulting product to the sum of the first, third, and fifth digits. The last digit of this number should equal the seventh digit of the DEA number. For example, the DEA number AR5472612 passes the check:

  The second, fourth, and sixth digits add up to 7 (4 + 2 + 1), and 7 times 2 is 14.
  The first, third, and fifth digits add up to 18 (5 + 7 + 6).
  The total of the two sums is 32 (14 + 18).
  The last digit of the total (2) is the seventh digit of the DEA number.

Prescription Label Requirements

The prescription label for schedule II through IV drugs contains all of the information discussed previously for a non-scheduled drug and "Caution: Federal law prohibits the transfer of this drug to any person other than the patient for whom it was prescribed." State law may require the address and DEA number of the prescriber.

Ordering Process

The ordering of controlled substances from a manufacturer or distributor is limited to those institutions registered with the DEA. The DEA tightly regulates both the ordering and record keeping regarding controlled substances.

Pharmacies must obtain and use special federal order forms (DEA form 222) to obtain schedule II drugs. These order forms must be requisitioned using DEA form 222d. Both the requisition and the order forms may be signed only by the person who signed the DEA registration or by the person given power of attorney. Each DEA form 222 contains 10 lines. The forms are in triplicate copies; copy one and two are forwarded to the supplier, and copy three is retained and filed by the pharmacy. The supplier retains copy one and sends copy two to the DEA for use in monitoring schedule II drug purchases. When completing the DEA form 222, the following requirements must be met:

- Use only a typewriter, pen, or indelible pencil.
- Forward copies one and two together to the supplier, with the carbon paper intact.
- Describe and order only one item per line.
- Make sure that the signature matches the one on the registration or power of attorney form.
- Make no erasures. Suppliers may not accept or fill an order if it contains any erasures or errors. Any forms with errors should be voided and kept in the pharmacy files.
- Keep the third copy in the pharmacy files separate from other pharmacy records.

When schedule II drugs are received, the number of containers received and the date of receipt must be written on the third copy of DEA form 222 and kept on file for 2 years. In case the supplier cannot supply a drug on the order, they may partially fill the order provided the remaining item(s) are supplied within 60 days.

Special order forms are not required for ordering schedule III through V drugs. However, pharmacies are required, as with all documents of controlled substances purchase and dispensing, to maintain ordinary business and professional records.

Record Requirements

Records of initial and subsequent inventory, receipt, dispensing, and disposal of controlled substances are required. Loss or theft of controlled substances must be reported, upon discovery, on a special form.

The federal requirement for maintaining controlled substance records for all types (schedule II order forms, invoices, prescriptions, records of schedule V dispensing, inventories) is that they be kept for at least 2 years. Most state pharmacy practice acts require that prescription dispensing records be kept for a longer period of time.

Poison Prevention Packaging Act (PPPA) of 1970

Intent

The Poison Prevention Packaging Act (PPPA) of 1970 regulates household substances and requires that they be packaged for consumer use in child-resistant packaging—special packaging that is significantly difficult for children under the age of five to open. PPPA standards do not require that all children be prevented from gaining access to child-resistant packaging, nor that all adults be able to gain entry into the package. Containers must be significantly difficult for 80% of children under five to open, and must allow 90% of adults to open them. In other words, child-resistant does not mean childproof.

One of the main purposes of the PPPA was to extend the special packaging requirements to nonprescription drugs as well as prescription drugs. The PPPA is particularly relevant to outpatient pharmacies, but also applies to clinic and emergency room dispensing, physician dispensing, and medications dispensed to patients upon being discharged from the hospital. Medications intended for administration to patients in an institution are exempt.

Exemption

In some situations prescription and nonprescription drugs may be exempt from the child-resistant container specifications of the PPPA. Three examples are given below, although there are many more.

Prescription drugs may be exempt if the prescriber or the consumer requests that noncompliant packaging be used. Federal law allows the consumer to make a blanket request that all medications be supplied in noncompliant packaging, but this request should be in writing.

A limited number of prescription drugs are exempt for various reasons. For example, sublingual nitroglycerin is exempt because quick access to the drug may be needed. Some drugs may be packaged in such small amounts that they would not be harmful to children under five. Others may be packaged to help the consumer comply with directions (e.g., oral contraceptives), thus child-resistant packaging would defeat the purpose.

Nonprescription drugs may be available in non-child-resistant packaging to aid elderly and handicapped individuals. Manufacturers are allowed to market one size of a product in noncompliant packaging provided the packaging contains the printed statement, "This package is for households without young children." Products that contain drugs such as aspirin, acetaminophen, elemental iron, and controlled substances are rarely, if ever, exempt from being dispensed in child-resistant containers.

Prescription drug containers supplied by manufacturers and intended for consumer use should also be child-resistant packaging.

Some customers bring in their prescription bottles to supply refill information. In addition, some customers may bring in their plastic bottles to literally be refilled (reused). Although the idea of refilling a prescription by reusing a customer's old bottle and applying a new label may be tempting, the PPPA prohibits reuse of plastic child-resistant containers because the wear and tear of normal use may decrease effectiveness. Some pharmacies do, however, save plastic prescription bottles (as well as plastic bulk containers from manufacturers) for recycling.

Enforcement

The enforcement functions of the PPPA are managed by the Consumer Product Safety Commission. If PPPA regulations are thought to be violated, Commission staff will investigate the complaint and take appropriate action, including criminal sanctions, as warranted. A state must have identical child-resistant packaging regulations as those developed by the Commission. They cannot be more or less strict than the Commission's. The state may require child-resistant packaging on a substance not regulated by the Consumer Product Safety Commission.[11]

Omnibus Budget Reconciliation Act of 1990 (OBRA 90)

History

With the advent of pharmaceutical care, many pharmacists began to provide cognitive services such as patient counseling and drug therapy review in addition to their distributive services. However, these services varied among pharmacists and were provided only when there was time. OBRA 90 mandated that pharmacists perform drug therapy review and provide counseling for individuals (or their caregivers) receiving Medicaid pharmaceutical benefits. It also provided guidelines for the pharmacist to follow.

Counseling Guidelines

OBRA 90 regulations state that the pharmacist or a designee (e.g., technician) must conduct an initial patient screening and must extend an offer for medication counseling to the patient. This should not be confused with the actual counseling session, which must always be performed by the pharmacist.

The patient may decline counseling, and if so, this should be documented. The offer to counsel may be made in numerous ways depending on specific state law. The offer may be written or oral. Written offers may be displayed materials, such as a sign. Mail-order pharmacies must also comply with the OBRA 90 patient counseling requirements, although an "in person" offer to counsel is not possible.

OBRA 90 and most state counseling regulations designate eight areas to be covered in patient counseling. They are the name and description of the medication; the route of administration, dosage, and dosage form; special directions and precautions for preparation, administration, and use by the patient; common severe side effects, adverse effects, interactions, and therapeutic contraindications that may be encountered; techniques for self-monitoring therapy; proper storage; prescription refill information; and action to be taken in the case of a missed dose. Written information may also be given to the patient but may not take the place of counseling. In addition, the above list represents the minimum standards; each patient needs to be evaluated individually to determine the amount of information they need to understand concerning how to take their medication correctly.

Documentation Requirements

When adding a drug to the patient's profile, pharmacists should review the seven screening tasks identified by OBRA 90 to determine if the added medication is rational. These are therapeutic duplication, overutilization or underutilization, drug-disease contraindications, drug-drug interactions, incorrect dosage or duration of treatment, drug-allergy interactions, and clinical abuse or misuse.

In order to do this, pharmacists must maintain current patient information. Minimal documentation required for Medicaid patients includes patient's name, address, telephone number, age, gender; disease state(s); known allergies/drug reactions; comprehensive list of medications; any relevant medical devices used; and the pharmacist's comments relative to a patient's therapy. Technicians can play a major role in gathering and documenting information that does not require professional judgment (e.g., name, address, telephone number) on the patient profile to allow pharmacists more time to counsel patients.

Documentation by pharmacists is not only required when patients refuse counseling, but it is critical anytime a potential drug therapy problem is discovered and professional judgment is exercised. Good documentation will help protect pharmacists when compliance and enforcement issues arise. The pharmacist's documentation indicates to the state board of pharmacy and Medicaid agency that the pharmacist did screen for drug therapy problems. Pharmacists should also document their actions if they discover patient behavior or drug therapy that is inappropriate; they counsel someone in a unique fashion; they provide a patient with unique information; or the patient refuses to provide the pharmacist with the information needed for the patient profile.

State inspectors use documentation to determine if the pharmacy is in compliance with OBRA 90 regulations and whether to take disciplinary action.

Extension of Standards

Although OBRA 90 standards apply only to Medicaid patients, it is likely that in cases involving non-Medicaid patients, the standards will be viewed by the courts to determine if the pharmacist has acted with reasonable care. Some states have passed laws or regulations that enact OBRA-type standards for all patients. For example, the laws/regulations may require that an offer be made to counsel all patients on *new prescriptions only* or that an offer be made to counsel all patients on *all prescriptions*.

Enforcement

OBRA 90 required each state to form a retrospective drug utilization review (DUR) program to examine claims and records on an ongoing basis in order to identify patterns of abuse, fraud, or inappropriate therapy among physicians, pharmacists, and Medicaid recipients. This program is intended to screen patients' drug profiles in the same manner set forth in the OBRA guidelines for the pharmacist. Each state must establish a DUR board composed of physicians and pharmacists to implement the program and review drug claims.

If a pharmacy is determined to have violated state laws or regulations regarding OBRA 90, the pharmacy could face disciplinary proceedings by either the state Medicaid agency, the state board of pharmacy, or both. Possible expulsion from the Medicaid program is possible if the pharmacy is found guilty of violations. In addition, violation of the state pharmacy practice act may result in licensure revocation or suspension and/or fines for the pharmacist(s) and pharmacy involved. The first step by most states will probably be educational intervention through the state DUR board when retrospective DUR problems are uncovered. When prospective DUR problems arise, warnings will be issued by the state board of pharmacy. Disciplinary proceedings will probably be reserved for intentional violations, situations when the above measures have not had a positive outcome, or when the pharmacy cannot prove their counseling activities through documentation.

SUMMARY

This chapter covers the laws and requirements that a pharmacy technician is likely to encounter in daily activities. This discussion is not inclusive of all laws governing the practice of pharmacy and should not be taken as such. As mentioned earlier, state laws vary and each reader should become familiar with those particular requirements. For additional information relating to pharmacy law, see the Recommended Reading section.

RECOMMENDED READING

Brown TR. *Handbook of Institutional Pharmacy Practice.* 3rd ed., Chapters 23 & 42. Bethesda, MD: American Society of Hospital Pharmacists; 1992.

Fink JL III, Marquardt KW, Simonsmeier JM, editors. *Pharmacy Law Digest.* St. Louis, MO: Facts and Comparisons, Inc.; 1993.

REFERENCES

1. Kaluzny, EL. *Pharmacy Law Digest.* Milwaukee, WI: Douglas-McKay, Inc.; 1979. p. 605.
2. Aspen Health Law Center. *Pharmacy Law Answer Book.* Gaithersburg, MD: Aspen Publishers, Inc.; 1996. p. 146.
3. Aspen Health Law Center. *Pharmacy Law Answer Book.* Gaithersburg, MD: Aspen Publishers, Inc.; 1996. p. 286.
4. Aspen Health Law Center. *Pharmacy Law Answer Book.* Gaithersburg, MD: Aspen Publishers, Inc.; 1996. p. 157,161.
5. ASHP guidelines for the use of investigational drugs in organized health-care settings. In: Hicks, WE, editor. *Practice Standards of ASHP 1994–95.* Bethesda MD: American Society of Hospital Pharmacists; 1994. p. 39–42.
6. Fortner CL. Investigational drugs in the hospital. In: Brown, TL, editor. *Handbook of Institutional Pharmacy Practice.* Bethesda, MD: American Society of Hospital Pharmacists; 1992. p. 250.
7. Fortner CL. Investigational drugs in the hospital. In: Brown, TL, editor. *Handbook of Institutional Pharmacy Practice.* Bethesda, MD: American Society of Hospital Pharmacists; 1992. p. 259.
8. Aspen Health Law Center. *Pharmacy Law Answer Book.* Gaithersburg, MD: Aspen Publishers, Inc.; 1996. p. 285.
9. Aspen Health Law Center. *Pharmacy Law Answer Book.* Gaithersburg, MD: Aspen Publishers, Inc.; 1996. p. 108.
10. Aspen Health Law Center. *Pharmacy Law Answer Book.* Gaithersburg, MD: Aspen Publishers, Inc.; 1996. p. 54.
11. U.S. Consumer Product Safety Commission; Poison Prevention Packaging: A Text for Pharmacists and Physicians. Washington, DC; 1993. p. 13.

SELF-ASSESSMENT QUESTIONS

1. True or False: Nonprescription drugs are able to be purchased without a prescription.

2. Which statement is false? Prescription drugs

a. may be obtained only with a prescription.

b. are not considered safe without medical supervision.

c. may be used for persons other than the one prescribed.

d. must be labeled by the manufacturer that dispensing without a prescription is prohibited.

3. Which of the following acts designated *The United States Pharmacopeia (USP)* and *The National Formulary (NF)* as official compendia?

a. The Federal Pure Food and Drugs Act of 1906

b. The Food, Drug, and Cosmetic Act

c. The Durham-Humphrey Amendment

d. The Kefauver-Harris Amendment

4. True or False: Investigational drugs have received marketing approval by the Food and Drug Administration (FDA) for human use.

5. Choose the correct statement. A generic drug

a. contains a different active ingredient than the brand name medication.

b. must meet required bioequivalence standards before it can be marketed.

c. is usually more expensive than the brand name version.

d. has to follow the same approval process as the brand name version.

6. True or False: The Food, Drug, and Cosmetic Act (FDCA) required product manufacturers to prove that their product is safe and effective for use under conditions stated on the label.

7. Which of the following statements is false? The Durham-Humphrey Amendment (DHA)

a. is also known as the prescription drug amendment.

b. requires that drugs not safely used without medical supervision be dispensed only on a written or oral prescription of a licensed practitioner.

c. considers a drug misbranded if a prescription drug is dispensed without a prescription.

d. limits the number of refills on a prescription.

8. True or False: The Kefauver-Harris Amendment (KHA) required manufacturers to

prove to the FDA that their drugs are competitively priced with other manufacturers.

9. Legal prescribers of medications may include:

a. medical doctors

b. dentists

c. pharmacists

d. all of the above

10. According to the Food, Drug, and Cosmetic Act (FDCA) the prescription label must contain all of the information listed below *except*:

a. name and address of the pharmacy

b. name of the prescriber

c. directions for use with precautions

d. the time it was filled

11. True or False: Some state laws may require that the address of the patient appear on the prescription label.

12. A prescription can usually be refilled:

a. more than what is indicated on the prescription.

b. within a specified time period determined by the state, usually one year from the date the prescription is written.

c. if it contains no refill information.

d. with a different medication.

13. True or False: An emergency supply of three days or less of medication may be dispensed to a patient if the pharmacist is unable to get refill authorization.

14. Record requirements under the FDCA deal with:

a. drug receipt

b. drug disposition

c. drug accountability

d. all of the above

15. How long should records of non-controlled substances by kept?

a. 1 year

b. as long as the state or federal statute of limitations on crime

c. 20 years

d. They do not have to be kept.

16. How many controlled substances schedules exist?

a. one

b. ten

c. five

d. three

17. True or False: A non-controlled substance may be designated a scheduled medication.

18. Which of the following statements about schedule I medications are true?
    a. They have accepted medical use in the United States.
    b. They have moderate potential for abuse.
    c. An example of a schedule 1 medication is heroin.
    d. They may be purchased over the counter.

19. True or False: Some state laws permit certain controlled drugs to be dispensed without a prescription.

20. Which of the following statements concerning schedules II to V prescription requirements is false?
    a. They must be written in ink or indelible pencil or typed.
    b. They must be issued for only legitimate medical purposes.
    c. The signature of the prescriber may be typed.
    d. It must contain the full name and address of the patient.

21. True or False: DEA number AR5432416 is valid.

22. When completing a DEA form 222 to obtain schedule II medications, which requirement must be met?
    a. Copies one and two together, with the carbon paper intact must be forwarded to the supplier.
    b. They may be handwritten in pencil.
    c. More than one item may be ordered per line.
    d. Suppliers may accept and fill an order with erasures or errors.

23. True or False: The universal requirement for maintaining controlled substances records of all types is that they be kept for a minimum of one year.

24. True or False: Under the Poison Prevention Packaging Act (PPPA), child-resistant and childproof are the same.

25. Which of the following statements concerning the Poison Prevention Packaging Act (PPPA) is false?
    a. It regulates household substances and requires that they be packaged for consumer use in child-resistant packaging.
    b. It extended the special packaging requirements to nonprescription drugs.
    c. Containers must be significantly difficult to open, but they must allow 75% of adults to open them.

    d. Medications intended for administration to patients in a hospital are exempt.

26. Which of the following drug(s) are likely to be exempt from packaging in child-resistant containers?
    a. nitroglycerin
    b. acetaminophen
    c. oral contraceptives
    d. a & c

27. True or False: The Poison Prevention Packaging Act (PPPA) allows consumers to use their old prescription bottles for medication refills.

28. What organization enforces the Poison Prevention Packaging Act (PPPA)?
    a. Illinois Council of Health-System Pharmacists
    b. Food and Drug Administration
    c. Drug Enforcement Administration
    d. Consumer Product Safety Commission

29. True or False: The Omnibus Reconciliation Act of 1990 (OBRA 90) mandates drug therapy review and counseling of individuals (or their caregivers) receiving Medicaid pharmaceutical benefits.

30. Which of the following people may conduct an initial patient screening and offer counseling related to the patient's medications under OBRA 90?
    a. pharmacist
    b. pharmacy technician
    c. cashier
    d. all of the above

31. Which one of the following is not a basic counseling guideline of OBRA 90?
    a. the name and description of the medication
    b. the route of administration
    c. adverse effects
    d. the cost of the medication

32. Which of the following is one of the seven screening tasks identified by OBRA 90 used in determining if an added medication is rational?
    a. therapeutic duplication
    b. ability to pay
    c. family history
    d. none of the above

33. Which of the following is not current patient information that must be kept as a result of OBRA 90?

a. known allergies/drug reactions
b. employment status
c. any relevant medical devices used
d. comprehensive list of medications

34. True or False: OBRA 90 standards only apply to Medicaid patients.

35. Which of the following agencies, if any, are responsible for enforcing OBRA 90 regulations.
    a. state board of pharmacy
    b. state Medicaid agency
    c. Consumer Product Safety Commission
    d. a & b

ANSWERS TO SELF-ASSESSMENT

1. True. Nonprescription drugs are recognized as safe and effective for use without a prescription. See Product Classification section, chapter 4.

2. c is false. Prescription drugs may only be used by the person for which the medication was prescribed. See Product Classification section, chapter 4.

3. a is correct. The Federal Pure Food and Drugs Act of 1906 designated these compendia as official. It also prohibits adulteration and misbranding of drugs. See Product Classification section, chapter 4.

4. False. Investigational drugs are being considered for marketing approval but have not yet received it. See Product Classification section, chapter 4.

5. b is correct. A generic drug must meet the same bioequivalency standards as the brand name product. Generic manufacturers may file an abbreviated new drug application (ANDA) and bypass clinical trials as long as the ANDA contains information that shows the new generic drug is bioequivalent to the previously approved brand name product. See Product Classification section, chapter 4.

6. True. The FDCA required this and also prohibits the introduction of misbranded or adulterated foods, drugs, and devices. See Basic Pharmacy Law section, chapter 4.

7. d is false. The DHA is only concerned with ensuring a medication requiring a prescription is not dispensed without one. It does not limit refills. See Basic Pharmacy Law section, chapter 4.

8. False. The KHA required that drug companies prove the effectiveness of their products to the FDA before marketing them. See Basic Pharmacy Law section, chapter 4.

9. d is correct. Each state decides who is authorized to prescribe medications and the latitude they have in doing this. See Legal Prescribers heading in FDCA section, chapter 4.

10. d is the correct answer. The prescription label must contain the date of the prescription or its date of filling, the name of the patient, and the serial number of the prescription in addition to a, b, and c. See Prescription Label Requirements heading in FDCA section, chapter 4.

11. True. Other items that a state may require on a prescription include initials or name of the dispensing pharmacist; telephone number of the pharmacy; drug name, strength, and manufacturer's lot or control number; expiration date of the drug; amount of drug dispensed, and refill information. See Prescription Label Requirements heading in FDCA section, chapter 4.

12. b is correct. A prescription that has no refill information or has exhausted its refills may be refilled only after the physician is contacted and additional refills are obtained. See Refill Requirements heading in FDCA section, chapter 4.

13. True. This may be done but the pharmacist must use his professional judgment to assess the situation and determine if it is warranted. See Refill Requirements heading in FDCA section, chapter 4.

14. d is the correct choice. These records provide evidence of the transactions involved and may be a valid defense in an alleged drug law violation. See Record Requirements heading in FDCA section, chapter 4.

15. b is correct. Records may be needed for defense purposes and should be kept as long as the statute of limitations, usually 5 or 6 years. See Record Requirements heading in FDCA section, chapter 4.

16. c is the correct answer. Controlled substances are divided into five schedules with abuse potential diminishing as the schedule increases. See Classification heading in Controlled Substances section, chapter 4.

17. True. Drugs with high abuse potential may be placed into a schedule for greater control. An example is certain anabolic steroids being placed into schedule III because of their potential for abuse. See Classification heading in Controlled Substances section, chapter 4.

18. c is correct. Schedule I medications have no accepted medical use in the United States and have a high potential for abuse. See Classification heading in Controlled Substances section, chapter 4.

19. True. This is usually limited to schedule V drugs, such as cough medicines with codeine and sales must be made by a pharmacist. There is also a limit on the quantity dispensed and the time period. See Classification heading in Controlled Substances section, chapter 4.

20. c is the false statement. Schedule II to V prescriptions must have a handwritten signature by the prescriber as he or she would sign a legal document. See Prescription Requirements heading in Controlled Substances Act section, chapter 4.

21. True. The rule for determining if a DEA number is valid is to add the second, fourth, and sixth digits and multiply by two (14); add the first, third, and fifth digits (12) and then add the two totals together (26). The last digit of the total (6) is the seventh digit of the DEA number. See Prescription Requirements heading in Controlled Substances section, chapter 4.

22. a is the correct answer. DEA 222 forms must be typed, written in pen or indelible pencil. Only one item is able to be ordered per line. Any forms with errors should be voided and kept in the pharmacy files. See Ordering Process heading in Controlled Substances section, chapter 4.

23. False. Controlled substances records should be kept for a minimum of two years. Most state pharmacy practice acts require prescription dispensing records to be kept for a longer period of time. See Record Requirements heading in Controlled Substances section, chapter 4.

24. False. Child-resistant means containers are significantly difficult for 80% of children under five to gain entry, while childproof means a child is not able to gain entry to the medication. See Intent heading in PPPA section, chapter 4.

25. c is the false statement. The PPPA requires that containers must be significantly difficult for 80% of children under five to open, but must allow 90% of adults to open them. See Intent heading in PPPA section, chapter 4.

26. d is the correct choice. Acetaminophen is rarely, if ever, exempt from being dispensed in a child-resistant container because of its overdose potential. Nitroglycerin is exempt because quick access may be necessary and oral contraceptives are packaged to help the consumer comply with directions. See Exemption heading in PPPA section, chapter 4.

27. False. The PPPA prohibits reuse of plastic child-resistant containers because the wear and tear of normal use may decrease their effectiveness. See Exemption heading in PPPA section, chapter 4.

28. d is the correct choice. The Consumer Product Safety Commission enforces the PPPA. It investigates complaints and takes appropriate action, including criminal sanctions, if warranted. See Enforcement heading in PPPA section, chapter 4.

29. True. This act forced pharmacists to counsel and perform drug therapy evaluations on this group of individuals. Although some pharmacists were doing this prior to the act, many were not. See History heading in OBRA 90 section, chapter 4.

30. d is the correct choice. The initial patient screening and offer to counsel may be performed by anyone. The actual counseling session must always be performed by the pharmacist. See Counseling Guidelines heading in OBRA 90 section, chapter 4.

31. d is the correct answer. In addition to a, b, and c, the other basic guidelines are: dosage and dosage form; special directions and precautions for preparation; administration and use by the patient; common severe side effects; interactions and therapeutic contraindications that may be encountered; techniques for self-monitoring therapy; proper storage; prescription refill information; and action to be taken in case of a missed dose. See Counseling Guidelines heading in OBRA 90 section, chapter 4.

32. a is the correct answer. The other six are overutilization or underutilization, drug-disease contraindications, drug-drug interactions, incorrect dosage or duration of treatment, drug allergy interactions and clinical abuse or misuse. See Documentation Requirements heading in OBRA 90 section, chapter 4.

33. b is the correct answer. a, c, and d are requirements. The other requirements are name, address, telephone number, age, gender, disease state(s) and the pharmacist's comments relative to a patient's therapy. See Documentation Requirements in OBRA 90 section, chapter 4.

34. True. Although OBRA 90 only applies to Medicaid patients, these standards will be applied by the courts to other patient groups to determine if the pharmacist has acted with reasonable care. Many states have enacted OBRA-type standards for all patients. See Extension of Standards heading under OBRA 90.

35. d is the correct choice. If OBRA regulations are violated, the pharmacy could face disciplinary proceedings from either the state board of pharmacy or the state Medicaid agency. Penalties range from expulsion from the Medicaid program to licensure revocation or suspension and/or fines.

Code of Ethics for Pharmacists

PREAMBLE

Pharmacists are health professionals who assist individuals in making the best use of medications. This Code, prepared and supported by pharmacists, is intended to state publicly the principles that form the fundamental basis of the roles and responsibilities of pharmacists. These principles, based on moral obligations and virtues, are established to guide pharmacists in relationships with patients, health professionals, and society.

PRINCIPLES

I.   A pharmacist respects the covenantal relationship between the patient and pharmacist.

II.   A pharmacist promotes the good of every patient in a caring, compassionate, and confidential manner.

III.   A pharmacist respects the autonomy and dignity of each patient.

IV.   A pharmacist acts with honesty and integrity in professional relationships.

V.   A pharmacist maintains professional competence.

VI.   A pharmacist respects the values and abilities of colleagues and other health professionals.

VII.   A pharmacist serves individual, community, and societal needs.

VIII.   A pharmacist seeks justice in the distribution of health resources.

Source: American Society of Health-System Pharmacists. Code of Ethics for Pharmacists. *Am J Health-System Pharm.* 1995;52(19):2131.

APPENDIX 4-B

ASHP Technical Assistance Bulletin on Use of Controlled Substances in Organized Health-Care Settings

Introduction

Federal regulation of controlled substances was consolidated by the enactment of the Comprehensive Drug Abuse Prevention and Control Act of 1970 (21 USC 801 et seq.). Enforcement of the Act is generally administered by the Drug Enforcement Administration (DEA), created in 1973 as an arm of the Department of Justice. While the Food and Drug Administration (FDA) retains the authority to regulate specified habit-forming drugs, such substances may be subject to regulation by both FDA and DEA. DEA regulations dealing with narcotic drugs in treatment settings appear in Title 21, *Code of Federal Regulations*, Part 1300 to the end. FDA regulations can be found in Title 21, Part 291.

Despite the comprehensiveness of the Act, its amendments, and its regulations, questions remain concerning their application to the practice of pharmacy in hospitals, long-term care facilities, health maintenance organizations (HMOs), ambulatory care centers, licensed residential care facilities, and other institutional and home health care settings. ASHP originally approved guidelines to the regulations in 1973 in order to provide assistance to institutional pharmacists in interpreting the regulations.

The purpose of this Technical Assistance Bulletin is to provide an interpretation of present legal requirements that will assist in establishing acceptable professional practices under the Controlled Substances Act (CSA). The guidelines should be used in connection with the law and regulations. They are not intended as a substitute for knowledge of the law and regulations.

Just as with patient care, accountability is the responsibility of every discipline within an institution. However, ASHP also recognizes that the pharmacist has primary responsibility for the distribution of drugs throughout the institution, including control methods designed to ensure accountability of controlled substances. The pharmacist is responsible for assuming the leading role in the control of drugs that are subject to diversion and misuse.

In adopting the following guidelines, the requirements of the CSA have been interpreted to ensure compliance with the law while still allowing the organized health-care setting to promote high quality patient care in accordance with acceptable legal and professional standards. ASHP believes that these guidelines provide effective controls against diversion or misuse while ensuring that a proper level of professional attention to the needs of patients is maintained.

Research, laboratory procedures, and instructional uses are dealt with separately under their own heading. Methadone is also discussed separately in its own section.

A final word of caution is in order. Some state laws are more stringent than federal laws. Where this is the case, the stricter law also must be followed.

Definitions

The following selected definitions are derived from the CSA or regulations of federal agencies. The definitions are presented here because they are critical to understanding the law or because of their effect on certain operative provisions of the law and its regulations. Most of the language contained in the definitions comes directly from the CSA or from DEA regulations. However, in certain instances, language has been added to assist in the understanding and application of the definitions.

1. **Person.** The term "person" is defined in the DEA regulations [21 CFR 1301.02(j)] but not in the CSA. It includes any individual, corporation, government or governmental subdivision or agency, business trust, partnership, association, or other legal entity. It would generally include a hospital but not the hospital pharmacy.

2. **Agent.** The term "agent" is defined in the CSA [CSA §102(3); 21 USC 802(3)] but not in the DEA regulations. It means an authorized person who acts on behalf of or at the direction of a manufacturer, distributor, or dispenser; such term does not include a common or contract carrier, public warehouseman, or employee of the carrier or warehouseman when acting in the usual and lawful course of the carrier's or warehouseman's business.

3. **Pharmacist.** The term "pharmacist" is defined in the DEA regulations [21 CFR 1304.02(g)] but not in the CSA. It means any individual licensed by a state to dispense controlled substances and also includes any other person (e.g., pharmacist intern) authorized by a state to dispense controlled substances under the supervision of a pharmacist licensed by that state.

4. **Practitioner.** The term "practitioner" is defined in the CSA [CSA §102(20); 21 USC 802(20)] but not in the DEA regulations. It means a physician, dentist, veterinarian, scientific investigator, pharmacy, hospital, or other person licensed, registered, or otherwise permitted, by the United States or the jurisdiction in which the practitioner practices or does research, to distribute, dispense, conduct research with respect to, administer, or use in teaching or chemical analysis, a controlled substance in the course of professional practice or research.

5. **Individual Practitioner.** The term "individual practitioner" is defined in the DEA regulations [21 CFR 1306.02(b)] but not in the CSA. It means a physician, dentist, veterinarian, or other individual licensed, registered, or otherwise permitted, by the United States or the jurisdiction in which he or she practices, to dispense a controlled substance in the course of professional practice. It does not include a pharmacist, pharmacy, or institutional practitioner.

6. **Institutional Practitioner.** The term "institutional practitioner" is defined in the DEA regulations [21 CFR 1306.02(c)] but not in the CSA. It means a hospital,

intermediate care facility, skilled nursing facility, federally qualified or state-licensed HMO, or other entity (other than an individual) licensed, registered, or otherwise permitted, by the United States or the jurisdiction in which it is located, to dispense a controlled substance in the course of professional practice. It does not include individual practitioners or a pharmacy.

7. *Dispense.* The term "dispense" is defined in the CSA [CSA §102(10); 21 USC 802(10)] but not in the DEA regulations. It means to deliver a controlled substance to an ultimate user or research subject by, or pursuant to the lawful order of, a practitioner, including the prescribing and administering of a controlled substance and the packaging, labeling, or compounding necessary to prepare the substance for delivery.

    Additionally, the term "dispenser," as defined in the CSA [CSA §102(10); 21 USC 802(10)] and the DEA regulations [21 CFR 1304.02(c)], means an individual practitioner, institutional practitioner, pharmacy, or pharmacist who dispenses a controlled substance.

8. *Administer.* The term "administer" is defined in the CSA [CSA §102(2); 21 USC 802(2)] but not in the DEA regulations. It means the direct application of a controlled substance to the body of a patient or research subject by either a practitioner (or in the practitioner's presence by the practitioner's authorized agent) or the patient or research subject at the direction and in the presence of the practitioner, whether such application be by injection, inhalation, ingestion, or any other route.

9. *Prescription.* The term "prescription" is defined in the DEA regulations [21 CFR 1306.02(f)] but not in the CSA. It means an order for medication that is dispensed to or for an ultimate user but does not include an order for medication that is dispensed for immediate administration to the ultimate user (e.g., an order to dispense a drug to an inpatient for immediate administration in a hospital is not a prescription). A medication order is not considered to be a prescription when it is dispensed from a pharmacy registered in the name of, and located at, an institution for an ultimate user who is a patient in the institution.

10. *Readily Retrievable.* The term "readily retrievable" is defined in the DEA regulations [21 CFR 1304.02(h)] but not in the CSA. It means that entries for controlled substances not maintained in separate written records are visually identifiable from other items appearing in the records (e.g., the use of asterisked or red-lined notations or, in the case of prescriptions, the letter "C" in red ink); or, where records are kept by automated data processing systems or other electronic or mechanized recordkeeping systems, the system possesses the capability to produce the controlled substance records in a reasonable time.

11. *Long-Term Care Facility.* The term "long-term care facility" is defined in the DEA regulations [21 CFR 1306.02(e)] but not in the CSA. It means a nursing home or a retirement care, mental care, or other facility or institution that provides extended health care to resident patients.

Registration

Persons Required to Register. Forms and fees. Every person who manufactures, distributes, dispenses, or conducts research with controlled substances, conducts narcotic maintenance or detoxification programs, or proposes to engage in any of these activities must obtain registration(s) unless exempted by law or DEA regulations. Dispensers may obtain registration for a period of up to 3 years, as determined by DEA. Manufacturers and distributors must obtain registration annually. Registration is accomplished by use of DEA Forms 224, 224a, 225, 225a, 363, and 363a, as required. The appropriate registration fee must be paid when the form is submitted to DEA. However, governmental registrants may claim exemption to the registration fee.

Types of Activities. Dispensing. Separate registration is required for dispensing. The hospital registration covers both inpatient and outpatient dispensing, unless outpatient dispensing is operated from a detached ambulatory care pharmacy.

Distribution. Separate registration is required for distribution of controlled substances to persons, other than employees or agents of the registrant, who will make final transfer to the ultimate user. If an institution regularly orders controlled substances for other facilities, it is in effect acting as a wholesaler and must register as a distributor.

An exception to the regulations allows for occasional distribution to other registrants without registration as a distributor, provided that the annual total number of dosage units of all controlled substances so distributed does not exceed 5% of the total number of dosage units of all controlled substances dispensed.

Place of Business. Separate registration is required for each principal place of business or professional practice. A principal place of business or practice is considered to be one general physical location. The hospital registration covers the entire institution. Separate registration is not required for satellite or decentralized pharmacy stations or outpatient pharmacies located onsite in the same institution. However, if the hospital has pharmacies that are physically removed from the main facility at different locations, each pharmacy may be required to register and obtain a separate DEA number depending on its distance from the main facility.

Contract pharmacy. A leased or contract pharmacy located on the premises of an existing DEA-registered hospital may operate under the hospital registration, provided that the hospital assumes full responsibility for the pharmacy operations and ensures full compliance with all applicable federal regulations governing the use of controlled substances. This would be permissible only if the hospital's responsibility for the operation is clearly set forth in the contract between the hospital and the contract pharmacy. Under these conditions, the pharmacy may perform all of the functions of a hospital pharmacy, including the dispensing of controlled substances pursuant to medication orders.

If the hospital does not wish to assume this responsibility, the contract pharmacy would be required to register with the DEA as a retail pharmacy, and a prescription would be required to dispense controlled substances to hospital patients.

A registered hospital is authorized to fill outpatient prescriptions without obtaining a retail pharmacy registration, provided that this practice is within its own use and allowed by state law. Outpatient "own use" includes the organized health-care setting's bona fide outpatients and its employees and medical staff and their families for their personal use. The same records as are required of a retail pharmacy must be maintained.

Pharmacy not onsite. Since registration is required for each principal place of business or professional practice where controlled substances are manufactured, distributed, or dispensed, a pharmacy not onsite at the institution must obtain a separate registration from the registration of the institution and must maintain all records required for a retail pharmacy.

Practitioners within Institution. Where the organized health-care setting is the registrant, its agents and employees are exempt from registration. The exemption permits institutional personnel to carry out functions of the institution with respect to controlled substances without being personally registered, provided that they are acting in the usual course of their business or employment. Thus, in this case, pharmacists do not need separate personal registration since DEA does not actually register pharmacists.

Additionally, a physician who practices only in a hospital that is itself registered with DEA as a practitioner need not apply for an additional personal registration. However, there are important limitations to the use of this exemption [21 CFR 1301.24(b)]. The employed physician (without a personal DEA registration) may not write prescriptions for controlled substances to be filled by

1. A pharmacy outside the hospital.
2. The hospital pharmacy if that pharmacy is itself registered as a practitioner.

The employed physician may administer or dispense controlled substances only while acting in the course of usual employment in the facility. (For application of this principle to unregistered interns, residents, or foreign-trained physicians, see the related subsection in the Prescriptions section of these guidelines.) State law determines for purposes of the CSA which agents or employees are authorized to have access to or responsibility for controlled substances. Institutions should have written policies that interpret state law and assign staff responsibility accordingly.

Termination of Registration.

1. The Administrator of DEA has authority under the CSA to suspend or revoke registration where the registrant
   a. Has materially falsified any application filed pursuant to or required by Title II or III of the CSA.
   b. Has been convicted of a felony under the CSA or of a felony under any other federal or state laws relating to controlled substances.
   c. Has had his or her state license or registration suspended, revoked, or denied and is no longer authorized by state law to manufacture, distribute, or dispense controlled substances, or has had the suspension, revocation, or denial of his or her registration recommended by competent state authority.

   The registration of a practitioner may now be denied if it is determined that such registration would be "inconsistent with the public interest." In determining the public interest, DEA may consider (1) the recommendations of the appropriate state licensing board or professional disciplinary authority, (2) the experience of the applicant in dispensing or conducting research with respect to controlled substances, (3) the applicant's conviction record under federal or state laws relating to the manufacture, distribution, or dispensing of controlled substances, (4) compliance with applicable state, federal, or local laws pertaining to controlled substances, and (5) such other conduct that may threaten the public health and safety.

   These considerations, along with the three existing grounds noted above, also allow for the input of competent state authority recommending the suspension, revocation, or denial of a registration.

   These factors expand DEA's authority to deal with problems of diversion at the practitioner level. Registrants have recourse to established administrative procedures under Section 1301.45 of the DEA regulations to ensure due process of law before suspension or revocation of registration.

2. The registration of any person is terminated if and when such person dies, ceases legal existence, discontinues business or professional practice, or changes his or her name or address as shown on the certificate of registration. The DEA must be promptly notified of the reason for termination. Where there is a change of name or address, the registrant is required to report this change.
3. Registration may not be assigned or transferred except in compliance with conditions designated in writing by DEA.

Records and Inventory

General. Every registrant under the Act must maintain, on a current basis, complete and accurate records of the receipt and disposition of all controlled substances. The records must include the following information for each controlled substance:

1. The name of the substance.
2. A description of each product in finished form (e.g., 10-mg tablet or 10-mg/ml concentration) and the number of units or volume of finished form in each commercial container (e.g., 100-tablet bottle or 3-ml vial).
3. The number of commercial containers of each such finished form received from other persons, including the date of receipt and number of containers in each shipment and the name, address, and registration number of the person from whom the containers were received.
4. The number of units or volume of products in finished form dispensed, including the name of the person to whom it was dispensed, the date of dispensing, the number of units or volume dispensed, and the written or typewritten name or initials of the individual who dispensed or administered the substance on behalf of the dispenser.
5. The number of units or volume of products in finished form of commercial containers disposed of in any other manner by the registrant, including the date of disposal and the quantity of the substance in finished form disposed.

All records must be kept for a 2-year period or longer if

state or other laws mandate. Records of Schedule I or II substances must be maintained separately from all other records of the registrant; those records of substances listed in Schedule III, IV, or V need not be kept separately, provided that the information is readily retrievable.

Inventory. To establish a starting point, the law requires a physical inventory of all controlled substances on the effective date of the Act or when the registrant first engages in business. A person registered to dispense controlled substances shall include in his or her inventory for each controlled substance in finished form the name and finished form of the substances (e.g., pentobarbital 100-mg tablets) and the number of containers and units per volume in each container. For substances that are damaged, outdated, awaiting disposal, being held for quality control, or maintained for extemporaneous compounding, the name, quantity, and reason for the continued maintenance of the substance are required. In determining units in an open commercial container, an exact count or measure of Schedule I or II drugs shall be made; an estimated count of Schedule III, IV, or V drugs shall be made unless the container holds more than 1000 tablets or capsules, in which case an exact count will be made.

An inventory must be taken every 2 years thereafter, on the date on which the initial inventory was taken, or on the registrant's regular physical inventory date, or on any other fixed date that does not vary by more than 6 months from the biennial date that would otherwise apply [21 CFR 1304.13]. For this biennial inventory and any other DEA-required inventories, the institution must record on that inventory record if it was taken at the beginning or end of that day's business and should note the name, initials, or signature of the person or persons taking that inventory. If the registrant elects to take the biennial inventory on his or her regular general physical inventory date or another fixed date, DEA must be notified of the election and of the date on which the biennial inventory will be taken.

The law specifically states that a perpetual inventory is not required. Nor does the law require periodic "audits." However, these procedures may be desirable in selected high risk areas or where diversion is suspected.

Records of Receipt. Order forms. To purchase substances in Schedule I or II, the law requires an official order form, DEA Form 222. After a substance purchased through Form 222 has been received, Copy 3 of the order form serves the requirement of a "separate" record and must be filed separately. No further record is needed. Order forms may be obtained only by registered persons. If the institutional pharmacist prepared and signed the registration application, he or she may obtain order forms on his or her own signature. If the institution's administrator signed the application for registration, the administrator should execute a power of attorney (to be retained on file) for DEA order forms to permit the pharmacist to obtain and execute order forms on his or her behalf. In a large institution, it may be desirable to designate more than one pharmacist on this power of attorney. The DEA regulations outline the form and substance of the power of attorney [21 CFR 1305.07].

The order form is prepared in triplicate. The purchaser submits Copy 1 and Copy 2 of the form to the supplier and retains Copy 3 in his or her own files to be used to record the quantity and the date on which the controlled substances are

received. As stated above, the order forms must be maintained separately from all other records of the registrant.

The requirements for completing Form 222 are specifically stated in the DEA regulations. Pharmacists must take great care to ensure that they literally follow the directions listed on the back of the form for completing it. Additionally, care should be taken in actually completing the form because the regulation does not allow suppliers to fill an order if the form shows "any alteration, erasure, or change of any description" [21 CFR 1305.11(2)]. If an error is made when completing Form 222, all copies of the form should be voided and kept on file.

The regulations also note that a supplier, not a purchaser, may void an item on a DEA Form 222 [21 CFR 1305.15(a)]. Consequently, the supplier is the only individual who has the authority to indicate the cancellation on an order form.

DEA policy does not preclude generic substitution for products ordered on Form 222, provided that the name and National Drug Code (NDC) number of the actual product shipped is reflected on the form. Therefore, it would be acceptable to make a substitution provided that the customer (pharmacy) agrees to accept a generic rather than a brand name product, the generic product of a manufacturer rather than the one specified on the form, or a brand name product rather than a generic one. The purchaser (pharmacist) is not required to submit a new DEA Form 222 to accommodate such an order change.

Purchase orders, invoices, and other forms. Purchase orders, invoices, packing slips, and other business forms may serve as records of receipt for substances in Schedule III, IV, or V, if they are accurately reconciled against the drugs actually received. If noncontrolled substances are listed on the same business form, controlled substances should be made readily identifiable by use of a red line, asterisk, or some other annotation to meet the requirement that the records be readily retrievable. An alternative to using business forms as the record of receipt is the maintenance of a log book or inventory card system. However, in order to meet the retrievability requirements of the regulations, a single system (not both) should be used.

Computer records. If a computer or other automated data processing equipment is used, separate written records as described above are not required for controlled substances in any schedule, provided that (1) DEA order forms are maintained in accordance with DEA regulations, (2) specific information in the data bank can be retrieved within a reasonable period of time, and (3) such information is retained for a period of 2 years and includes all of the information required by DEA as described earlier in this section under the General subheading.

Patient Records. Administration records. The basic records of disposition within the institution are patient medical records. Medical records contain physicians' original drug orders authorizing the dispensing and administration of medications. It is not necessary for the physician to sign and write his or her DEA registration number on each order for a controlled substance. However, the physician's registration number and signature should be kept on file in the pharmacy. If it is not on file in the pharmacy, the physician should enter the number in the medical record.

If the prescriber is an unregistered intern, resident, or

foreign-trained physician in the employ of the facility, he or she may use the institution's registration number in lieu of individual registration. To write outpatient prescription orders for controlled substances, he or she must be assigned a suffix code in addition to the institution's number. (See the related subsection in the section on Prescriptions.)

The medical record also contains nurses' entries indicating that drugs were administered to patients. This information may be contained in the nursing notes, in the progress notes, or on a medication treatment form.

Working solely from the medical record can be burdensome, especially with respect to reconciliation of medications issued and those administered. In addition, records for Schedule II substances must be maintained separately and those for Schedule III, IV, or V substances must be readily retrievable. Hence, it is desirable to maintain a derivative record from the medical record; such a record can be used for control purposes, with minimum interference to patient care. Adequate accountability does not require the use of any specific system or form. One type of effective and convenient to maintain record is a medication administration record (MAR). Variations of this record that achieve the same purpose may also be used. This record constitutes a separate section in the patient's chart, apart from the physicians' progress notes and nurses' notes.

For recordkeeping purposes, the MAR has a number of advantages. Most institutions already use, in one form or another, an MAR that contains the necessary information for patient-care purposes. Use of this record for control purposes eliminates the need to rewrite the same information on another record form, resulting in a significant savings of nursing and pharmacy time. If diversion does occur, the chances of discovery are increased because all clinical personnel are using the same records in caring for patients.

A second method of recordkeeping is a derivative record maintained by computer. Records of disposition used to provide information for computers or other automated data processing equipment need not conform to any particular format, provided that all required information (previously listed) is put into the system. The system must be designed so that records of Schedule II controlled substances can be retrieved separately from Schedule III, IV, and V records. As with other recordkeeping systems, computer records of disposition may be reconciled by comparing the quantities of controlled substances used and remaining against the quantities received.

A third form of record that could be used is the "certificate of disposition" or "proof of use" sheet. The same basic information is necessary as with other methods. Each time a dose of a controlled substance is administered, institutional personnel are required to make an entry on a manual form or in an automated control system. All controlled substances recorded as administered are reconciled against the physical inventory. One difficulty with this system is that these records do not contain the physicians' drug orders, complicating verification that drugs administered were in fact ordered. Patient charts are primary care records and are in constant use by physicians, nurses, pharmacists, and other personnel. Manual proof of use sheets are not used as often and, in fact, may not be used for many days for some seldom used drugs. Thus, falsification of proof of use sheets may go undetected for longer periods of time than with primary patient records such as the MAR. Automated systems with provisions for

additional levels of security and control can improve this type of record. DEA generally does not consider patient profiles to be acceptable documents for recordkeeping since required information is often not included.

Outpatient dispensing. Prescriptions for outpatients (see related section under Prescriptions) must be filed separately if for substances in Schedule I or II. Prescriptions for Schedule III, IV, or V substances may be kept with other prescriptions if they are stamped in red ink, in the lower right corner, with a letter "C" that is no smaller than 1 inch high [21 CFR 1304.04(h)(2)].

Transfers between pharmacies. The transfer of original prescription information for Schedule III–V controlled substances for the purpose of refill dispensing is permissible (if allowed under existing state or other applicable law) between pharmacies on a one-time basis provided that

1. The transfer is communicated directly between two licensed pharmacists.
2. The transferring pharmacist records "void" on the invalidated prescription and records the name, address, and DEA number of the pharmacy to which it was transferred, the name of the pharmacist receiving the information, the date of the transfer, and the pharmacist transferring the information.
3. The receiving pharmacist writes the following on the face of the prescription: the word "transfer"; the date of issuance of the original prescription; the original number of refills authorized; the date of original dispensing; the number of valid refills remaining; the date of the last refill; the name, address, DEA number, and original prescription number of the pharmacy from which it was transferred; and the name of the transferring pharmacist.
4. Both pharmacies maintain the required records for 2 years from the date of the last refill.
5. Pharmacies electronically accessing the same prescription record satisfy all information requirements of a manual mode of prescription transferral.

Waste and disposal. Controlled substances may be disposed of other than by administration to a patient. An ampul might be dropped and broken, the patient might refuse a dose of medication, the medication might become contaminated or decomposed, or the prescriber might cancel an order. Whenever possible, all such medications should be returned to the pharmacy for final disposition.

Each organized health-care setting should develop a policy to be followed when any quantity of controlled substances must be discarded as wastage. Pharmacies providing injectable drugs to patients receiving home care should develop a policy on appropriate waste and disposal of unused narcotics. In developing these policies, pharmacists should consult with their state board of pharmacy and the DEA's Special Agent in Charge (SAC) within the region. State and local regulations should be consulted, as jurisdictions differ on requirements within various types of institutions. Policies should contain provisions for a second signature to witness the destruction of any controlled substance. Authority to witness destruction of a controlled substance should be limited to those individuals who are given authority within the institution to administer or dispense controlled substances.

The DEA regulations require that a registrant who

desires or is required to dispose of controlled substances in his or her possession must request authority and disposal instructions from the SAC of the DEA office in the area where the registrant is located. If an institution is registered only as a dispenser of controlled substances and is not required to make periodic reports to DEA, then the request for disposal is made on DEA Form 41. The registrant must list the controlled substances for disposal and submit the form, in triplicate, to the SAC. The SAC shall authorize disposal by

1. Transferral to a person registered under the Act and authorized to possess the substance.
2. Delivery to an agent of the DEA or to the nearest office of DEA.
3. Destruction in the presence of an agent of DEA or other authorized person.
4. Other means determined by the SAC that ensure that the controlled substance does not become available to unauthorized persons.

The general method of disposal is incineration. Furthermore, DEA allows other reasonable types of disposal as long as the registrant receives approval of the disposal procedure from the SAC. However, flushing is no longer an appropriate method of disposal for controlled substances because of changes in the guidelines of the Environmental Protection Agency.

In lieu of disposal by DEA, authority has been granted for disposal of unwanted, outdated, controlled substances to agents of the individual states' narcotics control authorities and professional licensing board inspectors or investigators. In terms of disposal without a witness, DEA policy does not make a distinction between partially used controlled substances and other controlled substance waste. Partially used controlled substances should also be destroyed in accordance with DEA regulations. The local DEA office or state board of pharmacy should be contacted to determine if the state in which the institution is located performs these destructions. Contact the local DEA office to determine the conditions under which this can be done and the details for carrying out such disposal.

If the institution is required to dispose of controlled substances regularly, personnel may file a written request with the SAC to authorize the institution to dispose of those substances without prior authorization on the condition that records are maintained of such disposals and periodic reports are filed with DEA summarizing those disposals. Conditions may be placed on the disposal, such as the method of destruction and the frequency and details of the periodic reports. These requirements do not affect or alter any procedures established by the state in which the institution is registered. To ensure that the institution is in compliance with state laws and regulations regarding disposal, the registrant should also contact the appropriate state regulatory board before proceeding.

Additionally, in selected situations, the DEA may authorize more than one disposal annually without the presence of a witness from the DEA. Requests from an individual practitioner to destroy controlled substances in addition to the authorized annual disposal are handled on a case-by-case basis. Registrants must complete a legible Form DEA-41 listing all drugs to be destroyed and submit it to the nearest DEA office, with a letter requesting permission to destroy the drugs. The letter must be received by the DEA at least 2 weeks before the proposed destruction.

Prescriptions

General. Substances in Schedule II, III, or IV (and, in some states, V) may be dispensed or administered only pursuant to a written or oral prescription from a prescribing individual practitioner or pursuant to an order for medication made by an individual practitioner that is dispensed for immediate administration to the ultimate user. All such orders, or direct copies thereof, should be received and interpreted by the pharmacist before administration. The practitioner's order is the keystone to any control system. Without it, the entire system is rendered useless since counterfeit administration records could be entered as the means for diverting controlled substances. Administration of emergency medications from floor stock or emergency supplies should be provided for in written policies and procedures. In a small facility without onsite pharmaceutical services, all controlled substances must be dispensed pursuant to prescriptions.

Outpatients. Controlled substances may not be dispensed to outpatients for home use unless all of the prescription and labeling requirements of the law are met. Prescriptions for controlled substances in all schedules must include the name and strength of the drug to be dispensed, the dosage form, quantity prescribed, directions for use, the name and address of the patient, and the name, address, and registration number of the prescriber. Further, they must be dated as of, and signed on, the day they are issued [21 CFR 1306.05(a)].

For injectable products administered in the home, the prescription should include the concentration, rate of administration, and route of administration. If the medication is to be administered through patient-controlled analgesia devices, then other pertinent variables (e.g., dose, amount and frequency of bolus doses, and lockout period) should be included on the prescription.

Dispensing of Prescriptions. A prescription for controlled substances may be dispensed by a pharmacist acting in the usual course of his or her professional practice. The pharmacist must be employed in either a registered institution or a registered retail pharmacy.

Schedules II, III, IV, and V. Requirement of prescription. A pharmacist may dispense a controlled substance listed in Schedule II only pursuant to a written prescription signed by the prescribing individual practitioner. An exception occurs in an emergency situation [21 CFR 1306.11(d)]. Then, a pharmacist may dispense a controlled substance listed in Schedule II upon oral authorization provided that

1. The quantity prescribed and dispensed is limited to the amount needed to treat the patient during the emergency period.
2. The prescription is immediately reduced to writing by the pharmacist and contains all information required except for the signature of the prescriber.
3. The pharmacist makes a reasonable effort to determine that the oral authorization came from a registered individual practitioner. This may include a call to the prescriber using the telephone number listed in an appropriate directory or other good faith efforts to

establish identity.

4. The prescribing individual practitioner delivers or mails a written prescription to the pharmacist within 72 hours. The phrase "Authorization for Emergency Dispensing" and the date of the oral order should be written on the prescription. Upon receipt, the pharmacist should attach the written prescription to the oral emergency prescription. If a written prescription is not received, the pharmacist should notify the nearest office of the DEA or risk forfeiture of the authority to dispense without a written prescription conferred by the regulations [21 CFR 1306.11(d)].

Controlled substances listed in Schedules III–V, however, may be dispensed pursuant to either a written prescription or a telephoned order. An original prescription for a Schedule III or IV controlled substance received via the telephone may be entered directly into the computer system, provided that the computer system provides the necessary documentation required by law. A hard copy record may be required; it may be provided by the computer system.

Refills. Refills of prescriptions for Schedule II controlled substances are prohibited, except as stated below, but partial filling is permitted if the pharmacist is initially unable to supply the full quantity called for in a written or emergency oral prescription and a notation is made of the quantity supplied on the face of the written prescription. However, the remaining portion may be filled only within the 72-hour period. If the remaining portion is not filled within the 72-hour period, the pharmacist must notify the prescribing individual practitioner. No further quantity may be supplied beyond 72 hours without a new prescription.

Partial filling. A prescription for a Schedule II controlled substance written for a patient in a long-term care facility or for a patient with a medical diagnosis documenting a terminal illness may be filled in partial quantities [21 CFR 1306.13]. If there is any question whether a patient may be classified as having a terminal illness, the pharmacist must contact the prescribing practitioner before partially filling the prescription. The pharmacist must record on the prescription whether the patient is terminally ill or a patient in a long-term care facility.

For each partial filling, the dispensing pharmacist shall record on the prescription (or on another appropriate record, uniformly maintained and readily retrievable) the date of the partial filling, the quantity dispensed, the remaining quantity authorized to be dispensed, and the identification of the dispensing pharmacist. Schedule II prescriptions for patients in a long-term care facility or patients with a medical diagnosis documenting a terminal illness shall be valid for a period not to exceed 60 days from the issue date unless earlier terminated by the discontinuance of the medication. Information pertaining to current Schedule II prescriptions for patients in a long-term care facility or for patients with a medical diagnosis documenting a terminal illness may be maintained in a computerized system if this system has the capability to permit

1. Output (display or printout of the original prescription number).
2. Date of issue.
3. Identification of individual prescribing practitioner.
4. Identification of patient.

5. Address of the long-term care facility or address of the institution or residence of the patient.
6. Identification of medication authorized (including dosage form, strength, and quantity).
7. Listing of the partial fillings and quantities that have been dispensed under each prescription.
8. Identification of the prescribing pharmacist.

Refills for Schedule III or IV controlled substances may not be made more than 6 months after the date of issue and may not be refilled more than five times.

Refills for Schedule III–V controlled substances may be made only if expressly authorized by the prescribing individual practitioner on the prescription. Each refilling of a prescription shall be entered on the prescription or on another appropriate document. The practitioner may authorize additional refills of Schedule III or IV controlled substances on the original prescription through an oral refill authorization transmitted to the pharmacist if the total quantity authorized, including the amount of the original prescription, does not exceed five refills or extend beyond 6 months from the date of issue of the original prescription. The practitioner must execute a new and separate prescription for any additional quantities beyond the five-refill, 6-month limitation.

Interns, Residents, or Foreign-Trained Physicians. Interns, residents, or foreign-trained physicians on the institution's staff who do not have their own registration numbers may use the number of the institution plus a suffix code assigned to each by the institution.

The use of the institution's registration in lieu of personal registration is contingent on the practitioner being authorized under the law of the jurisdiction to prescribe, dispense, or administer drugs. The institution must also verify the practitioner's status under local law.

The practitioner must be authorized by the institution to use its number to dispense or prescribe, and the practitioner's activities must be within the scope of employment and in the usual course of professional practice.

A current list of the internal suffix codes must be kept by the institution and made available to other registrants and law enforcement agencies upon request for the purpose of verifying authority to prescribe. The list must identify each practitioner with the appropriate individual suffix code.

Labeling

Intrahospital Distribution. Controlled substances, as with all medications, must be properly labeled before distribution within the institution. In this manner, nursing personnel should know what items need identification in charting. In addition to the usual identifying information, the controlled status of such products may be indicated on the label by the use of a symbol or color code.

Outpatient Dispensing. The labeling for all schedules of controlled substances dispensed to outpatients must contain the date of filling, the pharmacy's name and address, the serial number of the prescription, names of patient and prescriber, directions for use, and the statement "Caution: Federal Law prohibits transfer of this drug to any person other than the patient for whom it was prescribed."

Where injectable drugs are used in the home and dosages may change frequently, each department of pharmacy should develop policies and procedures for reprogramming pumps, notifying caregivers of changes, and documenting dosage changes.

Offsite Pharmacy Services. The DEA regulations provide an exception to the labeling requirements in cases where controlled substances are prescribed for administration to an institutionalized patient and dispensed from a separately registered pharmacy serving the institution [21 CFR 1306.14 and 1306.24]. The controlled substance must not be in the possession of the patient, appropriate safeguards and records must be maintained, and the labeling system used must be adequate to identify the supplier, the product, and the patient and to set forth proper directions for use. No more than a 7-day supply of Schedule II controlled substances or, in the case of Schedules III and IV, no more than a 34-day supply or 100 dosage units, whichever is less, may be dispensed at one time under this labeling system.

Automated Systems. An automated distribution system can be used to assist in inventory control of controlled substances, but conformance with state and federal regulations must be ensured.

According to current DEA policy, automated data processing systems may be used to produce a backup record of the original, hard copy prescription. However, the original, hard copy prescription must be maintained even after entry into the computerized system. As such, prescriptions for Schedule II controlled substances could be entered into a computerized system as a backup record; however, the original, hard copy prescription must serve as the primary record of the prescription. The same would apply to a Schedule V controlled substance in states that require a prescription. However, in states that allow the purchase of a Schedule V controlled substance without a prescription, applicable state record-keeping requirements apply.

An automated data processing system may be used for the storage and retrieval of original and refill information for prescription orders for Schedule III and IV controlled substances. The conditions listed below for such a system are most applicable to outpatient prescriptions. A hospital order for medication is not a prescription and, therefore, is not required to meet requirements of that particular format [21 CFR 1306.02(f)]. However, all records must meet the requirements for accountability of the controlled substances dispensed or administered by institutional personnel. Additionally, the hospital records must be maintained in a readily retrievable manner [21 CFR 1304.03]. Automated data processing systems must meet the following requirements:

1. Any such computerized system must provide on-line retrieval (via display or hard copy printout) of original prescription order information. This shall include the original prescription number; date of issuance of the original prescription order by the practitioner; name and address of the patient; name, address, and DEA registration number of the practitioner; name, strength, dosage form, and quantity of the controlled substance prescribed (and quantity dispensed if different from the quantity prescribed); total number of refills authorized by the prescribing practitioner; and name or initials of the dispensing pharmacist. A unique numeric identifier (such as an NDC number) may be used in place of the name, strength, and dosage form. When requested by an authorized official, the information must be provided by name, strength, and dosage form.

2. At the end of each month, a record shall be generated that documents all original prescriptions and refills of Schedule III and IV controlled substances dispensed during that month. This record must segregate the original and refill information for Schedule III and IV controlled substance prescriptions from other prescriptions in the same data system. This record shall include the prescription number, date of issuance, name and address of the patient, name and address and DEA number of the practitioner, initials of the dispensing pharmacist, and name, strength, dosage form, and quantity of the controlled substance prescribed. The quantity dispensed must be listed if different from the quantity prescribed. The monthly printouts must be provided upon request from an authorized official.

3. Accuracy and completeness of the original and refill information entered into an automated system must be verified each time by the individual pharmacist who fills an original prescription or refill order for a Schedule III or IV controlled substance (i.e., a thorough check of the data screen before the actual entry into the database). The system must be designed to protect against unauthorized access to and use of the automated system and associated data and must be able to identify the pharmacist filling the original prescription or refill. Such protection shall be accomplished as follows:

    a. Each authorized pharmacist shall be assigned a unique access code to be entered before each and every original prescription, refill order, or edit of data. The knowledge of assigned access codes and the ability to change, delete, or add them shall be strictly limited to a few individuals (e.g., pharmacy director, manager, or corporate security officer).

    b. Any such computerized system shall have the capability to produce a printout for the current month's original and refill data for Schedule III and IV controlled substance prescriptions. Such a printout must include all of the information required for the monthly printouts. The printout must be produced upon request of an authorized official.

    c. In the event that a pharmacy using such a computerized system experiences system downtime, the pharmacy must have an auxiliary procedure that will be used for documentation of original and refill prescriptions of Schedule III and IV controlled substances.

    d. A backup copy of original prescriptions and refill information must be made daily for that day's transactions. The backup copy can be stored on electronic media in lieu of a printed copy. The copy must be stored on an entirely separate storage medium distinct from the operating medium normally used and must be kept for 2 years after the transaction date.

Security

General. Only personnel authorized by written policies of the institution may have access to medication storage areas and supplies.

Central Storage Areas. Controlled substances in the pharmacy or other central storage areas should be stored in a securely locked, substantially constructed cabinet, vault, closet, or similar enclosure. As an alternative, controlled substances, except Schedule I drugs, may be dispersed throughout the stock of noncontrolled substances in such a manner as to obstruct theft or diversion. Controlled substances of any schedule that require refrigeration should be stored in a refrigerator within the locked storage room where other controlled substances are maintained, or within a lock box that has been secured to the inside of the refrigerator within the nursing station, or in a locked refrigerator in the pharmacy or nursing station.

Other Hospital Areas. Nursing units. When controlled substances kept as floor stock are stored on nursing units for extended periods of time, they should be in a securely locked, substantially constructed storage unit.

Carts. Medication carts containing controlled substances should be locked if they are used for storage or left unattended at nursing units.

Surgical, delivery, or special procedure areas. Increased emphasis should be placed on management of wasted narcotics (e.g., unused portions of syringes or ampuls) in these areas because they are frequently sources of higher amounts of diversion. There are a number of solutions for the control and security of controlled substances routinely used in these areas. Security in these areas may include the following:

1. Use the same physical security as at nurses' stations for floor stock and the same beginning and end of shift inventories; use the same type of record of administration as used for floor stock. (Record identifies drug, physician or anesthetist, date, adequate patient identification, notation made in patient chart as to medications received, date, and specific operating room.)
2. Maintain no stocks of controlled substances in the area. Instead, the anesthesiologist or anesthetist should take to the area the assigned stocks for each operation, delivery, or other procedure. The anesthesiologist or anesthetist would maintain the stock and all appropriate records for controlled substances, and the stock would be replenished on an as needed basis.
3. Locate a satellite pharmacy in the immediate area of the operating rooms. This annex could stock supplies that would routinely be necessary for the anesthesiologist or anesthetist. Medication could be signed out to the individual anesthesiologist or anesthetist before each operation or for all procedures scheduled for a given date.

Emergency vehicles and mobile dispensaries. If permitted by state or other applicable law, controlled substances needed for emergency vehicles may be supplied in small quantities as an extension of the hospital if the service is operated by the hospital. If it is a private ambulance service, small quantities may be supplied based on a written agreement with one hospital to supply the medications for the emergency kit. In either of these two instances, the institution is responsible for the controlled substances supplied. Local authorities should be consulted regarding basic and advanced life-support units because regulations may differ.

As an alternative, the emergency vehicle may acquire controlled substances under the registration of a consulting practitioner who must be registered at the central office location of the owner or operator of the emergency service.

The institution must develop recordkeeping and security measures that will minimize diversion potential. When the institution supplies controlled substances to a private service, no more than one kit per vehicle will be supplied; subsequent distributions will be on a replacement basis only.

The SAC may supply written approval of emergency vehicles. A written request outlining scope of operations, proposed security, and recordkeeping is required of the registrant by the SAC. If the request is adequate, written approval will be granted.

Proper state authorization for either method is required; if the operation is disapproved by the state, DEA approval will not be given.

If diversion does occur, the SAC will determine if additional safeguards are needed or if DEA approval is to be withdrawn. In either case, the registrant will be notified in writing.

Home-care setting. When injectable controlled substances are ordered in as needed doses for home-care patients, appropriate storage of large amounts of scheduled drugs in the home should be evaluated. Pharmacies providing injectable drugs to home-care patients should develop a policy on appropriate storage of injectable drugs in the home setting.

Loss or theft. Inventories of controlled substances should be performed regularly. This task is facilitated by the use of a perpetual inventory system; in that case, an audit of all purchase and issue records would identify a shortage. If the inventory shows a shortage of a particular controlled substance, it must be reported to the DEA upon discovery of such theft or loss. The federal regulations require that theft or "significant" losses of controlled substances must be reported to the DEA's Field Division Office. However, the regulations do not specifically define the term "significant." The loss or theft of controlled substances must be reported to the agency on DEA Form 106 (Report of Loss or Theft). Thefts must be reported whether or not the controlled substances are subsequently recovered or the responsible parties are identified and action is taken against them.

Pharmacies should take care not simply to file the forms and neglect procedural changes that may be indicated. Frequent filing of the forms for the same reason (e.g., consistent unexplained losses) could be a signal that actions should be taken to change departmental procedures. These reports should be analyzed and departmental procedures should be modified to attempt to avoid the problems in the future.

Placement of emergency kits containing controlled substances in (unregistered) long-term care facilities. The placement of emergency kits containing controlled substances in nonfederally registered long-term care facilities is in compliance with CSA if the appropriate state agency or regulatory authority specifically approves such placements and promulgates procedures for their use, security, recordkeeping, and accountability. The individual state authorities should be contacted to determine if such procedure is permissible in the state in which the institution is located.

Employee Screening. Registrants must screen employees

who have access to controlled substances for any prior convictions or for histories of drug abuse, and employees with knowledge of illicit drug diversion by fellow employees are responsible for reporting the illicit activity to the employer. The registrant shall not employ, as an agent or employee who has access to controlled substances, any person who has been convicted of a felony offense related to controlled substances or who, at any time, had an application for registration with DEA denied, had a DEA registration revoked, or surrendered a DEA registration for cause [21 CFR 1301.76(a)].

Research, Laboratory Procedures, and Instructional Uses

Registration. General. Persons engaged in research, laboratory procedures, or instructional uses with controlled substances are required to register under the CSA and follow laws and regulations in place in their state or locality.

Use of Schedule I drugs. The conduct of research with controlled substances listed in Schedule I requires separate registration. Institutional registrations do not suffice.

Separate locations. If research or related activities are conducted with controlled substances in more than one principal place of business or professional practice at one general physical location, a separate registration is required for each principal place of business or professional practice.

Records and Reports. General requirement. Each person registered or authorized to conduct research or related activities with controlled substances is required to keep records. A registered person using a controlled substance in preclinical research or in teaching at a registered establishment does not have to maintain separate records if the establishment maintains records. The registered person must notify DEA of the name, address, and registration number of the establishment maintaining the records. Notice to DEA should be given in the form of an attachment to the application for registration or reregistration.

Inventory. The inventory requirements of a person registered to dispense or authorized to conduct research or related activities with controlled substances shall include the same information required for the inventories of dispensers (see Records and Inventory section).

Receipt and dispensing. Receipt and dispensing records must be kept by the registrant. If the registrant is a hospital, the required records should be kept by the pharmacist in the same manner as records for other controlled substances (see Records and Inventory section). It should be noted that records for substances used in chemical analysis or other laboratory work are not required. However, records must be maintained for controlled substances transferred to the laboratory and those distributed or destroyed by the laboratory.

Research. When research is conducted on human subjects, informed consent forms signed by the patients are required and must be retained in the patients' records.

Security. In a registered institution, the pharmacist should be the custodian of all controlled substances. Controlled substances may be dispensed only to or for authorized investigators, laboratory personnel, or instructors. The pharmacist should be responsible for the security of controlled substances used in research and related activities.

Methadone

Methadone for Analgesic Purposes. The allowances under DEA regulations for a registered hospital or clinic to use methadone for analgesic purposes are stated in CFR Section 1306.07, Parts (b) and (c). Section 1306.07(b) addresses physicians who are not specifically registered and allows them to administer (but not prescribe) narcotic drugs to a person for the purpose of relieving acute withdrawal symptoms when necessary while arrangements are being made for referral for treatment. Such emergency treatment may not be carried out for longer than 3 days and may not be renewed or extended.

Section 1306.07(c) notes that these regulations are not intended to impose any limitations on a physician or authorized hospital staff to administer or dispense narcotic drugs in a hospital or to maintain or detoxify a person as an adjunct to medical or surgical treatment of conditions other than addiction, or to administer or dispense narcotic drugs to persons with intractable pain in which no relief or cure is possible or none has been found after reasonable efforts.

Methadone for Narcotic Treatment Programs: Registration and Approval. General. The use of methadone in an institution for maintenance or detoxification of narcotic addicts is controlled jointly under FDA and DEA regulations. The FDA methadone regulations [21 CFR 291.501 and 291.505] provide for approved uses of methadone in institutions, medication units, and methadone treatment programs. If an institution desires to establish a methadone treatment program for detoxification and maintenance of drug-dependent persons, separate approval is required. In any case, the institution must be separately registered with DEA as a narcotic treatment program to dispense Schedule II controlled substances in addition to receiving approval under the FDA methadone regulations. Programs must submit to DEA an application for registration as a narcotic treatment program, using DEA Form 363.

Hospital use of methadone in a narcotic treatment program. The hospital shall submit to FDA and the appropriate state authority a general description of the hospital, including number of beds, specialized treatment facilities for drug dependence, and nature of patient care undertaken. The hospital shall permit FDA and the state authority to inspect supplies of these drugs at the hospital and evaluate the uses to which the drug is being put. For a hospital pharmacy lawfully to receive or dispense methadone for its approved hospital use for detoxification, the hospital must submit Form FDA-2636, Hospital Request for Methadone for Detoxification and Temporary Maintenance Treatment. The application must be approved by the responsible state authority and FDA. The form requires detailed information about the hospital, including the name of the pharmacist responsible for receiving and securing supplies of methadone.

In addition to requirements that hospitals have separate DEA registrations for narcotic treatment programs, the programs must maintain separate inventories, appropriate DEA forms, and patient records.

Program approval. Before a narcotic treatment program may be lawfully operated, the program, whether an inpatient facility, an outpatient facility, or a private practitioner, must submit the appropriate applications to FDA and the state authority and must receive the approval of both. At the time of the application for approval, the program sponsor shall indicate whether medication will be administered or dispensed at the facility.

Medication unit. A program may establish a medication unit to facilitate the needs of patients who are stabilized on an optimal dosage level. To operate a medication unit lawfully, the program shall, for each separate unit, obtain approval from FDA, DEA, and the state authority. A medication unit is limited to administering or dispensing a narcotic drug and collecting samples for drug testing or analysis for narcotic drugs.

Description of facilities. A program must have ready access to a comprehensive range of medical and rehabilitation services so that the services may be provided when necessary. The name, address, and description of each hospital, institution, clinical laboratory, or other facility available to provide the necessary services must be provided in the application submitted to FDA and the state authority. The application is also required to include the name and address of each medication unit.

Methadone treatment programs. To obtain approval to establish a methadone treatment program, the sponsor must submit Form FDA-2632, Application for Approval of Use of Methadone in a Treatment Program. The application must receive the approval of the responsible state authority and FDA with the concurrence of DEA. To ensure that each participating physician in a methadone treatment program is aware of his or her professional and administrative responsibilities, FDA requires that Form FDA-2633, Medical Responsibility Statement for Use of Methadone in a Treatment Program, be completed by each physician licensed to dispense or administer methadone in an approved program. These statements must accompany the program application. All patients in the program are required to give their consent for treatment by signing Form FDA-2635, Consent for Methadone Treatment.

Dispensing. *Authorized dispensers.* Only a licensed practitioner or an agent of the practitioner may administer or dispense methadone. The agent must be a pharmacist, registered nurse, licensed practical nurse, or other health-care professional authorized by federal and state law to administer or dispense narcotic drugs. The licensed practitioner assumes responsibility for the amounts of methadone administered or dispensed, and the licensed practitioner shall record and countersign all changes in dosage schedule.

Form. Methadone may be dispensed or administered only in an oral liquid formulation when it is used in a treatment program. Hospitalized patients under care for a medical or surgical condition are permitted to receive methadone in injectable form when the physician determines that it is needed.

Take-home medications. There are stringent requirements establishing the frequency and quantity of methadone permitted for take-home use. Take-home medication is required to be labeled with the treatment center's name, address, and telephone number. It is recommended that the liquid formulation of methadone be nonsweetened and contain a preservative so that the program staff may instruct patients not to refrigerate the product to minimize accidental ingestion by children and others or fermentation of the product.

Records and Reports. *Hospital use of methadone.* All records must be kept in compliance with the DEA requirements for Schedule I and II controlled substances. Hospitals must also maintain accurate records traceable to specific patients, and they must include dates, quantity, and batch or code marks of the drug dispensed. Methadone records must be retained for a 3-year period instead of the 2-year period required for other controlled substances. The hospital does not have to submit a detailed annual report.

Methadone treatment programs. All records must be kept in compliance with the DEA requirement for Schedule I and II controlled substances. The FDA methadone regulations require also that there be accurate records traceable to specific patients, and they must include dates, quantity, and batch or code marks of the drug dispensed. Methadone records must be retained for 3 years. The methadone treatment program is required to file an annual report with the responsible state authority and FDA. The content of the annual report is detailed in Form FDA-2634, Annual Report for Treatment Program Using Methadone.

Security. The regulations note that adequate security is required over stocks of methadone and over the manner in which it is (1) administered or dispensed, (2) distributed to medication units, and (3) stored to guard against theft and diversion of the drug. The methadone program is required to meet the security standards for the distribution and storage of controlled substances as required by DEA.

Approved by the ASHP Board of Directors, November 18, 1992. Developed by the ASHP Council on Legal and Public Affairs. Supersedes the "ASHP Technical Assistance Bulletin on Institutional Use of Controlled Substances," which was approved on November 19, 1986.

This Technical Assistance Bulletin was developed in collaboration with the staff of the Liaison and Policy Section of the Office of Diversion Control of the Drug Enforcement Administration (DEA). It is an interpretation of the Controlled Substances Act and Title 21, *Code of Federal Regulations,* for use in health-care settings and is not official DEA policy.

Reprinted from the *Am J Hosp Pharm.* 1993; 50:489–501.

5 | Interpreting Medication Orders and Prescriptions

Linda Y. Fred, R.Ph.

This chapter will describe the technician's role in evaluating and processing medication orders and prescriptions from the time they are received until the medications leave the pharmacy. The differences between the process in the inpatient and outpatient settings will be discussed as well. Additional information specific to one setting or the other is offered in the Institutional Pharmacy Practice and Ambulatory Pharmacy Practice chapters.

Typically, the term "medication order" refers to a written request on a physician's order form in an inpatient setting. This order becomes part of the patient's medical record. The term "prescription" is used to describe a medication order on a prescription blank that is intended to be filled in an outpatient or ambulatory care setting. In this chapter, the terms may be considered interchangeable unless specific reference is made to one setting or the other.

LEARNING OBJECTIVES

After reading this chapter, the reader will be able to
1. Identify the components of a complete prescription or medication order.
2. Prioritize prescriptions and medication orders on the basis of pertinent criteria.
3. Identify the necessary steps in processing a prescription or medication order.
4. List information normally contained in a patient profile.
5. Identify the proper language to be used on medication labels.
6. List the information needed to make a medication label complete.

Although achieving these objectives will give the reader a basic understanding of medication order processing activities, actually performing these functions requires specialized training in the procedures of the specific practice site, such as the use of the organization's computer system.

RECEIVING MEDICATION ORDERS AND PRESCRIPTIONS

Medication orders and prescriptions come to the pharmacy in various ways. They are delivered to the pharmacy in person or via some mechanical method

The contributions of Robert S. Guynn and Kevin W. Zajac to this chapter are gratefully acknowledged.

such as fax transmission or a pneumatic tube system. Orders and prescriptions may also be telephoned to the pharmacy by either the prescriber or an intermediary such as a registered nurse. There are some legal restrictions on who may telephone in a prescription and who may receive that information in the pharmacy—particularly when controlled substances are involved. Technicians should consult their employer's policy and procedures or job description to see what restrictions apply in their practice setting. Many states require that prescriptions be phoned in by the prescriber or licensed professional operating under the prescriber's authority. It is also commonly required that telephone prescriptions be received by a pharmacist or another licensed professional.

Upon receipt of a prescription, there are two steps that should be taken. The first step is to review the order for clarity and completeness. The second step is to prioritize the order based on a number of factors, including the time the medication is needed, the seriousness of the condition that is being treated, and the urgency of the other medication orders waiting to be processed. Although these processes differ in the inpatient versus the outpatient setting, the fundamental responsibility of getting the right medication to the right patient at the right time remains the same.

Clarity and Completeness

When a new order is received, the first step is to ensure that the order is clear and complete. Ideally, every medication order and prescription should contain the following elements:
- Patient name
- Generic drug name (it is recommended that generic drug names be used and many institutions have policies to this effect)
- Brand drug name (if a specific product is required)
- Route of administration (with some injectables, the site of administration should also be included)
- Dosage form
- Dose
- Strength
- Quantity and frequency of administration
- Dilution, rate, and time of administration (in some cases)
- Indication for use of the medication
- Prescriber's name and signature
- Date

Some of this information is required by state law or by policy. In addition, inpatient orders often include allergy and patient demographic data, such as an account number and a room and bed location. However, as demonstrated in Figures 5-1 and 5-2, not all of the elements previously described are always included.

In an ambulatory care practice, additional clarity and completeness issues must be considered. When the prescriber uses "Dispense as written," or DAW, on the prescription blank, the brand name drug written on the prescription must be dispensed. Substituting the generic equivalent is not allowed when DAW is used. Depending on state law, institutional policy, or both, some prescription blanks come preprinted with areas the prescriber can use to designate DAW or, alternatively, "generic substitution acceptable." In some practice settings the prescriber must write DAW; preprinted prescription blanks are not recognized as official. Outpatient orders should also include refill information, a space for the patient's address, and may, depending on the drug ordered, need the physician's Drug Enforcement Agency (DEA) registration number.

Another outpatient issue is prescription forgeries. Screening prescriptions, particularly those for controlled substances, for potential forgeries should be part of the routine. Prescription forgeries may be easy to identify, such as erasure or overwriting of the strength or dispensing quantity of the drug (e.g., changing a 3 to an 8). Some forgeries are much more subtle and may involve theft of preprinted prescription pads and legitimate looking prescriptions. The technician should screen prescriptions for anything that looks unusual, such as a dispense quantity in excess of normal quantities or an unusual or unrecognizable signature. Any suspicious prescription should be *discreetly* presented to the pharmacist for further evaluation.

If information is missing, for example the patient's name, the technician may be able to clarify the order without pharmacist intervention. However, some clarifications should involve the pharmacist. When an order is set aside for clarification it is important to make the patient or the caregiver aware of any anticipated delays. In an outpatient pharmacy, for example, the patient may be asked to return at a later time or wait in the pharmacy. Estimates of how long patients may have to wait for their prescriptions should be based on the completeness and clarity as well as the priority of the prescriptions in relation to the other prescriptions waiting to be filled.

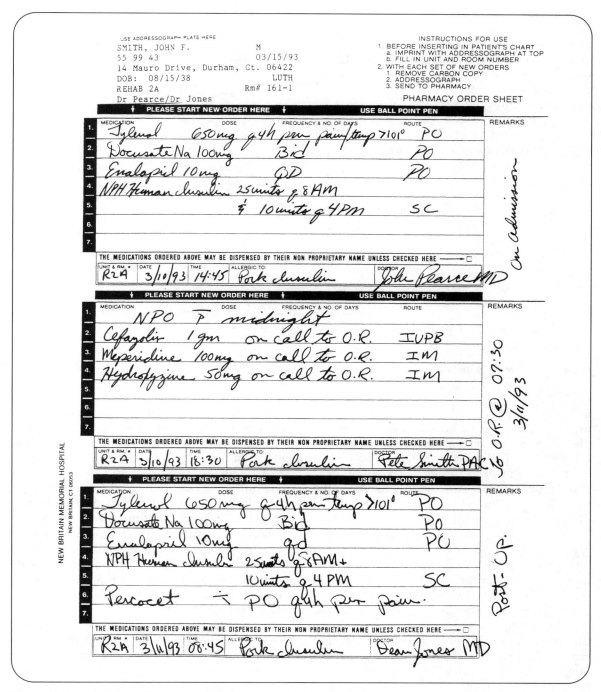

Figure 5-1. Sample inpatient medication order from the medical chart.

Prioritization

Once orders are deemed clear and complete, they must be prioritized so that the most urgent prescriptions or orders are filled first. Prioritizing orders means comparing the urgency of new orders against the urgency of existing orders.

This ensures that those prescriptions needed the most will be processed first. Technicians can prioritize prescriptions by evaluating the directions for use, type of drug, intended use of the drug, and patient-specific circumstances.

Some orders are designated as "stat" (abbreviation of *statim*, Latin for immediately), which

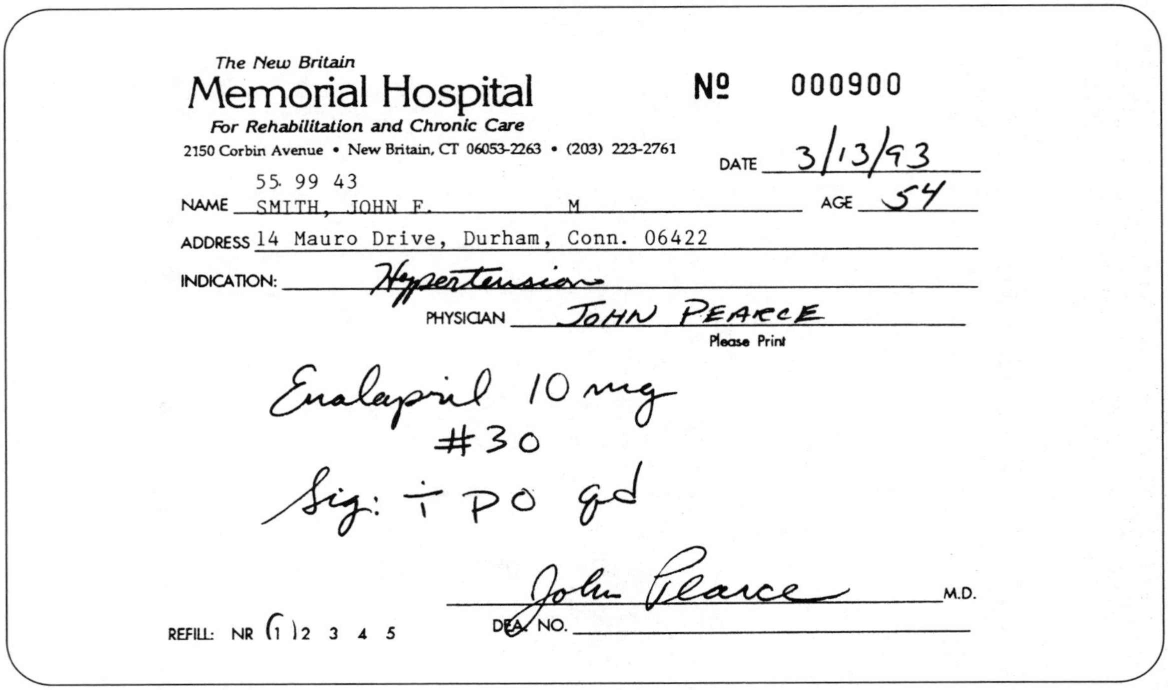

The New Britain
Memorial Hospital
For Rehabilitation and Chronic Care
2150 Corbin Avenue • New Britain, CT 06053-2263 • (203) 223-2761

№ 000900

DATE 3/13/93

55 99 43
NAME SMITH, JOHN F. M AGE 54

ADDRESS 14 Mauro Drive, Durham, Conn. 06422

INDICATION: Hypertension

PHYSICIAN JOHN PEARCE
Please Print

Enalapril 10 mg
#30
Sig: i PO qd

John Pearce M.D.

REFILL: NR (1) 2 3 4 5 DEA NO.

Figure 5-2. Sample ambulatory prescription.

indicates an urgent need. Additional clues about urgency can be gleaned from orders. For example, when surgery or some diagnostic procedure is indicated—as in this order: "Give 1 g cefazolin IVPB 1 hour prior to surgery." You might consult the operating room schedule to determine the priority of the order. A prescriber may also designate that a medication is to be started "now" or "ASAP" (As Soon As Possible), or simply state "start today" or "start this morning." If there is no apparent urgency or specific time denoted in the order or prescription, it may receive a lower priority. Most pharmacies, however, designate a standard amount of time it should take to process and deliver an order to the patient or caregiver. A typical turnaround time for filling an order in an institutional setting might be 10–15 minutes for a stat order and 1 hour for a routine order.

If there is no specific designation about the urgency of a medication in the body of the order, technicians can use some assumptions to prioritize orders properly. Medications ordered for the initial treatment of pain, fever, or nausea and vomiting are generally high priority because of the need to relieve the discomfort of the patient. A regularly scheduled vitamin, on the other hand, would be a lower priority. Most of the decisions involved in prioritizing orders require some basic knowledge of the drugs and common sense. It is also helpful for technicians to be familiar with their pharmacy's specific policies regarding prioritization of orders. Some hospitals, for example, treat all orders from a particular unit—such as an intensive care unit—as stats, regardless of the order type or perceived urgency. Many hospitals have designated administration times for certain drugs, such as warfarin, that may alter prioritization of the order depending on the time the order is received. Policies vary from pharmacy to pharmacy, and technicians need to become familiar with the system of prioritization used at their institution.

In the outpatient setting, although stat orders are known, the patient-service aspect of prioritizing prescriptions is a primary concern. Many outpatient pharmacies employ some sort of take-a-number system to maintain order in the waiting area as well as to provide an additional means of patient identification. All outpatient pharmacy personnel would do well, however, to be sensitive to patient needs rather than to rely on the first-come, first-served system. For example, a prescription for a patient with an infectious disease or a child who has been vomiting should receive some special attention. It is also just good common sense to fill prescriptions for patients who are waiting in the lobby before you complete the prescriptions to be sent in tomorrow's mail. Most outpatient pharmacies, like institutional pharmacies, have a standard for the maximum amount of time a patient should have to wait for a prescription. Fifteen minutes is a fairly common wait.

PROCESSING MEDICATION ORDERS AND PRESCRIPTIONS

After the order has been received, determined to be clear and complete, and prioritized, the order is ready to be processed. Processing involves identifying the patient; establishing, reviewing, and updating the patient profile; selecting the drug product; scheduling the medication administration times; documenting the directions for use; inputting the prescriber information; labeling the medication; dispensing the appropriate amount of medication; and checking the completed prescription to ensure accuracy. Processing usually involves a computer, but some pharmacies still use a manual system (e.g., typewriters, pen and paper, and notebooks).

Identifying the Patient

Identification of the patient entails comparing the patient identification on the prescription or medication order against the one chosen in the patient profile system (i.e., the patient's computer record) to make sure they match. Although it sounds like a very elementary task, the importance can not be overestimated, and an appropriate level of attention must be paid to this detail—particularly when dealing with very common names.

In an institutional setting, patient identification numbers are generally used. Most commonly, patients are identified by two numbers: a unique medical record number that distinguishes patients from one another and an account number that is specific to a transaction or set of transactions such as an individual hospitalization. A patient's medical record number never changes, but account numbers change every time a patient is admitted to an institution. The account number may also be known by other names, such as a billing number or an admission number. Many institutions are now using bar codes or magnetic strips to facilitate accuracy and verify patient identification numbers. As more hospitals employ electronic charting, a computerized mechanism of document-

ing patient care, bar-coded or magnetic strip patient identifiers will play a larger role. In the mean time, most hospitals continue to rely on a printed name that is generated by an addressograph (a raised-letter registration card similar to a credit card) or preprinted on adhesive labels that are affixed to documents.

It is important to make sure the patient name matches the number and vice versa. It is easy to make errors when keying numbers, and some patients may have the same names. Occasionally, orders get marked with the wrong patient name, and checking the profile may prevent this error from causing any harm to the patient involved. For this reason, it is also vital to ensure that each order makes sense for the patient by checking the order against the patient profile.

In the outpatient setting, prescription blanks may be imprinted by addressograph or marked with a bar-coded label—particularly if it is a prescription issued when a patient was released from the hospital. More often, the patient's name will be handwritten by the prescriber. In this case, the spelling of the patient's name should be verified. This will facilitate finding the correct patient profile in the computer or, in the case of a new customer, will allow you to accurately establish a new patient profile. Most ambulatory care pharmacies will also use some type of numerical identifier such as an account number.

Creating, Maintaining, and Reviewing Patient Profiles

The patient profile is a fundamental tool that pharmacists use to provide pharmaceutical care. It is vital that pharmacists and technicians build and review patient profiles while they are processing medication orders and prescriptions. The following information is usually found in the pharmacy's patient profile:

- Patient name and identification number
- Date of birth, or age
- Sex
- Height and weight
- Diagnosis, problem list, or both
- Name of parent or guardian, if applicable
- Patient address and phone number
- Names of practitioners (e.g., physicians, dentists, podiatrists, physician assistants, nurse-practitioners)
- Medication allergies
- Third-party payer information (e.g., medical insurance information)

- Medication history (profiles may include current and discontinued medication; outpatient profiles will include history of medication refills)
- Special considerations (e.g., foreign language, disability)
- Clinical comments (e.g., therapeutic monitoring, counseling notes)

Before prescriptions are entered into a patient's profile, the profile should be reviewed in relation to the changes indicated on the new orders. In some cases, information in the profile may raise questions about whether the patient should receive the medication as it is prescribed. For example, the patient may be allergic to the medication or may already be on a similar medication. In addition, the profile may contain information that changes how the order will be processed or prioritized. For example, the patient may require directions in a foreign language or may have received a supply of the medication recently and will not need more medication for some time. If a technician suspects that the prescribed medication is inappropriate for the patient, he or she should consult the pharmacist or follow the pharmacy's standard procedure.

Processing medication orders and prescriptions involves adding a medication to a patient's regimen or modifying or deleting a previously ordered medication. Computerized systems facilitate the speed and accuracy of processing prescriptions because patient profiles can be created or modified easily and prescription labels can be printed quickly, all within a single step. In manual systems, this is done in two separate steps: the modifications to the patient's profile are handwritten and the prescription label is typed.

Selecting Drug Products

Once the order has been compared against the profile, it is time to proceed with selecting the drug product indicated on the medication order or prescription. It is recommended that prescribers order drug products by generic name instead of brand name. However, drug products are often prescribed by either or both names, which can result in confusion for patients and staff. Selecting drug products requires a working knowledge of both brand names and generic names.

With most inpatient and outpatient computer systems, drug products can be reviewed by scrolling through an alphabetical listing of the brand or generic names, or by entering a code or mnemonic of the product name. For example, to enter an order for ampicillin 250 mg, at the drug name prompt you might enter the mnemonic or drug code "amp250" and the following choices would appear:

1. amp250c ampicillin 250 mg capsule each
2. amp250s1 ampicillin 250 mg/5 ml oral suspension. 100 ml bottle
3. amp250s2 ampicillin 250 mg/5 ml oral suspension. 200 ml bottle

Note that once the correct drug is located, the correct strength and dosage form must be selected. If the order was for a 250 mg/5 ml suspension to be given four times daily for 10 days, the proper choice would be number three (i.e., 5 ml four times a day equals 20 mls per day for 10 days is a total of 200 ml).

In institutions, only those drugs approved for use in the institution (i.e., formulary drugs) may be selected by technicians. Input from the pharmacist is usually required to process an order for a medication not approved for use in the institution (i.e., nonformulary drugs). Outpatient pharmacies generally have more brands available and may or may not use a formulary system. A more detailed discussion of the formulary system is offered in the chapter on Institutional Pharmacy Practice.

Many computer systems alert the operator if he or she attempts to enter medications that interact with pre-existing orders, conflict with the patient's drug allergies, represent therapeutic duplications, or are nonformulary drugs. Many systems also check the dosage range and alert the pharmacist or technician if he or she entered a dose that exceeds the recommended dose for that patient. Although these alert systems help prevent errors, they are not always correct given the patient's unique situation. Therefore, it is important to consult the pharmacist when the alert is posted. The pharmacist may by-pass the alert based on his or her professional judgment or the pharmacist may call the prescriber and ask to change the order. Technicians should be familiar with and follow the procedure at their practice site regarding computer alerts.

Scheduling Medication Administration Times

Scheduling medication administration times has a large effect on patient outcomes. In institutions, standard medication administration times are set. These times are often defined by institutional policy or by a drug therapy protocol. Such protocols may define times for common dosing frequencies such as "every day" (e.g., qd = 0800, bid = 0900 and 1700) or a specific administration time for certain drugs (e.g., warfarin may be administered at a set time to coincide with laboratory blood draws). These protocols are usually based on therapeutic issues, nursing efficiency, or designed to coordinate services. Standard administration schedules and protocols are usually agreed upon by pharmacy, nursing, and the medical staff (i.e., physicians). Pharmacy personnel involved in order entry are often informed about these policies during their orientation to the pharmacy computer system. Many pharmacies have a written document that staff can refer to when the appropriate administration time is unclear. Because these times are usually conveyed on the pharmacy's patient profile, on medication labels, and on the Medication Administration Record (MAR), pharmacy technicians should be sure to choose the correct medication administration schedule.

Standardized administration times usually appear as default entries associated with a particular drug or administration schedule that was selected in the computer during the order entry process. This means that if a "bid" administration schedule is entered for a particular drug, the computer would automatically assign its standard administration times, which could be 0900 and 1700.

Default time schedules may differ on some specialized nursing units, such as intensive care units. Generally, scheduling for "qd" may default to 0800; however, intensive care units may require administration scheduling for certain drugs to start when the order is received. During order entry, the technician must be aware of such protocols and change the default entries when necessary.

Outpatient pharmacies do not usually use default administration times. Instead, they consider the convenience and habits of the patient when assigning an administration schedule. To make sure that outpatients know when and how to take their medications properly, instructions are provided on the container label, and are commonly conveyed verbally to the patient or a family member at the time the medication is delivered. It is important to make sure the administration schedule is one the patient can maintain. If you suspect that it is not well understood or compatible with the patient's life style, it is important to alert the pharmacist. It's possible that a more suitable administration schedule can be used.

When scheduling medication administration times for a new medication pharmacists also consider other medications the patient is taking. This consideration is critical in both inpatient and outpatient settings and technicians should keep it in mind as well. For example, if a patient is taking both digoxin and milk of magnesia there must be an adequate amount of time between the doses of each agent. If these medications are taken too close together, the milk of magnesia can reduce the amount of digoxin that the patient absorbs. The resulting reduced absorption of digoxin could render therapy ineffective. Another good example is estrogen and progesterone hormone replacement therapy in postmenopausal women. The start and stop dates for both medications must be clear. An example of a good approach is "Take conjugated estrogens 0.625 mg by mouth on days 1–25 of each month. Take medroxyprogesterone 5 mg by mouth on days 15–25 of each month."

Documenting Directions for Use

In both the inpatient and outpatient environments, the prescriber's directions for proper use of the medications must be conveyed clearly and accurately. The style used to convey the prescriber's directions differs between the two practice settings because the labels are read, generally speaking, by non-health care professionals in the outpatient setting and health care professionals in the inpatient setting.

In institutions, physicians' orders are input into the pharmacy's patient profile. Then, pharmacy technicians generate MARs for nursing documentation (Figure 5-3), medication profiles and fill lists (for pharmacy use) and labels (for updating MARs and for placement on medications to be issued to patient care areas), (Figure 5-4). Because this information will be used only by health care personnel, the directions for use may contain only the name of the medication, strength, dose and schedule, and administration times, all of which may be written using medical terminology and Latin abbreviations.

In the outpatient setting, directions for use must be translated from the prescriber's abbreviated notation into plain English. The medical terminology and Latin abbreviations that are used in directions for nursing and pharmacy personnel are clearly not acceptable for use in directions

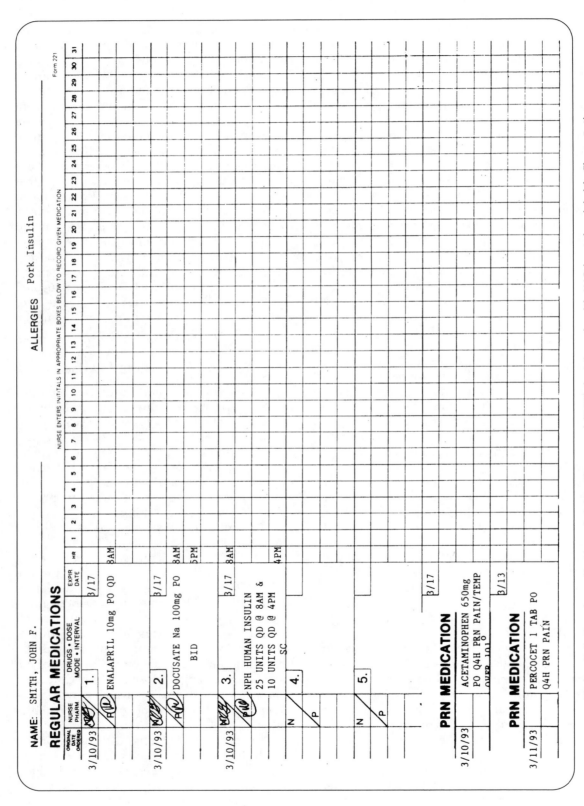

Figure 5-3. Sample medication administration record (MAR) (not to scale with MAR/container label in Figure 5-4).

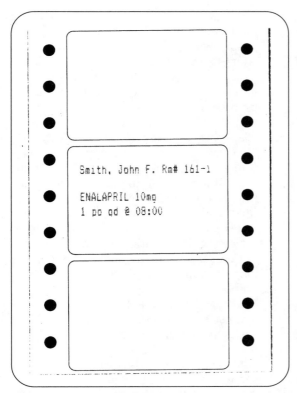

Figure 5-4. Inpatient label that can be used on the medication container sent to the patient care area or to update the MAR. Note that the label is for use by health care personnel and contains Latin and abbreviated information that a patient is not likely to understand.

to patients who self-administer their medications. It is the responsibility of the pharmacy personnel to make sure that when patients leave the pharmacy with medication they have a clear understanding of how to safely and effectively use it. Many therapeutic failures are thought to be attributable to unclear, inadequate, or misunderstood directions. In addition, the patient's compliance with the prescribed regimen can be affected significantly by the quality of the directions the patient received. For this reason, verbal communication with the patient is recommended whenever possible. This gives the pharmacist the opportunity to evaluate the patient's understanding of the therapeutic plan.

Labeling for an outpatient prescription (Figure 5-5); (also refer to the chapters on Pharmacy Law and Ambulatory Pharmacy Practice) should include the following:

- Administration directions (e.g., "Take," "Insert," "Apply")
- Number of units constituting one dose and the dosage form (e.g., 2 tablets)
- Route of administration (e.g., "by mouth," "vaginally")
- How frequently or at what time (e.g., "twice daily," "daily at 9 a.m.")
- Length of time to continue (e.g., "for 10 days," "until finished")
- Indication of purpose (e.g., "for pain," "for blood pressure")

Many outpatient pharmacies also use auxiliary labels to reinforce some points of use, storage, or scheduling (see Figure 5-5). Many computer systems even indicate which auxiliary stickers should be applied.

Clinical Comments

Most pharmacies have a field or location in the patient profile system where pharmacists can note clinical comments. Such comments may include indications for use, incidents of adverse drug reactions, laboratory values, or any other information that may help the pharmacist provide pharmaceutical care. During the initial screening and evaluation of the drug order, for example, the pharmacy technician might note in the clinical comments field that therapeutic monitoring may be needed or that recent monitoring parameters are outside normal limits. To ensure optimal safety and efficacy of drug therapy, it's best to alert the pharmacist to such situations as early in the processing as possible.

Prescriber Information

Because treatment is often provided by mid-level practitioners such as nurse practitioners and physician's assistants, or medical residents, medication orders are often written by someone

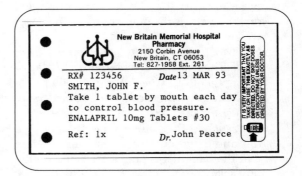

Figure 5-5. Outpatient prescription label with auxiliary label affixed.

other than the physician named in the medical record. It is important to accurately record the physician prescriber, even if a mid-level practitioner wrote the order, because it is the physician's authority that provides the legal basis for dispensing medications to a patient.

Filling and Labeling Medications

Once the computer entry has been completed and labeling materials generated, the prescription order must be filled with the correct quantity of the correct drug. During this step, it is important to carefully review the label against the order and the product to be used in filling the order to make sure the correct product has been chosen.

Sample Order Entries

In this section, the steps involved in processing medication orders are reviewed and illustrated for inpatient and outpatient settings. The intent is to help the reader put all the information together and to provide a brief, general overview of the processing routine.

The reader should assume the orders have been checked for clarity and completeness to the extent possible without the patient profile, and prioritized.

Inpatient Setting

Inpatient order entry usually goes as follows (using the enalapril example, Figure 5-1):

1. *Enter the patient's name or medical record number and verify them.* To enter patient John Smith, key in the medical record number, 559943, or the name. Compare the patient profile with the written medication order to verify that the patient represented on the screen is the one for whom the order was written.

2. *Compare the order with the patient profile in detail.* The order to be entered is "Enalapril 10 mg QD PO." Check for general appropriateness of the order; it should make sense in regard to patient profile information, such as the patient's age, allergy profile, and drugs currently being taken. Note that the patient's allergies are listed on the physician's order form. It is useful to check this information against the patient's profile to make sure they agree.

3. *Enter the drug.* Go into the order entry mode and type in the drug mnemonic. For example, typing "enal" might give you a short list of enalapril products to select from, while typing "enal10" might give you the specific product. After a specific product has been selected (enalapril 10 mg tablet), most systems check for drug interactions, therapeutic duplication, and drug allergies. If any of these problems are found, the system may "lock up" and require input from the pharmacist. Once interaction checks are cleared, the computer will show the drug on the screen, and order entry may proceed. Also note, in reviewing the medications ordered for this patient, that most are ordered by generic name although one (Tylenol) is ordered by brand name.

4. *Verify the dose.* Check the dose on the order against the drug product entered. Most computer systems have a field that allows for some modifications here. In the enalapril example, the drug product chosen was a 10 mg tablet, and the dose is 10 mg, so no adjustments are necessary. However, if we were entering the Tylenol (acetaminophen) order (Figure 5-1), we would only find a 325 mg tablet in the computer. Therefore, the dose field would have to be modified to 650 mg, or two tablets. It is important to review all the available products and become familiar with drug product dosages. For example, if a patient needs 100 mg of a drug and it comes in 10, 25, and 50 mg tablet strengths, it would be preferable to give the patient two 50 mg tablets as opposed to ten 10 mg tablets. Also be aware that odd dosages may indicate a prescribing error. In the previous example, if the only available tablet strength was 10 mg, a 100 mg dose is odd and should be verified by the pharmacist.

5. *Enter the administration schedule.* Type in the scheduling mnemonic (qd). Verify that the default administration time is appropriate for the patient and medication.

6. *Enter any comments in the clinical comments field.* There may be nothing to add for enalapril. In the Tylenol example, an entry of "for temp > 101" would be appropriate.

7. *Verify the prescriber name.* Depending on the computer system, the accuracy of the prescriber name may need to be verified. Most systems default to the admitting or attend-

ing physician, but some allow or require changing to the actual prescriber. Note in the example that orders were written at three different times by three different prescribers. This information would need to be updated with each entry.

8. *Fill and label the medication.* The correct product (e.g., enalapril 10 mg tablets) must be obtained and supplied in the correct quantity with proper labeling. In this case, one or two tablets might be sent in a typical inpatient setting, depending on the time of day and the time the next dose was due. This is the final opportunity for the technician to check the medication against the label and the order to ensure accuracy.

Outpatient Setting

This section highlights how the outpatient order entry process differs from inpatient order entry. Refer to the prescription in Figure 5-2.

1. *Enter the patient's medical record number or name and verify them.* (Same as for inpatients.) On the basis of the prescription or by questioning the patient directly, verify that the rest of the patient information is also correct (address, date of birth, insurance information, etc.).
2. *Compare the order with the patient profile in detail.* (Same as for inpatients.)
3. *Enter the drug.* (Same as for inpatients.)
4. *Enter the label direction mnemonic.* This step will encompass steps four and five of the inpatient procedures. Remember, outpatient directions must be in a language the patient can understand, so they must go beyond giving a milligram dose and a scheduled time to take the medication. The enalapril mnemonic might be t1tpoqd, which consists of encoded characters for all of the major elements of the directions ("sig" text): *t* = take, *1* = one, *t* = tablet, *po* = by mouth, *qd* = daily. The translation onto the patient label is "Take one tablet by mouth each day."
5. *Enter comments.* For example, add "to control blood pressure" to the enalapril label and medication profile.
6. *Enter the prescriber's name.* Depending on the computer system, you might enter either the full name, a mnemonic, or a numeric code. In this case, "John Pearce" should be entered.

7. *Enter the amount to dispense and the refill information.* The amount dispensed is 30 and one refill is authorized in the example.
8. *Fill and label the prescription.* This step is similar to the process for inpatient orders, but differs on one point. In an outpatient setting, the quantity to be dispensed to the patient is specified in the prescription. In this case, 30 tablets would be dispensed. As in the inpatient setting, this is the final opportunity for the technician to ensure the accuracy of the process by checking the chosen product against the original order.

Physician Order Entry

In some hospitals physicians are entering orders directly into the hospital's computer system instead of writing orders and sending them to nursing or pharmacy to be entered into the computer system. In this situation, the pharmacy still reviews the order prior to dispensing the medications. Generally, physician order entry is advantageous because it promotes the submission of more complete orders and it prevents errors due to illegible handwriting among other reasons.

Filling and Checking Orders

Typically, when orders are entered into a computer, the patient profile is updated and a label is generated indicating that an order needs to be filled. It is important when filling orders that labels and medication profiles are carefully compared to one another to prevent errors. When possible, the medication order or prescription should accompany the label during the filling process. If a label doesn't look right, it may not be right. The accuracy of the label should be checked before the medication order or prescription is filled. If an order is filled from an inaccurate label and the pharmacy system of checking fails, the wrong product could be inadvertently dispensed.

When a label seems to indicate an error, the first step is to review the label against the order and profile. From the example in Figure 5-1, if the label indicated a 100 mg enalapril dose, and it was reviewed against the original order it would be clear that an error was made when the order was entered. The label would be discarded and the entry in the computer would have to be corrected. If, however, the original order did specify a 100 mg dose, the order should be brought to the attention of the pharmacist. The pharmacist can then evaluate the order and take action to get it corrected if necessary.

Medication orders and prescriptions may need to be filed after they are filled. Policies and legal requirements differ as to how orders are filed and how long the files have to be maintained. Consult state law and your organization's policies for a better understanding of these requirements.

CONCLUSION

As a member of the pharmaceutical care team, the technician provides considerable assistance in operations of the pharmacy. The technician's ability to evaluate and assist in processing orders adds another measure of safety and efficiency to the system and provides the individual technician with the opportunity to contribute significantly to the welfare of patients.

RECOMMENDED READING

1. Employer's policy and procedure manual and orientation materials regarding order receiving and processing, filling and labeling medication orders, use of the computer system, error prevention, standard administration times, delivery expectations and turnaround time, and duties of the technician involved in dispensing functions.

2. Rules and Regulations for the Administration of the Pharmacy Practice Act for the state in which the technician is employed. (These may generally be obtained from the regulating body in the state).

SELF-ASSESSMENT QUESTIONS

1. Anyone who has worked in a pharmacy for a minimum of one year may receive a telephone prescription from a physician.
   a. True
   b. False

2. Generally, the first step to take place when a prescription is received, is a review of the prescription for completeness and accuracy, and then it should be prioritized in relation to the other work to be done.
   a. True
   b. False

3. Which of the following pieces of information should be on a prescription in an outpatient pharmacy, but would not be required on a medication order for a hospitalized patient?
   a. Patient's address
   b. Physician's address and telephone number
   c. Refill information
   d. All of the above would appear on an outpatient prescription but not an inpatient order.

4. "Dispense as written" on a prescription means:
   a. the brand name product ordered by the physician must be used to fill the prescription.
   b. generic substitution is prohibited, but an alternative brand name product may be used if the one ordered is not available.
   c. generic substitution may occur only if the patient insists upon it.
   d. none of the above

5. Any suspicious prescription should be brought to the attention of the pharmacist because it may be a forgery.
   a. True
   b. False

6. Considerations in determining an order's priority include all of the following *except*:
   a. the type of medication prescribed and what it is used to treat.
   b. whether or not the technician likes to process the type of drug ordered.
   c. the patient's expectation for the time of delivery.
   d. specific instructions from the prescriber as to the delivery time.

7. A typical "turnaround time" for a stat order in a hospital is 10–15 minutes.
   a. True
   b. False

8. Common methods of identifying patients on medication orders in institutional settings include:
   a. addressograph cards.
   b. bar-coded name labels.
   c. patient account number.
   d. all of the above.

9. Once a bar-coded account number system is instituted in an organization, less attention may be paid to patient identification since these systems are basically foolproof.
   a. True
   b. False

10. A thorough review of a well kept patient profile when entering new medication

orders will generally allow the technician to identify all of the following problems *except:*
a. existing orders for the same medication.
b. allergies which may indicate the medication should not be used.
c. a disability such as blindness, which requires special attention.
d. how the patient will make payment for the amount the insurance company does not pay (i.e., the co-pay).
e. the patient's date of birth or age.

11. Which of the following drug file options would be the best choice for a prescription for 250 mg of cephalexin suspension four times daily for 10 days?
a. cep125s100—cephalexin suspension 125 mg/5 ml, 100 ml
b. cep125s150—cephalexin suspension 125 mg/5 ml, 150 ml
c. cep250c—cephalexin capsules 250 mg
d. cep250s100—cephalexin suspension 250 mg/5 ml, 100 ml
e. cep250s150—cephalexin suspension 250 mg/5 ml, 150 ml

12. Common screening options during a pharmacy or nursing operated computerized order entry process in a hospital include all of the following *except:*
a. therapeutic duplication.
b. price range checking.
c. allergy screening.
d. dose range checking.
e. drug interactions with existing orders.

13. Medication administration times are generally standardized without exception within hospitals.
a. True
b. False

14. Scheduling medication administration times must be discussed with the patient or family member in the outpatient setting, to ensure optimal benefit.
a. True
b. False

15. In the case of a prescription with complex directions such as "tid for 3 days, bid for 3 days, qd for 3 days and dc," it is acceptable to use the Latin abbreviations on the label as long as they are carefully explained to the patient.
a. True
b. False

16. Which of the following best incorporates all recommended components of label directions for outpatient use?
a. Take one tablet three times daily.
b. Take one tablet by mouth three times daily.
c. Take one tablet three times daily for pain.
d. Take one tablet by mouth three times daily for 10 days.
e. Take one tablet by mouth three time daily for 10 days for infection.

17. In some hospitals, physicians are now entering medication orders into the hospital's computer system instead of writing orders on paper.
a. True
b. False

18. Although a prescription or medication order may be written by a mid-level practitioner such as a physician's assistant, the physician himself is the legal authority for dispensing medications and it is his name that should appear in the records as the prescribing physician.
a. True
b. False

19. When a filling label seems to indicate an error, which of the following would be an appropriate initial action for the technician?
a. Alert the pharmacist that an error has been made.
b. Check the label against the original order to determine if an error was made.
c. Call the physician to clarify the order.
d. Call the nursing unit (institutional setting) or notify the patient (outpatient setting) that an error was made on the prescription order and that delays will result.
e. Any of the above would be appropriate as a first step.

20. The final step in processing a prescription or medication order is filing the order in compliance with the requirements of the state the pharmacy is located in and the policies of the organization.
a. True
b. False

ANSWERS TO SELF-ASSESSMENT

1. False. State laws vary in their requirements for telephone prescriptions—particularly when controlled substances are involved. It

is not uncommon that only a pharmacist can receive telephone prescriptions.

2. True. An initial review of the prescription for completeness and accuracy will identify problems and facilitate their efficient resolution. Prioritization will help ensure that the most urgent work is done first.

3. d. All of the listed information would appear on an outpatient prescription but not on an inpatient order. Several other pieces of information would appear on inpatient orders but not outpatient prescriptions—most commonly a room and bed location for the patient and an admission number or account number of some type.

4. a. A dispense as written order must be filled with the brand listed by the prescriber.

5. True. Prescription pads may be lost or stolen and can then be used in attempts to obtain controlled drugs. It is also possible for forged prescriptions to be called in to the pharmacy. Although they may be more difficult to spot than when presented with a written document, the technician should consider anything unusual in a phone order as potentially indicating an attempt to illegally obtain medications. These calls should be directed to the pharmacist.

6. b. Although the pharmacist or technician may have a preference for one type of work over another, the indication of the drug and the needs and expectations of the patient and caregiver should determine the priority of orders.

7. True. Stat is derived from the Latin word *statim*, meaning immediately. Most hospitals have a designated time limit on these orders—typically 10–15 minutes.

8. d. Institutions rely heavily on a patient account number that is reproduced by an addressograph system or on a self-adhesive label that may or may not be bar coded.

9. False. No identification system is completely free from potential error. Patient identification is one of the most important steps in the order processing sequence.

10. d. The patient profile should contain a full range of patient information, including patient demographics such as date of birth, allergies, medical conditions, and disabilities, as well as a complete list of currently prescribed medications. Although it would typically contain information regarding the type of insurance coverage the patient has and the amount of any required deductible or co-pay, how the patient chooses to meet that requirement would not usually be indicated.

11. d. The best choice in this example would be the 100 ml bottle of 250 mg/5 ml suspension. Two full bottles would be required and would have to be transferred to another properly labeled container. Answer "e" would be an alternative, but is less desirable, because it would result in more suspension than needed.

12. b. There is no screening for prices of drugs, although price information may be available. Some outpatient systems may offer price information for generic equivalents.

13. False. Although it is true that the majority of administration times are standardized, there may be numerous exceptions to such a policy. It is not uncommon, for example, for pediatric or neonatal units to have specialized administration schedules that differ from other units. This is also true of many intensive care areas. Exceptions may be based on individual drug characteristics as well. One example is a "tid" order for a medication that should be given before meals. Standard "tid" administration times may be 0900, 1300, and 1800. The schedule might be automatically altered to 0730, 1130, and 1700 to be timed for 30 minutes before each meal.

14. True. Because there are fewer controls on medication administration in the outpatient setting, scheduling should be discussed with the patient or a family member to make sure the instructions are clear and that the patient will not have difficulty using the medication as intended.

15. False. Latin abbreviations should never be used on labeling for home use. Although the patient may fully understand the directions when he or she leaves the pharmacy, they may be forgotten by the time the patient gets home. If detailed instructions do not fit on the prescription label itself, it would be more appropriate to give the patient a separate piece of paper with instructions written in plain English.

16. e. There are six pieces of information that are recommended for inclusion in outpatient labeling. They are (1) the administration direction, (2) the number of units constituting one dose, (3) the route of administration, (4) frequency of administration, (5) duration of therapy, and (6) indication or purpose.

17. True. Physician order entry is not yet widespread but is becoming more common. It offers some advantages since it allows that physician to make timely responses to potential problems with the order without having to wait for the technician to discover the issue and refer it to the pharmacist, who must then contact the prescriber for clarification.

18. True. Many prescribers now employ mid-level practitioners such as physicians' assistants and nurse practitioners. Some states also allow pharmacists to write medication orders within the constraints of physician approved protocols. The physician remains the prescriber of record in most situations, but the mid-level practitioner may be the person generating the order and therefore more appropriate for clarifying issues than the physician he or she represents. It is still the physician though, who is the legal prescriber.

19. b. Checking the label against the original order is a good initial step because the error may have been a simple keystroke error in the computer which could be easily corrected, eliminating the need for many of the other options listed.

20. True. Once the dispensing activities have been completed, the order should be filed. State laws differ in their requirements for filing. Individual organizations will develop their own policies dictating how orders are to be filed and for how long. The technician should be familiarized with those requirements during training and orientation.

Drug Classification and Pharmacologic Actions

Gail Bernstein, Pharm.D., BCPS

A drug can be defined as any substance that, when introduced into the body, alters the body's functions. An ideal drug would have several characteristics: it would be effective for its therapeutic use, be safe even if large quantities are ingested, and not have any adverse effects. Obviously, the ideal drug does not exist. All drugs have some adverse effects, and many drugs are toxic when more than the recommended dose is taken. Therefore, the decision to use any drug therapy is made after weighing the benefits of the drug against the risks involved with its use.

Drugs discussed in this chapter have been arranged according to the body organ systems in which they have their major effects. Drugs often have actions in more than one part of the body and may be mentioned in several areas. The major actions or uses of drugs, their major adverse effects, and important characteristics particular to specific drugs, especially where these characteristics are important in dispensing activities, will be discussed. Table 6-1 lists some of the abbreviations commonly used in practice. A list of Recommended Reading is included for readers who desire more in-depth information.

LEARNING OBJECTIVES

After completing this chapter the reader will be able to
1. Describe the important actions and/or therapeutic uses for the major classes of drugs.
2. Describe the most common or most serious adverse effects for the major classes of drugs.
3. Describe special dispensing precautions for the major classes of drugs.

TOPICAL MEDICATIONS

Ophthalmic Medications

Diseases of the surface or near the surface of the eye can often be treated with topical medications. The most common ophthalmic diseases are conjunctivitis, glaucoma, and dryness of the eyes. Topical treatment of eye diseases is advantageous because the side effects that might occur with systemic medication can be avoided.

Table 6–1

Abbreviations

ACE	— Angiotensin converting enzyme	HMG-CoA	— Hydroxymethylglutaryl-Coenzyme A
ACTH	— Adrenocorticotropic hormone	LDL	— Low density lipoprotein
ADH	— Antidiuretic hormone	MAOI	— Monoamine oxidase inhibitor
AIDS	— Acquired immunodeficiency syndrome	NSAID	— Nonsteroidal anti-inflammatory
AQ	— Aqueous	NPH	— Isophane zinc
AV	— Atrial-ventricular	PZI	— Protamine zinc
BPH	— Benign prostatic hyperplasia	PUD	— Peptic ulcer disease
CMV	— Cytomegalovirus	RSV	— Respiratory syncytial virus
COPD	— Chronic obstructive pulmonary disease	SSKI	— Saturated solution of potassium iodide
DDAVP	— Desmopressin acetate	SSRI	— Selective Serotonin reuptake inhibitor
FDA	— Food and Drug Administration	T3	— Triiodothyronine
GERD	— Gastroesophageal reflux disease	T4	— Levothyroxine
HCG	— Human chorionic gonadotropin	TB	— Tuberculosis
HDL	— High density lipoprotein	TMP/SMX	— Trimethoprim/sulfamethoxazole
HIV	— Human immunodeficiency virus		

Eye drops and ointments must be used properly to obtain the desired benefit. The tears that lubricate and cleanse the eye naturally drain out of the eye through ducts. If eye products are not used correctly, the drug can drain out of the eye without producing the desired effect. If too much drug is used, systemic side effects can be produced by drug that has drained out of the eye. The external coat of the eye is resistant to infection. Once this surface is broken, the eye is very susceptible to infection. For this reason, ophthalmic products must be made and kept sterile. Ophthalmic preparations should be labeled "For the eye."

Medications for Conjunctivitis

Conjunctivitis is the most common eye disease in the Western hemisphere.[1] Conjunctivitis is an inflammation of the conjunctiva, which is a membrane covering the inside of the eyelids and the white part of the eye. Conjunctivitis can be caused by infection, allergy, chemical irritation, or other diseases. The signs and symptoms of conjunctivitis include redness, tearing, secretions, drooping of the eyelid, itching, a scratchy or burning sensation, sensitivity to light, and the sensation that a foreign body is present in the eye. The treatment of conjunctivitis depends on the cause.

Conjunctivitis that is caused by infection can be treated with antibiotics or antiviral eye drops. Newborn infants are routinely given erythromycin ophthalmic ointment to prevent conjunc-

tivitis caused by bacteria that might have entered the eye during birth. Some other antibiotics commonly used to treat infectious conjunctivitis are gentamicin, tobramycin, bacitracin, sodium sulfacetamide, ciprofloxacin, and ofloxacin. Combinations of antibiotics such as neomycin, polymyxin, and bacitracin are commonly used. Antibiotics combined with steroids to provide an anti-inflammatory action are used in some cases. Cortisporin® and Maxitrol® are examples of antibiotic and steroid combination products. Antiviral ophthalmic preparations are effective against herpes simplex viruses and cytomegalovirus. Cytomegalovirus infections occur in patients whose immune systems have been compromised by drugs used to prevent transplant organ rejection or by acquired immunodeficiency syndrome (AIDS). The anti-viral drugs used in these situations are vidarabine, trifluridine, idoxuridine, foscarnet, and ganciclovir.

Two agents are available for the treatment of allergic conjunctivitis. These agents are lodoxamide tromethamine and levocabastine. They work by preventing the release of chemicals that lead to an allergic response. Their use should be limited to 3 months and 2 weeks, respectively.[2]

Medications for Glaucoma

Glaucoma is a disease caused by increased pressure within the eye. Untreated glaucoma can damage the optic nerve resulting in partial to total loss of sight. Many drugs are used to treat glaucoma by lowering the pressure in the eye by two basic mechanisms: decreasing the rate of production of the eye fluid or increasing the drainage of eye fluid. Sympathomimetic drugs used to treat glaucoma include epinephrine, dipivefrin, and apraclonidine. Epinephrine may cause stinging upon instillation into the eye, and epinephrine and dipivefrin may cause blurred vision temporarily. Beta-blocking drugs are effective antiglaucoma drugs. They include metipranolol, carteolol, levobunolol, betaxolol, and timolol. Because of the systemic effects of these drugs, caution is advised in patients with lung disease, heart failure, and diabetes. Miotic drugs, such as carbachol, pilocarpine, physostigmine, demecarium, echothiophate iodide, and isoflurophate, constrict the pupil size. Patients using these drugs to treat glaucoma can experience difficulty in seeing at night. Patients should be cautioned about night driving and performing hazardous tasks in poor light. In addition to eyedrops, pilocarpine is also available in a controlled release unit that is placed under the lower eyelid and releases medication for 1 week. The antiglaucoma drug echothiophate is available as a powder that must be reconstituted before dispensing and labeled with an expiration date.

Medications for Dryness

A large number of ophthalmic preparations are available as artificial tear solutions for the relief of dry eyes. These products contain salts in the same concentrations as that found in the tissues and fluids of the eye. They also contain buffers to maintain the same acidity as the eye tissues and thickening agents to prolong the time they stay on the surface of the eye. All of these products are available over the counter. A prescription-only insert, Lacrisert®, is available that provides relief from dryness with once-daily insertion as opposed to application of drops multiple times daily.

Ophthalmic vasoconstrictors are commonly used to reduce redness in the eyes from minor irritations. Several products are available over the counter for this purpose. These products are also used to dilate the pupil for eye examinations and surgery. The over-the-counter products should not be used for more than 72 hours without consulting a physician. Products include phenylephrine, oxymetazoline, naphazoline, and tetrahydrozoline. Some of these drugs are available in combination with antihistamines or with zinc sulfate as an antiseptic for minor eye irritations.

Corticosteroids are available in topical ophthalmic preparations. They are indicated for inflammatory conditions such as allergic conjunctivitis, selected infections of the eye, chemical and other burns, and penetration of foreign bodies. Prednisolone and dexamethasone are available as single drugs and in combination with many different anti-infective agents.

Otic Medications

The anatomy of the ear is divided into three sections: the external ear, the middle ear, and the inner ear. The external ear consists of the auricle and the external auditory canal. The auricle is the protruding part of the ear, which is cartilage covered with skin. The external auditory canal is a tube leading from the auricle to the ear drum. The auditory canal conducts sound to the ear drum and protects the ear drum from injury. The canal contains hair follicles and glands that secrete oils and ear wax (cerumen).

Topical otic medications are effective for treating conditions of the external ear. Conditions involving the middle or inner ear require systemic treatment. Topical ear treatments are most commonly used for impacted ear wax and minor infections or irritation of the auditory canal. Otic preparations should be labeled "For the ear." Several products have names similar to ophthalmic products, and care should be taken to avoid confusion and mistakes. Topical otic products should not be used if the ear drum is perforated.

The antibiotic chloramphenicol is available as an otic preparation for infections of the auditory canal. Antibiotic combinations of neomycin and polymyxin B with the corticosteroid hydrocortisone are also used to treat these infections. Acetic acid, M-cresyl acetate, boric acid, benzalkonium chloride, benzethonium chloride, and aluminum acetate are antibacterial or antifungal ingredients in ear drops.

Otic preparations that contain carbamide peroxide, triethanolamine, and glycerin are used to soften and disperse ear wax. After instilling these agents, the wax is removed by irrigating the ear with a syringe. Warming solutions will help relieve pain in the ear. Any wax not responding to these drugs after 4 days should be removed by a physician.

Intranasal Products

The nose is the entrance to the respiratory tract. It warms and humidifies air and filters out particles. The presence of many blood vessels is necessary to provide the warming function. The secretion of mucus keeps the nasal cavity damp and traps dust, bacteria, and other particles. Small hairs called cilia then transport the mucus to the throat where it is expectorated or swallowed. Nerves control the blood vessels and mucus production.

The major ailment of the nose that is treated with topical products is rhinitis. Rhinitis may also be treated with oral drugs. Rhinitis is a hyper-reactivity of the lining of the nose to stimuli. The stimuli may include seasonal allergens such as pollen, perennial allergens such as animal dander, or nonallergic stimuli such as stress, temperature changes, and other environmental factors. Rhinitis also occurs during infections such as the common cold and the flu. Symptoms of rhinitis are nasal congestion, runny nose, post nasal drainage, sneezing, itching, redness of the membrane lining the nose, watery eyes, dark circles under the eyes, and inability to breathe through one's nose.

Intranasal corticosteroids are used for rhinitis and other allergic or inflammatory conditions of the nose. If the nasal passages are blocked, use of a decongestant nasal spray before the corticosteroid spray may allow better penetration of the corticosteroid spray. With doses that exceed the recommended range and occasionally in recommended doses, systemic effects may occur. These effects of corticosteroids are discussed under the musculoskeletal system and anti-inflammatory drugs. Intranasal corticosteroids include dexamethasone, flunisolide, beclomethasone, triamcinolone, and budesonide. These drugs are also available as oral inhalers with similar names, so care must be taken to dispense the product for the correct route of administration. Some aqueous (AQ) preparations sting less than other preparations.

Cromolyn sodium and nedrocromil sodium are intranasal products used to treat allergic rhinitis. These drugs prevent the allergic response to stimuli. Both are also available as oral inhalers, so care should be taken to avoid confusion in dosage forms.

Decongestant drugs are available in intranasal sprays, drops, or inhalers. These drugs act on the nerves of the blood vessels in the nose. They cause the blood vessels to constrict, which decreases swelling and stuffiness in the nose. Topical agents are associated with rebound congestion when used for more than 3 to 5 days. Essentially, the nasal lining becomes more congested as the effect of the drug wears off. This increased stuffiness may cause the patient to increase the use of the decongestant, creating a cycle that is difficult to break.

Phenylephrine, naphazoline, oxymetazoline, tetrahydrozoline, and xylometazoline are topical decongestants. Xylometazoline and oxymetazoline are long acting and can be used every 8 to 10 hours and every 12 hours, respectively. Reactions such as stinging, burning, and sneezing may occur. Patients with hypertension or other cardiovascular disease, overactive thyroid, diabetes mellitus, or an enlarged prostate gland should not use these products because of possible detrimental effects.

Dermatological Agents

The skin is the largest organ of the body. It protects the body from invasion by foreign materials and organisms. The skin also has many other functions. It contains glands and sensory nerves, influences metabolism, helps maintain fluid and electrolyte balance and temperature control, and produces metabolites, and excretes waste products.[3]

The skin is made of three layers. The outer layer, the epidermis, has no blood supply and is a layer of cells that are constantly shed and regenerated. The middle layer, the dermis, is thicker than the epidermis. It contains blood vessels, nerves, lymph vessels, elastic and connective tissue, sweat and scent glands, hair follicles, and sebaceous glands that secrete an oily film. The innermost layer, the hypodermis, contains a layer of fat that insulates, cushions, and gives the skin pliability.

Dermatitis and hypersensitivity reactions are common diseases of the skin. Contact dermatitis can be an acute or chronic reaction to irritants or allergens. Symptoms of contact dermatitis are redness, oozing, hives, swelling, and scaling. Poison ivy rash is an example of contact dermatitis. Sunburn is a dermatitis that results from overexposure to the sun. Normal exposure to the sun can also result in a sunburn in patients who are taking drugs that sensitize the skin. Drug reactions and hives caused by foods and inhalants are other forms of dermatitis. Psoriasis is a non-infectious, chronic dermatitis that is characterized by white scale over red patches of skin, most commonly on the elbows, knees, scalp, lower back, genitalia, and feet. The cause of psoriasis is unknown. Generally, psoriasis may improve and then relapse.

Coal tar and salicylic acid have been used for many years to treat psoriasis. These products are available as ointments, creams, lotions, shampoos, and bath additives. They have an unpleasant odor and can stain clothing and hair. They should not be applied to broken skin. Salicylic acid is also used to remove warts, calluses, and corns. Some newer drugs for treating psoriasis include anthralin and calcipotriene. Anthralin also can stain clothing and hair.

Corticosteroid creams, ointments, and lotions can be used for psoriasis. Other uses for corticosteroid topical products include other skin conditions involving itching and inflammation such as contact dermatitis, reactions to insect and spider bites, burns and sunburns, diaper rash, and inflammation associated with fungal infections of the skin. Corticosteroids vary in potency and the strengths available. When topical steroids are being dispensed, the correct formulation (ointment, cream, or lotion) and strength must be carefully selected. Hydrocortisone and hydrocortisone acetate are available over the counter in 0.5% and 1% strengths. Many combinations with antifungals, antibiotics, and antibacterial agents are available. Such products should be applied sparingly. Very high and high potency steroids should not be applied on large areas, the face, scrotum, or areas with skin folds or used in children. Very high potency steroids include clobetasol, diflorasone, halobetasol, and augmented betamethasone diproprionate; and high potency steroids are betamethasone diproprionate, betamethasone valerate, desoximetasone, fluocinolone, fluocinonide, halcinonide, and triamcinolone acetonide. Medium potency steroids are betamethasone benzoate, betamethasone valerate, hydrocortisone butyrate, hydrocortisone valerate, and mometasone furoate. Low potency steroids are desonide, dexamethasone, hydrocortisone, and hydrocortisone acetate. Systemic effects can occur if a significant amount of the corticosteroid is absorbed through the skin. Significant absorption of corticosteroids is more likely to occur when patients use more potent steroids, apply them to large surface areas, use them for prolonged periods of time, and apply occlusive dressings over the steroid.[2]

Skin may be infected by numerous organisms. Parasites, such as lice and mites, can cause rashes and itching by biting or laying eggs in the skin. Fungal and yeast infections are most common in skin folds such as under the breasts and in the groin areas. Fungal infections can also occur on the feet (athlete's foot), on the scalp or body (ringworm), around the nails, or in the mouth. Viral infections that involve the skin include warts, cold sores, sexually transmitted herpes simplex, and herpes zoster rash (shingles). Bacterial infections that involve the skin include impetigo, a honey-colored crust commonly seen around the mouth and nose in children, and various sexually transmitted diseases.

Many topical anti-infective agents are available. Mupirocin, tetracycline, chloramphenicol, erythromycin, gentamicin, bacitracin, neomycin, and combinations of polymyxin B, neomycin, and bacitracin are examples of topical anti-infective agents. Many of the antifungal agents are marketed for athlete's foot: undecylenic acid, miconazole, econazole, ciclopirox olamine, clotrimazole, triacetin, and tolnaftate. Undecylenic acid, miconazole, clotrimazole, nystatin, and amphotericin B can also be used for more generalized fungal infections of the skin, including diaper rash. Acyclovir is available as an antiviral ointment.

Acne is a chronic condition in which lesions called comedones appear on the skin. Comedones are commonly called whiteheads and blackheads. Acne is most common in teenage years. Hormones, friction, sweating, and stress can all cause and influence the severity of acne.[4]

A large number of topical products are available for treating acne. Most acne products work to prevent breakouts by one of four mechanisms: increasing the rate of turnover of skin cells, killing bacteria on the skin, inhibiting inflammation, and decreasing the production by the skin of oily substances.[5] Tretinoin, benzoyl peroxide, azelaic acid, and sulfur are examples of topical preparations. Combinations of sulfur drugs, salicylic acid, and resorcinol are also available. Antibiotics such as tetracycline, meclocycline, erythromycin, and clindamycin are available to treat acne topically. In more severe cases of acne, systemic treatment with antibiotics or isotretinoin can be used. In some cases, both topical and systemic therapies are used.

CENTRAL NERVOUS SYSTEM DISORDERS

The central nervous system is made up of the brain and the nerves that carry information to and from the brain. Nerves carry information about the environment (e.g., the stove is hot) from all the parts of the body into the spinal cord and up to the brain. The brain interprets the information received and decides on any action (e.g., remove hand from stove) and then sends the appropriate response back down the spinal column nerves and out to the tissues, such as muscles, which will create the correct response (e.g., hand is moved away from stove).

Throughout this system, including within the brain, impulses are sent from nerve to nerve. The impulse is sent from one nerve to the next by chemicals produced at the junction of the two nerves. These chemicals are called neurotransmitters. Almost all drugs that act on the central nervous system do so by affecting the amounts of these chemicals within the brain or at the nerve junctions in the spinal cord, and throughout the body.

Psychoactive Drugs

The true causes of most mental illnesses are unknown. The drugs used in the treatment of these disorders work by altering the various chemicals found at the nerve junctions in the brain. The following types of drugs have this kind of activity: antidepressants, antipsychotics, anxiolytics, sedatives, and hypnotics.

Antidepressants

Depression is a common illness in the United States. Depression may be reactive (in response to a stimulus such as grief) or endogenous (a chemical disorder in the brain). Antidepressant medications can be used in either type of depression but are most often used for endogenous depression. Depression can also be caused by drugs. If this is the case, the suspected drug should be withdrawn. Symptoms of depression include a depressed mood, the inability to experience pleasure in activities, changes in sleep habits, loss of energy, changes in appetite, inability to concentrate, and thoughts of suicide.

Antidepressants can be divided into several classes based on their chemical structures and chemical actions in the brain. Tricyclic antidepressants, monoamine oxidase inhibitors (MAOIs), and selective seratonin reuptake inhibitors (SSRIs) have been the most frequently used drugs. Several of the drugs, such as bupropion, venlafaxine, nefazadone, trazodone, and mirtazapine, do not fit into these classifications. All of the classes of antidepressants are effective treatments for depression. The adverse effects associated with a drug are a factor in the choice of a particular drug for a patient.

Tricyclic Antidepressants

Tricyclic antidepressants were the most widely used antidepressants for many years. The mechanism of action is unclear, but they are thought to potentiate the action of several different neurotransmitters in the brain. They are effective but have a large number of bothersome side effects that include dry mouth, blurred vision, constipation, difficulty urinating, dizziness upon standing, sedation, and sexual dysfunction. These side effects may be so bothersome that patients stop taking their medication. Overdose with these drugs can be lethal because of their effects on the heart or because they can cause convulsions. Since depressed patients often have suicidal tendencies, the overdose potential of drugs used for treatment is an important consideration. Some examples of tricyclic antidepressants are amitriptyline, doxepin, imipramine, desipramine, and nortriptyline.

Monoamine Oxidase Inhibitors

The three monoamine oxidase inhibitors are phenelzine, isocarboxazid, and tranylcypromine. These drugs are thought to work by preventing the natural breakdown of neurotransmitters. The most common side effect of MAOIs is postural hypotension, which is a drop in blood pressure upon arising (moving from a sitting or lying position to a standing position) that results in dizziness. Hypertensive crisis, an extreme elevation of blood pressure that can be fatal or produce organ damage, is a potential adverse reaction with MAOIs. This event most often occurs when certain foods or drugs are taken with the MAOI. Therefore, patients must be fully informed of the foods (e.g., aged cheeses, sausages, and red wine) and medications (e.g., pseudoephedrine in decongestants or diet pills) they should avoid.

Selective Serotonin Reuptake Inhibitors

The selective serotonin reuptake inhibitors are the newest class of antidepressants. Tricyclics and MAOIs affect several neurotransmitters, but SSRIs affect only one neurotransmitter, serotonin. This class includes fluoxetine, paroxetine, and sertraline. These drugs gained quick acceptance because the side effect profile is more tolerable when compared with the previous classes of antidepressants, and the SSRIs are less dangerous at normal or excessive doses. The side effects that are common with the SSRIs are nausea, anorexia, diarrhea, anxiety, nervousness, and insomnia. Sexual dysfunction does occur frequently.

Miscellaneous Agents

Nefazadone, trazodone, venlafaxine, bupropion, and mirtazapine do not fit into the usual classes of antidepressants. Nefazadone and trazodone share some of the adverse effects of the tricyclic antidepressants, such as sedation and postural hypotension, but they are less likely to cause heart rhythm disturbances or anticholinergic effects, such as dry mouth, blurred vision, constipation, and difficulty urinating. Like the tricyclic antidepressants, bupropion can cause constipation and dry mouth. The most serious adverse reaction of bupropion is seizures. Venlafaxine's most common adverse effects are nausea, drowsiness, insomnia, dry mouth, dizziness, nervousness, sweating, and sexual dysfunction. An increase in blood pressure can occur in patients taking venlafaxine. Mirtazapine is not likely to cause heart rhythm disturbances or seizures, but it can cause agranulocytosis, a decreased production of all types of blood cells, and neutropenia, a decreased production of white blood cells.

Antidepressants are usually started at low doses and gradually increased. It may take 3 to 4 weeks of therapy before a patient will respond to antidepressants.[5] Caution must be used when discontinuing one antidepressant and starting another so that adverse effects are avoided. Antidepressants should be discontinued over a period of several weeks. During this time the dose should be tapered gradually. Drug interactions are common with most antidepressants. Patients should be warned to check with their doctor or pharmacist before taking other prescription or nonprescription medications.

Antipsychotics

Psychosis is a mental disorder in which a person's capacity to recognize reality is distorted. Schizophrenia is one type of psychosis. Common symptoms include hallucinations (hearing or seeing things that are not real), delusions (fixed beliefs that are false), and thought processes that are not logically connected.

Antipsychotics are also known as neuroleptics and major tranquilizers. Although the precise mechanism of action is not known, antipsychotics are thought to act by blocking the action of the neurotransmitter dopamine. Examples of commonly used antipsychotics are chlorpromazine, thioridazine, trifluoperazine, perphenazine, fluphenazine, thiothixene, haloperidol, and loxapine. Three drugs, clozapine, olanzepine, and risperdone, are often used in patients who have not responded to other medications.

Most of the antipsychotics are available as injections and oral tablets. Oral solutions, which should be diluted with liquids such as fruit juice, are available for patients who refuse tablets. Fluphenazine and haloperidol are available as long-acting injections for patients who may not be compliant with daily medication regimens. The effectiveness of haloperidol decanoate injections lasts 1 month. Long-acting fluphenazine is available in two different salts, fluphenazine enanthate and fluphenazine decanoate. One dose of fluphenazine enanthate will last approximately 1 to 3 weeks, while 1 dose of fluphenazine decanoate will last more than 4 weeks.

Adverse effects of the antipsychotics can be divided into four types: sedation, extrapyramidal, anticholinergic, and cardiac. Extrapyramidal symptoms include abnormal muscle contractions and restlessness. Some muscle contractions can be life threatening (such as when the throat muscles contract). Anticholinergic side effects are common with many drugs and include dry mouth, blurred vision, constipation, difficulty urinating, and increased heart rate. The cardiac side effects associated with antipsychotic drugs include postural hypotension and heart rhythm changes. Antipsychotic drugs vary in their tendency to cause each of these adverse effects.

Drugs for Bipolar Disorder

Bipolar disorder, also called manic-depressive disorder, is characterized by mood swings. Patients cycle between an agitated or overexcited and a depressed state. Manic episodes have traditionally been treated with lithium. Lithium is also taken as a maintenance drug to prevent episodes. Two other drugs are now commonly used for bipolar disorder, carbamazepine and valproic acid. These drugs are both generally used to prevent seizures (anticonvulsants). They are discussed in more detail in the section on neurological disorders.

The mechanism of action of lithium is unclear. Lithium affects many of the salts in the blood, leading to adverse effects such as increased thirst and urination. Tremors are a common side effect of lithium, which can be alleviated with propranolol. Lithium also decreases thyroid function in a high percentage of patients and causes kidney toxicity. The amount of lithium in the blood can be measured to ensure that the dose is high enough to be effective but still low enough to avoid adverse effects.

Sedatives, Hypnotics, and Anxiolytics

Sedative-hypnotic drugs are used for the treatment of anxiety and sleep disorders. Sedatives are used to reduce anxiety or produce a calming effect. Hypnotic drugs are used to produce sleep or drowsiness. Some drugs have sedative effects at lower doses and hypnotic effects at higher doses.

Drugs used for anxiety (anxiolytics) include the benzodiazepines, barbiturates, and buspirone. Phenobarbital is the main barbiturate used for anxiety, but since the development of the benzodiazepines, barbiturates are rarely used for that indication. Barbiturates have a higher risk of adverse effects and toxicity than the benzodiazepines.

Benzodiazepines are the most commonly used drugs for anxiety and sleep. Examples of benzodiazepines used mainly for anxiety are alprazolam, chlordiazepoxide, clorazepate, diazepam, lorazepam, midazolam, and oxazepam. Injectable forms of midazolam and diazepam are frequently used for sedation for procedures such as an endoscopy and the setting of a fractured bone.

The most common side effects of benzodiazepines are drowsiness and slowed reactions. These effects are enhanced when drugs such as alcohol or narcotics are used simultaneously. All patients on benzodiazepines should be counseled about possible impairment of driving abilities, ability to operate machinery, and judgment. Amnesia, or memory loss, is often considered an adverse effect but is desirable when these drugs are used for sedation during painful medical procedures. Withdrawal symptoms may occur when patients who have taken drugs for a long time abruptly stop therapy. People who deliberately overdose often choose benzodiazepines. However, a drug called flumazenil is available to reverse some of the effects of benzodiazepines.

Buspirone is chemically unlike the benzodiazepines. Its advantage over benzodiazepines is that it is less likely to cause drowsiness and slowed reactions. It also has a low potential for abuse and no withdrawal symptoms.

Hypnotics may be used to treat a variety of sleep problems: difficulty in falling asleep, frequent awakening during the night, early morning awakening, and not feeling rested even after what should be an adequate amount of sleep.

Nondrug therapies are usually tried first, such as establishing a regular bedtime and wake-up time and reducing the use of alcohol, caffeine, and nicotine. General guidelines for the use of hypnotics include using the lowest effective dose for the shortest duration possible.

Hypnotic drugs, like sedatives, include barbiturates, benzodiazepines, and nonbarbiturate, nonbenzodiazepine drugs. Because of their potential for the development of tolerance, fatality in overdose, dependence, withdrawal symptoms, and drug interactions, barbiturates are used as hypnotics less often since the development of benzodiazepines.[5] Amobarbital, pentobarbital, and secobarbital are the barbiturates most often used as hypnotics.

Benzodiazepines commonly used as hypnotics include estazolam, quazepam, flurazepam, temazepam, and triazolam. A drug that is chemically not a benzodiazepine but has similar actions is zolpidem. The effects of some hypnotics carry over into daytime. This carryover of drowsiness and decreased concentration, called a hangover, is an important consideration in the use of hypnotics. Benzodiazepines that are metabolized and excreted rapidly are less likely to produce a hangover.[5] Tolerance, a loss of effectiveness over time, may occur with all benzodiazepines.

Nonbenzodiazepine and nonbarbiturate hypnotics include several groups of drugs. Some drugs are used as hypnotics because drowsiness is one of their most common side effects. The antihistamine diphenhydramine is used for sleep because of the frequency with which it causes drowsiness. Many nonprescription sleep aids contain diphenhydramine. Antidepressants such as amitriptyline, doxepin, and trazodone are often used for patients who complain that they do not feel rested after adequate sleep or who should not take benzodiazepines. Chloral hydrate has many of the same disadvantages as the barbiturates and is rarely used today as a hypnotic.

Drugs for Neurological Disorders

Anticonvulsants

Epilepsy is a disorder of the central nervous system characterized by recurrent seizures. Seizures are brief episodes of brain dysfunction that result from abnormal firing of nerves in the brain. The sudden sharp muscle contraction and rigidity that many people think of as a seizure is only one type of seizure. Other seizures consist of a sudden cessation of ongoing activities and a blank stare or muscle contractions of isolated parts of the body such as the face or arms.

Seizures may be caused by some type of central nervous system damage or have no discernible cause. Strokes and tumors are common causes of seizures in the elderly. Head trauma, fever, changes in certain blood constituents, and the sudden withdrawal of certain drugs (antidepressants, alcohol, benzodiazepines) are other causes of seizures.

Anticonvulsant drugs, also called antiepileptics, are used to reduce the frequency of seizures. They do this by reducing the excitability of the nerve cells in the brain. All anticonvulsants have adverse effects, so their use is only called for when the probability of recurrent seizures is more worrisome than the adverse effects of the drugs.

The four major drugs used to control seizures are phenytoin, carbamazepine, phenobarbital, and valproic acid. Ethosuximide is an antiepileptic drug with efficacy in one special type of seizure. Several benzodiazepines are used for epilepsy. The newest anticonvulsants available are lamotrigine, felbamate, and gabapentin.

Phenytoin has been available for over 50 years. It effectively prevents many types of seizures. Dosing phenytoin is complicated. Under some circumstances small changes in the dose result in large changes in the drug's effects. Phenytoin blood levels are usually measured to ensure that enough phenytoin is present to prevent seizures but not enough to cause side effects related to the dose, such as double vision, loss of muscle coordination, and sedation. Side effects that are common but are not affected by decreasing the dose are overgrowth of the gums and excessive body hair. Phenytoin also has many drug interactions. Patients should be warned not to take extra doses or other drugs without checking with their doctor or pharmacist first. Phenytoin is available in capsule, tablet, oral suspension, and injectable form. A new injectable drug, fosphenytoin, is converted to phenytoin in the body.

Carbamazepine is effective for many of the same seizure types as phenytoin. Carbamazepine has other therapeutic uses such as for psychiatric disorders, for a painful facial nerve condition called trigeminal neuralgia, and for restless leg syndrome. Like phenytoin, blood levels of carbamazepine are measured to ensure that the dose is producing therapeutic blood levels but not levels high enough to result in adverse effects. The dose-related side effects of carbamazepine are similar to phenytoin: double

vision, muscle incoordination, and drowsiness. Liver function and red blood cell production must be monitored. Carbamazepine can cause a rare serious adverse effect called pancytopenia, which is a depression of the production of all types of blood cells (red cells, white cells, and platelets). Like phenytoin, carbamazepine has many drug interactions. This drug is only available in oral forms: a chewable tablet, a regular tablet, and a suspension.

Valproic acid, like phenytoin and carbamazepine, is used to treat many types of seizures. Like carbamazepine, valproic acid is also used for many psychiatric disorders. Blood levels of valproic acid are used to guide effective dosing and avoid dose-related side effects. The dose-related side effects are nausea and vomiting and tremor. Nausea and vomiting can be avoided by gradually increasing the dose. Liver toxicity is the most serious side effect but is reversible if the drug is stopped. Other side effects are weight gain, increased appetite, and hair loss. Like phenytoin and carbamazepine, drug interactions are common. Oral capsules of valproic acid and syrup of sodium valproate are available. Divalproex sodium is available as a slow-release tablet and as coated pellets in a capsule that can be swallowed whole or sprinkled on soft foods. Sodium valproate is available as an injection.

Benzodiazepines are used for status epilepticus, a condition of repetitive seizures with little or no interruption between them. Injectable forms of diazepam and lorazepam are commonly used initially to stop the repetitive seizure activity, then longer acting drugs, such as phenytoin, are given to prevent the recurrence of seizures. Clonazepam is a benzodiazepine used orally as a maintenance medication for several types of seizures. Sedation is a prominent side effect.

Phenobarbital is effective against fewer seizure types than some of the newer drugs. The adverse effects of phenobarbital, mainly excessive sedation, and the potential for dependence and withdrawal symptoms limit its usefulness today.

Lamotrigine, gabapentin, and felbamate are newer antiepileptics. These drugs have been studied more in combination with older drugs than when used alone. Their role in the therapy of epilepsy remains to be determined. An advantage of gabapentin is that it has few drug interactions. After being marketed, felbamate was found to have an unacceptable occurrence of serious blood reactions. It should not be used except for patients whose seizures cannot be controlled with other drugs. Lamotrigine has been associated with several kinds of rash that may be mild or may be severe enough to require discontinuation of the drug.

Antiparkinson Drugs

Parkinson's disease is a nervous system disorder characterized by movement abnormalities: tremor, extreme slowness in movement, and rigidity or stiffness of joints. Common movements seen in these patients are "pill rolling" with the thumb and index finger, a cogwheel or ratcheting appearing movement of the arms or legs, a stooped posture, and a blank stare due to decreased blinking.

The cause of Parkinson's disease is unknown, but the basis of drug therapy is to correct an imbalance of two chemicals in the brain, dopamine and acetylcholine. The available drug therapies only control symptoms; despite therapy the disease will progress with further debilitation.

Levodopa is the major drug used in Parkinson's disease. It increases the amount of a chemical, dopamine, in the brain and other areas of the body. The increased amount of dopamine in the brain helps to reduce the Parkinson's symptoms, but the increases in dopamine in the rest of the body can cause adverse reactions. Therefore, levodopa is usually given in combination with carbidopa. Carbidopa inhibits the conversion of levodopa to its active form outside the brain and thus reduces the adverse effects.

Nausea and vomiting and effects on the heart rate and rhythm can be caused by levodopa but are not major problems when carbidopa is combined with levodopa. However, certain movement disorders are more common in patients taking the combination product than in those taking levodopa alone. A variety of other side effects, including depression, anxiety, agitation, inability to sleep, confusion, and hallucinations, can occur with both. Levodopa should not be given to psychotic patients. Its actions are the opposite of the antipsychotic drugs, so it may make psychotic patients worse and most antipsychotics may worsen symptoms of Parkinson's disease.

Other agents used in Parkinson's disease, amantadine, bromocriptine, pergolide, and selegiline, mimic or increase the actions of dopamine. These drugs are usually used in combination with levodopa but may be used alone.

Their side effects are similar to those of levodopa: mental changes and movement disorders.

Anticholinergic drugs used in Parkinson's disease are benztropine, biperidin, procyclidine, trihexyphenidyl, ethopropazine, and diphenhydramine. Their mechanism of action is related not to dopamine but to the other chemical involved in Parkinson's disease, acetylcholine. Anticholinergics are more useful for patients with tremor and rigidity than those with slowed movement. These drugs have many side effects. Mental side effects include drowsiness, confusion, restlessness, and hallucinations. Other common side effects are dry mouth, blurred vision, difficulty urinating, constipation, nausea and vomiting, and rapid heart rate.

RESPIRATORY SYSTEM

Oxygen is essential to body tissues. The functions of the various tissues are made possible by the energy produced when oxygen combines with chemical substances. Carbon dioxide is one byproduct of these chemical reactions. Oxygen is inhaled as air through the mouth and nasal passages, down the windpipe and the trachea, and into the lungs. In the smallest passages, the lung tissue and blood vessels are separated by only a thin membrane that allows gases (i.e., oxygen, carbon dioxide) to pass back and forth. At this membrane, oxygen passes into the blood and carbon dioxide passes from the blood back into the lungs to be exhaled.

Some common diseases of the pulmonary system are pneumonia, asthma, and chronic obstructive pulmonary disease (COPD). Pneumonia is a lung infection. Antibiotics for the treatment of pneumonia are discussed in the section on infectious disease. Asthma is characterized by a reversible narrowing of the air passages caused by over-responsiveness of the airways to various stimuli and inflammation of the airways. The stimuli that can cause inflammation and airway narrowing include viruses, cold air, exercise, pollens, dust, cigarette smoke, and animal dander. Airway narrowing is responsible for the symptoms of asthma, which are wheezing, difficulty breathing, and coughing. Chronic obstructive pulmonary disease is an irreversible chronic obstruction of airways. Emphysema and chronic bronchitis are examples of COPD. The symptoms of asthma and COPD are similar (i.e., wheezing, difficulty breathing, and coughing). These diseases differ in their cause, development, and reversibility. Similar drugs are used to treat both.

Bronchodilators

Bronchodilators are drugs that open up, or dilate, the bronchioles (large passageways in the lungs). There are three types of bronchodilators: β_2 agonists, xanthines, and anticholinergics.

The β_2 agonists are bronchodilators that act on the nerves that control the smooth muscles in the bronchial airways. These agents are available in several dosage forms: metered-dose inhalers, solutions for inhalation via a nebulizer machine, oral tablets, oral liquids, and injections. Most patients use metered-dose inhalers. The proper use of inhalers is critical to the success of treatment with these drugs. Since proper use of inhalers is not always intuitive, patients should be counseled on the correct use of their inhaler.

Common side effects of β_2 agonists are a rapid heartbeat, tremors, anxiety, and nausea. These effects are less likely to occur with inhaled products because they act locally on the airways. Most of these side effects will disappear as the body adjusts to the medication. Rare, but more serious side effects, are chest pain, fast or irregular heartbeat, severe headache, dizziness, and severe nausea and vomiting. Overuse of β_2 agonists can result in decreased effectiveness of the agents. The beta-blockers used in cardiovascular diseases and glaucoma should not be used together with bronchodilators because the drugs have opposite effects.

Examples of β_2 agonists are salmeterol, albuterol, metaproterenol, isoetharine, terbutaline, pirbuterol and bitolterol. These drugs differ primarily in their duration of action, with salmeterol acting longer than the others. All of these drugs except salmeterol are used to resolve an acute attack of bronchoconstriction, that is, narrowing of airways that causes shortness of breath. Salmeterol should be used for prevention of attacks. Epinephrine, isoproterenol, and ephedrine are drugs that produce bronchodilation similarly to the β_2 agonists, but they act on more than just the lungs. This lack of selectivity increases the number of side effects these agents cause. Epinephrine and ephedrine are available in over-the-counter formulations but should not be used without medical supervision. Since asthma, emphysema, and bronchitis are serious diseases, self-treatment is not recommended.

The xanthines are another class of bronchodilators. The exact mechanism of action of these drugs is not known, but may be related to an anti-inflammatory effect. The xanthines most commonly used are aminophylline and theophylline. Aminophylline is a salt of theophylline. If theophylline is substituted for aminophylline, the dose should be 80% of the aminophylline dose.

Theophylline has a high incidence of side effects that often occur at therapeutic doses. Nausea and vomiting are common. Other side effects include irritability, restlessness, headache, insomnia, muscle twitching, and rapid heartbeat. Too much xanthine in the blood after rapid intravenous injection or excessive doses can lead to serious side effects, such as causing the heart to stop or beat irregularly and seizures.

The metabolism of theophylline varies greatly from patient to patient, which means the amount of theophylline a patient needs also varies. Age, diet, smoking, other medications, and illnesses are all factors that can change the amount of theophylline a patient needs to achieve and maintain therapeutic theophylline blood concentrations. Blood levels are often measured periodically to ensure that patients achieve and maintain therapeutic concentrations.

Theophylline and aminophylline are available in many dosage forms. Theophylline is the drug most commonly used orally, although it can be given intravenously. It is usually given in sustained-release forms but is also available in regular-release oral liquids, tablets, and capsules. Aminophylline is the drug most commonly used intravenously. It is also available as oral tablets and liquids and as a rectal suppository.

Anticholinergic drugs are the third class of bronchodilators. These drugs act on different nerves than the β_2 agonists but have the same result of relaxing the muscles in the airways. The anticholinergic drugs are more useful in chronic obstructive pulmonary disease than in asthma, but patients with either disease can benefit from them. Combined use with a β_2 agonist may increase the benefit. There are oral and inhaled formulations of anticholinergic agents. Because of the side effects associated with the oral formulations, such as atropine, the inhaled formulations (e.g., metered-dose inhalers and nebulization solutions) are commonly used. Atropine nebulization solution has been used as a bronchodilator for many years. However, since it is absorbed well through the airways, it causes systemic effects, such as flushing, dry mouth, difficulty urinating, constipation, rapid heart rate, and confusion, in addition to dilating the bronchioles. Ipratropium is a newer anticholinergic drug that has fewer systemic side effects. Ipratropium is available in metered-dose and nebulization formulations.

Since asthma is an inflammatory reaction, preventing or reducing the inflammation can eliminate or lessen the severity of acute asthma attacks. Corticosteroids, cromolyn sodium, and nedocromil sodium are often used for this purpose.

Cromolyn sodium and nedocromil sodium are used to prevent asthma attacks. They are not useful for resolving acute asthma attacks. Adverse reactions are rare but include irritation and dryness of the throat, cough, and bronchospasm (spasmodic narrowing of the airways). These drugs may take up to 8 weeks to be effective. These drugs are especially effective for asthma in children. Cromolyn is available as a solution for nebulizers, as a metered-dose inhaler, and as a capsule used in a special inhaler device. An oral capsule form is available but is not indicated for respiratory diseases. The oral capsule and the capsule for the inhaler are not interchangeable. Nedocromil is available as a metered dose inhaler.

Corticosteroids are used to prevent acute asthma attacks and, in combination with bronchodilators, to interrupt ongoing acute attacks. The inhaled route of administration is useful in pulmonary diseases to prevent the numerous side effects these drugs can cause when given systemically (see Musculoskeletal System). Inhaled corticosteroids can suppress the function of the adrenal gland, retard growth and cause bone loss in children, induce a hyperactive mental state, cause cataract formation in the eyes, cause fungal overgrowth in the throat and hoarseness. The latter two effects can be prevented by using a spacing device with the inhaler and rinsing the mouth with water after use. Corticosteroids available as metered-dose inhalers are beclomethasone, dexamethasone, triamcinolone, and flunisolide. Some patients may require oral corticosteroids to control their symptoms. Injectable corticosteroids are used in combination with β_2 agonists for acute attacks requiring emergency room treatment.

Patients with pulmonary diseases may use combinations of these drugs. Patients should be able to identify which inhalers are to prevent an attack (i.e., their "preventors") and which are to abort an acute attack (i.e., their "helpers"). If a corticosteroid and a bronchodilator inhaler are both used, it is recommended that the bronchodilator be used first to open up the airways to allow better penetration of the corticosteroid.

Antihistamines, Decongestants, Expectorants, and Antitussives

The common cold remains one of the most bothersome illnesses. More than 120 strains of viruses are responsible for causing the common cold. Most colds are self-limiting and can be self-treated. Treatment is aimed at reducing the symptoms: runny nose (rhinitis), sore throat (pharyngitis), and cough. These symptoms are produced by an inflammatory response of the lining of the nose, throat, and lungs to the viral invasion. Influenza (flu) viruses cause similar symptoms but may cause more damage to the lining of the respiratory tract. A lasting cough is common after the flu.

Many of the same symptoms occur with allergic rhinitis, a reaction of the nasal lining to allergic stimuli (called allergens). Similar products are used to treat symptoms of both diseases. Decongestants are used to reduce the swelling of the lining of the nose. Antihistamines prevent the release of histamine, which is responsible for symptoms of allergic rhinitis. Antitussives are drugs that reduce the frequency of cough. Expectorants are drugs used to decrease the thickness and ease expulsion of sputum from the lungs.

Decongestants can be used topically in the nose (see Intranasal Products) or taken orally. They constrict blood vessels in the nose, which decreases nasal swelling and congestion. Topical decongestants are often preferred because they reduce congestion better, last longer, and have fewer side effects than oral decongestants. However, when topical decongestants wear off, the returning congestion is usually worse than before the decongestant was used. This rebound congestion does not occur with oral decongestants. Patients with hypertension, heart disease, overactive thyroid, diabetes mellitus, or an enlarged prostate gland should not take oral decongestants and should use the topical formulation with caution. The oral decongestant drugs, phenylpropanolamine and pseudoephedrine, are available as sustained-release preparations and regular-release tablets. They are available in many over-the-counter cold, sinus, and allergy preparations and are frequently combined with antihistamines, expectorants, and antitussives.

During the initial part of an allergic reaction, cells release histamine. Antihistamines block the body's response to histamine and thus reduce or prevent symptoms of allergic rhinitis, such as sneezing, nasal congestion, mucus secretion, and itching and tearing of the eyes. Reducing mucus secretion is a side effect of antihistamines. However, antihistamines often help stop the runny nose associated with a common cold because of the side effect.

Antihistamines have many side effects. The side effect that concerns most people is drowsiness. This effect varies among antihistamines and is the reason they are sometimes used as sleep aids. In children and the elderly, a paradoxical reaction, excitation rather than drowsiness, is sometimes seen. Anticholinergic effects such as dry mouth, blurred vision, difficulty urinating, and constipation occur with many antihistamines. Patients with glaucoma, peptic ulcer, or an enlarged prostate gland should avoid most antihistamines. Astemizole, loratadine, and fexofenadine do not cross into the central nervous system and are not sedating. Some serious drug interactions are possible with astemizole.

Many antihistamines are available over the counter and in combination with decongestants, expectorants, and antitussives. Promethazine, hydroxyzine, and cyproheptadine require a prescription, as do the nonsedating antihistamines.

Cough can be classified as productive or nonproductive depending on whether or not phlegm is expectorated with the cough.[4] A productive cough is helpful if it removes phlegm from the airways. This type of cough should only be treated if the coughing is frequent enough to disturb sleep or is unbearable to the patient. A nonproductive cough without chest congestion can be treated with an antitussive (cough suppressant). A nonproductive cough with chest congestion can be treated with an expectorant to try to facilitate the expectoration of phlegm. Persistent cough or any cough with chest congestion could indicate a serious condition such as asthma or pneumonia.

Antitussives are drugs that reduce the frequency of cough. Codeine, hydrocodone, dextromethorphan, and diphenhydramine suppress the cough center in the brain. Codeine and hydrocodone are narcotic drugs that can depress breathing and have addiction potential. Their most common side effects in doses used for cough suppression are nausea, drowsiness, lightheadedness, and constipation. Dextromethorphan is chemically related to codeine and has similar antitussive efficacy but does not have pain-relieving properties, cause respiratory

depression, or have addictive potential. It is widely used in over-the-counter cough medicines instead of narcotics because of these advantages. Drowsiness and gastrointestinal upset are the most common side effects. Diphenhydramine is an effective cough suppressant that is used in many over-the-counter cough and cold remedies. The sedative and anticholinergic side effects of this drug are discussed with the antihistamines.

Expectorants are controversial because there is little scientific evidence to show that they effectively decrease the thickness of phlegm and thus aid in its expectoration, which may indirectly treat a cough. Guaifenesin is the only expectorant recognized as safe and effective by the FDA.[2] Other agents require more testing to draw sound conclusions. Increased intake of fluids and humidification of air may be effective in treating cough.

Guaifenesin is available over the counter as a single drug and in combination with bronchodilators, antihistamines, decongestants, and antitussives. It is available in liquid forms and as regular- and sustained-release capsules and tablets. There are no absolute contraindications to the use of guaifenesin. Nausea and vomiting, dizziness, headache, and rash are rare side effects. It is recommended that patients drink plenty of fluids, since fluid intake is important in decreasing the viscosity of phlegm.

Other expectorants are ammonium chloride, iodides, and terpin hydrate. The first two of these may have serious side effects if over used. All of these have questionable effectiveness.[2]

CARDIOVASCULAR SYSTEM

The major components of the cardiovascular system are the heart and the blood vessels. The right side of the heart pumps blood to the lungs where carbon dioxide is exchanged for oxygen. The left side of the heart then pumps the oxygenated blood throughout the body. Blood is pumped away from the heart through large arteries into progressively smaller vessels until it reaches the smallest vessels, the capillaries. At the capillary level, nutrients and oxygen are provided to tissues and waste products and carbon dioxide are picked up. Blood then flows into larger vessels again, the veins, until it returns to the right side of the heart. The heart itself is muscle tissue in need of oxygen and nutrients, which are supplied by the coronary arteries.

Common diseases of the cardiovascular system are angina pectoris, heart attack, and stroke. Angina pectoris is characterized by episodes of chest pain caused by decreased oxygen supply to heart muscle. Heart attack (myocardial infarction) occurs when heart muscle dies from lack of oxygen. A stroke is most often caused by blockage of the arteries supplying the brain with blood and oxygen. The area of the brain that is deprived of oxygen is damaged. Less often, stroke may be caused by bleeding that occurs in the brain. Atherosclerosis, the deposition of fatty plaques in the blood vessels, leads to narrowing of these vessels and subsequent reduction in the volume of oxygen-carrying blood they deliver to the heart and/or brain. Thus atherosclerosis can result in angina pectoris, heart attack, or stroke. High blood cholesterol is a significant risk factor for atherosclerosis, angina pectoris, heart attack, and stroke.

Hypertension is high blood pressure, an increase in the pressure the blood exerts on the blood vessels as it circulates. Although hypertension rarely produces any symptoms in patients, when it remains untreated, it is a major cause of heart disease and stroke by worsening atherosclerosis and stimulating an increase in heart size.

Arrhythmias are disturbances in the conduction of nerve impulses in the heart that disrupt the rhythm or rate of heart muscle contraction. When the heart rate is too fast, too slow, or irregular inadequate amounts of blood are pumped.

Antihyperlipidemic Agents

Heart attack and stroke are caused by blockage of blood vessels to the heart and brain. Hyperlipidemia, increased levels of cholesterol in the blood, is a risk factor in the development of these diseases. Lowering of blood cholesterol has been shown to decrease the number of people who die from strokes and heart attacks.

Cholesterol and triglycerides are the fats implicated in heart disease. Cholesterol is measured as total cholesterol; low density lipoprotein (LDL), the so-called "bad" cholesterol; and high density lipoprotein (HDL), the "good" cholesterol. Drugs have differing effects on these various components of blood cholesterol and triglycerides. Drugs are selected based on the type of fats that are elevated as well as the side effect profiles of the drugs.

Initially, hyperlipidemia is treated with diet and exercise. If these methods fail, drugs may be added. The agents used today are bile acid sequestrants, hydroxymethylglutaryl coenzyme A (HMG-CoA) reductase inhibitors, clofibrate, gemfibrozil, and nicotinic acid. Since drug therapy always has unwanted effects, the patient's risk factors for heart disease and degree of blood cholesterol elevation are considered before drug treatment is started.

Bile Acid Sequestrants

Bile is secreted by the liver and gallbladder into the intestine to aid the absorption of fats from food in the intestines. The bile secreted into the intestine is reabsorbed back into the blood. Bile acid sequestrants bind the bile in the intestines and prevent it from being reabsorbed. Instead, it is excreted in the feces. The loss of bile stimulates production of more bile, which requires cholesterol. Since the body uses cholesterol to make more bile, which is then bound and excreted, this cycle leads to a decrease in LDL and total cholesterol. The bile acid sequestrants are cholestyramine and colestipol. The most common side effects with these drugs are constipation, aggravation of hemorrhoids, abdominal cramping, gas, nausea and vomiting, diarrhea, and heartburn. These effects often disappear with continued use. Patients who take bile acid sequestrants can have abnormal liver function tests. This does not necessarily indicate liver damage, but the drug is often discontinued if this occurs. Tablet forms of these drugs are available, but for convenience these drugs are usually given as a powder mixed in juice. If insufficient fluid is given with the bile acid sequestrants, they can form a solid mass in the esophagus or the intestines resulting in blockage of these parts of the digestive tract. In the same way that these drugs bind bile acids, they can also bind other medications. Other drugs should be taken 1 hour before or 4 to 6 hours after the bile acid sequestrants. Cholesterol can be decreased further when these drugs are combined with HMG-CoA reductase inhibitors or nicotinic acid (niacin).

HMG-CoA Reductase Inhibitors

Much of the cholesterol in the body is not ingested as cholesterol but is made in the body from fats. This is the basis of the dietary recommendations to avoid not only foods high in cholesterol but foods high in fat. The HMG-CoA reductase inhibitors prevent the formation of cholesterol from fats. They effectively increase the good cholesterol, HDL, and decrease the bad cholesterol, LDL, as well as decreasing total cholesterol and triglycerides. The most common side effects are muscle and joint pain, headache, and gastrointestinal distress. The most serious effects include abnormalities of liver function tests, although liver damage does not usually occur. A more serious muscle disease, rhabdomyolysis, can occur, usually in patients taking these drugs in combination with other drugs. These drugs may cause increased sensitivity to sunlight. Sunscreen should be used when exposure to the sun cannot be avoided.

The drugs in this class are lovastatin, simvastatin, pravastatin, fluvastatin, and atorvastatin. Lovastatin should be taken with meals, but the others may be taken without regard to meals. Atorvastatin is more effective than the other drugs at lowering triglycerides.[2]

Other Lipid-lowering Agents

Clofibrate lowers LDL and total cholesterol but is more useful for its triglyceride-lowering effect. The mechanism of action is unknown. The most common side effects are nausea and other gastrointestinal symptoms, muscle and joint aches, skin rash, fatigue, and weakness. More serious effects are a possible increased risk of liver cancer, gallstones, and decreased white and/or red blood cells.

Gemfibrozil decreases triglycerides and raises HDL. Its effects on total cholesterol and LDL vary. Common adverse effects are GI symptoms, dizziness, blurred vision, fatigue, and taste disturbances. Like clofibrate, gemfibrozil may be associated with increased risk of liver cancer and gallstones. When given with HMG-CoA reductase inhibitors, a form of muscle breakdown may rarely occur.

Nicotinic acid (niacin) is a form of vitamin B that reduces serum cholesterol and triglycerides. Another form of this vitamin, nicotinamide (niacinamide), does not affect blood cholesterol levels. The most bothersome adverse effect of nicotinic acid is a flushing sensation or a feeling of warmth, as well as itching, tingling, or headache. An aspirin tablet 30 minutes before the niacin dose can alleviate this effect. GI upset can also occur. More serious effects include abnormal liver function tests. Liver damage is more likely to occur with sustained-release preparations. Decreased blood pressure can occur, causing dizziness, especially upon suddenly rising to a sitting or standing position. Larger doses are needed for treatment of high blood cholesterol than for vitamin supplementation.

Antihypertensives

When the heart pumps blood through the blood vessels, the blood exerts pressure on the walls of the blood vessels. This is blood pressure. The pressure is highest when the heart squeezes blood out and lower when the heart rests. This is why blood pressure is expressed with two numbers (130/90). The systolic pressure is the higher number and represents the pressure during heart contraction. The diastolic pressure is the lower number and represents the pressure when the heart is resting and filling. Some factors that affect blood pressure are constriction or dilation of blood vessels, the volume of blood in the vessels, and the rate and strength of heart contractions.

High blood pressure can be caused by other diseases or medications, but 90% of high blood pressure is essential hypertension, of unknown cause.[6] Hypertension usually has no symptoms but is important to treat because it is a risk factor for heart attack and stroke. Additionally, untreated hypertension can lead to blindness, kidney damage, and blood vessel diseases that affect the arms, hands, legs, and feet. Compliance with medication regimens is a problem in hypertension because patients have no symptoms. Patients may actually feel worse with medication because they were never aware of their hypertension and now have side effects from the drugs. They may also see no reason to continue medication because they don't feel any different when they take it.

Like hyperlipidemia, the primary treatment for hypertension is lifestyle changes such as diet, weight loss (if overweight), and exercise. If these changes do not control blood pressure, then drug therapy may be indicated in addition to these changes.

There are many classes of drugs used to treat hypertension. Diuretics and beta-blockers have been shown in controlled studies to reduce the number of people who die from heart attacks and strokes.[6] Angiotensin converting enzyme inhibitors (ACE inhibitors), calcium channel blockers, and alpha-blockers are other drugs that have advantages in certain types of patients. Other agents used are central alpha-2-agonists, peripheral adrenergic antagonists, and direct vasodilators.

Diuretics

Diuretics decrease blood pressure by decreasing the blood volume. They are commonly called water pills and work on the kidneys to increase urinary excretion of sodium, chloride, and water. Since all diuretics increase urination, they should be taken as early in the day as possible so that the need to urinate does not interrupt the patient's sleep.

There are three types of diuretics used to treat hypertension: thiazides, loop diuretics, and potassium-sparing diuretics. Thiazide diuretics in low doses are usually effective for hypertension. Loop diuretics are more effective in patients with mild kidney failure. Potassium-sparing diuretics are weak diuretics but are often added to other diuretics to prevent potassium loss. Both the thiazide and loop diuretics cause decreased potassium in the body. Potassium is essential for nerve conduction and muscle contraction throughout the body and in the heart. Potassium-sparing diuretics, as their name implies, do not decrease potassium.

Commonly used thiazide diuretics are hydrochlorothiazide, indapamide, metolazone, and chlorthalidone. Metolazone and indapamide may be more effective in patients with mild kidney failure. Potassium loss caused by diuretics may require potassium supplements. Blood glucose control in diabetics may be altered by thiazide diuretics. Patients who are taking thiazide diuretics may be more sensitive to sun, so they should be warned to avoid exposure or use sunscreen. Drug interactions may occur, usually because of changes in excretion of drugs or changes in the electrolytes (chemical salts) in the body. Patients allergic to sulfonamides may also be allergic to thiazide diuretics.

Loop diuretics are more potent diuretics and may affect electrolytes such as sodium, potassium, chloride, calcium, and magnesium to a greater degree than the thiazides. Commonly used drugs are furosemide, ethacrynic acid, bumetanide, and torsemide. Adverse effects similar to those of the thiazides may occur, including altered blood glucose control in diabetics, sun sensitivity, drug interactions, and allergic reactions in sulfonamide-allergic patients. Hearing loss and kidney damage have occurred. Hearing loss is most likely in patients using high doses, in patients with kidney failure, in patients taking other drugs that cause hearing damage (such as aminoglycoside antibiotics), and in patients who receive furosemide by rapid injection.

Potassium-sparing diuretics used alone do not cause potassium loss like the other diuretics. Commonly used drugs are spironolactone, amiloride, and triamterene. Used alone, they may cause increased potassium levels in patients with kidney failure or who are taking other drugs, such as ACE inhibitors, that decrease potassium excretion. Increased potassium levels, like decreased levels, can adversely affect the heart. Potassium-sparing diuretics are often used with other diuretics to combine the greater potency of a loop or thiazide diuretic with their potassium-sparing effects. Combination drugs are Dyazide®, Maxzide®, Moduretic®, and Aldactazide®.

Beta-blockers

Beta-blockers block the action of certain nerves in cardiac muscle, lungs, and the smooth muscles of the blood vessels. As a result, the heart rate decreases, heart muscle contraction is less forceful, the airways in the lungs constrict, and the dilation of blood vessels is blocked. They lower high blood pressure by decreasing the volume of blood pumped by each contraction of the heart. Beta-blockers are first-line drugs for treatment of hypertension and, like diuretics, have been shown to reduce the number of people who die from heart attack or stroke. They have many other indications, including angina pectoris, cardiac rhythm disturbances, heart attack, migraine headache, tremor, and anxiety.

Beta-blockers that are more selective for the nerves in the heart are called cardioselective. These drugs are metoprolol, acebutalol, bisoprolol, esmolol, betaxolol, and atenolol. The selectivity is dose dependent and action on the nerves in the lungs and blood vessels may also occur with these drugs at higher doses. The noncardioselective drugs are propranolol, pindolol, carteolol, nadolol, penbutolol, sotalol, timolol, and labetalol.

Beta-blockers should usually be avoided in conditions in which the heart rate is slow, in the presence of lung diseases such as asthma or chronic obstructive pulmonary disease, and in the presence of diseases in which the blood supply to the extremities (hands, feet, arms, and legs) is insufficient. Beta-blockers also block the symptoms of low blood sugar, which can be life threatening. Therefore, diabetics should not take beta-blockers because they would not be able to tell if their blood sugar was dangerously low. Beta-blockers may increase blood cholesterol. Undesirable side effects include central nervous system effects such as dizziness, tiredness, and depression. Some patients may develop tingling,

Table 6–2

Commonly Prescribed Drugs

Trade Name	Generic Name	Trade Name	Generic Name
Amoxil, Trimox	Amoxicillin	Micronase, Diabeta Glynase	Glyburide
Ativan	Lorazepam		
Atrovent	Ipratropium	Motrin, Nuprin, Advil	Ibuprofen
Augmentin	Amoxicillin and Clavulanic acid	Naprosyn	Naproxen
		Nitrostat	Nitroglycerin
Axid	Nizatidine	Norvasc	Amlodipine
Bactrim, Septra	Sulfamethoxazole/ trimethoprim	Ortho-Novum 7/7/7	Norethindrone/ethinyl estradiol
Biaxin	Clarithromycin	Paxil	Paroxetine
Calan, Isoptin, Verelan	Verapamil	Pepcid	Famotidine
		Pravachol	Pravastatin
Capoten	Captopril	Premarin	Conjugated Estrogens
Cardizem	Diltiazem	Prilosec	Omeprazole
Ceclor	Cefaclor	Procardia	Nifedipine
Ceftin	Cefuroxime Axetil	Proventil, Ventolin	Albuterol
Cipro	Ciprofloxacin	Provera	Medroxyprogesterone
Claritin	Loratidine	Prozac	Fluoxetine
Coumadin	Warfarin	Relafen	Nabumetone
Darvocet N	Propoxyphene napsylate with acetaminophen	Synthroid	Levothyroxine
		Tagamet	Cimetidine
Dilantin	Phenytoin	Timoptic	Timolol (ophthalmic)
Duricef	Cefadroxil	Toradol	Ketorolac
Dyazide	Triamterene/ hydrochlorothiazide	Triphasil	Levonorgestrel/ethinyl estradiol
Ery-tab, E-mycin, PCE	Erythromycin	Tylenol with Codeine	Acetaminophen with Codeine
Estraderm	Estradiol (patch)		
Glucotrol	Glipizide	Vasotec	Enalapril
Hytrin	Terazosin	Veetids, Pen-Vee-K	Penicillin V Potassium
K-dur, Micro-K, Slow K	Potassium Chloride	Vicodin, Lortab	Hydrocodone with acetaminophen
Keflex	Cephalexin		
Klonopin	Clonazepam	Voltaren	Diclofenac
Lanoxin	Digoxin	Xanax	Alprazolam
Lasix	Furosemide	Zantac	Ranitidine
Lodine	Etodolac	Zestril, Prinivil	Lisinopril
Lopressor	Metoprolol	Zoloft	Sertraline
Mevacor	Lovastatin	Zovirax	Acyclovir

Adapted From: *Blue Book, Essential Directory of Pharmaceuticals.* New York: Hearst Corporation; 1995.

loss of sensation, or intolerability to cold in the hands and feet. Weight gain or loss and impotence are also possible.

As with all drugs for hypertension, compliance is very important. Patients who receive counseling about their disease and medication are more likely to be compliant with their drug and dietary regimens. Beta-blockers should not be abruptly discontinued. Patients should be screened for potential drug interactions as well

as for drug-disease contraindications, such as diabetes, asthma, COPD, heart failure, and high blood cholesterol.

Metoprolol, propranolol, and labetolol are available as oral and injectable preparations. Esmolol is only available as an injection. All the other agents are available for oral use. A few beta-blockers are available as ophthalmic products for the treatment of glaucoma (see the section on ophthalmic products).

ACE Inhibitors

Angiotensin-converting enzyme inhibitors (ACE inhibitors) prevent the production of certain chemicals in the blood that cause the constriction of blood vessels and retention of sodium and water. By blocking blood vessel constriction and salt and water retention, these drugs can lower blood pressure. Like the beta-blockers, they have many other uses. ACE inhibitors may slow or prevent the development of kidney disease in diabetic patients and increase survival, alleviate symptoms to some extent, and decrease hospitalization in patients with heart failure.

Adverse reactions to ACE inhibitors are uncommon and usually mild. Some patients experience temporary dizziness and fainting when they begin therapy. ACE inhibitors can also cause skin rashes, abnormal taste in the mouth, potassium retention, and a bothersome dry cough that can lead to discontinuation of the medication. Patients who are taking potassium supplements may no longer need them when they begin ACE inhibitors.

More serious side effects include an allergic reaction characterized by swelling of the face, lips, extremities, tongue, and throat. If the swelling is in the throat, it can be fatal. Although ACE inhibitors are used to treat or prevent kidney disease in some patients, they can also cause kidney disease in a small number of patients. ACE inhibitors should not be used in pregnant women; they can cause injury or death to the fetus.

Calcium Channel Blockers

The movement of calcium in and out of cells is essential to nerve conduction and muscle contraction. Calcium channel blockers inhibit this movement. The result is a decreased force of contraction of the heart, blocked contraction of smooth muscle in the blood vessels resulting in dilation of blood vessels, and slowed conduction of nerve impulses throughout the heart resulting in a slowed heart rate. The drugs in this class vary in the selectivity of their actions on heart rate, blood vessel dilation, or heart contraction.

Calcium channel blockers are first-line agents for hypertension but are also used for angina pectoris, heart rhythm disturbances, migraine headache, and diseases of the heart muscle. One drug, nimodipine, has a special indication for reducing nerve damage caused by bleeding in the brain, which is called subarachnoid hemorrhage.

The drugs in this class are grouped by their chemical structure. In general, drugs with similar structure have similar uses and side effects.

Verapamil is an example of a phenylalkylamine structural type of calcium channel blocker. It can be given by mouth or injected. It is used to treat angina, hypertension, arrhythmias, migraine headache, and cardiomyopathy, a degenerative disease of heart muscle. Patients who are taking beta-blockers or digoxin can experience problems taking verapamil because it may slow the heart down too much. Verapamil should also be avoided in patients who have heart failure. Adverse reactions include dizziness, headache, and constipation. Verapamil must be give three times daily, so sustained-release forms are often used to simplify dosing to once daily.

Diltiazem is a benzothiazepine structural type of calcium channel blocker. It affects heart rate and heart contraction less than verapamil. It is most often used to treat angina pectoris and hypertension. Like verapamil, diltiazem can slow the heart rate excessively, especially when given with beta-blockers or digoxin. It should also be used with caution in patients who have heart failure. Adverse effects include dizziness, headache, and occasionally swelling of the legs or feet. Diltiazem must be taken three times a day, although sustained-release forms allow for once- or twice-daily dosing. An injectable form is available for treating rapid heart rate. An intravenous bolus dose is given and can be followed by an intravenous infusion for continued reduction of heart rate.

Amlodipine, felodipine, isradipine, nicardipine, nifedipine, nimodipine, and nisoldipine are calcium channel blockers of the dihydropyridine structural group. These drugs have little or no effect on the nerve impulse conduction in the heart but can cause an increase in heart rate as a reflex reaction to their greater effect in dilating blood vessels. These drugs have less effect on heart contraction and can be used with caution in patients who have heart failure. They are used to treat angina and hypertension. Nifedipine has been used for migraine headaches, cardiomyopathy, and Raynaud's syndrome. Nimodipine is used mainly for subarachnoid hemorrhage, as mentioned above, and for migraine headache. Adverse effects include dizziness, headache, swelling of the legs or feet, rapid heartbeat, and flushing.

All of the dihydropyridine drugs are available in oral dosage forms. Nifedipine is available as a liquid-filled capsule. Although the capsule has been punctured and swallowed or squirted under the tongue to quickly treat dangerously high blood pressure, recent research demonstrates that the drug is not absorbed from under the tongue.[2] The safety of rapidly lowering high blood pressure with this medicine is questionable, according to recent research.[8] Felodipine and amlodipine are eliminated from the body slowly and can be used once daily without sustained-release forms. Nicardipine is available for oral use and as an injection.

Miscellaneous Anti-hypertensives

The alpha-1 blockers, alpha-2 agonists, peripheral acting adrenergics, and direct vasodilators are other classes of drugs used to treat hypertension. They act through various effects on nerve pathways to dilate the blood vessels and reduce blood pressure. All of these drugs except hydralazine and minoxidil frequently cause postural hypotension. Because these drugs block the ability of blood vessels to constrict, people who take them often get dizzy or feel faint when they stand up after sitting or sit up after lying down. This is called postural hypotension.

The alpha-1 blockers are doxazosin, prazosin, and terazosin. In addition to postural hypotension, they can cause weakness, rapid heartbeat, and headache.

The alpha-2 agonists are clonidine, guanabenz, guanfacine, and methyldopa. Common side effects in addition to postural hypotension are drowsiness, sedation, dry mouth, and fatigue. Clonidine is available as a patch that is changed weekly. The Catapres-TTS® patch system consists of an active patch containing drug and an inactive overlay; both patches must be dispensed. The patient must be taught to apply the patches properly, being sure to use both. Since the patches are only changed weekly, a patient would go a full week without medicine if the inactive overlay were applied alone.

The peripherally acting adrenergics are guanadrel, guanethidine, and reserpine. In addition to postural hypotension, guanadrel and guanethidine can cause diarrhea. Reserpine can cause lethargy, nasal congestion, and mental depression.

The direct vasodilators hydralazine and minoxidil can cause headache, rapid heartbeat, and fluid retention. They are usually used with a beta-blocker to counteract the rapid heartbeat and a diuretic to counteract the fluid retention. It is rare, but hydralazine can cause drug-induced lupus erythematosus. Symptoms associated with lupus erythematosus include joint pain, rash, fever, enlarged spleen, and kidney dysfunction. This syndrome usually regresses when the drug is discontinued. Hydralazine is available for oral or injectable use. Minoxidil was found to increase the growth of body hair in patients and is now available as a topical product (Rogaine®) for stimulating hair growth in people with balding or thinning hair.

Drugs Used for Angina Pectoris

Angina pectoris is chest pain of short duration that is due to a lack of oxygen in the cardiac muscle cells. The pain subsides when the imbalance between the amount of oxygen needed by the cells and the amount of oxygen supplied to the cells is corrected. The pain of angina pectoris may not be limited to the chest. The pain is frequently felt in the arm or neck, usually on the left side of the body. An acute angina pectoris attack not relieved within 30 minutes by the use of two or three nitroglycerin tablets should receive medical attention for possible heart attack. Drugs used to treat angina pectoris include those used to abort an acute attack and those used on a daily basis to prevent attacks. Such drugs include nitrates, beta-blockers, and calcium channel blockers.

Nitrates

The nitrates are the most commonly used medicines for treating angina pectoris. Nitrates help resolve acute angina attacks by increasing the amount of oxygen delivered to the heart and by decreasing the oxygen needs of the heart. The amount of oxygen needed by heart muscles depends mainly on the workload of the heart. Nitrates decrease the workload by reducing the amount of blood presented to the heart and the pressure the heart must pump against. This is accomplished by dilating the arterial and venous blood vessels. Dilating the coronary arteries also allows more oxygen to flow to the heart. Pumping less blood against a lower pressure and delivering a larger supply of oxygen to the heart balance the oxygen demand and supply and may resolve the acute angina attack.

Nitrates are available in many dosage forms. For acute attacks, sublingual tablets, inhalants, translingual (on or under the tongue) spray, and buccal tablets are used. In the hospital setting, nitroglycerin may be used as an intravenous infusion. For prophylaxis of angina, oral sustained-release tablets and capsules, oral regular-release tablets and capsules, topical ointment, and transdermal patches are used. The nitrates used are amyl nitrate (inhalant only), nitroglycerin, isosorbide dinitrate, isosorbide mononitrate, erythritol tetranitrate, and pentaerythritol tetranitrate.

An important concern in choosing dosage forms and dosage regimens for nitrates is the development of tolerance. After 24 hours of continuous therapy, nitrates no longer work. Increasing the dose does not restore efficacy, but a nitrate-free period does. For this reason, nitrates are not usually dosed around the clock. Regular-release tablets may be given between 8 a.m. and 7 p.m. with no drug given at night. Long-acting tablets and capsules may be given orally once daily or at 8 a.m. and 2 p.m. Isosorbide mononitrate regular release is frequently given as two doses 7 hours apart during the day. Nitroglycerin patches are often applied in the morning and removed at night. All of these schedules provide a nitrate-free period at night.

Common side effects of nitrates include headaches, postural hypotension, dizziness, or flushing. Headache may be an indicator of the drug's activity and may be treated with aspirin or acetaminophen.

Patients should be provided with instructions on the use of the various dosage forms. They need to understand which products to use routinely and which to use for an acute attack. The importance of the dosage schedule to prevent tolerance must also be understood.

Beta-blockers

Beta-blocking agents, discussed in more detail under antihypertensive agents, are also used to prevent angina attacks. By decreasing blood pressure, slowing the heart rate, and decreasing the force of the heart contraction, they decrease the heart's demand for oxygen. This effect makes the existing supply of oxygen closer to adequate. Both cardioselective and non-cardioselective beta-blockers are effective for angina prophylaxis.

Calcium Channel Blockers

Calcium channel blockers, also discussed under antihypertensive agents, are used to prevent angina attacks. They reduce the heart's demand for oxygen by decreasing blood pressure and reducing the contractile force of the heart. They may also dilate the vessels that supply blood to the heart. Thus, they may increase oxygen supply and decrease oxygen demand in the heart. These drugs must be chosen carefully based upon the patient's condition because of the ability of some dihydropyridine calcium channel blockers to increase heart rate and of diltiazem and verapamil to decrease the force of heart contraction.

One other drug commonly used in patients with angina is aspirin. In doses from 81 mg to 325 mg daily, it is prescribed for patients to prevent heart attacks. Heart attacks involve the formation of a clot in an already-narrowed blood vessel supplying the heart. Aspirin inhibits the aggregation of certain blood cells called platelets, preventing clot formation.

Cardiac Glycosides and Drugs Used for Heart Failure

Heart failure is a condition in which the heart does not function adequately as a pump. Symptoms of weakness and fatigue result from an inadequate oxygen supply to tissues. When the left side of the heart cannot pump all the blood presented to it, fluid backs up into the lungs, causing shortness of breath and cough. With reduced pumping of blood, less blood is presented to the kidneys. The end result is retention of fluid and sodium causing weight gain and swelling in the legs and feet. These symptoms may be mild to severe depending upon the degree to which the pumping ability of the heart is decreased.

Like many cardiac diseases, diet modification is part of the treatment. Fluid restriction and a low sodium diet will be prescribed to reduce the amount of fluid retention.

Drug therapy includes several types of drugs: ACE inhibitors, the combination of hydralazine and isosorbide dinitrate, diuretics, beta-blockers, and cardiac glycosides. The choice of drugs will be based upon the severity of disease and the symptoms the patient experiences. An ACE inhibitor, discussed under antihypertensive agents, is the first drug used in most patients. They are useful for patients with mild to severe disease. In patients with mild disease and no symptoms, they have been shown to reduce mortality and worsening of disease. The combination of hydralazine and isosorbide dilates both arterial and venous blood vessels like the ACE inhibitors do. This combination is used in patients who cannot take ACE inhibitors.

Diuretics are used to reduce fluid retention in patients with fluid overload. Beta-blockers were previously thought to be contraindicated in heart failure but have been found to have a role in some patients. The role of cardiac glycosides is not well defined presently, but they have been shown to increase the force of heart muscle contraction in selected patients.[5]

Cardiac glycosides have been used for over 200 years to treat heart failure and are still recommended for patients with symptomatic disease. The three currently available cardiac glycosides are digoxin, deslanoside, and digitoxin. Digitoxin and deslanoside are rarely used. Digitoxin differs mainly in its onset, length of action, and route of elimination from the body. Its actions are otherwise similar to digoxin.

Digoxin acts on both the heart muscle and the nerve conduction system of the heart. It increases the rate and force of heart muscle contractions. It slows the conduction of the nerve impulses that prompt contraction of the heart muscle. The end result is improved pumping of blood and a slower heart rate. Digoxin is used to treat heart failure and rhythm disturbances of the heart.

Digoxin has serious toxicities. Effects on nerve impulses in the heart can cause rhythm disturbances that can be fatal. The difference between a therapeutic and a toxic dose of digoxin is relatively small. Therefore, digoxin blood levels are monitored to help ensure safe dosing. Patients or caregivers should be aware of the early symptoms of toxicity: loss of appetite, nausea, vomiting, diarrhea, headache, weakness, confusion, and visual disturbances (particularly blurred vision, yellow or green vision, or a halo effect). An antidote, digoxin immune fab, is administered intravenously to treat life-threatening digoxin intoxication.

Digoxin is available as an injection, a tablet, an elixir, and a capsule. The amount absorbed from the different preparations varies, so the dose may need to be adjusted when dosage forms are switched. Since the amount absorbed from different brands can also vary, patients should always use the same brand. A loading dose may be given for more immediate effects, but loading doses increase the risk of toxicity. Many drug interactions are possible that result in increased or decreased blood levels of digoxin.

Antiarrhythmics

Disturbances in the rate or rhythm of the heartbeat are called arrhythmias. Arrhythmias are often classified by where they occur in the heart. Common arrhythmias originating in the upper chambers of the heart, the atria, are atrial fibrillation and atrial flutter. Common arrhythmias occurring in the lower chambers of the heart, the ventricles, are premature ventricular contractions, ventricular tachycardia, ventricular fibrillation, and torsades de pointes. The atrial ventricular (AV) node is the point at which nerve impulses are conducted from the atria to the ventricles. A common rhythm disturbance at the AV node is called heartblock. Arrhythmias may cause too rapid, too slow, or unsynchronized heart muscle contractions. The result is a decrease in the amount of blood pumped by the heart. Symptoms include dizziness, fatigue, and palpitation (forcible and rapid heartbeats that are usually noticed by the patient).

Antiarrhythmic drugs are classified according to their effects on the conduction of impulses through the heart and their mechanism of action. Drug therapy of arrhythmias is limited by the serious toxicities associated with the drugs. Many of the drugs used to treat arrhythmias can also cause arrhythmias. Drug therapy is used only when patients have life-threatening arrhythmias or intolerable symptoms.

Class I, group IA, antiarrythmic drugs, quinidine, procainamide, and disopyramide, are used for both atrial and ventricular arrhythmias. They all affect cardiac nerve conduction in a similar way. Procainamide can be given as an intravenous infusion and orally. Quinidine is given by IM or IV injection or orally. Disopyramide is given orally. All of these drugs can cause arrhythmias. Severe gastrointestinal disturbances (e.g., nausea, vomiting, abdominal pain, and diarrhea) are common side effects of quinidine. When dispensing this drug, be careful not to use *quinine* by mistake. The milder side effects of procainamide include gastrointestinal side effects (similar to quinidine), dizziness, and mood changes. Procainamide has two serious side effects, lupus erythematosus and neutropenia. Lupus erythematosus is a syndrome of joint pain, rash, fever, and possible kidney dysfunction. Neutropenia is a decrease in white blood cells resulting in a higher susceptibility to infection. Side effects of disopyramide include dry mouth, difficulty urinating, dizziness, constipation, and blurred vision. The most serious side effects are low blood pressure and heart failure.

Another subset of class I antiarrhythmics, class IB, includes lidocaine, tocainide, and mexilitine. The anticonvulsant phenytoin can also be used as an antiarrhythmic drug and has properties similar to these drugs. Class IB drugs are useful for ventricular arrhythmias. Like the IA drugs, they can cause as well as treat arrhythmias. Lidocaine is given intravenously. Its side effects are related to its effects on the central nervous system: dizziness, confusion, mood changes, hallucination, drowsiness, vision disturbances, muscle twitching, and seizures. The side effects of tocainide are similar to lidocaine but it can also cause blood disorders and lung disease. The side effects of mexilitine are also similar to lidocaine, plus some gastrointestinal disturbances (e.g., nausea, vomiting, and heartburn).

Flecainide and propafenone are class IC antiarrhythmics. Drugs in this class have been found to increase mortality in patients with asymptomatic, non-life-threatening arrhythmias. These drugs are now used only to treat life-threatening ventricular arrhythmias and some life-threatening atrial arrhythmias. Both of these drugs are available only as oral dosage forms and have mild side effects that are similar: gastrointestinal disturbances (e.g., nausea, vomiting, taste disturbances), dizziness, tremor, and blurred vision.

Several beta-blockers, such as propranolol, esmolol, and acebutalol, have antiarrhythmic properties and are used as class II antiarrhythmics. They are described in more detail in the antihypertensive drugs section of this chapter.

The class III antiarrhythmics are bretylium, amiodarone, and sotalol. They are used to treat ventricular arrhythmias. Bretylium is given intravenously. Low blood pressure is common with bretylium, and nausea and vomiting may also occur. Adverse reactions are common with amiodarone. Less serious side effects are visual disturbances, increased sensitivity to sunlight, blue discoloration of the skin, fatigue, tremor, gastrointestinal disturbances (e.g., nausea, vomiting, constipation, loss of appetite), and changes in thyroid gland function. More serious side effects are microdeposits in the cornea of the eye resulting in visual halos or blurred vision, lung toxicity, and liver toxicity. Amiodarone is given both orally and intravenously, and dosing of both forms involves a higher initial loading dose and a lower maintenance dose. Sotalol is a beta-blocking drug with antiarrhythmic properties similar to bretylium and amiodarone. Sotalol is only given orally.

The calcium channel blocker verapamil is used as an antiarrhythmic drug. It is discussed in the antihypertensive agents section of this chapter.

Also, digoxin is used for atrial arrhythmias and is discussed in the cardiac glycosides section of this chapter.

Anticoagulants

Coagulation of blood (clot formation) is essential to prevent bleeding to death from cuts. But abnormal blood clot formation within blood vessels can cause heart attack, stroke, or pulmonary embolism (a blood clot in the lung), all potentially fatal conditions. Clots forming in the vessels that supply the heart with blood can result in heart attack. Blood clots forming in veins in the leg or in the upper chambers of the heart can migrate to the brain or lungs. Anticoagulants are used to prevent these potentially fatal clots from forming. Anticoagulants are commonly called blood thinners.

Heparin is the injectable drug used intravenously or subcutaneously to prevent clot formation. It is frequently given as an intravenous infusion. The dose is adjusted based on a blood test that measures its effectiveness. Because anticoagulants slow clot formation, the main concern with anticoagulant therapy is excessive bleeding. Blood tests are used to maintain a level of heparin that should prevent clot formation but not allow excessive bleeding. A possible adverse reaction to heparin is a decrease in the number of platelets, a type of blood cell involved with clot formation. A blood test is also used to monitor for this side effect. Intramuscular injections should be avoided while a patient is receiving heparin because of the possible development of small bleeds, hematomas, that could develop at the site of injection. When the effects of heparin need to be reversed, protamine sulfate can be given.

Recent additions to anticoagulant therapy in the United States are two low-molecular weight heparins, enoxaparin and dalteparin. These drugs are derived from heparin but have different actions on the clotting mechanism and more reliable activity by subcutaneous injection. They are currently used to prevent clot formation after orthopedic or abdominal surgeries but may be used for other purposes in the future. Bleeding and reduction in platelets may be less common with these drugs but can still occur. An advantage of these drugs is that it is not necessary to monitor blood tests as it is with heparin.

Warfarin is the most commonly used oral anticoagulant. The maximal effect of warfarin takes 3 to 5 days to occur, so heparin is often given until warfarin takes effect. When the full effect of warfarin is present, according to a blood test used to measure it, the heparin is discontinued. As with other anticoagulants, bleeding is the most serious adverse effect. Nausea, diarrhea, skin rashes, mouth ulcers, and red-orange urine are other effects that can be seen. Many drug interactions as well as changes in diet can alter the effectiveness of warfarin. Patients should always inform health professionals of all the drugs they take or have taken to avoid drug interactions. Patients should also be instructed to watch for signs of bleeding, to take their medication at the same time every day, to avoid major diet changes, and to have blood tests taken as instructed. The effects of warfarin can be reversed with vitamin K.

GASTROINTESTINAL SYSTEM

The function of the gastrointestinal system is to transfer nutrients from food into the body. The gastrointestinal system consists of the mouth, esophagus ("food pipe"), stomach, intestines, colon, rectum, gallbladder, biliary tract, liver, and pancreas. This section focuses on the mouth, esophagus, stomach, and intestines.

The digestion of food begins in the mouth. The food is physically broken down into smaller pieces when it is chewed. At the same time, enzymes in the saliva chemically break down the food. As the food is swallowed it passes through the esophagus to the stomach. In the stomach, acid and pepsin break down the food further. When the food is passed from the stomach to the intestines it continues to be broken down and the nutrients are absorbed. Nonabsorbable products, bacteria, and water pass through the intestine and are excreted as feces.

The most common disorders of the gastrointestinal system are peptic ulcer disease (PUD), gastroesophageal reflux disease (GERD), nausea and vomiting, diarrhea, constipation, and inflammatory bowel disease. Drugs used to treat peptic ulcer disease, gastroesophageal reflux disease, diarrhea, and constipation will be discussed. Drugs used to treat nausea and vomiting are discussed in the section on oncology.

Peptic ulcer disease and gastroesophageal reflux disease are both related to the acid secretion of the stomach. The lining of the stomach has several mechanisms to protect it from the digestive substances it secretes. Mucus acts as a physical barrier between the stomach acid and the stomach lining. Cells of the stomach secrete bicarbonate into the mucous layer, which neutralizes acid. Chemicals called prostaglandins, which increase the mucus and bicarbonate production and also decrease the secretion of acid, are produced by the stomach. When these protective mechanisms are not enough and the stomach acid erodes the stomach lining, it results in a gastric ulcer. When such an ulceration occurs in the small intestine it is called a duodenal ulcer. Gastroesophageal reflux disease is a condition in which acid from the stomach moves backwards (refluxes) into the esophagus. The esophagus is not normally exposed to acid and does not have a protective barrier like the stomach, so ulceration of the esophagus can occur.

Most gastrointestinal ulcer treatments work by reducing the acid content of the stomach. The most commonly used agents are antacids, histamine-2 receptor antagonists, proton pump inhibitors, a prostaglandin drug, and sucralfate.

Antacids

Antacids neutralize existing acid in the stomach. They do not reduce the secretion of acid. They cannot decrease the acid in the stomach to the same extent as the newer drugs but may still be effective therapy. Sodium bicarbonate (baking soda) has been a household heartburn remedy for generations. It reacts with acid to create sodium chloride (ordinary table salt), water, and carbon dioxide, which reduces stomach acid but causes other problematic effects. The production of carbon dioxide, a gas, may result in flatulence and distention of the abdomen. The sodium, chloride, and bicarbonate are absorbed and can cause undesirable electrolyte changes in patients with disorders such as kidney disease, swelling of the ankles or feet, heart failure, liver failure, or hypertension.

Calcium carbonate (the ingredient in Tums®) similarly reacts with acid in the stomach to produce calcium chloride, water, and carbon dioxide. The calcium is not absorbed as well as sodium is, so systemic effects are less likely. Patients with renal failure may develop high blood levels of calcium. Calcium carbonate and other calcium salts are also used as a nutritional supplement to provide calcium. Use of calcium antacids may result in the milk-alkali syndrome, which consists of high blood levels of calcium, a low blood acid content, irritability, headache, vertigo, nausea, vomiting, weakness, and muscle aches. Calcium salts may bind phosphates in food and make them unable to be absorbed. Calcium salts are used for this purpose in patients with kidney failure to prevent the absorption of too much phosphate.

Aluminum hydroxide is a commonly used antacid. It reacts with acid to produce aluminum chloride and water. Although the aluminum chloride is poorly absorbed, it can cause problems in patients with kidney failure. If used in large amounts, the unabsorbed aluminum may prevent the absorption of phosphates. Aluminum hydroxide is used, as are the calcium salts, in patients with kidney failure for this purpose. Aluminum antacids commonly cause constipation.

Magnesium hydroxide may be used as an antacid. It reacts with stomach acid to form magnesium chloride and water. Little magnesium is absorbed, but like the other salts, accumulation may occur in patients with kidney failure. Magnesium products commonly cause diarrhea. Therefore, combinations of aluminum and magnesium hydroxides are used to try to avoid either constipation or diarrhea. The diarrhea effect tends to predominate in these combinations.

Alginic acid is combined with the antacids sodium bicarbonate, aluminum hydroxide, and magnesium trisilicate in a product called Gaviscon®. This product is useful in gastroesophageal reflux disease. The alginic acid does not neutralize acid but floats on the surface of the stomach contents as a thick solution. It may function to prevent reflux of the stomach acid or act as a barrier between the esophagus and the acid when reflux occurs.

Antacid preparations differ in potency (acid-neutralizing ability). They must be taken in adequate amounts to treat peptic ulcer disease or gastroesophageal reflux disease. Timing of doses is important because the duration of effect of antacids is only 15 to 30 minutes. They are often given before and after meals and at bedtime.

Antacids are implicated in many drug interactions. For the most part, antacids affect how well drugs are absorbed. They either react with the drug itself or the changes in the acidity of the stomach inhibit the absorption.

Sucralfate is an aluminum salt that functions differently from the antacids. In an acid environment, sucralfate binds to an ulcer forming a protective barrier between it and the acid environment. Adverse effects are similar to other aluminum compounds: constipation, nausea,

dry mouth, dizziness, and a metallic taste. The same cautions with regard to accumulation in kidney failure and binding of phosphates apply. Similar drug interactions occur as with aluminum antacids.

Histamine-2 Receptor Antagonists

The histamine-2 receptor antagonists (H_2 antagonists) were a significant discovery in the treatment of peptic ulcer disease and GERD. These drugs block a different histamine receptor than the antihistamines used for allergic conditions. When histamine binds to the histamine-2 receptor on cells in the stomach it stimulates the secretion of acid. H_2 antagonists reduce the output of acid from stomach cells by blocking this receptor.

The H_2 antagonists are similar in action and side effects. The agents currently available are cimetidine, ranitidine, famotidine, and nizatidine. They are safe and well-tolerated drugs. The most common side effects are gastrointestinal disturbances. Central nervous system effects such as drowsiness and headache may occur. More severe central nervous system effects such as confusion, agitation, and hallucinations occur most often in severely ill patients.[9] All of these drugs are available as oral or injectable formulations except nizatidine, which is only available in capsules. All products are available over the counter as well as in prescription-only strengths. Drug interactions are common with this class of drugs.

Proton Pump Inhibitors

Proton pump inhibitors act within the stomach cells to prevent the production of acid. They can lower the stomach's acid output more than the H_2 antagonists. Two proton pump inhibitors are available: omeprazole and lansoprazole. These drugs are similar in action and side effects. Adverse reactions are similar to the H_2 antagonists, with nausea, diarrhea, and headache predominating. These drugs are administered as capsules containing enteric coated pellets to protect them from the acid environment of the stomach. The coating protects the drug until it passes into the less acidic duodenum, where the coating breaks down and the drug is absorbed. If a patient cannot swallow the whole capsule, the pellets can be administered. However, if they are crushed or put into an alkaline substance (such as antacids), the coating will break down and the drug will be destroyed by the acid in the stomach.

The prostaglandin misoprostol is indicated to prevent gastric or duodenal ulcer caused by the nonsteroidal anti-inflammatory drugs (NSAIDs). The NSAIDs prevent inflammation and swelling in some areas of the body by inhibiting prostaglandins. In the stomach, prostaglandins protect the lining of the stomach by stimulating increased mucus and bicarbonate production and inhibiting acid secretion. Inhibition of prostaglandin synthesis may be one of the mechanisms by which NSAIDs cause peptic ulcer disease.

Although misoprostol is effective in preventing NSAID-induced ulceration, it is often not tolerated because of the abdominal pain and diarrhea it causes. In some patients, lowering the dose eliminates side effects but still provides protective effects. Other side effects are nausea, flatulence, headache, vomiting, and constipation. Misoprostol can stimulate uterine contractions, so female patients must be sure that they are not and will not become pregnant while taking this drug.

Recent findings suggest that a bacterium common to the lining of the stomach, *Helicobacter pylori*, causes peptic ulcer disease. This bacterium produces an enzyme that degrades the mucus barrier and allows acid to come in contact with the stomach lining. Treatment of peptic ulcer disease is now directed at elimination of this bacterium. Drug regimens directed at eradicating *H. pylori* include various combinations of antibiotics such as amoxicillin, metronidazole, tetracycline, and clarithromycin with histamine-2 receptor antagonists or proton pump inhibitors and bismuth subsalicylate (see antidiarrheals).

Antidiarrheals

The frequency of normal bowel movements varies from one stool every two or more days to greater than three stools per day. Diarrhea therefore is hard to define but is usually considered to be an increased frequency of loose, watery stools. Diarrhea can be acute or chronic and a symptom of another disease.

The intestine is a hollow tube composed partly of layers of smooth muscle. Nerves regulate the normal motion of the muscles in the intestine. The large intestine absorbs water from the contents passed to it from the stomach and small intestine. It also stores feces for excretion. The feces normally consist of unabsorbed food, minerals, bacteria, and electrolytes. The presence of bacteria is normal for this part of the body. The bacteria produce enzymes to degrade waste products, and they synthesize vitamins.

Diarrhea may result when the operation of the large intestine is disrupted. Decreased absorption of water, increased secretion of electrolytes into the intestinal contents, excessive amounts of mucus production, bleeding into the intestine, or alteration of the movements of the intestine can all result in diarrhea. These disruptions of intestinal function may be caused by infection, toxins, drugs, diet, laxative abuse, or other diseases. Persistent diarrhea should be referred to a physician.

Antiperistaltic drugs treat diarrhea by inhibiting the propulsive movements of the intestine. Slowing passage of the intestinal contents allows absorption of water and electrolytes. Cramping and stool frequency are reduced. Loperamide and diphenoxylate are antiperistaltic drugs. High doses of diphenoxylate have some narcotic effects, including euphoria. Atropine is added to diphenoxylate to discourage, through unpleasant side effects, the abuse of large doses of diphenoxylate. Antiperistaltic agents should not be used to treat diarrhea caused by bacteria because doing so may result in prolonged diarrhea. Diarrhea accompanied by fever may have a bacterial cause.

Adsorbent antidiarrheal drugs adsorb bacteria and toxins. They also adsorb nutrients, digestive enzymes, and drugs. Kaolin, pectin, attapulgite, and polycarbophil are adsorbent antidiarrheals. Polycarbophil absorbs water and treats both diarrhea and constipation. The other adsorbent drugs do not have proven efficacy.

Bismuth subsalicylate has been used for indigestion, nausea, and diarrhea. Its use for peptic ulcer disease has already been discussed. Bismuth appears to have an antisecretory action that blocks the copious fluid flow in diarrhea. It has been used to treat infectious diarrhea, including diarrhea common in travelers to foreign countries. Bismuth subsalicylate does contain salicylate, so patients taking aspirin, which also contains salicylate, may inadvertently take too much salicylate if not warned. The signs of high levels of salicylate are ringing in the ears, nausea, and vomiting.

Laxatives

As mentioned previously, the frequency of bowel movements varies. The common misconception that daily bowel movements are necessary for good health leads to the misuse of laxatives and worsens bowel problems. A wide range of diseases, as well as drugs and diet, may cause constipation. Treatment of constipation with laxatives should only occur after causative diseases have been identified, causative drugs have been discontinued, and dietary adjustments have been tried.

Laxatives are used to increase patient comfort and also to prevent complications. Hemorrhoids may be aggravated by constipation. In some cases of constipation, the bowel may become so distended with fecal content that perforation of the bowel or loss of blood supply to the bowel may occur. Laxatives are also commonly used to empty the bowel before various diagnostic procedures.

Bulk-forming laxatives dissolve or swell as they mix with the fluid in the intestine. The increased bulk in the intestine stimulates the movement of the intestine. Because this is the natural method of stimulating bowel movement, these laxatives are usually the first choice. Bulk laxatives do not act quickly. They take 12 to 24 hours or longer to act. They must be given with adequate water to prevent them from forming an obstruction in the esophagus, so they are not useful for patients on fluid restrictions. Examples of bulk-forming laxatives are polycarbophil, methylcellulose, and psyllium.

Emollient laxatives are also known as stool-softeners. They facilitate the mixing of fatty and watery substances in the intestine to soften the fecal contents. These drugs are better suited to preventing constipation than treating it. They are not fast-acting in treating constipation; they may take up to 5 days to act. As with bulk laxatives, fluid intake should be increased. These drugs are commonly used in heart attack patients to prevent straining with stool passage, in maternity patients after delivery, and in patients taking narcotic pain relievers. Examples of emollient laxatives are docusate sodium, docusate calcium, and docusate potassium.

Saline laxatives contain salts that are not absorbed. These salts draw water into the intestines. The increased pressure in the intestine from this water stimulates movement in the intestine. These drugs are indicated for acute evacuation of the bowel. Examples of saline laxatives are milk of magnesia, magnesium citrate, and sodium phosphates. These drugs act within 30 minutes to several hours.

Hyperosmotic laxatives draw water into the intestine. The onset of action is within one-half hour. Glycerin suppositories are a hyperos-motic laxative. Their effect may be enhanced by the irritant effect of sodium stearate in the suppository.

Stimulant laxatives irritate the lining of the intestine or the nerves in the wall of the intestine, which causes the intestines to excrete their contents. Another way by which they may act is to increase the amount of water and electrolytes the body secretes into the intestine. These drugs produce thorough evacuation of contents within hours of administration. They also may produce cramping, colic, mucus secretion, and excessive loss of fluid. Their chronic abuse may result in a poorly functioning colon. If signs of appendicitis are present (abdominal pain, nausea, vomiting, fever), these drugs should not be used. Examples of stimulant laxatives are cascara sagrada, phenolphthalein, senna, castor oil, and bisacodyl. Bisacodyl tablets are coated to prevent action in the stomach. Administering these tablets with antacids or milk of magnesia may cause the coating to dissolve, which may result in vomiting.

Gastrointestinal Stimulants

Drugs that increase gastrointestinal tract motility have a number of therapeutic uses. In GERD, these drugs appear to increase the tone of the muscle separating the stomach and esophagus so that reflux is prevented. They are also used in a complication of diabetes called gastroparesis. Gastroparesis is a reduced motility of the stomach that results in delayed emptying of the stomach contents into the intestine. Symptoms of gastroparesis are nausea, vomiting, and abdominal distention.

Metoclopramide and cisapride are gastrointestinal stimulants. Metoclopramide has other effects, which make it useful as an antiemetic drug but also account for some side effects. Metoclopramide can cause drowsiness, nervousness, fatigue, dizziness, weakness, depression, diarrhea, and rash. An uncommon possible reaction is extrapyramidal symptoms, movement disorders that are common with antipsychotic drugs (see Central Nervous System) and include involuntary movements of the limbs, head, neck, and eyes and facial grimacing. Cisapride does not have the antiemetic activity of metoclopramide or the extrapyramidal symptoms. The most common adverse effects with cisapride are abdominal cramping, rumbling noises in the stomach, and diarrhea.

MUSCULOSKELETAL SYSTEM

The musculoskeletal system consists of the bones, which support the body, and muscles, which allow movement of the body. Muscles are attached to bones by tendons. Bending of the limbs and other parts of the body is allowed by the joints, where two or more bones meet. Within joints, bones are held in place and limited to a particular range of movement by ligaments and cartilage. Many diseases of the musculoskeletal system cause pain or inflammation of the muscles or joints.

Anti-inflammatory and Antipyretic Agents

Inflammation is the body's response to infection or trauma. The blood vessels send fluid, dissolved substances, and cells into areas of tissue injury or death. This reaction is intended to protect and aid in the healing of tissue. However, a prolonged or unneeded response produces unnecessary pain or discomfort.

The signs of inflammation include redness, heat, pain, swelling, and altered function of the involved tissue. These signs of inflammation are common symptoms of inflammatory diseases such as rheumatoid arthritis, lupus erythematosis, tendonitis, bursitis, and gout. Anti-inflammatory agents do not cure these diseases; they just relieve the symptoms.

Fever is a systemic reaction (involving the entire body) to inflammation caused by infection or other inflammatory diseases. The white blood cells that the body sends to areas of tissue injury release substances, called pyrogens, which reset the temperature regulating area of the brain to increase the body's temperature. Fever is especially beneficial in infection because the increased body temperature may be too high for the bacteria or viruses causing the infection to thrive. Like inflammation, this protective response may cause discomfort.

The nonsteroidal anti-inflammatory drugs are a large class of agents commonly abbreviated as NSAIDs. The term nonsteroidal is used to differentiate these agents from corticosteroid hormones, which also have anti-inflammatory properties and are discussed later in this chapter. NSAIDs also have analgesic (pain relieving) and antipyretic (fever reducing) properties. Aspirin is the oldest of this class of drugs. Other drugs in this class include fenoprofen, flurbiprofen, ibuprofen, ketoprofen, naproxen, oxaprozin, diclofenac, etodolac, indomethacin, ketorolac, nabumetone, sulindac, tolmetin, meclofenamate, mefenamic acid, and piroxicam.

All NSAIDs can cause serious bleeding and ulcers in the stomach. Many of the drugs used to treat ulcers (see section on Gastrointestinal System) can be given to prevent damage to the stomach lining. Most NSAIDs can also cause kidney dysfunction. Platelets, blood cells involved in the formation of blood clots, are inhibited by NSAIDs. Aspirin has a longer-acting effect on platelets than the other NSAIDs.

There are two special cautions concerning aspirin use in children. The first is the occurrence of Reye's syndrome, which can result in liver disease and central nervous system damage, when aspirin is used to treat fever in children with chicken pox and influenza. The second is the frequency with which aspirin is a cause of poisoning in children. The similarity of chewable aspirin tablets to candy probably contributes to its potential as a poison.

Several NSAIDs are now available without prescription. In addition to oral tablets or capsules, several are available as liquids and suppositories. Only ketorolac is available in an injectable form.

Analgesics

Control of pain (analgesia) is an important part of medicine. Analgesics are drugs that relieve pain by altering the way the brain receives and interprets the sensation of pain from the nerves. Effectively controlling pain puts patients at ease and promotes quicker recovery.

Opioid analgesics (also called narcotic analgesics) all act on the same types of receptors in the brain to control pain. These drugs do not reduce inflammation or lower fever but do have other therapeutically useful properties such as the suppression of cough. There are a large number of opioid analgesics, most of which are available in injectable and oral forms. Butorphanol is available as a nasal spray. Morphine, hydromorphone, meperidine, and fentanyl are some of the most potent opioid analgesics. Some less potent agents are codeine, oxycodone, propoxyphene, nalbuphine, butorphanol, buprenorphine, dezocine, and tramadol. The choice of drug depends on factors such as the site, duration, and severity of the pain.

Similar adverse effects occur with all opioid analgesics. Depression of the breathing reflex is the most important. Overdose may result in death. Combining analgesic with other drugs, such as alcohol, that also depress breathing may have additive effects on breathing. Opioid analgesics also produce drowsiness, so patients must be warned about driving and other activities that require them to be alert. Nausea and constipation are other common side effects. Patients on several days of therapy may need to take a stool softener to prevent constipation.

The most popular nonopioid analgesic is acetaminophen. This drug is similar to aspirin in its ability to relieve pain and reduce fever, but it has no anti-inflammatory properties. It is a useful alternative to aspirin in children with chicken pox or other viral illnesses, in patients with stomach or intestinal ulcers, in patients with conditions likely to cause bleeding, and in patients with aspirin allergies. In usual doses acetaminophen rarely causes side effects, but in larger doses it can cause liver damage. Acetaminophen is available without prescription and is widely used in oral and rectal dosage forms. It is often combined with stronger opioid analgesics.

Skeletal Muscle Relaxants

There are two main groups of drugs that have skeletal muscle relaxant effects: those given intravenously and those given orally. Intravenous drugs are used to relax muscles during medical procedures. Oral drugs include those used for painful muscle conditions such as sprains or strains and those used mainly for muscle spasms.

The intravenous drugs are called neuromuscular blocking agents. Their mechanism of action is to block the nerve impulse at the point where it is transmitted from the nerve to the muscle. Neuromuscular blocking agents prevent muscles from moving when movement would interfere with the medical treatment or procedure. For example, they are used to relax muscles during surgery, in patients who are on mechanical ventilators (breathing devices), and when broken bones are being set. Since these drugs have no effect on pain or level of consciousness, other agents must be used to control pain and anesthetize the patient. Neuromuscular blocking agents include succinylcholine, tubocurarine, mivacurium, rocuronium, pancuronium, atracurium, vecuronium, and doxacurium. Drugs are chosen for different types of procedures according to how quickly they start to act and how long their effects last. At the end of the pro-

cedure, the actions of these drugs are commonly reversed with drugs such as neostigmine, pyridostigmine, or edrophonium. Adverse effects of neuromuscular blocking agents are usually extensions of their action: slow recovery of breathing and muscle weakness.

Another group of skeletal muscle relaxants is used orally for painful muscle conditions such as sprains and strains. It is not known whether these drugs actually relax muscles or relieve pain as a result of their sedative properties. Drugs in this group include carisoprodol, chlorzoxazone, cyclobenzaprine, metaxalone, methocarbamol, and orphenadrine. Drowsiness is a shared adverse effect. These drugs are commonly given with pain relievers, which may add to the drowsiness. Patients should be warned about driving or other activities that require them to be alert.

Two drugs are used mainly for muscle spasticity, which is seen in diseases such as cerebral palsy and multiple sclerosis and following stroke. Diazepam, a sedative-hypnotic drug, is used for its muscle relaxant properties in these diseases. Baclofen is also used in these diseases and has the advantage of producing less sedation than diazepam.

Systemic Corticosteroids

Corticosteroids are hormones secreted by the adrenal gland, a part of the endocrine system. These drugs are discussed under this section because they are commonly used to suppress inflammation and the immune response, which is useful in a wide spectrum of diseases including rheumatoid arthritis, bursitis, asthma, allergic reactions, lupus erythematosis, inflammatory bowel disease, ulcerative colitis, psoriasis, and organ transplantation.

Other names for the corticosteroids are adrenocorticosteroids, glucocorticosteroids, and, simply, steroids. Drugs available include hydrocortisone, prednisone, prednisolone, methylprednisolone, triamcinolone, dexamethasone, betamethasone, and flunisolide. Dosage forms available include topical creams, ointments, and lotions; eye drops; injectable products for intramuscular, intravenous, and intra-articular (into the joint) injections; enemas; oral inhalers; nasal sprays; and tablets.

While short-term use of corticosteroids carries little risk of adverse effects, long-term use is only indicated when the benefits outweigh the risks. Long-term corticosteroid use can lead to

Cushing's syndrome, which is characterized by a rounded, puffy face; thinning of the skin; osteoporosis (bone weakening); muscle loss; and high blood glucose. Therapeutic use of corticosteroids suppresses natural adrenal gland function, which is essential to the body in times of physical stress. The dose of corticosteroids must be tapered when they are to be discontinued so that the adrenal gland can recover and begin to secrete natural hormones. Tablets are available in special packaging that provides a high initial daily dose for treatment of the disease followed by gradually decreasing doses over several days. Another method of dosing is to use alternate-day therapy (alternating days with and without drug) to allow the recovery of natural adrenal function on the drug-free days.

ENDOCRINE SYSTEM

The endocrine system consists of three components: hormone producing cells, circulating hormones, and target cells or tissues. Hormone producing cells are located in glands such as the thyroid, the adrenal, or the pituitary. Nonglandular endocrine tissue may also produce hormones; one example is the pancreas, which produces insulin. Hormones are chemical substances produced by one part of the body that help control some function elsewhere in the body. Hormones control body functions in several ways. They regulate metabolism, the process by which the body converts food into energy and tissue; control growth from infancy to adulthood; control the maturation and function of the reproductive system; keep the appropriate amount of water and salts in the blood stream; control the body's response to anger, fright, injury, and stress; and control the production of other hormones.

An important feature of the endocrine system is the feedback loop. The amount of hormones produced is increased or decreased depending on the effect of the hormone. This feedback loop keeps the hormones at a level that will control the body's functions. An example of this loop is the production of insulin. The presence of high blood sugar after a meal causes the production of insulin. The insulin attaches to receptors on the cells and allows the sugar to enter the cells. The lower blood sugar is sensed and insulin production is decreased so that the blood sugar does not fall too low. When all the processes are properly functioning, blood sugar stays within the range that the body needs.

Endocrine drugs can be either natural or synthetic. Endocrine drugs are used to compensate for a deficiency or excess of a specific hormone, to block the production or effects of a hormone, and to treat a non-endocrine disease. Examples of the latter would be corticosteroid therapy for asthma or the use of vasopressin to minimize bleeding in the esophagus (food tube) of alcoholics. The indications for endocrine drugs that will be discussed are diabetes mellitus, thyroid diseases, oral contraception, fertility agents, osteoporosis, benign prostatic hypertrophy, and pituitary functions.

Diabetes

Diabetes mellitus is the most common endocrine disease. It is characterized by disturbed metabolism and inappropriate blood sugar levels. As a result of poor blood sugar control, diabetics may develop kidney disease; heart disease; painful nerves in the hands, feet, and legs (peripheral neuropathy); and gastrointestinal problems. Diabetics are more likely than the general population to die of heart disease.

There are two types of diabetes mellitus, Type I (also called insulin dependent diabetes mellitus) and Type II (also called noninsulin-dependent diabetes mellitus). Type I is characterized by decreased production of insulin and therefore must be treated with insulin. This type of diabetes is the least common of the two and is more commonly diagnosed in children and adolescents than in adults. Type II may be characterized by either decreased production of insulin or normal amounts of insulin with abnormal sensitivity of the tissues to the insulin that is present. This type of diabetes may be treated with diet alone, with oral hypoglycemic agents, or with insulin. Type II is the more prevalent type and is more commonly diagnosed in adulthood.

Insulin is one of the two treatments for diabetes mellitus. Insulin can be given only by injection, either subcutaneous or intravenous. There are many types of insulin, but only regular insulin can be given intravenously. The types of insulin differ in the time that they take to work (onset of action) and the length of time after the injection that the effects last (duration of action).

- The rapid-acting insulins are regular insulin, Semilente insulin, and insulin lispro. These work quickly after injection but have a short duration of action.
- The intermediate-acting insulins are NPH (isophane) and Lente insulin. These take

longer to have an effect than regular or Semilente insulin, but their effects last longer.

- The long-acting insulins are PZI (protamine zinc) and Ultralente insulin. As would be expected, these insulins take the longest time to start to work but also last the longest.
- Some insulins can be mixed together to achieve the desired effect such as quick action but a longer duration of action. The most common mixture is regular insulin with NPH insulin, and a premixed form of 70 units of NPH and 30 units of regular insulin per milliliter is available. Other insulins can be mixed, but not all insulins are compatible with each other.

Insulin is available from animal sources (beef and pork) and as human insulin. Human insulin is now used most commonly because it causes fewer side effects than animal source insulin. The animal source insulins used today are very purified and cause fewer side effects than the products available years ago.

Insulin doses are measured in units. Special insulin syringes should be used to properly measure the dose. Insulin may be dosed only in the morning or may be given two to four times a day. A sliding scale dose is commonly used in hospitals when blood sugar is uncontrolled. Blood sugar will be measured by a finger-stick method four or more times daily and a dose of regular insulin given according to the amount of sugar measured.

Oral hypoglycemics are used to lower blood sugar in Type II diabetes and can be taken by mouth. The oral hypoglycemics are thought to act by increasing the ability of the pancreas to secrete insulin by reducing levels of another hormone (glucagon) that increases blood sugar, by reducing the production of glucose by the liver, and by increasing the ability of cells to respond to insulin. The oral hypoglycemic agents are of three chemical types: sulfonylureas, biguanides, and thiazolidinediones. The most commonly prescribed drugs are the sulfonylureas. Commonly used sulfonylureas are tolbutamide, chlorpropamide, glyburide, glipizide, and glimepiride. There is only one biguanide drug available, metformin, and only one thiazolidinedione, troglitazone.

Thyroid Diseases

The thyroid gland influences the rate of metabolism in the body and the development of the body from youth to maturity. Diseases of the thyroid gland include hypothyroidism, underproduction of thyroid hormone, and hyperthyroidism, overproduction of thyroid hormone.

Hypothyroidism has many causes such as autoimmune disease (the immune system attacks the body's own cells), radiation or surgical treatment of hyperthyroidism, iodine deficiency, and pituitary disease. Goiter, an enlargement of the thyroid gland causing a lump in the neck, may occur. Symptoms of hypothyroidism are related to decreased metabolism. These symptoms include fatigue; hoarseness; cold intolerance; decreased sweating; cool, dry skin; facial puffiness; and slow movement.

Hypothyroidism is treated by the administration of thyroid hormone. Naturally produced thyroid hormone actually consists of several substances, including triiodothyroxine (T_3) and levothyroxine (T_4). Levothyroxine is the most commonly prescribed drug for hypothyroidism. Thyroid USP is dried animal thyroid gland that contains both T_3 and T_4. Thyroid USP is often prescribed in grains, while all the other preparations are prescribed in milligrams or micrograms. Liotrix is a combination of T_3 and T_4. All of these drugs are usually given once daily. Liothyronine must be given more often than once daily, so it is used more often for thyroid function tests than for treatment.

Adverse effects related to thyroid hormone replacement include increased heart rate, which can be dangerous in patients with heart disease. Therefore, older patients or those with heart disease should begin therapy with low doses. Other adverse effects include nervousness, heat intolerance, heart palpitation, and weight loss. These effects usually indicate that the patient should have a blood test to evaluate the appropriateness of the dose.

Hyperthyroidism is most often caused by an immune system disorder such as Graves' disease. Symptoms of hyperthyroidism are usually the opposite of hypothyroidism. Heat intolerance, weight loss, increased sweating, palpitations, swelling of the feet, diarrhea, tremor, and nervousness are common symptoms. Hyperthyroidism is most often treated with nondrug therapies, surgery or radioactive iodine, to remove the gland. Often hypothyroidism will occur after removal of the gland, and thyroid hormone replacement will be necessary.

Antithyroid drugs block the synthesis of thyroid hormones. They are used most often in children and young adults who do not need permanent removal of the gland. Methimazole and propylthiouracil are the primary antithyroid drugs. The most common adverse effect associated with these drugs is a raised, itchy rash. A rare but serious side effect is agranulocytosis, which is a pronounced decrease in blood cells. This effect is usually reversible if the drug is discontinued. Antithyroid drug therapy, like surgery and radioactive iodine, can cause hypothyroidism.

Iodides were the major antithyroid drugs many years ago, but today they are infrequently used to inhibit thyroid hormone release. Forms of iodine used include Lugol's solution, containing 8 mg of iodide per drop, and saturated solution of potassium iodide (SSKI), containing 50 mg of iodide per drop. Both of these products are dosed in drops, not teaspoonfuls, and diluted in juice or other liquid. Pharmacy personnel must alert patients and caregivers to the proper dose to avoid overdose.

Oral Contraceptives and Fertility Agents

A woman's menstrual cycle is controlled by hormones released in sequence that cause ovulation and prepare the uterus for implantation of a fertilized egg. Manipulating the levels of these hormones can prevent pregnancy (contraception) or make pregnancy more likely.

Oral contraceptives include two types of preparations: estrogen and progestin combinations and progestin-only preparations. The combination pills work largely by inhibiting ovulation. They also change the lining of the uterus, slow the movement of the egg through the fallopian tubes to the uterus, and thicken the cervical mucus so that it is more difficult for sperm to penetrate it. These effects make fertilization of the egg and implantation of the fertilized egg less likely, should ovulation occur. The progestin-only pills do not inhibit ovulation as reliably and are more reliant on the other mechanisms to prevent pregnancy.

Combination pills contain either ethinyl estradiol or mestranol as the estrogen component and norethindrone, norgestrel, or ethynodiol diacetate as the progestin component. When oral contraceptives were first developed, they contained high doses of both estrogen and progestin. Since that time, the doses of both hormones have been greatly decreased, improving the safety of oral contraceptives and reducing the number of side effects.

Today there are three types of combination oral contraceptives in use: monophasic, biphasic, and triphasic. Monophasic pills contain the same amounts of estrogen and progestin in each of the 21 pills taken per cycle. Biphasic pills contain a different ratio of estrogen to progestin for the first 10 days and the last 11 days of the cycle. Triphasic pills vary the amount of hormones three times during the 21 days. The biphasic and triphasic pills are designed to more closely mimic normal hormonal changes and therefore have fewer side effects. Progestin-only oral contraceptives contain the same amount of progestin (norethindrone or norgestrel) in each tablet.

Although the oral contraceptive pills used today are very effective and much safer than the earlier high dose pills, there are still risks. The risks associated with these pills occur rarely and are higher for women who smoke or take higher-dose preparations. Blood clots may occur which travel through the blood stream and block the vessels in the lungs. Gallbladder disease, strokes, and heart attacks may be more common in women who use birth control pills. Researchers are not sure if oral contraceptive use can result in an increased risk of breast or cervical cancer.

Side effects that are less serious but bothersome include irregular vaginal bleeding or spotting, change in vision in contact lens wearers, water retention, and patchy darkening of the skin. Progestin-only pills have a higher incidence of abnormal bleeding but do not have the risk of blood clots associated with estrogen.

Use of oral contraceptives may also provide some health benefits such as lighter menstrual flow, which reduces the likelihood of anemia due to iron deficiency; less menstrual pain; reduction in the development of noncancerous breast lumps in women who are prone to developing them; decreased likelihood of pelvic inflammatory disease, an infection in the pelvis of sexually active women; and they provide some protection against cancer of the ovaries and the lining of the uterus.

Birth control pills are packaged in containers that are designed to make it easy to remember to take the pills at the same time and daily. Combination pills come in packages of 21 (21 active pills, so the patient takes them for 21 days, waits 7 days, and begins another 21 days) or 28 pills (21 active pills and 7 inactive pills, so that the patient takes a pill every day). The progestin-only pills come in packages of 28 active pills and the patient takes one tablet every day. Included with each package is a patient package insert, which should be given to the patient with each refill. This insert includes information about the risks and side effects of the pills as well as instructions on how to take the pills and what to do if a dose is missed.

Two other forms of progestin hormones, medroxyprogesterone and levonorgestrel, are used as long-acting contraceptives. Medroxyprogesterone acetate is given as an injection every three months. Levonorgestrel is implanted under the skin in the upper arm. This set of progestin capsules slowly releases progestin in a manner that provides birth control for 5 years. The advantage of these forms is that patients do not have to take a pill every day. The disadvantages include the long duration of action. If adverse effects occur, they cannot be quickly discontinued like other forms of contraception. The injection requires an office or clinic visit every 3 months for another injection as opposed to the once a year visit required with oral contraceptives. Levonorgestrel is expensive and the insertion can be uncomfortable.

Fertility agents are used to increase the likelihood of pregnancy in patients having difficulty conceiving. They stimulate the pituitary hormones that release the egg from the ovary (ovulation). Clomiphene, urofollitropin, and menotropins are the drugs used to stimulate ovulation. An injection of human chorionic gonadotropin (HCG) is given after a cycle of urofollitropin and menotropins. Timing the doses of these drugs to coincide with the woman's cycle is important to success in inducing ovulation. Therefore, pharmacy personnel must ensure that HCG will be available for the patient when she needs it. Women should be seen frequently by their physicians while taking fertility agents so that adverse effects are noticed early. Multiple births occur more commonly in women who have taken fertility agents. Otherwise, adverse effects are not common.

Osteoporosis

Bone, the hard substance that forms the framework of the body, is one of the body's most active tissues. Bone consists of living cells that continually perform metabolic functions and control the amount of calcium and phosphorus in the blood. The calcium and phosphorus salts that form bone are constantly being absorbed out of the bone into the blood and deposited back into bone again. Osteoporosis, a disease characterized by the loss of bone, occurs when more salts

are absorbed into the blood from bone than are deposited back into the bone. Osteoporosis can result in misshapen bone, such as curvature of the backbone seen in the elderly, or in easily broken bones.

Drugs used to treat osteoporosis can be grouped into those that decrease the reabsorption of calcium and phosphorus and those that increase the deposition of calcium and phosphorus. Drugs that decrease reabsorption of calcium and phosphorus are estrogens, calcium, calcitonin, vitamin D, and biphosphonates. A drug that stimulates bone formation (deposition) is sodium fluoride.

Estrogens are used both to prevent and to treat osteoporosis. Ethinyl estradiol and conjugated estrogens are the drugs most commonly used for this purpose. For prevention, they are taken at the time of menopause, either natural menopause or menopause caused by removal of the ovaries. Progesterone is also commonly given to postmenopausal patients, who have not had a hysterectomy, to decrease the risk of cervical cancer. When estrogens are used alone, they are given for 21 to 25 days a month. When estrogens are given with progesterone, the progesterone may be added for 5 to 10 days of the cycle or given all 25 days with the estrogen. Estrogens are available as pills and patches.

Adequate calcium intake is essential to the prevention and treatment of osteoporosis. The various calcium salts provide different amounts of elemental calcium, which is the active part of the salt. Calcium carbonate, calcium lactate, calcium phosphate, calcium chloride, and calcium acetate are commonly given orally. Most calcium salts will include on the label the amount of the salt and the amount of calcium in each tablet (e.g., calcium carbonate 500 mg, 200 mg calcium). Calcium carbonate has a high calcium content and a low cost. Taking calcium salts between meals may increase calcium absorption.[5] Constipation is the most common side effect.

Calcitonin is a hormone that inhibits calcium reabsorption from bone. Human source calcitonin is available as an injection. Calcitonin from salmon is available as injection and as a nasal spray. Development of antibodies (neutralizing substances produced by the body) to salmon calcitonin limits its effectiveness. Antibody development is less likely when salmon calcitonin is used in low doses, intermittently, or intranasally.

Etidronate, alendronate, and pamidronate are examples of biphosphonates. These drugs are potent inhibitors of the reabsorption of calcium from bone, but they also impair the formation of new bone. An intermittent regimen of 2 weeks of etidronate followed by 11 to 13 weeks of calcium is currently used to obtain the greatest benefit. Alendronate is the newest biphosphonate. It is a more potent inhibitor of reabsorption of calcium from bone than etidronate or pamidronate. Alendronate is given orally. To prevent damage to the esophagus (food tube) and to promote its absorption, alendronate should be taken immediately upon arising with a full glass of water. Patients should remain upright and not eat for at least 30 minutes after taking alendronate.

Benign Prostatic Hypertrophy

Benign prostatic hypertrophy (BPH) is a noncancerous enlargement of the prostate gland that develops in older men. Because the prostate gland encircles the urethra and urine leaves the body through the urethra, enlargement of the prostate can cause difficulties in urinating.

Surgery has been the mainstay of treatment for BPH but alpha-adrenergic blocking drugs and finasteride are viable alternatives. The alpha-adrenergic blocking drugs prazosin, doxazosin, and terazosin are used to relieve the urinary symptoms of BPH, but do not affect the growth of the prostate tissue. These drugs are discussed in more detail in the section on antihypertensives.

Finasteride reduces the size of the prostate by inhibiting production of the hormone that causes enlargement of the prostate gland. Finasteride does not work in all patients and may take up to 6 months to produce a noticeable effect. The adverse effects of finasteride include impotence, decreased sex drive, and headache. Finasteride may cause abnormalities in a male fetus. Therefore, women who are or may become pregnant should not be exposed to this drug, including contact with crushed tablets or contact with semen from a sexual partner taking finasteride. Whole tablets are film coated to protect against exposure to the drug.

Pituitary Hormones

The pituitary gland controls some of the body's functions by producing hormones that control the production of other hormones. For example, the production of thyroid, adrenocortical, and reproductive hormones are controlled by other hormones produced in the pituitary gland. The pituitary gland also regulates growth in children, water retention by the kidneys, and uterine contraction. The pituitary hormones that are available as pharmacological agents are oxytocin, vasopressin, and adrenocorticotropin.

Oxytocin is a pituitary hormone used to induce or augment labor and to control bleeding after birth. Two other synthetic versions of oxytocin, ergonovine and methylergonovine, are used to control uterine bleeding after birth. A synthetic version of oxytocin is administered as a nasal spray to help milk flow in nursing mothers.

Vasopressin, also called antidiuretic hormone (ADH), has an important role in blood pressure regulation. This hormone increases water reabsorption by the kidneys. A lack of vasopressin results in diabetes insipidus, a disease that is different from, and much less common, than diabetes mellitus. In diabetes insipidus too much water and sodium are lost in the urine. Vasopressin and a synthetic agent, desmopressin acetate (DDAVP), are used to treat diabetes insipidus. Because vasopressin also constricts blood vessels, it is used to stop bleeding from blood vessels in the esophagus (food tube) and stomach in alcoholic liver disease. DDAVP has also been useful to treat bedwetting in children and to prevent blood clotting in certain blood disorders. DDAVP can be given by injection or by nasal spray.

The function of adrenocorticotropin (ACTH) is to stimulate the release of hormones from the adrenal gland. ACTH and a synthetic version, cosyntropin, are used most often to diagnose diseases of the adrenal gland. Because ACTH causes the release of cortisol, a corticosteroid, from the adrenal gland, it can be used to treat diseases such as asthma, rheumatoid arthritis, inflammatory bowel disease, and neurological diseases. However, giving corticosteroids is usually preferred in these diseases. ACTH is sometimes used for flare-ups of multiple sclerosis.

INFECTIOUS DISEASES

The term infection refers to the invasion of tissue by a foreign substance such as a microorganism. In response the body sends white blood cells to destroy the microorganisms. Invading microorganisms include bacteria, viruses, fungi, protozoa, and parasites such as amoebas, flukes, and worms. The emphasis of this section is on drugs used to treat bacteria with some discussion of antivirals and antifungals. Tissue damage can occur directly from the invading organisms or from the white blood cells sent to fight the organisms. The body can also increase its temperature to help kill the invaders. Therefore, common symptoms of infection are similar to those of inflammation: fever, pain, heat, redness, and swelling.

The body is invaded by organisms from the environment every day. Some of these organisms are not harmful and some are even helpful, such as the bacteria that normally live in the gastrointestinal tract. When too many organisms are encountered or when the body's defenses cannot overcome the organism, signs of the infection may occur. Even when this happens, the body's defenses eventually overcome most infections. Examples of this are the common cold and chicken pox. But antibiotics are used when the body's defenses need help fighting an infection or if there may be serious long-term effects of the infection. Many of the infective organisms acquired by patients in hospitals or long-term care facilities are more difficult to kill than those acquired by patients at home.

Antibiotics are used three different ways: empirically, definitively, and prophylactically. The selection of an antibiotic depends on the way it will be used and the type of infection. It is not uncommon for patients in hospitals to receive prophylactic, empirical, and definitive antibiotic therapies within a short period of time.

Empirical antibiotic therapy is used when the organism causing the infection is unknown. The choice of drug is based upon the organisms usually found at the site of infection (e.g., urine, sinus, lungs). Samples of fluid or tissue from the site of infection will be grown (cultured) in the laboratory to try to identify the infecting organism.

When cultures have identified the organism, definitive therapy is started. Drugs used for definitive therapy are those known to be effective against the organism. When cultures are done, various antibiotics may also be tested to see which ones kill the organism (sensitivities). Antibiotic therapy can then be based on these sensitivities.

A third type of antibiotic use is prophylactic or preventive. Antibiotics may be used to prevent infection from occurring in situations such as surgery. In surgery, cutting open tissues may expose these tissues to bacteria from the skin or the environment. Antibiotics are given prior to surgery to prevent the few organisms that enter the body from multiplying and causing an infec-

tion. Patients with weakened immune systems such as cancer patients and patients with acquired immunodeficiency syndrome (AIDS), may receive antibiotics to prevent infections that are common in these populations. Patients planning to travel to areas with diseases that are not prevalent in the United States, such as malaria, may take antibiotics to prevent contracting such diseases.

Antibiotics are divided into classes based on their chemical structures. Antibiotics may differ between classes and within classes in several ways:

- The bacteria they are effective against
- If they actually kill bacteria (bactericidal) or just prevent the multiplication of bacteria (bacteriostatic)
- Adverse effects
- The sites of infection they are most effective against (e.g., skin, lungs, kidneys, bone)
- How they are removed from the body
- Routes by which they are given (oral, IV, IM)

The infection, characteristics of the antibiotic, and characteristics of the patient are all considered when an antibiotic is selected.

Beta-lactam Antibiotics

Beta-lactam antibiotics have a common chemical structure but vary widely in the organisms against which they are effective and in how easily organisms develop resistance to them. The beta-lactam drugs have relatively few adverse effects and are distributed well into many body tissues. Beta-lactam antibiotics are further broken down into penicillins, cephalosporins, carbapenems, and monobactams.

Penicillin

Penicillin was one of the first antibiotics developed. The original penicillin G was effective against limited organisms. Since penicillin G was introduced, many bacteria developed enzymes that destroy the drug. Therefore, it is of limited use now. The next group of penicillins developed, ampicillin and amoxicillin, are effective against more organisms but can also be destroyed by the enzymes some bacteria produce. Oxacillin, dicloxacillin, nafcillin, and methicillin were developed to be stable against the enzymes produced by *Staphylococcus aureus*, a common organism. These antibiotics are used when this organism is suspected. The newest penicillins are broad spectrum, meaning that they are effective against many types of bacteria. Broad spectrum antibiotics include carbenicillin, mezlocillin, ticarcillin, piperacillin, and azlocillin. Some of these penicillins are also combined with a beta-lactamase inhibitor, a substance that inactivates the enzymes bacteria produce and prevents the destruction of the antibiotic.

Penicillin allergies are estimated to occur in 5 to 8% of the population and can be fatal.[10] All patients should be carefully questioned about their allergy histories before they are given any drug of this class. Technicians should be sure to record this information accurately.

Cephalosporins

Cephalosporins are another group of beta-lactam antibiotics. These drugs are resistant to some of the bacterial enzymes that destroy penicillins. Some patients who are allergic to penicillin can also be allergic to cephalosporins. This is called cross-sensitivity.

Cephalosporins are divided into generations based on their spectrum of activity (i.e., how many different types of bacteria they are effective against). First generation cephalosporins have the most limited activity but are effective against many bacteria that cause skin infections and urinary tract infections. Examples of first generation cephalosporins are cefazolin (injectable), cephalexin (oral), and cefadroxil (oral). Second generation cephalosporins have broader activity than first generation cephalosporins. Examples are cefotetan and cefoxitin (injectable); cefaclor, cefpodoxime, loracarbef, cefprozil (oral); and cefuroxime (oral and injectable). Third generation cephalosporins have the broadest spectrum of activity. Some of them are used to treat serious hospital-acquired infections. Examples are cefotaxime, ceftizoxime, ceftriaxone, ceftazidime, and cefoperazone (injectable), and cefixime (oral).

Carbapenems and Monobactams

There are two other types of beta-lactam antibiotics. Imipenem-cilastatin and meropenem are carbapenems with activity against many bacteria that have developed resistance to other antibiotics. Some patients who are allergic to penicillin will also be allergic to imipenem-cilastatin and meropenem. Aztreonam is a monobactam with good activity against some of the hospital-acquired organisms but not as many as the third generation cephalosporins and carbapenems. Patients who are allergic to penicillin can usually take aztreonam without a reaction.

Macrolides

Macrolides are antibiotics that are especially useful against several organisms that cause respiratory infections. Patients who are allergic to penicillin can usually take any of the macrolides. Erythromycin, the oldest drug in this group, frequently causes diarrhea and gastrointestinal cramping. The newer drugs in this group, clarithromycin and azithromycin, are effective against more bacteria and cause less diarrhea.

Sulfonamides

Sulfonamides are effective against many bacteria which cause respiratory, urinary tract, and ear infections. The most frequently used sulfonamide is a combination of the sulfonamide, sulfamethoxazole, and trimethoprim. This combination is often abbreviated as TMP/SMX or called cotrimoxazole. Since the two drugs act in different ways to inhibit bacteria, the development of resistance is less likely than it is with a single drug. Sulfisoxazole and sulfamethoxazole are two other commonly used sulfonamides.

Allergic reactions to sulfonamides are common but are usually not fatal. A serious skin reaction occurs only rarely. Patients with penicillin allergies can usually take sulfonamides. Sulfonamides can precipitate in the urinary tract, so patients should be told to drink plenty of water while taking them. Also, a patient may sunburn more easily when taking sulfonamides. Patients should be told to avoid sun exposure, use sunscreens, and not use artificial tanning lamps.

Tetracyclines

Tetracyclines have a broad spectrum of activity, but they only inhibit the reproduction of organisms. Despite their broad spectrum, their inability to kill organisms limits their usefulness to mild infections. Tetracyclines are useful against some of the organisms involved in sexually transmitted diseases, mild respiratory infections, and acne. The most commonly used drugs are tetracycline hydrochloride, doxycycline, and minocycline. Although doxycycline is sometimes given intravenously, most tetracyclines are given by mouth.

Since tetracyclines combine with metals such as iron, aluminum, calcium, and magnesium, they should not be given with iron tablets, antacids, or milk products. The large molecule formed when they combine with these metals prevents their absorption and renders the drug ineffective.

Because tetracyclines react with calcium, they can be deposited in newly formed bone and teeth. The complex they form with calcium can be weaker than normal tooth and bone and discolor tooth enamel. Since this reaction is of more concern in children or the developing fetus, who are actively forming bone and teeth, these drugs should not be given to children or pregnant women.

Allergies are uncommon to tetracyclines, and these drugs can be given to people with penicillin allergies. However, sun sensitivity may occur as with sulfonamides, and the same precautions should be urged.

Aminoglycosides

Aminoglycosides are able to kill many organisms, including most of the hospital-acquired organisms. These drugs include gentamicin, tobramycin, amikacin, netilmicin, streptomycin, kanamycin, and neomycin. The first four drugs are almost always given intravenously. These four drugs are commonly used for serious infections and in combination with other antibiotics, both to broaden the spectrum of bacteria that will be killed and to lessen the development of resistance in bacteria. None of the aminoglycosides are absorbed well when given orally. This poor absorption and resulting high gastrointestinal concentration makes neomycin a useful agent for cleansing the gastrointestinal tract prior to intestinal surgery. Neomycin and erythromycin are often used together for this purpose.

Allergies to aminoglycosides are uncommon, and these drugs can be used in patients with penicillin allergies. Damage to the ear nerves and the kidneys are serious side effects that can be avoided by careful dosing. Many hospitals have pharmacokinetics programs to help improve the dosing of aminoglycosides and prevent side effects.

Miscellaneous Antibiotics

Clindamycin

Clindamycin is effective against many organisms found on the skin and in the mouth. Because of its activity against mouth organisms, it is used in pneumonias that occur in patients who inhale their mouth secretions because of poor swallowing reflexes. It is also used in combination with other antibiotics for some abdominal infections. There is no cross sensitivity in penicillin-allergic patients. Diarrhea is a common side effect.

Metronidazole

Metronidazole is the most effective antibiotic against anaerobic bacteria, bacteria that grow without oxygen. Anaerobic bacteria cause infections primarily in the abdomen and vagina. To cure vaginal infections, both the woman and the sexual partner must be treated. Metronidazole is also used to treat an anaerobic bacterium that frequently causes diarrhea. Metronidazole is not effective against other bacteria, so it is often given in combination with other antibiotics.

Vancomycin

Vancomycin is effective against certain bacteria that are resistant to most of the penicillins. It is also useful for treating infections in patients who are allergic to penicillin. Infections acquired in the nursing home or the hospital are more likely to be caused by bacteria that are resistant to penicillins than are infections acquired at home. Patients, such as cancer patients, who have long-term intravenous lines also are likely to develop infections that will be resistant to penicillins. Vancomycin is often used in these situations and to treat infections of the heart or heart valves.

Vancomycin is usually given intravenously. It should be well diluted and given slowly. A reaction referred to as Red Man Syndrome may occur if the drug is given too rapidly. This syndrome is characterized by low blood pressure (hypotension) with or without a rash on the upper trunk, face, and arms. Older preparations of vancomycin were impure and damaged hearing and kidney function. Preparations available today are purified and rarely cause this damage unless combined with other drugs that are toxic. To prevent these toxicities, blood levels of vancomycin have been measured and pharmacokinetics programs have been established to promote dosing regimens unlikely to result in toxicity. Since these toxicities are less common with the improved preparations, many hospitals are no longer checking blood levels for vancomycin in all patients.

Fluoroquinolones

Fluoroquinolones act by a different mechanism than beta-lactam or aminoglycoside antibiotics, and may be useful against bacteria that have developed resistance to other antibiotics. Fluoroquinolones may also be useful in treating infections in penicillin-allergic patients. Currently available fluoroquinolones are norfloxacin, ofloxacin, ciprofloxacin, sparfloxacin, levofloxacin, and lomefloxacin. Ciprofloxacin, levofloxacin, ofloxacin are available as oral and intravenous preparations. They attain similar blood levels by either route, which allows them to be used orally for some serious infections that are usually treated with intravenous antibiotics. Fluoroquinolones are particularly useful for prostate gland infections because they penetrate this tissue better than most antibiotics. Fluoroquinolones are also used to treat urinary tract infections, respiratory infections, and gastrointestinal infections and as single-dose therapy for some sexually transmitted diseases.

Common side effects of fluoroquinolones are nausea and vomiting, skin rashes, and headache. In large doses or when drug accumulation occurs because of renal failure, seizures can occur. Fluoroquinolones are contraindicated in pregnant women and children because of possible effects on bone growth.

Antitubercular Drugs

Tuberculosis (TB) was a common and dreaded disease prior to the development of effective diagnosis and treatment practices in the 1940s and 1950s. Currently in the United States, groups such as drug addicts, patients with end-stage renal disease, homeless shelter residents, nursing home residents, and patients with AIDS, are more likely to acquire active TB.[11]

Antitubercular drugs are used for prevention and treatment of TB. Preventive therapy is used for people with a positive skin test for TB or in people exposed to patients with active cases of TB. Treatment is given to patients with active TB. Because therapy with just one drug often leads to the development of bacterial resistance, TB treatment regimens consist of multiple drugs that are effective against tuberculosis. The use of two or more drugs simultaneously minimizes the development of resistance to the other drugs.

The Centers for Disease Control and Prevention, an agency of the U.S. Government, has published guidelines for the prevention and treatment of TB. The major drugs included in these guidelines are isoniazide, rifampin, pyrazinamide, ethambutol, and streptomycin.

Isoniazid is the mainstay of preventive therapy and is one of the drugs used in treatment when drug resistance is not suspected. Patients receiving isoniazid may also receive vitamin B_6 (pyridoxine) to prevent side effects such as numbness or tingling in the hands or feet. Liver failure is the most dangerous adverse effect but it rarely occurs.

Rifampin and pyrazinamide are the other drugs recommended for the treatment of tuberculosis and are also given for prevention if isoniazid resistance is suspected. Rifampin has also been added to antibiotic therapy of other infections to prevent the development of resistance. Rifampin imparts a harmless orange color to urine, sweat, and tears and can stain contact lenses orange. Patients should be forewarned of this possibility. Rifampin also has many significant drug interactions. Pyrazinamide can cause hypersensitivity reactions such as rash, fever, and joint pain. Like isoniazid, its most serious adverse effect is liver damage.

Combination tablets of isoniazid with rifampin, and isoniazid with rifampin and pyrazinamide are now available. These combinations are intended to make compliance with long-term therapy easier for some patients. Because tuberculosis drugs must be taken for at least 6 months and resistance development is more likely if patients take medication erratically, directly observed therapy is recommended. Directly observed therapy means that the patient comes to an office or clinic and takes the medicine in front of the health care worker.

Addition of a fourth drug to the treatment regimen is now recommended by the Centers for Disease Control. The fourth drug improves the likelihood that a resistant strain will be covered and thus enhances the effectiveness of the regimen. This increased effectiveness also allows the patient to take the medication twice a week instead of daily, which is more convenient for directly observed therapy. The fourth drug is usually ethambutol, although streptomycin is used sometimes. The disadvantages of streptomycin are that it must be given intramuscularly and that it can damage the nerves involved with hearing and balance.

When patients cannot tolerate one or more of the drugs used in the regimens described above, or when different types of tuberculosis occur, regimens that include capreomycin, kanamycin, amikacin, cycloserine, ethionamide, ciprofloxacin, ofloxacin, or clofazimine can be used instead.

Antivirals

Until the 1980s, many drugs were available that were effective against bacteria, but few were effective against viruses. The emergence of viral diseases, such as AIDS and genital herpes, and the increased severity of common viral infections like chicken pox in patients with weakened immune systems spurred the development of many new antiviral drugs.

Herpes simplex virus is the cause of fever blisters. Another strain of the herpes simplex virus causes genital herpes, characterized by painful lesions on the genitalia that are spread by sexual contact. Even the less serious herpes, which causes fever blisters, can cause more serious, painful lesions in patients with weakened immune systems, such as cancer patients. Several drugs—acyclovir, famcyclovir, and valacyclovir—are now available that can decrease the symptoms caused by these viruses. These same drugs are also used to reduce the severity of the symptoms caused by herpes zoster virus. Herpes zoster causes the very painful symptoms of shingles and the potentially serious cases of chicken pox in children with weakened immune systems (e.g., children with leukemia).

Amantadine and rimantidine have limited usefulness against the influenza virus. These drugs are reserved to prevent infection after exposure to influenza or are used to reduce symptoms in some patients who develop infection. There are several types of influenza viruses, but these drugs are only effective against Influenza A. The side effects associated with amantadine are hallucinations, blurred vision, and difficulty urinating. Rimantadine has fewer side effects. Amantadine has some effects that rimantadine does not, which has made it useful in Parkinson's disease (see Central Nervous System Drugs).

Ribavirin is an antiviral drug used for a respiratory virus that is common in infants and small children called respiratory syncytial virus (RSV). This drug can also be used for Influenza A and B infections. Ribavirin is administered as an aerosol in an oxygen hood or tent. Ribavirin can cause fetal harm, so women who are or who may become pregnant should avoid contact. Nursing or respiratory care personnel, as well as visitors, who are in the patient room where the drug is being aerosolized should be made aware of this precaution.

The emergence of AIDS has prompted the development of several new antiviral drugs.

Some of these agents are designed to inhibit the human immunodeficiency virus (HIV) which causes AIDS while others are designed to treat opportunistic infections. Opportunistic infections occur in patients with abnormally weak immune systems (immunocompromised), such as AIDS and leukemia patients. People are exposed every day to organisms that can cause opportunistic infections. But most people do not develop opportunistic infections because they have competent immune systems.

There are three classes of antivirals available to treat the HIV virus. The nucleoside reverse transcriptase inhibitors are zidovudine, stavudine, lamivudine, zalcitabine, and didanosine. Protease inhibitors include indinavir, ritonavir, nelfinavir, and saquinavir. The only non-nucleoside reverse transcriptase inhibitor currently available is nevirapine. These classes of antivirals work on different enzymes involved with replication of the virus. Because they work on different enzymes, a combination of drugs from different classes enhances their effectiveness and delays the emergence of resistant strains of HIV. Scientists continue to develop more effective agents or more effective ways to use these agents to treat AIDS.

Zidovudine, a nucleoside reverse transcriptase inhibitor, was the first drug available with activity against HIV. It is currently used alone or in combination with other drugs to treat patients with AIDS, to treat patients with HIV infection but no symptoms, and to decrease the likelihood of transmission of the HIV virus from mother to fetus. The major side effect of zidovudine is decreased white blood cells, which increases the likelihood of infection.

The other nucleoside reverse transcriptase inhibitors are often added to zidovudine or substituted for it in various combinations. Stavudine, zalcitabine, and didanosine can all cause significant peripheral neuropathy, which is numbness or tingling in the hands, feet, arms, or legs. Serious side effects of zalcitabine and didanosine include pancreatitis and liver damage. The adverse effects of lamivudine, pancreatitis and peripheral neuropathy, are more likely to occur in children than in adults. All the drugs in this class except didanosine can be taken with or without food. Didanosine must be taken on an empty stomach for optimal absorption. Didanosine is inactivated by stomach acid, so formulations contain buffers to neutralize the stomach acid. Patients must take two tablets per dose to provide enough buffer to effectively neutralize the stomach acid.

The protease inhibitors are the most potent anti-HIV drugs available. All the drugs in this class have many drug interactions. Indinavir can cause nausea, abdominal pain, and elevated liver function tests. To avoid the formation of kidney stones, patients should drink six glasses of water daily. To increase absorption, indinavir should be taken on an empty stomach. The most frequently reported adverse effects among patients taking saquinavir are diarrhea, abdominal discomfort, and nausea. For optimal absorption, saquinavir should be taken within 2 hours after a full meal. The most frequent adverse effect of nelfinavir is diarrhea. Nelfinavir, like saquinavir, should be taken with food. Weakness, nausea, vomiting, diarrhea, altered taste, and tingling or numbness around the mouth or in the hands and feet are adverse effects associated with ritonavir. For optimal absorption, ritonavir should be taken with food. A low starting dose of ritonavir, with gradual increase to the full dose, minimizes nausea.

Nevirapine, the only non-nucleoside reverse transcriptase inhibitor, should always be used in combination with other antiviral drugs. The most common adverse effects of nevirapine are rash, fever, nausea, headache, and abnormal liver function tests. The rashes associated with nevirapine can be severe and life threatening. Nevirapine can be taken with or without food.

Antivirals used to treat other viral infections in AIDS patients include acyclovir, famcyclovir, and valacyclovir (the drugs mentioned above to treat herpes viruses). Ganciclovir and foscarnet are antivirals used to treat another virus, cytomegalovirus (CMV), which can cause infections in the eye, colon, lungs, and liver. These drugs can also be used for the treatment or prevention of these same infections in patients who have had a kidney or liver transplant. Ganciclovir may decrease white blood cells. Patients also taking zidovudine may have greatly decreased white blood cells because of the combination of drugs. Foscarnet's major adverse effect is kidney toxicity. Since foscarnet does not affect white blood cells, it can be useful for treating AIDS patients who have decreased white blood cells. Ganciclovir causes less kidney toxicity than foscarnet, which makes it useful for kidney transplant patients. Because ganciclovir has the ability to cause tumors and changes in cellular chromosomes, it is advisable to handle and dispose of ganciclovir according to guidelines for cancer chemotherapy drugs.

Antifungals

Antifungals are often used for skin or vaginal infections. This section will focus on antifungal agents used for internal fungal infections.

Like many other types of infections, fungal infections have increased in recent years because of the increased number of patients whose immune systems are not able to control the growth of fungi (e.g., AIDS, cancer, and transplant patients). Additionally, the widespread use of antibiotics kills the bacteria that normally control the growth of fungi.

Amphotericin B is the "gold standard" antifungal drug. It can be given by intravenous injection and as a bladder irrigation for fungal bladder infections. Although amphotericin B is effective against most of the fungi that cause disease in humans, its usefulness is limited by its adverse effects. These effects include fever, chills, vomiting, and headache. These reactions can be limited by the administration of acetaminophen, diphenhydramine, methylprednisolone, or meperidine. More serious reactions include kidney toxicity, decreased red blood cells, and changes in the salts normally found in the blood.

The search for effective agents without the side effects of amphotericin B led to the development of ketoconazole, fluconazole, and itraconazole. These drugs can be used to treat both topical and internal infections.

Ketoconazole is available as an oral agent. It is an inexpensive, effective agent for thrush, a fungal infection of the mouth and throat. Thrush is common in cancer patients treated with drug therapy or radiation. An acidic environment is necessary for the absorption of ketoconazole, so antacids or histamine-2 blockers, such as ranitidine and cimetidine that decrease stomach acidity, should not be given with ketoconazole because they will decrease its absorption.

Fluconazole is an antifungal that can be given orally and intravenously. It is just as effective orally as intravenously, so IV use is necessary only in patients who cannot take the oral formulation or absorb the oral form reliably. Like ketoconazole, fluconazole is useful for thrush and esophageal infections but is more effective than ketoconazole for fungal infections in the lungs, blood, abdomen, and urinary bladder. A single dose of fluconazole can be used to treat vaginal yeast infections. Some patients may prefer a single oral dose to the use of topical creams. Fluconazole is well absorbed even in a non-acidic stomach. It has fewer side effects than amphotericin B, but amphotericin B is more effective for some infections. Serious side effects are rare with fluconazole, but it can cause liver damage and severe skin disorders.

Itraconazole is the newest antifungal agent. It is useful because it is effective against some fungal infections that fluconazole cannot treat. Like fluconazole, itraconazole can cause liver damage. For optimal absorption, itraconazole should be taken with a full meal or with a cola beverage.

ONCOLOGY

Cancer can occur in any tissue of the body. It is not a single disease but rather a set of over 100 disorders occurring in different tissues.[5] Cells in the body are constantly dividing to replace cells that have died. In cancer, a change occurs in some cells causing them to disregard the normal controls that stop cellular growth after a certain number of cells have developed. Therefore, cells multiply out of control and are generally nonfunctional. They can form a large mass called a tumor that compresses healthy cells around it and steals nutrition from the healthy cells. This results in a decrease in the number of cells that are functional. Cancerous cells can also break off from the primary site and migrate through blood or the lymphatic system to other tissues. This process is called metastasis. The ability of cancer to spread is the reason early detection is so important. It is much easier to treat cancer in one area than cancer that has spread throughout the body.

Three types of treatment are used for cancer: surgery, radiation, and chemotherapy (drug therapy). Surgery is usually performed to remove large masses of cancer cells. To make sure that all the cancerous cells are removed, surgeons also remove some healthy tissue around the tumor. Hopefully, this will prevent regrowth of the tumor due to a small number of remaining cancer cells. Radiation is a way of reducing tumor size. X-rays, or particles from radioactive materials, bombard the cancerous tissue to kill cells. Technology is constantly improving the capability to target radiation at the cancerous cells only and thus reduce damage to normal tissue. Chemotherapy is administered to kill cells in large tumors as well as cancer cells that remain after the bulk of the tumor is removed by surgery and/or killed by radiation therapy. Different cancers are treated with different combinations of these three treatments or therapies. Combinations tailored to specific can-

cers allow for more successful elimination of cancerous cells and less damage to normal tissue.

Several factors contribute to the success of chemotherapy regimens. These include the growth cycle of the cancerous cells during therapy, the mechanism by which chemotherapeutic agents kill cancer cells, the combination of agents used for therapy, and the severity of the adverse effects the agents cause. Chemotherapy can work better if the tumor is small and the cells are in a phase of rapid division. Debulking with surgery or radiation helps reduce the tumor size. Because it is hard to know what phase tumor cells are in, using combinations of chemotherapy drugs that act in different ways will kill more tumor cells than using a single agent. Because chemotherapy is more effective against rapidly dividing cells, chemotherapy is given in cycles that allow rest periods during which the normal tissue is allowed to recover and tumor cells are allowed to re-enter a rapid division phase for the next cycle of therapy. The risk-benefit ratio of chemotherapy must be favorable. In other words, the benefits of therapy must out-weigh the harm caused by the adverse effects.

Chemotherapeutic agents are divided into classes on the basis of how they kill cells. Common chemotherapeutic agents are listed below. The toxic effects of these agents on healthy cells can be the limiting factor in the effectiveness of chemotherapy. Many chemotherapy drugs have several commonly used names, which can lead to confusion and medication errors. Because these drugs have so many dose-related adverse effects, mistakes with chemotherapy (e.g., giving the wrong drug or dose) can be fatal.

Common Chemotherapeutic Agents

Alkylating Agents

Mechlorethamine, Chlorambucil, Cyclophosphamide, Lomustine, Carmustine, Busulfan, Cisplatin, Carboplatin

Antimetabolites

Methotrexate, Fluorouracil, Floxuridine, Cytarabine, Mercaptopurine

Hormones

Megestrol Acetate, Medroxyprogesterone, Diethystilbestrol, Estramustine, Tamoxifen, Leuprolide

Antibiotics

Bleomycin, Doxorubicin, Daunorubicin,
Mitoxantrone, Mitomycin, Dactinomycin,
Idarubicin

Mitotic Inhibitors

Etoposide, Vincristine,
Vinblastine, Vinorelbine

Miscellaneous

Hydroxyurea, Procarbazine, Dacarbazine,
Interferon alpha 2a and 2b, Asparaginase,
Paclitaxel

Combinations of chemotherapeutic agents usually leads to higher response rates and a longer period of remission than therapy with a single agent. The selection of drugs for combination is based upon different mechanisms of action, responsiveness to dosage schedules, and the toxicity of the agents. Combination therapy often allows decreased doses of each drug, which may decrease the incidence and severity of toxicity. Chemotherapy combinations are called regimens and they are abbreviated with the initials of the drug names. The initials stand for trade and generic names, and the same letters do not always stand for the same drugs in different regimens. Orders without the drug names can be confusing. An example of a chemotherapy regimen is MAC, used for ovarian cancer. MAC stands for mitomycin, Adriamycin® (doxorubicin), and cyclophosphamide. In the MOPP regimen for Hodgkin's disease, the "M" stands for mechlorethamine, "O" stands for vincristine (Oncovin®), and the "P"s stand for Procarbazine and Prednisone. Never guess what the abbreviations stand for. As shown here, "M" in one abbreviation is not the same as "M" in another abbreviation. Mistakes with chemotherapy can be fatal.

Chemotherapeutic agents cause many severe adverse effects. The bone marrow, where new blood cells are produced, is inhibited by many agents. This leads to decreased numbers of white blood cells, which makes the patient vulnerable to infection. Filgrastim and sargramostim can be used to stimulate the production of white blood cells and minimize the risk of infection due to low white blood cell counts. Decreased numbers of platelets in the blood can result in bruising or bleeding. Other common side effects are hair loss, kidney damage, nerve damage, lung damage, heart damage, inflammation of the bladder, diarrhea, and nausea and vomiting.

Nausea and vomiting is one of the major adverse reactions to chemotherapy. Patients can lose so much fluid through vomiting that they must be admitted to the hospital to receive intravenous fluids. Additionally, many cancer patients cannot maintain adequate nutrition because of nausea. This lack of nutrition is especially devastating because cancer cells are stealing nutrition from healthy cells. Perhaps most important, nausea and vomiting adversely affect the patient's quality of life. Drug therapy to control vomiting is therefore an important part of chemotherapy.

Antiemetics prevent nausea and vomiting. Which antiemetic drug is used will depend upon how common and how severe nausea and vomiting are with the chemotherapy regimen. Combinations of antiemetics are used to increase the total effectiveness. Granisetron and ondansetron are given either orally or intravenously with chemotherapeutic agents that cause the most severe emesis (vomiting). Dexamethasone and lorazepam are often given in combination. Other antiemetic drugs include metoclopramide, droperidol, haloperidol, dronabinol, prochlorperazine, trimethobenzamide, and diphenhydramine.

NUTRITIONAL PRODUCTS

Vitamins

Vitamins are compounds involved in the cellular chemical reactions that are essential to normal tissue growth, maintenance, and function. Vitamin D can be synthesized by the body upon exposure to sunlight, but the rest of the essential vitamins must be supplied by the diet. The recommended dietary allowance (RDA) is the daily level of intake needed to meet the nutritional needs of most healthy people.

Vitamins are classified as fat-soluble or water-soluble. The fat-soluble vitamins are vitamins A, D, E, and K. These are absorbed with fats in the diet, so very low fat diets and conditions that impair fat absorption may decrease amounts of these vitamins in the body. Excessive use of mineral oil as a laxative may cause decreased absorption of the fat-soluble vitamins. These vitamins are stored in fats in the body when excess amounts are ingested. Toxic effects may occur when large amounts are taken. The water-soluble vitamins are C, folic acid, and the B vitamins. With normal kidney function, excess of these vitamins is excreted in the urine and toxic levels do not accumulate.

Many vitamins have more than one name. Knowing the alternate names may be helpful for dispensing the correct product. Listed below are some duplicate names:

Vitamin A = Retinol
Vitamin E = Tocopherol
Vitamin B_1 = Thiamine
Vitamin B_2 = Riboflavin
Vitamin B_5 = Pantothenic Acid
Vitamin B_6 = Pyridoxine
Vitamin B_{12} = Cyanocobalamin
Vitamin B_3 = Niacin = Nicotinic Acid

Several forms of vitamin D are available but are not substitutable in all patients. These forms include cholecalciferol, 25-hydroxycholecalciferol, 1,25-dihydroxycholecalciferol, and ergocalciferol.

Vitamins are used therapeutically in some situations. Vitamin A may be used for certain skin disorders. Vitamin D is used for patients with bone malformation caused by kidney disease. Vitamin K may be given to reverse the effects of the blood thinner warfarin. Niacin (vitamin B3) is used to treat high blood cholesterol.

Vitamins are also given as supplements. Supplements are indicated when a patient's diet is poor, such as with some elderly patients and alcoholics. Vitamin supplements also may be given during periods of increased metabolic requirements such as pregnancy, major surgery, or cancer. Poor absorption is another indication for vitamin supplementation. Some patients lack a substance necessary for the absorption of vitamin B_{12} and must receive B_{12} by injection. Some drugs may affect absorption or requirements for some vitamins. Patients taking the anti-tuberculosis drug isoniazid may have an increased need for pyridoxine to avoid adverse effects on nerves.

Vitamins can be given as individual products or as multivitamin preparations. The multivitamins vary in the quantities of vitamins provided. Few patients require high-potency vitamins. Most patients' needs will be met with inexpensive supplements that provide approximately the recommended dietary allowance of the major vitamins.

Minerals

Minerals are small molecules found in nature that are essential to both the composition and the function of the body. They are present in the body as compounds with other substances or as free ions. Minerals are constituents of enzymes, hormones, and vitamins and are essential to processes such as muscle contraction, nerve conduction, and water and acid balance.

The minerals present in the body in larger amounts are calcium, phosphorus, potassium, chloride, magnesium, and sulfur. The minerals present in small amounts (trace elements) are iron, zinc, iodine, chromium, selenium, fluoride, copper, manganese, and others.

Diets may vary in their mineral content to a greater extent than vitamin content. Plants take up minerals from soil, so the mineral content of the soil where they are grown influences the amount of minerals present in foods. Deficiencies of certain food groups in the diet may cause deficiencies in certain minerals. For instance, dairy products are the most important source of calcium. Patients who are intolerant of dairy products or are strict vegetarians may require calcium supplements to get adequate amounts of calcium.

Some drugs affect body stores of minerals and minerals may also affect the absorption of drugs. Diuretics may decrease body levels of sodium, potassium, and magnesium. Antacids may decrease phosphorus levels. Calcium and iron particularly interfere with the absorption of a number of drugs such as norfloxacin, ofloxacin, ciprofloxacin, and tetracycline.

Minerals, like vitamins, may be given individually when only one is needed. For instance, to prevent the bone disease osteoporosis, postmenopausal women are frequently given calcium supplements. The four minerals that are most commonly administered as single entities are calcium, iron, potassium, and magnesium. Minerals, especially iron, are also added to many multivitamin preparations.

Calcium is a component of bone. It is also essential for nerve conduction and muscle contraction. Calcium is available as many different salts that all vary in the amount of calcium provided. For example, 650 mg of calcium carbonate provides 260 mg of calcium. Calcium gluconate 650 mg provides only 58.5 mg of calcium. Therefore, four times as many tablets of calcium gluconate compared to calcium carbonate would be required to provide one gram of calcium. Calcium is also available as injectable salts for intravenous use.

Iron is a component of hemoglobin, the molecule in red blood cells that carries oxygen. Iron deficiency anemia can result from poor absorption of iron, inadequate intake of iron, or iron loss secondary to bleeding. Iron is administered as many different salts that contain varying amounts of iron. Both the amount of the iron salt and the amount of elemental iron may be listed on the product. Iron products are most often prescribed as the desired salt (e.g., ferrous sulfate) and the amount of the salt (325 mg). If the prescription does not clearly state which product to dispense, the technician should consult with the pharmacist. Iron is also available in an injectable preparation for intramuscular or intravenous use.

Potassium is the primary mineral found inside cells. Potassium imbalance adversely affects cellular metabolism and nerve and muscle function. Potassium replacement is often necessary in patients taking diuretics. Patients with vomiting and diarrhea may lose excessive amounts of potassium in these gastrointestinal fluids. Potassium salts are available as tablets and liquids for oral use. The amount of potassium present may be expressed as milli-equivalents (mEq) rather than milligrams (mg). Potassium chloride is the salt most commonly prescribed. Liquid forms have an unpleasant taste. One tablet form, K-Dur®, is a tablet of pressed pellets which can be suspended in liquid to provide a tasteless liquid form. Potassium salts are irritating to the stomach, so they are usually given as wax or polymer forms that minimize irritation by slowly releasing potassium in the gut. Potassium chloride and potassium phosphate can also be given intravenously. Overly concentrated intravenous potassium solutions are irritating to veins. Intravenous solutions must be administered slowly to avoid heart rhythm disturbances.

Magnesium is important to many of the body's enzymes, nerves, and muscles. It is the second most abundant mineral found inside cells. Magnesium may be lost similarly to potassium through gastrointestinal illnesses or the use of diuretics. Cisplatin and amphotericin B are two other drugs that can cause magnesium losses. Magnesium may be administered as oral tablets and liquids, and injection. As with the other minerals, the amount of magnesium in different salts varies. The amount is often expressed as mEq. Magnesium sulfate is the salt used for intravenous administration. Various salts are used for oral replacement. Diarrhea is a common side effect of oral formulations.

Enteral Nutrition

Enteral nutrition is the provision of food or nutrients using the gastrointestinal tract. While parenteral nutrition is available, use of the gastrointestinal tract is the preferred route of feeding when it is available. When patients are not able to eat adequate amounts of food but do have a functional gastrointestinal tract, enteral nutrition products may be administered. These may be given by mouth if the patient can swallow. Often patients cannot swallow adequately. For these patients various tubes placed into the stomach or intestine through the nose or abdominal skin can be used to administer enteral nutrition products.

Enteral nutrition products contain protein, carbohydrates, and fats. The sources of these nutrients may be intact entities similar to regular food, partially digested products, or simple entities that require little digestion before absorption. Electrolytes, vitamins, and minerals are added to most products to provide complete nutrition. Fiber may also be added to regulate bowel function. The balance of these ingredients differs as does the thickness and amount of calories in a formulation. Products are chosen for specific patients based upon these differences. Some products are meant to be supplements rather than a complete diet. These are usually taken by mouth and taste becomes an important criterion for choice.

One important consideration is drug-nutrient interactions. A number of drugs are less effective when administered with enteral tube feedings. Lists of drug incompatibilities with enteral nutrition products are available and should be consulted when patients are receiving drugs that will come in contact with enteral nutrition products.

RECOMMENDED READING*

USPDI, Volume II, *Advice for the Patient*. Rockville, MD: United States Pharmacopeia Convention, Inc; 1997.

USPDI, Volume I, *Drug Information for the Health Care Professional*. Rockville, MD: United States Pharmacopeia Convention, Inc.; 1997.

Merck Manual of Diagnosis and Therapy. 16th ed., Rahway, NJ: Merck Research Laboratories; 1992.

Facts and Comparisons. St. Louis, MO: Facts and Comparisons, Inc.

Basic and Clinical Pharmacology. 6th ed. Norwalk, CT: Appleton & Lange; 1995.

*See chapter 7 for more information about medication references.

REFERENCES

1. Principles of management of common ocular disorders In:Vaughan D, Asbury T, editors. *General Ophthalmology*. 11th ed. Los Altos, CA: Lange Medical Publications; 1986. p.54–65.
2. *Facts and Comparisons*. St. Louis, MO: Facts and Comparisons, Inc.; 1995.
3. The Skin: Assessment. Syntex Laboratories, Inc.; 1986.
4. Covington T, et al., editors. *Handbook of Nonprescription Drugs*. 10th ed. Washington, DC: American Pharmaceutical Association; 1993.
5. DiPiro J. et.al., editors. *Pharmacotherapy A Pathophysiologic Approach*. 2nd ed. New York: Elsevier Science Publishing Co., Inc.; 1992.
6. The Fifth Report of the Joint National Committee on Detection, Evaluation and Treatment of High Blood Pressure (JNC V). *Arch Intern Med.* 1993; 153:154–183.
7. vanHarten J, Burggraaf K, Danhof M, et al. Negligible sublingual absorption of nifedipine. *Lancet* 1987;2:1363–5.
8. Immediate-release nifedipine labeling will warn against off-label uses, FDA indicates following calcium channel blocker advisory committee review. F-D-C Reports 1996;58(5):3–5.
9. McEvoy G. et al., editors. *AHFS 97 Drug Information*. Bethesda, MD: American Society of Health-System Pharmacists; 1997.
10. Katzung B, editor. *Basic and Clinical Pharmacology*. 6th ed. Norwalk, CT: Appleton & Lange; 1995.
11. Des Prez RM, Heim CR. Mycobacterium tuberculosis. In: Mandell GL, Douglas RG, Bennett JE, editors. *Principles and Practice of Infectious Diseases*. New York: Churchill Livingstone, Inc; 1990; p.1877–82.

SELF-ASSESSMENT QUESTIONS

1. Which of the following antibiotics can be prescribed for a patient who is allergic to penicillin?
   a. ticarcillin
   b. erythromycin
   c. amoxicillin
   d. dicloxacillin

2. Which of the following drugs is used in the treatment of Parkinson's disease?
   a. dobutamine
   b. oxytocin
   c. levodopa/carbidopa
   d. ciprofloxacin

3. Insulin cannot be given by which of the following routes?
   a. oral
   b. intravenous
   c. subcutaneous
   d. intravenous drip

4. Several of the most commonly prescribed drugs are used for depression. Which of the following is not an antidepressant?
   a. fluoxetine
   b. sertraline
   c. amitriptyline
   d. diazepam

5. Which of the following is not an action of ibuprofen?
   a. anti-inflammatory
   b. fever reduction (antipyretic)
   c. pain relief (analgesic)
   d. nausea relief (antiemetic)

6. Which of the following statements is true about chemotherapy agents (drugs used for cancer)?
   a. The naming of chemotherapy regimens (such as MAC, MOPP, CHOP, etc.) has been standardized so that the same letter always stands for the same drug.
   b. Chemotherapy drugs frequently have similar-sounding names that can be easily confused.
   c. Chemotherapy drugs are very safe and have few adverse effects.
   d. Chemotherapy drugs are the only treatment available for cancer.

7. A drug that inhibits ovulation and is used in birth control pills is:
   a. conjugated estrogens
   b. ethinyl estradiol
   c. clomiphene
   d. oxytocin

8. Corticosteroids may be used to treat all but which of the following diseases?
   a. rheumatoid arthritis
   b. asthma
   c. allergic reactions
   d. peptic ulcer disease

9. When corticosteroids are no longer needed, how should the drug be discontinued?
   a. The drug should be stopped immediately and all extra tablets washed down the sink.
   b. The drug should be gradually stopped by reducing the dose over days to weeks.
   c. The drug should never be discontinued.
   d. The oral form should be changed to injectable.

10. Which of the following drugs is to treat AIDS (Acquired Immunodeficiency Syndrome)?
    a. glyburide
    b. enalapril
    c. zidovudine
    d. albuterol

11. Conjunctivitis (inflammation of the eye) can be treated with all of the following *except:*
    a. corticosteroid eye drops.
    b. anti-allergy agents.
    c. antibiotic eye drops.
    d. beta-blocker eye drops.

12. Bronchodilators for asthma
    a. are often used as oral metered-dose inhalers.
    b. are obsolete since the introduction of nedocromil.
    c. include theophylline, β_2 agonists, and corticosteroids.
    d. are ineffective by the inhaled route.

13. Lovastatin
    a. lowers blood pressure in patients with angina pectoris.
    b. lowers the bad cholesterol and raises the good cholesterol.
    c. prevents the absorption of fat in food.
    d. commonly causes a dry cough.

14. Drugs used to treat hypertension include all of the following *except:*
    a. verapamil.
    b. hydrochlorothiazide.
    c. atenolol.
    d. digoxin.

15. Effects of warfarin include all *except:*
    a. decreasing the formation of blood clots.
    b. nose bleeds.
    c. red-orange urine.
    d. ringing in the ears.

16. If a patient has a feeding tube into the stomach and is taking omeprazole,
    a. empty the capsule, crush the pellets and dissolve them in Maalox® to flush down the tube.
    b. consult the pharmacist for the correct action to take.
    c. give omeprazole in the intravenous fluid.
    d. tell the nurse to discontinue the drug.

17. The minerals calcium and iron
    a. are needed by the body in trace amounts.
    b. may interfere with the absorption of tetracycline.
    c. are only available in vitamin/mineral combinations.
    d. must be given as supplements because they are not found in food.

18. Levothyroxine and Thyroid USP are used to replace natural thyroid hormone in hypothyroidism. True or False.

19. Ciprofloxacin and tetracycline are good drugs for pediatric infections because they are available in liquid forms. True or False.

20. Acetaminophen is preferred to aspirin to lower fever in children with chicken pox. True or False.

21. Prescriptions for opioid analgesics should have a label affixed to the bottle to warn patients against the use of alcohol with these drugs. True or False.

22. Intranasal beclomethasone is used to treat asthma. True or False.

23. If relief of the common cold does not occur with an intranasal decongestant, increase the dose and use the drug more often. True or False.

24. Nitrates are only effective if they are used every day, around the clock. True or False.

25. Emollient laxatives (stool softeners) are effective drugs for preventing constipation. True or False.

26. Large doses of vitamins might not help you, but they won't hurt you. True or False.

27. Match the trade name with the appropriate generic name.

Trade Name	Generic Name
1. ___Premarin	A. Alprazolam
2. ___Lanoxin	B. Captopril
3. ___Prozac	C. Phenytoin
4. ___Zantac	D. Albuterol
5. ___Mevacor	E. Conjugated Estrogens
6. ___Capoten	F. Ranitidine
7. ___Ceclor	G. Digoxin
8. ___Xanax	H. Fluoxetine
9. ___Proventil	I. Lovastatin
10. ___Dilantin	J. Cefaclor

ANSWERS TO SELF-ASSESSMENT

1. b. Erythromycin. All of the other answers are penicillins and would cause a similar allergic response. Erythromycin is safe to use in penicillin-allergic patients. Cephalosporins should be used with caution, as cross-sensitivity does occur.

2. c. Levodopa/carbidopa. Levodopa/carbidopa is the mainstay of therapy of Parkinson's disease. Dobutamine is used for cardiac conditions and shock. Oxytocin is a hormone which causes uterine contractions and milk flow. Ciprofloxacin is an antibiotic.

3. a. Oral. Insulin is destroyed in the stomach when given orally. Regular insulin can be given intravenously either as a bolus injection or a drip. Other forms of insulin are given subcutaneously.

4. d. Diazepam. Diazepam is a sedative-hypnotic that is also used sometimes as an antispasmolytic and as an antiepileptic. Fluoxetine, sertraline, and amitriptyline are all antidepressants.

5. d. Nausea relief. Ibuprofen may have nausea as an adverse effect. Ibuprofen is a non-steroidal anti-inflammatory agent, so it provides all three of the other actions: anti-inflammatory, antipyretic, and analgesic.

6. b. Chemotherapy drugs frequently have similar-sounding names that can be easily confused. Vinblastine and vincristine sound so much alike that they have been the source of fatal drug errors. The letters in chemotherapy regimens do not always stand for the same drug, so confusion is likely. Chemotherapy drugs have many serious adverse effects. Chemotherapy is only one of three medical treatments for cancer. Radiation and surgery are other treatments.

7. b. Ethinyl estradiol. Ethinyl estradiol is found in many combination birth control pills. Conjugated estrogens are a type of estrogen, but they are used only for postmenopausal estrogen replacement and osteoporosis prevention and treatment. Clomiphene is used to stimulate ovulation to enhance fertility. Oxytocin is a hormone that stimulates uterine contraction during and after labor and stimulates milk flow.

8. d. Peptic ulcer disease. Corticosteroids suppress inflammation and suppress the immune system. They are useful for diseases characterized by inflammation such as rheumatoid arthritis, asthma, and allergic reactions. Corticosteroids have no role in the treatment of peptic ulcer disease.

9. b. The drug should be gradually stopped by reducing the dose over days to weeks. Gradually reducing the dose allows the adrenal gland to recover its important function. Corticosteroids can only be stopped immediately if a very low dose has been taken for a short time. "c" is incorrect because corticosteroids should only be taken as long as the benefit outweighs the risks. The oral form would not be changed to injectable. Usually the opposite is done-injectable drug is given for greater effect, then changed to oral, and finally oral drug is gradually discontinued.

10. c. Zidovudine. Zidovudine is an antiviral drug with activity against human immunodeficiency virus (HIV), which is the cause of AIDS. Glyburide is an oral hypoglycemic agent for Type II Diabetes mellitus. Enalapril is an angiotensin converting enzyme inhibitor (ACEI) used for high blood pressure. Albuterol is a drug used to relax the lungs in asthma and other breathing disorders.

11. d. Beta-blocker eye drops are used to treat glaucoma but have no role in the treatment of conjunctivitis.

12. a. Nedocromil is not a bronchodilator and plays a different role in asthma treatment than the bronchodilators. Corticosteroids are not bronchodilators. Bronchodilators except theophylline are used by the inhaled route.

13. b. is correct. Lovastatin has no effect on blood pressure and does not prevent absorption of fat. It prevents the formation of cholesterol from fats after they are absorbed. ACE inhibitors are the drugs associated with dry cough.

14. d. is correct. Digoxin is used to treat heart failure and atrial fibrillation but has no role in the treatment of hypertension. Verapamil, hydrochlorothiazide, and atenolol are all used to treat hypertension.

15. d. Decreasing the formation of blood clots is the therapeutic effect of warfarin. Nose bleeds and red-orange urine are side effects of warfarin. Ringing in the ears is associated

with aspirin, salicylates, quinine, and quinidine, but not with warfarin.

16. b. is correct. The pharmacist will need to assess how to give the drug and whether there are any drug-nutrient interactions. Crushing the pellets and mixing with Maalox will destroy the coating and expose the drug to the acid in the stomach. Omeprazole is destroyed by acid. Omeprazole does not have an injectable dosage form. Telling the nurse to discontinue the drug would be inappropriate for a technician. The pharmacist or nurse could consult the physician about alternative therapies.

17. b. is correct. Iron is a trace element, but calcium is needed in larger amounts. Calcium and iron are available in single ingredient tablets, as well as in some combination products. A normal diet provides adequate amounts of these minerals in most people.

18. True. Hypothyroidism is the underproduction of thyroid hormone. It is treated with replacement hormone such as levothyroxine or Thyroid, USP.

19. False. Ciprofloxacin and tetracycline should not be used in children because of adverse effects.

20. True. Aspirin should not be used in children with chicken pox or viral illnesses because they are at increased risk of developing Reye's syndrome.

21. True. Alcohol can add to the sedative effect and depression of breathing that can occur with opioid analgesics.

22. False. Orally inhaled beclomethasone is used to treat asthma. Intranasal beclomethasone is used to treat allergic rhinitis.

23. False. Overuse of intranasal decongestants can lead to rebound congestion.

24. False. Tolerance develops to nitrates. A daily "nitrate-free" period improves their effectiveness.

25. True. Stool softeners are preferred for preventing rather than treating constipation.

26. False. The water-soluble vitamins in large doses are excreted by the kidney in healthy people. But fat-soluble vitamins, even in healthy people, accumulate in body fat and may cause toxic effects.

27. Answers: 1-E; 2-G; 3-H; 4-F; 5-I; 6-B; 7-J; 8-A; 9-D; 10-C

7 | Introduction To Drug Information Resources

Charmaine Hunt, Pharm.D.
Melissa Hogan, Pharm.D.

Technicians are frequently challenged with drug information questions throughout the workday, and are called upon to become more knowledgeable about the handling, availability, and uses of medications. The pharmacy technician certification examination questions may ask the technician to identify the best textbook to help answer specific practice-related questions. Also, knowledge of basic textbook content will make the technician more resourceful and less reliant on the pharmacist for drug information.

Pharmacy reference books that are available in all practice settings often hold answers to typical day-to-day practice-related questions. These resources may also be used as study aids for the technician certification examination or to expand the technician's general knowledge about medications. Therefore, it is essential that the technician understands the basics about the frequently used, reputable pharmacy references.

The purpose of this chapter is to describe the key information held in the pharmacy textbooks available in most practice sites. With time and practice, technicians will be able to find the information that they need quickly and efficiently, and in doing so, will become even more valuable members of the healthcare team.

LEARNING OBJECTIVES

After reading this chapter, the technician should review the drug information references at the pharmacy and discuss the potential uses of each with a pharmacist. Further, the technician should be able to

1. Describe the key features of each textbook.
2. Identify the best resource to use when answering a specific pharmacy-related question.
3. Distinguish between questions that may be answered by a technician and those which should be answered only by a pharmacist.
4. Successfully answer the questions at the end of this chapter and be able to locate answers to drug information questions at the workplace.

DRUG INFORMATION QUESTIONS

Before responding to a drug information question, technicians must clearly differentiate questions that fall within their scope of practice, and may be answered by a pharmacy technician, from those that must be answered only by a pharmacist. In many situations, the distinction between the two situations may not be apparent.

As a professional guideline, the technician should recognize that questions that have only one factual, exact answer may usually be answered by a pharmacy technician. Examples of questions that may be answered by a technician include the following:

Q. What is the brand name of warfarin?
A. Coumadin®

Source: *American Drug Index, Drug Facts and Comparisons*

Q. Do Naprosyn® and Alleve® contain the same active ingredient?
A. Yes, both are brand names of naproxen, a NSAID. Naprosyn® is available as a prescription product, and Alleve® is available over the counter.

Source: *American Drug Index, Drug Facts and Comparisons*

Q. In what controlled substance schedule is zolpidem (Ambien®)?
A. Schedule IV.

Source: *Drug Facts and Comparisons*

Q. What dosage forms of clonidine are available in your pharmacy?
A. Clonidine comes as tablets, transdermal patches, and now as an injection (epidural).

Source: Your pharmacy formulary, computer systems, or products on shelves.

Q. An ounce contains how many milliliters?
A. 30 milliliters

Source: *American Drug Index, Physicians' GenRx*

Q. Who manufactures Transderm Scop®? In what text can the manufacturer's phone number be found?
A. Ciba (or its new company name, Novartis)

Source: *American Drug Index, Drug Facts and Comparisons*

Q. Is Augmentin® available as a suspension? If so, what size and concentration is available?
A. Yes, Augmentin® comes as a 125 mg/5 ml and 250 mg/5 ml suspension; in 75 ml and 150 ml sizes.

Source: *American Drug Index, Drug Facts and Comparisons*

Technicians should not interpret a patient specific question or provide information that may require professional judgment. At times, a simply stated question can turn into a complex patient specific situation. Many times, the person requesting the information may be indirectly asking for a pharmacist's point of view or interpretation of a situation, and require an in-depth analysis and recommendation from the pharmacist. Attempting to interpret or answer such a question could result in miscommunication and delivery of inaccurate information. Both scenarios could be potentially harmful to the patient. Examples of questions that require a pharmacist's interpretation and that should not be answered by a technician are listed below. The rationale as to why a pharmacist must be involved is also provided.

Q. My patient is allergic to codeine. What narcotic would be safe for him to take?

Rationale: This is a patient specific situation. To answer such a question, the pharmacist will have to find out more about the patient's specific problems and apply clinical judgment in choosing a safe alternative.

Q. Is Primaxin® compatible with dopamine?

Rationale: What this person wants to know is, can it be piggybacked into a dopamine infusion? Much more information is needed to appropriately answer this question. For example, the pharmacist must know the concentrations of both drugs, the admixture solutions, the infusion routes (y-site vs. central line vs. admixture) and rates, etc. Then the pharmacist must interpret the information found in The *Handbook on Injectable Drugs* and apply it to the specific situation. Therefore, this question should be deferred to a pharmacist.

Q. What is a normal dose of propranolol?

Rationale: Propranolol is used for many indications, at many different doses. Therefore, the normal dose depends on the patient and indication. More detailed information is needed, so a pharmacist should answer this question.

Q. Do erythromycin and fexofenadine (Allegra®) interact? Can they be given together safely to a patient with allergies and an upper respiratory tract infection?

Rationale: This is a patient specific situation, and requires interpretation and a recommendation from a pharmacist.

Q. Can ibuprofen cause renal failure?

Rationale: Questions worded this specifically suggest that there is much more going on in this situation that requires further probing by a pharmacist. This question should be deferred to a pharmacist.

Q. What are the side effects of fluoxetine (Prozac®)?

Rationale: Adverse reaction information in textbooks often provides a list of adverse effects that are often difficult to interpret and convey. Also, it is possible that the requestor wants to apply the information to a specific patient. Therefore, adverse reaction questions should be answered by a pharmacist.

Q. How long should my patient receive cotrimoxazole (Bactrim®) for the treatment of a urinary tract infection?

Rationale: This question calls for a pharmacist's analysis and interpretation of the events surrounding the situation. To answer such a question, the pharmacist will have to ask many more questions to understand the patient's specific problems.

When answering the telephone, technicians should identify themselves as pharmacy technicians, so that the person asking the question will know the type of information that may be appropriately conveyed. If there is any doubt about the nature of the question, the technician should defer the question to the pharmacist.

CHOOSING THE RIGHT REFERENCES

There are a number of drug information resources available to the pharmacy technician.

The key to answering questions quickly and accurately is knowing where the necessary information is likely to be found. Not all references contain every possible answer to every drug information question. At times, it may be difficult to find a reference that contains the information that you are seeking. Pharmacists usually search for information until they exhaust all possible resources. As part of a normal search strategy, a pharmacist is taught to first consult tertiary references, then secondary references, and finally, primary references.

Tertiary references are general references that present documented information in a condensed and compact format and may include a textbook, a computerized system such as Micromedex® (to be discussed later), or review articles. Most of the information that a technician needs can usually be found in tertiary references. Therefore, this chapter will focus on tertiary references.

Secondary references include indexing systems such as Medline that provide a list of journal articles on the topic that is being searched. Secondary systems are used when new or very up-to-date information is required, or when no information can be located in tertiary references.

Primary references are research articles published in journals (or "medical magazines").

If the information cannot be found in a tertiary reference, then, the technician should consult a pharmacist who may advise an alternative search strategy or consult a secondary reference if that is the practice at the particular site. It is recommended that if time permits, the technician consult as many resources as possible and compare information between resources. Most questions that are appropriate for a technician to answer should be available in a tertiary reference.

COMMON REFERENCE BOOKS

This section highlights common, reputable drug information resources. A brief discussion of the resource, features, and questions that the reference will help answer are provided. The following discussion may not apply equally to the various practice settings and does not include all the information resources that are used. Technicians should familiarize themselves with the references in their practice settings to determine which sources best fit their needs.

Drug Facts and Comparisons
Threlkeld DS, Hagemann RC, Brantley AJ, *et al.*, editors.
St. Louis, MO: Facts and Comparisons, Inc.
(updated monthly – loose leaf edition)
(updated yearly – hard cover edition)

Drug Facts and Comparisons is a comprehensive, general drug information reference. This textbook provides complete drug monographs that are organized by therapeutic class (e.g., calcium channel blockers, corticosteroids). It includes tables that allow quick comparisons of drugs. Information that may be found in this textbook includes the following:

Drug Facts

- general drug information: pharmacology, drug interactions, admixture information, normal doses, adverse effects, drug safety in pregnancy, etc.
- product availability: dosage form, brand/ generic names, manufacturer, etc.
- generic drugs when they are available
- active ingredients and strengths of multiple-ingredient products
- controlled substance schedules
- distinguishes over-the-counter (otc) vs. prescription medications
- sugar-free products
- ethanol-free products
- abbreviation tables
- drug company phone numbers and addresses
- color coded pictures that may assist tablet/product identification (hard-bound edition only)

Drug Comparisons

Tables allow comparisons of drugs within the same therapeutic class (e.g., penicillins, beta-blockers, calcium channel blockers). Tables may include drug or class comparisons of:
- pharmacokinetic parameters (i.e., compares time of onset, metabolism, durations of drug action)
- adverse effects
- drug interactions
- dose conversions (i.e., roughly equivalent doses of morphine to other narcotics, or steroid equivalencies, etc.)

- multiple ingredient preparations (i.e., lists the individual ingredients of the cough and cold preparations, analgesic combinations, etc.)

Using *Drug Facts and Comparisons*

Drug Facts and Comparisons contains information that may be used to answer the following questions:

Questions that may be answered by a technician:
- Nifedipine is in what therapeutic class?
- Is ranitidine available as an over-the-counter product?
- What are the available dosage forms of nicotine (for smoking cessation)? Is nicotine nasal spray available yet?
- Is tramadol available as a generic drug?
- What is a non-alcohol containing decongestant syrup?
- What company manufactures Roxanol®? What is the manufacturer's phone number?

Summary of *Drug Facts and Comparisons* Features

- general drug monographs (i.e., indications, pharmacology, normal doses, adverse effects, etc.)
- tables allow rapid comparisons of drugs in the same class
- product availability: dosage form and strength of a product, brand and generic names, manufacturer, ingredients
- monthly updates for the loose leaf version (This is the most up-to-date drug information textbook.)
- pharmaceutical manufacturer phone numbers and addresses

Questions that should be answered by a pharmacist:
- What are the adverse effects of ganciclovir (Cytovene®)?

- What disease(s) does nifedipine treat?
- How do the adverse effects of captopril (Capoten®) compare to those of enalapril (Vasotec®)? (Both are angiotensin converting enzyme inhibitors.)

- Do the tricyclic antidepressants have the same onsets of action, metabolism, and durations of action? How do their adverse reaction profiles compare?
- What dose of oral codeine is equivalent to 30 mg of oral morphine?

United States Pharmacopeia Drug Information (USP DI)
Rockville, MD: United States Pharmacopeial Convention.
(updated yearly)

The *United States Pharmacopeia Drug Information (USP DI)* is a three volume set that provides medication information that suits the needs of health care providers (Volume I) and patients (Volume II). The third volume (*Approved Drug Products and Legal Requirements*) provides information on laws affecting pharmacy practice.

Volume I (*Drug Information for the Healthcare Professional*) provides comprehensive, general drug information. The drug monographs are arranged alphabetically, but discuss similar medications in a single section. The monographs provide a brief discussion on how medications work, their indications and other uses, adverse effects, potential drug interactions, admixture information, storage requirements, auxiliary label recommendations, etc.

Volume II (*Advice to the Patient*) provides a more general discussion of the medications in language that patients will understand. This volume answers questions that patients may ask such as how to take the medication; special considerations about whether to take during pregnancy and breastfeeding; or common adverse effects that may occur when taking the medicine. This information may be photocopied and given to patients to reinforce issues that were discussed during patient counseling.

All volumes contain a section with color coded pictures that may assist tablet/product identification.

Using the *USP DI*

USP DI contains information that may be used to answer the following questions:

Questions that may be answered by a technician:

- For another health care professional, identify a brown, coated tablet with the imprint "Geigy" on one side and 140 on the other side.
- Provide a pharmacist with a patient information sheet for the drug verapamil.
- Nifedipine (Procardia®) is in what therapeutic class?
- Which auxiliary labels should be placed on a captopril (Capoten®) vial?

Summary of *USP DI* Features

- three volumes: drug monographs for health care professionals, patient information, and information on pharmacy law
- product availability: dosage forms and strengths, brand/generic names, etc.
- auxiliary label suggestions
- color coded pictures for tablet/product identification
- updated yearly

Questions that should be answered by a pharmacist:

- What disease(s) or medical condition(s) is sucralfate (Carafate®) used to treat?
- What are the adverse effects of foscarnet (Foscavir®)?
- Does cisapride (Propulsid®) interact with ketoconazole (Nizoral®)?
- What are the indications and major uses of Toprol®?

The Physicians' Desk Reference (PDR)
Montvale, NJ: Medical Economics.
(published yearly)

A package insert is a manufacturer's product information sheet that provides general drug information such as how it works, indications, adverse effects, drug interactions, dosage forms, stability, and dosing information, etc.

The *Physicians' Desk Reference (PDR)* is a book of package inserts. It also contains other useful information such as colored pictures of tablets, capsules, or packaging that may be used for product identification. It lists manufacturer phone numbers and addresses.

The *PDR* should not be considered a primary source of drug information as it has many limitations. It is not comprehensive and only contains information on select brand name drugs. The information is written by the manufacturer and approved by the FDA. It only contains information about FDA-approved uses of the drug. It does not provide comparative information of that drug with similar medications. Therefore, using the *PDR* to compare products is not as straight-forward as with other reference books. Information about generic medications is not available.

Using the *Physicians' Desk Reference*

The *PDR* contains information that may be used to answer the following questions:

Questions that may be answered by a technician:

- What dosage forms of clonidine (Catapres®) are available?
- What company manufactures Roxanol®? What is the manufacturer's phone number?

- How is intravenous amiodarone (Cordarone®) prepared (with what diluent, solution)? How long is it stable?
- Does amphetamine/dextroamphetamine (Adderall®) contain lactose or tartrazine as an inactive ingredient?
- What is the address and phone number of Abbott Laboratories?

Questions that should be answered by a pharmacist:

- What are the adverse effects of ganciclovir (Cytovene®)?
- How is enoxaparin (Lovenox®) dosed for deep venous thrombosis prophylaxis?
- Methylprednisolone sodium succinate is used to treat what condition(s)?

Summary of the *Physicians' Desk Reference* Features

- a book of package inserts (manufacturer monographs)
- lists only major drugs manufactured by a particular company
- provides information on how a drug works, indications, adverse effects, and dosing information, and guidelines for drug preparation (i.e., dilution, stability) and storage
- pharmaceutical manufacturer addresses and phone numbers
- inactive ingredients—(i.e., sulfites, tartrazine, lactose; preservatives, coloring agents, fillers)
- pictures of selected tablets/capsules and products to assist in product identification
- does not contain generic drugs or comparative information

Mosby's Complete Drug Reference: Physicians' GenRx
BeDell LS, editor. St. Louis, MO: Mosby-Year Book, Inc.
(updated yearly with 2 supplements)

Physicians' GenRx is a comprehensive, general drug information reference. This textbook provides complete drug monographs that are organized alphabetically by generic drug names. While the textbook is called *GenRx*, it contains extensive information about prescription brand and generic products when available.

The monographs are fairly extensive and provide information to assist the pharmacist and health care professional in using the drugs clinically. Information provided in each monograph includes medication names (i.e., generic, brand, chemical names), manufacturer, dosage forms, general uses of agents, and clinical trial information when available, adverse reactions and precautions, costs, and therapeutically equivalent products. This textbook is much more comprehensive than the *PDR*, but less comprehensive than *American Hospital Formulary Service (AHFS)*. A key feature of *Physicians' GenRx* is its indexing system, that allows identification of all drugs within a therapeutic class, schedules of controlled substances, pregnancy categories, etc.

Physicians' GenRx will be useful when pharmacists and technicians need to identify a brand or generic product or determine product availability information. It does not provide comparisons between agents within a therapeutic class and does not have comparative tables. It is updated yearly (with two supplements) but will not contain up-to-date information or information about newly marketed drugs.

Using the *Physicians' GenRx*

The *Physicians' GenRx* contains information that may be used to answer the following questions:

Questions that may be answered by a technician:

- What dosage forms of nitroglycerin are available?
- What company manufactures Revia®? What is its phone number?
- How is fosphenytoin (Cerebxy®) prepared (with what diluent, solution)?
- What is the address and phone number of GlaxoWellcome?

- Is there a generic drug for donepezil?
- What is a brand name for hyoscyamine?
- Can Prevacid® be crushed?
- An ounce contains how many milliliters?
- Does Zoloft® come as a 25 mg tablet?
- Does Calan® have a therapeutically equivalent generic product?
- What is the generic name of Pertofrane®?
- Identify a tablet with the markings I-2.

Questions that should be answered by a pharmacist:

- What are the adverse effects of acarbose (Precose®)?
- What drugs does itraconazole (Sporanox®) interact with?
- How do you dose methylprednisolone for spinal cord injuries?

Summary of *Physicians' GenRx* Features

- general drug monographs (i.e., indications, dosage information, adverse effects, etc.)
- product availability: dosage form and product strength, brand and generic names
- generic drug listings, and therapeutic equivalency information
- pharmaceutical manufacturer phone numbers and addresses
- extensive indexing system
- list of drugs that should not be crushed
- published yearly (two supplements)
- brief guidelines for drug preparation (i.e., dilution, stability) and storage
- pictures of tablets/capsules and products to assist in product identification

---

American Drug Index
Olin BE, Hebel SK, Dombek CE, Kastrup EK, editors
St. Louis, MO: Facts and Comparisons, Inc.
(updated yearly)

The *American Drug Index* is an alphabetical listing of drugs that provides brief monographs of each agent. Information provided includes drug name (i.e., generic, brand, chemical name), manufacturer, dosage form, strength and packaging information, and general uses (i.e., general anesthetic, narcotic, antitussive). Its extensive cross indexing is useful when pharmacists and technicians need to quickly identify a brand or generic product or determine product availability information.

Using the *American Drug Index*

The *American Drug Index* contains information that may be used to answer the following questions:

All of the following questions may be answered by a technician.

- What dosage forms of clonidine (Catapres®) are available?
- What company manufactures Roxanol®?
- What is methylprednisolone sodium succinate generally used for?
- What is the address and phone number of Abbott Laboratories?
- What is the brand name of amiodarone?
- Can TheoDur® be crushed?
- A teaspoon contains how many milliliters?
- Does desipramine come as a 25 mg capsule?

- What is the generic name of Pertofrane®?

Summary of *American Drug Index* Features

- product availability information (strength, dosage from, manufacturer)
- cross-indexed alphabetically by brand, generic, or chemical names
- pharmaceutical manufacturer phone numbers and addresses
- weight and measuring conversions
- list of drugs that should not be crushed
- published yearly

Handbook on Injectable Drugs
Trissel LA. Bethesda, MD:
American Society of Health-System Pharmacists.
(published biannually;
updated with biannual supplements)

The *Handbook on Injectable Drugs* is a textbook often used in hospital and home health care pharmacies. As the title states, it focuses solely on injectable medications. Information provided by this reference includes data on the solubility, compatibility, and stability of many different medications. Specifically, it is useful to determine when two medications may be safely mixed together in an IV bag, a syringe, or at a Y-site on an administration set. This reference also addresses special handling requirements of certain agents (i.e., glass vs. plastic container, light restrictions, filters, refrigeration requirements, expiration, etc.).

When assessing questions regarding injectable drugs, careful attention must be paid to the concentrations of both drugs, the admixture solutions, infusion rates and routes, and dosing frequency. It must not be assumed that medications listed as compatible under specific conditions will also be compatible at higher concentrations or in different solutions. Technicians should ask the pharmacist to help them learn how to interpret the tables provided in this text, and should always consult with the pharmacist before applying information learned or before providing another healthcare professional with this information.

Summary of *Handbook On Injectable Drugs* Features

- injectable medications only
- tables denote if certain combinations of drugs are compatible or incompatible
- tables denote the time period that medication combinations are stable
- drug dilution information (specifies solutions and concentrations)
- includes special packaging and handling information (i.e., glass vs. plastic container, light restrictions, filters, refrigeration requirements, expiration, etc.)

Using the
Handbook On Injectable Drugs

The *Handbook on Injectable Drugs* contains information that may be used to answer the following questions:
Most of these questions should be answered by a pharmacist; however, the technician may wish to use this textbook under the supervision of a pharmacist.

- Is vancomycin (Vancocin®) stable in normal saline? If so, for how long?

Table 7-1

Reference Review	
Type of information needed	**Reference likely to have such information**

Product Availability
• dosage form
• product strength
• brand and generic name
• manufacturer
• indication
	American Drug Index
	Drug Facts and Comparisons
	Physicians' Desk Reference
	Physicians' GenRx
	United States Pharmacopeia Drug Information
	    (does not provide manufacturer information
	    consistently)
	Micromedex

Product Identification
• dosage form
• product strength
• brand and generic name
• manufacturer
• colored pictures of tablets/capsules
	Drug Facts and Comparisons (only hardbound
	    edition contains color pictures of tabs/caps)
	Physicians' Desk Reference
	Physicians' GenRx
	United States Pharmacopeia Drug Information
	    (does not provide manufacturer information
	    consistently)
	Micromedex

Drug Uses • FDA approved indications • other uses of the agent	*American Hospital Formulary Service* *American Drug Index* *Drug Facts and Comparisons* *Physicians' Desk Reference* (FDA approved indica- tions only) *Physicians' GenRx* *United States Pharmacopeia Drug Information* Micromedex
Drug Monographs • general drug information • pharmacology • indications and uses • drug interactions • admixture information • doses • adverse effects • drug interactions	*American Hospital Formulary Service* *Drug Facts and Comparisons* *Physicians' Desk Reference* *Physicians' GenRex* *United States Pharmacopeia Drug Information* Micromedex

Injectable Drug Compatibility/
Stabiliity Information
• drug diluent and solution compatibilities
• drug compatibility
• states conditions for handling products (i.e.,
    glass vs. plastic container, protection from
    light, filters, refrigeration, expiration, etc.)
	American Hospital Formulary Service
	Drug Facts and Comparisons
	Handbook on Injectable Drugs
	Package inserts
	Physicians' Desk Reference
	United States Pharmacopeia Drug Information
	Micromedex

Hazardous Chemicals or Drugs
• specifies hazards of the chemicals or drugs
    used at the work site
• guidelines for their safe use
• recommendations to treat or clean up an
    exposure
	Material Safety Data Sheets
	Micromedex

- Is 30 units of regular insulin stable in total parenteral nutrition solutions (D20/7% amino acids)?
- Is 100 mg iron dextran compatible with total parenteral nutrition solutions?
- Can 2 g nafcillin (Unipen®) be infused into the Y-site of a heparin infusion (25,000 u/500 ml infusing at 15 ml/h)?
- Are cisplatin, cyclophosphamide, and etoposide stable in the same solution? With what concentrations of each drug? With what solution? Under what conditions? For how long?
- Is famotidine (Pepcid®) stable in syringes? In what solution? For how long? Under what conditions?
- Should nitroglycerin be prepared in plastic or glass containers?
- Can lipid emulsions be filtered?
- Is sodium nitroprusside (Nipride®) stable under light?
- Under what conditions should mannitol be stored?

Material Safety Data Sheets

Material Safety Data Sheets (MSDS) are information sheets provided by manufacturers for chemicals or drugs that may be hazardous in the workplace. The primary purpose of the MSDS is to provide information about the specific hazards of the chemicals or drugs used at the work site (i.e., to describe acute and chronic health effects), to provide guidelines for their safe use, and to provide recommendations to treat an exposure or clean up a spill. Materials commonly encountered in pharmacies that require MSDS information at the workplace site include cytotoxic chemotherapy agents (i.e., adriamycin, methotrexate), hormonal agents (i.e., diethylstilbesterol), and volatile or explosive agents (i.e., isopropyl alcohol, ethyl alcohol).

Using Material Safety Data Sheets

Material Safety Data Sheets contain information that may be used to answer the following questions:

- What precautions must be taken when preparing and dispensing adriamycin?
- Where should isopropyl alcohol be stored?
- How should an employee exposed to a adriamycin be immediately treated?
- How should a chemotherapy spill be cleaned?

Summary of Material Safety Data Sheets Features

- written information for handling chemicals or drugs which may be hazardous in the workplace
- outline the specific hazards of the chemicals or drugs used at the work site
- provide guidelines for their safe use
- provide recommendations to treat or clean up a spill or chemical exposure

---

American Hospital Formulary Service Drug Information (AHFS DI)
McEvoy GK, editor. Bethesda, MD:
American Society of Health-System Pharmacists
(updated annually, plus three supplements)

American Hospital Formulary Service (AHFS) is a detailed, comprehensive, general drug information reference. This textbook provides complete drug monographs that are organized by therapeutic class (e.g., calcium channel blockers, corticosteroids). The text provides detailed information about the use of a drug, its side effects, dosing considerations, etc., and its coverage is not limited to FDA approved uses of medications. *AHFS* is widely used by pharmacists as it provides in-depth, un-biased, evaluative reviews of medications. This resource is extensively reviewed by editors and contains information from many reputable sources.

AHFS does not provide many tables to allow direct comparisons of agents within a therapeutic class. Neither does it provide extensive product availability information as seen with *Drug Facts and Comparisons*. Also, *AHFS* is exhaustively reviewed and information about new drugs may not be incorporated immediately. Therefore, it is not the best source of information about drugs that were recently approved. This text is updated yearly, and has three supplements annually. The technician will see this reference in all pharmacy practice areas. Technicians would best use this textbook to educate themselves about medications.

Summary of *AHFS* Features

- comprehensive drug monographs (i.e., FDA approved and nonapproved indications, pharmacology, normal doses, adverse effects, etc.)
- detailed, in-depth, unbiased evaluative reviews
- updated yearly (with 3 supplements)

Micromedex® Healthcare Series
Englewood, CO: Micromedex, Inc.
(updated quarterly)

Other resources that may become widely available include *Micromedex® Computerized Clinical Information Systems* and other CD-ROM or information system software. *Micromedex®* is a comprehensive reference system that can be accessed with a personal computer. One advantage is that the computer increases search efficiency. It contains comprehensive drug information, poison information, pregnancy information, patient information, therapeutic information, and more. It is also updated every 3 months, which is faster than most textbook updates. A disadvantage is the cost of the subscription and the technology needed to run this system.

Advancing technology is quickly changing the media on which information is available. It is conceivable that soon all references will be only accessible from computers. Therefore, the technician is urged to begin to become familiar with personal computers and computer information systems in the workplace.

Summary of *Micromedex* Features

- computerized referencing system
- provides complete, comprehensive clinical information including but not limited to:
  toxicology information
  drug information (domestic and foreign)
  tablet/capsule identification
  disease and trauma information
  patient information
  reproductive risk information
  adverse drug reactions information
  diagnostic and monitoring information
  formulations and manufacturers information
  occupational and environmental exposure information
  therapeutic information

SELF-ASSESSMENT QUESTIONS

1. If you are asked, "Fluvastatin (Lescol®) is available as what strengths?" which is the best reference(s) to find this information?
   a. *Drug Facts and Comparisons*
   b. *American Drug Index*
   c. *Physicians' Desk Reference*
   d. all of the above
   e. b and c only

2. If you want to know the diseases or conditions that propranolol (Inderal®) treats, which of the following reference(s) would you consult?
   a. *Handbook on Injectable Drugs*
   b. MSDS
   c. *Drug Facts and Comparisons*
   d. all of the above
   e. none of the above

3. If question #2 was a question from a nurse, this question should be answered by:
   a. a pharmacy technician.
   b. Only a pharmacist should answer this type of question.

c. The technician may answer this question after discussing it with the pharmacist.

d. all of the above.

e. a or c

4. A nurse would like a chart or list that compares the ingredients of cough and cold products. She states that this will be used as a reference in a physician's office. Where would the technician find such a chart?

a. *Handbook on Injectable Drugs*

b. MSDS

c. *Drug Facts and Comparisons*

d. *American Drug Index*

e. none of the above

5. A nurse wants to identify a non-codeine, non-alcohol containing cough formula that can be bought over the counter. She states that the patient has diabetes. Which reference could help answer this question?

a. *Handbook on Injectable Drugs*

b. MSDS

c. *Drug Facts and Comparisons*

d. *American Drug Index*

e. none of the above

6. Question #5 should be answered by:

a. a pharmacy technician.

b. a pharmacist only.

c. The technician may answer this question after discussing it with the pharmacist.

d. all of the above

e. a or c

7. The question "What is the generic name of Prolixin®?" could be most quickly answered with which textbook?

a. *Handbook on Injectable Drugs*

b. *Physicians' Desk Reference*

c. *Drug Facts and Comparisons*

d. *American Drug Index*

e. none of the above

8. The question "Parnate® is in what therapeutic class?" may be best answered with which textbook?

a. *Handbook on Injectable Drugs*

b. MSDS

c. *Drug Facts and Comparisons*

d. *American Drug Index*

e. none of the above

9. Which reference(s) would provide information to answer the following question: What dosage forms of beclomethasone are available?

a. *Physicians' Desk Reference*

b. *Drug Facts and Comparisons*

c. *American Drug Index*

d. *United States Pharmacopeia Drug Information*

e. all of the above

10. Which reference(s) would provide information to answer the following questions:

What company manufactures Roxanol®? What is its phone number?

a. *Physicians' Desk Reference*

b. *Drug Facts and Comparisons*

c. *American Drug Index*

d. *Handbook on Injectable Drugs*

e. a, b, and c only

11. Which reference(s) would provide information to answer:

What are the adverse effects of methotrexate?

a. *Physicians' Desk Reference*

b. *Drug Facts and Comparisons*

c. *United States Pharmacopeia Drug Information*

d. *American Drug Index*

e. a, b, and c

12. Which reference(s) would provide information to answer the following questions:

How is injectable amiodarone (Cordarone®) prepared (with what diluent, solution)? How long is it stable?

a. *Physicians' Desk Reference*

b. MSDS

c. *American Drug Index*

d. *Handbook on Injectable Drugs*

e. a and d only

13. Which reference(s) would provide information to answer the following question:

Does troglitazone (Rezulin®) contain lactose or tartrazine as inactive ingredients?

a. *Physicians' Desk Reference*

b. *Drug Facts and Comparisons*

c. *United States Pharmacopeia Drug Information*

d. *American Drug Index*

e. all of the above

14. Which reference(s) would provide information to answer the following question:

How should a cytarabine spill be cleaned?

a. *Physicians' Desk Reference*

b. MSDS
c. *American Drug Index*
d. *Handbook on Injectable Drugs*

15. Which reference(s) would provide information to answer the following question:

    Is ranitidine (Zantac®) stable in syringes?
    a. *Physicians' Desk Reference*
    b. MSDS
    c. *American Drug Index*
    d. *Handbook on Injectable Drugs*
    e. *Drug Facts and Comparisons*

16. A physician calls and states he needs to know the identification of a pink capsule with imprint code "Geigy 22." Which reference(s) would provide information to answer this question?
    a. *Handbook on Injectable Drugs*
    b. *United States Pharmacopeia Drug Information*
    c. *American Drug Index*
    d. all of the above
    e. a and c only

17. Which references would provide information to answer the following question:

    Risperidone (Risperdal®) is in what therapeutic class?
    a. MSDS
    b. *American Drug Index*
    c. *Handbook on Injectable Drugs*
    d. *Drug Facts and Comparisons*
    e. none of the above

18. A technician may answer the question "What is the infusion rate of vancomycin?" without consulting the pharmacist.
    a. True   b. False

19. A technician may answer the question "What is the brand name of gabapentin?" without consulting the pharmacist.
    a. True   b. False

20. A technician may answer the question "Does your pharmacy carry ProStep® or Nicoderm®?" without consulting the pharmacist.
    a. True   b. False

21. A technician may answer the question "Can lipid emulsions be filtered?" without consulting the pharmacist.
    a. True   b. False

22. To check if Augmentin® 500 mg tablets contain lactose, you should consult:
    a. the package insert.

b. MSDS.
c. *American Drug Index*.
d. *Handbook on Injectable Drugs*.
e. *United States Pharmacopeia Drug Information*.

23. If you want to know if ciprofloxacin (Cipro®) interacts with Mylanta®, you should consult:
    a. the package insert.
    b. *Drug Facts and Comparisons*.
    c. *United States Pharmacopeia Drug Information*.
    d. all of the above
    e. none of the above

24. If you want to know the dose of alendronate (Fosamax®) for the treatment of osteoporosis, you should consult:
    a. the package insert.
    b. *Drug Facts and Comparisons*.
    c. *United States Pharmacopeia Drug Information*.
    d. all of the above
    e. none of the above

25. If you want to know if nitroprusside (Nipride®) is compatible with normal saline, you should consult:
    a. the package insert.
    b. MSDS.
    c. *Handbook on Injectable Drugs*.
    d. a and c
    e. *Drug Facts and Comparisons*.

26. Which reference contains tablet/capsule photographs?
    a. *Physicians' Desk Reference*
    b. *Drug Facts and Comparisons*
    c. *United States Pharmacopeia Drug Information*
    d. *Physicians' GenRx*
    e. all of the above

27. If you want to know all of the drugs available in the ophthalmic antiglaucoma therapeutic class, you should consult:
    a. the package insert.
    b. *Drug Facts and Comparisons*.
    c. *Handbook on Injectable Drugs*.
    d. MSDS.

28. If you want to know the mechanism of action of naloxone (Narcan®), you should check:
    a. the *Physicians' Desk Reference*.
    b. *Drug Facts and Comparisons*.
    c. *United States Pharmacopeia Drug Information*.

d. *American Hospital Formulary Service.*
e. all of the above

29. Which reference contains information developed specifically to help with patient education and counseling?
    a. *Physicians' Desk Reference*
    b. *Drug Facts and Comparisons*
    c. *United States Pharmacopeia Drug Information*
    d. all of the above

30. If you are looking for information about a new drug, and cannot find information in the many references available in your pharmacy, you should:
    a. assume the information does not exist.
    b. consult a pharmacist to help you redefine your search strategy.
    c. make up information.
    d. none of the above

31. Which reference does **not** contain a pharmaceutical manufacturer's directory?
    a. *Physicians' Desk Reference*
    b. *Drug Facts and Comparisons*
    c. *Handbook on Injectable Drugs*
    d. *American Drug Index*

32. The technician's best use of *American Hospital Formulary Service*, or *AHFS*, is:
    a. as a study aid or for general, in-depth information about drugs.
    b. for stability information.
    c. to find information about how to clean up cytotoxic drug spills.
    d. for tablet identification.

33. In which drug information reference would you most likely find information about a **newly** marketed beta-blocker?
    a. the *PDR*
    b. *Drug Facts and Comparisons*
    c. *Physicians' GenRx*
    d. *AHFS*

34. If you want to use the most efficient reference to find the brand name of metformin quickly, which of the following reference(s) would you consult?
    a. *American Drug Index*
    b. *Physicians' GenRx*
    c. *Drug Facts and Comparisons*
    d. *PDR*

35. Which reference could be checked for auxiliary label suggestions?
    a. *American Drug Index*

b. *Physicians' GenRx*
c. *United States Pharmacopeia Drug Information*
d. *PDR*

36. Which reference would help answer the question: Does Calan® have a therapeutically equivalent generic product?
    a. *American Drug Index*
    b. *Physicians' GenRx*
    c. *United States Pharmacopeia Drug Information*
    d. *PDR*
    e. *Drug Facts and Comparisons*

37. The question "Can Asacol® be crushed?" should be answered by which of the following references?
    a. *American Drug Index*
    b. *Physicians' GenRx*
    c. *Handbook on Injectable Drugs*
    d. a and b

38. The available flavors of Bactrim® suspension can be determined by checking:
    a. the package insert.
    b. MSDS.
    c. *American Drug Index.*
    d. *Handbook on Injectable Drugs.*

39. Nicotine patches come as what strengths? Which reference will provide a quick comparison of the available agents? These questions may be answered by checking:
    a. *American Drug Index.*
    b. *AHFS.*
    c. *PDR.*
    e. *Drug Facts and Comparisons.*

ANSWERS TO SELF-ASSESSMENT

1. d. All resources provide availability information for fluvastatin and any of the listed references may be used to answer this question.

2. c. The answer is *Drug Facts and Comparisons* which lists both FDA approved uses and nonapproved uses of both oral and injectable propranolol. The *Handbook on Injectable Drugs* does not give a complete list of indications and only provides information about injectable drug uses; it will provide the reader with select uses. The MSDS does not list indications.

3. b. A nurse would probably have a very specific reason for asking this type of question and it is likely to be a patient-related question. Because propranolol is used for a variety of medication conditions, the pharmacist involvement and interpretation of the circumstances is likely required.

4. c. *Drug Facts and Comparisons* is the only resource that provides lists of combination products. The *American Drug Index* lists all products separately. The MSDS does not contain this type of information.

5. c. The MSDS, *American Drug Index*, and *Handbook on Injectable Drugs* do not contain this type of information. *Drug Facts and Comparisons* lists individual ingredients (to determine alcohol and sugar free products), as well as over the counter versus prescription status of agents.

6. b. This question requires a pharmacist's interpretation of the patient specific situation and interpretation of the pharmacy textbook information. When the pharmacist is conveying the information, the nurse may have more patient specific questions; therefore, this question should be answered by a pharmacist.

7. d. The *Handbook on Injectable Drugs* will not contain this information because it provides information on injectable products only. The *Physicians' Desk Reference* and *Drug Facts and Comparisons* will provide this information, but the index must be used first to find the page on which the product is listed (and may not be very efficient). The *American Drug Index* lists products alphabetically and would be the fastest reference to use to find this information.

8. c. Of the listed references, only *Drug Facts and Comparisons* classifies agents by therapeutic class.

9. e. All of the listed resources provide dosage form information.

10. e. The *Physicians' Desk Reference, Drug Facts and Comparisons,* and *American Drug Index* all provide information about manufacturers and provide company phone numbers also. The *Handbook on Injectable Drugs* does not contain information about Roxanol® or provide phone numbers.

11. e. The texts listed as a, b, and c provide drug monographs which include information about adverse drug reactions. The *American Drug Index* does not provide information about adverse effects of drugs, it is an index of drug names.

12. e. Both the *PDR* (the package insert) and *Handbook on Injectable Drugs* provide information on preparation of injectable products. Material Safety Data Sheets provide information about the hazards of certain medications or chemicals and the *American Drug Index* is an index or alphabetical list of drug brand, chemical, and generic names.

13. a. The *PDR* (the package insert) provides an up to date and detailed list of all drug inactive ingredients. *Drug Facts and Comparisons* at times will list the major inactive ingredients (such as tartrazine, lactose, etc.); however, it does not do this consistently with all products. The *United States Pharmacopeia Drug Information (USP DI)* does not list this information. The *American Drug Index* is an index or alphabetical list of drug brand, chemical, and generic names.

14. b. Material Safety Data Sheets (MSDS), as the name implies, provide information about the hazards of certain medications. They specify hazards of the chemicals or drugs used at the work site, and provide guidelines for their safe use and recommendations to treat an exposure or clean up a spill.

15. d. While the *Physicians' Desk Reference* (package insert) may provide stability information, it rarely provides information about drug stability in syringes. Stability is not within the content of the MSDS and the *American Drug Index* textbooks. The *Handbook on Injectable Drugs* may provide syringe stability information, if such information exists. Therefore, the *Handbook on Injectable Drugs* is a reasonable place to check for such information.

16. b. Resources for product identification (pictures) are not available within the context of the *Handbook on Injectable Drugs* (which discusses injectable drugs only) and the *American Drug Index* (drug list). The *United States Pharmacopeia Drug Information* (Volumes I–III) has photographs that may help you identify this capsule.

17. d. The *Handbook on Injectable Drugs* discusses injectable drugs only and is arranged alphabetically. The *American Drug Index* is a drug list arranged alphabetically. Material Safety Data Sheets (MSDS), as the name implies, provide information about the hazards of certain medications; this resource does not identify therapeutic classes of agents. *Drug Facts and Comparisons* arranges drug names by therapeutic class.

18. False. The infusion rate of vancomycin will depend on the drug dosage, and the patient's past history for tolerating a specific rate of infusion. Because interpretation of this question is needed, it is best answered by a pharmacist. Most infusion rate questions should be answered by a pharmacist.

19. True. The technician may answer this question as no interpretation of patient specific information is required, and the question is without ambiguity.

20. True. The technician may answer this question as no interpretation of patient specific information is required, and the question is without ambiguity.

21. False. While it is clear that lipid emulsions should not be filtered (*Handbook on Injectable Drugs*), the pharmacist should be involved with this question. In this case, the pharmacist should determine the circumstances in which the question is being asked, as he/she may offer other solutions to the problem at hand. Because interpretation of this question is needed, it must be answered by a pharmacist.

22. a. The *Physicians' Drug Reference* (and the package insert) provides an up-to-date and detailed list of all drug inactive ingredients. The *United States Pharmacopeia Drug Information (USP DI)* and the *Handbook on Injectable Drugs* do not list this information. The *American Drug Index* is an index or alphabetical list of drug brand, chemical, and generic names.

23. d. Any of the listed references may be used to answer this question. The texts listed as a, b, and c provide drug monographs which include information about drug interactions. This type of question should be answered by a pharmacist.

24. d. Any of the listed references may be used to answer this question. The texts listed as a, b, and c provide drug monographs which include information about dosing. This type of question should be answered by a pharmacist.

25. d. The package insert, *Handbook on Injectable Drugs* and *Drug Facts and Comparisons* provide specific compatibility information for Nipride®. The *Handbook on Injectable Drugs* will generally have more information about compatibility than the package insert. *Drug Facts and Comparisons* has limited compatibility information. Compatibility information is not within the context of the MSDS.

26. e. Any of the listed references may be used to answer this question. The *United States Pharmacopeia Drug Information*, the *Physicians' Desk Reference*, and the bound edition of *Drug Facts and Comparisons* have tablet/capsule photographs. *Drug Facts and Comparisons* is probably more useful as the information is arranged by color and size, whereas, the *PDR* arranges the photographs by manufacturer (and you essentially must know the product before you can identify it). The *United States Pharmacopeia Drug Information* and *Physicians' GenRx* arrange the photographs alphabetically by generic drug name.

27. b. *Drug Facts and Comparisons* organizes information by therapeutic class, and has lists of all agents within that class (to allow comparisons of agents). The package insert contains information about the specific product only. This therapeutic class is not within the context of the MSDS or *Handbook on Injectable Drugs*.

28. e. The texts listed as a, b, c, and d provide drug monographs which include information about the mechanisms of action of medications.

29. c. The *United States Pharmacopeia Drug Information* was specifically developed in lay language to be used as an aid to patient counseling. These sheets are best used to reinforce information discussed during patient counseling.

30. b. Information about newly marketed drugs is, many times, hard to find. Asking the pharmacist about a different search strategy

may be helpful. Never assume the information doesn't exist unless you have run an exhaustive search and consulted the drug's manufacturer. Of course, never make up information.

31. c. Only the *Handbook on Injectable Drugs* does not have a manufacturer's directory.

32. a. *AHFS* is not the best source for drug stability. It does not contain information about cytotoxic agent clean up or tablet identification. It is an excellent source for comprehensive, in-depth drug information and is an excellent educational tool.

33. b. *Drug Facts and Comparisons* (the loose leaf version) provides monthly updates and is most likely to contain information about newly marketed drugs. The *PDR, AHFS* and *Physicians' GenRx* are updated yearly and will not reflect newly marketed drugs. *AHFS* and *Physicians' GenRx* do have periodic supplements; however, *Drug Facts and Comparisons* is the most up-to-date reference.

34. a. The *American Drug Index* is a concise alphabetical handbook that allows quick information retrieval. *Physician's GenRx* is alphabetized and may be efficient also. However, it is a bulky, cumbersome textbook that may not be as easily handled. Both the *PDR* and *Drug Facts and Comparisons* require using an index to find the page numbers of the drug monograph and will take that one extra step to find the needed information.

35. c. The *United States Pharmacopeia Drug Information* is the only reference which provides specific suggestions for auxiliary labels.

36. b. Only *Physicians' GenRx* provides information about generically equivalent products.

37. d. Both the *American Drug Index* and *Physicians' GenRx* contain tables of drugs that cannot be crushed. Also, even though it is not listed as an answer, the product's package insert or the *PDR* may provide specific instructions about not crushing a drug whose properties would be destroyed by crushing.

38. a. In this case, product-specific information from the package insert will answer this question. The MSDS, the *American Drug Index*, and the *Handbook on Injectable Drugs* would not provide information about drug flavoring.

39. e. *Drug Facts and Comparisons* provides the best resources for comparing agents within a drug class. The *American Drug Index* only indexes drug names separately and does not group them as a class. The *PDR* will list each nicotine patch brand name separately and typically does not compare products.

8 | Nonsterile Compounding and Repackaging

Linda Y. Fred, R.Ph.
Dennis M. Fruin, R.Ph.

The medicine used today has changed greatly from that described in the first English pharmacopoeia, published in 1778. Brews of animal drugs, elixirs, spirits, and various powders have been replaced by modern synthetic and semi-synthetic manufactured products regulated by the United States Food and Drug Administration. Historically, institutional pharmacies have been responsible for formulating and packaging pharmaceuticals for patient use. In early institutional practice, the packaging process was the end result of the process of formulating and compounding medications. As pharmaceutical manufacturers began to prepare, package, and distribute commonly prescribed medications, the role of the pharmacist has partly changed from formulator and packager to repackager of commercially prepared medications. The availability of a large percentage of products in unit-of-use packaging has allowed pharmacists to focus more energies on ensuring the proper use of medications rather than formulating and compounding. Although many pharmaceuticals used today arrive at the pharmacy in a ready to use form, there are still medications that require repackaging into unit-of-use dosage forms. In addition, there are drugs that need to be compounded or manipulated into a dosage form that is suitable for a specific patient or group of patients. Since pharmacists are focusing more on clinical activities, much of the compounding and dosage form manipulation is performed by technicians.

LEARNING OBJECTIVES

After completing this chapter the reader will be able to
1. Define batch repackaging and explain the importance of batch repackaging.
2. Identify nine key areas that define good manufacturing practices.
3. Summarize the criteria to consider when choosing drug product containers and closures.
4. Understand the importance of written procedures for production and process control.
5. Describe the essentials of record keeping in the repackaging process.

6. Understand the importance of quality control and end-product testing programs for extemporaneous preparations.

GOOD MANUFACTURING PRACTICES

Basic guidelines for good manufacturing practices (GMP) for finished pharmaceuticals were established by the U.S. Food and Drug Administration (FDA) in 1963. *United States Pharmacopeia—National Formulary (USP XXII)* states that "while these regulations are directed primarily to the drug manufacturers, the principles embodied therein may be helpful to those engaged in the practice of pharmacy..." [1]

USP XXII lists nine key areas that define GMP and the requirements of each:

- Organization and personnel
- Facilities
- Equipment
- Control of components and drug product containers and closures
- Production and process controls
- Packaging and labeling controls
- Holding and distribution
- Laboratory controls
- Records and reports[1]

Organization and Personnel

The organization and personnel are responsible for ensuring that the entire process yields a product of acceptable and desirable quality. Some organizations establish a quality control unit to take responsibility for the quality of products. This unit has the authority to approve or reject materials that will be used in packaging and labeling the drug products. Quality control units may be informal and exist only in the expectation that all technicians and pharmacists will check the products they produce, or they may be formal in that a staff member is dedicated to ensuring a certain level of quality. Another aspect of quality control is educating the personnel involved with drug product production.

Pharmacies may educate their staff by using an in-house program that is given by professional staff; a certified community college program; a program produced by professional associations; on the job training; or any combination of these methods. The intent is to ensure that each technician involved in the processing, packaging, or holding and distributing a drug product has the knowledge necessary to perform the compounding and repackaging tasks appropriately.

Education and training programs teach technicians about the attire they should wear, precautions that should be taken to keep the compounding and repackaging environment clean, and how to avoid contact with products when they have open wounds or communicable diseases.

Facilities

An appropriately designed area helps reduce the chances of a medication being contaminated or unintentionally altered while it is being compounded or repackaged. The area should be clean and well lighted, with adequate ventilation, humidity and temperature controls. The area should be located away from high traffic areas such as front line dispensing and counseling sections. The area should be isolated from chemical contaminants and sources of particulate matter. To minimize chemical contaminants, the immediate area and work counter should be free of drugs and chemicals used for previous tasks. To minimize dust and particulate matter, stock cartons and boxes should not be stored or opened in this area. The area should be free of dust containing overhangs (e.g., ceiling utility pipes, hanging light fixtures) and ledges (e.g., window sills). At least one sink with hot and cold water for hand washing should be in the immediate area.

Work areas should be constructed of materials that allow for frequent cleaning and disinfecting. All work surfaces should be level and clean. The work surfaces should be smooth, free of cracks and crevices (preferably seamless), and nonshedding. Surfaces should be cleaned with the appropriate cleaner or solvent at both the beginning and at the end of each distinct operation.[2] If another product needs to be prepared before the work surfaces air dry, the surfaces can be dried with a lintless cloth.

Trash and waste materials should be separated from the process and immediately removed from the production area. Smoking, food, and beverages should not be allowed in the area.

The processing area should be large enough to eliminate the possibility of cross-contamination of products, that is, the placement of products in the wrong containers, mislabeling, or contaminating with microbes or particulate. Cross-contamination resulting from drug product residue on equipment and work surfaces will not occur if written policies regarding cleaning and maintenance are followed and documented. Large containers or "set up" trays should be used to consolidate each repackaging or compounding project's components, labels, production logs, and packaging materials to decrease the chance of cross-contamination or the mislabeling of products.

Personnel working in this area should wear clothing appropriate for these duties. Protective apparel, such as head, face, hair, hand, and arm coverings, should be worn as necessary to preclude contamination of products and to protect workers. Generally, a clean laboratory jacket or a hospital cover gown are considered appropriate body covering for most personnel involved with these activities. For tasks that involve hazardous materials, protective gear such as goggles, gloves, masks, respirators, double gowns, and foot covers may also be required depending upon the substances being handled.[2]

Equipment

Pharmacies may use equipment similar to that used by manufacturers. Hospitals commonly use various strip packaging machines to package single units of oral solid medication and liquid-pumping devices for placing oral liquid medications into glass and plastic vials.

Most automatic, mechanical, electronic, or other types of equipment have written programs for maintenance and cleaning to ensure proper performance. Technicians should familiarize themselves with these programs and document that these procedures have been completed as part of an ongoing quality assurance program. Routine cleaning of reusable equipment prevents cross-contamination of products.

Control of Components and Drug Product Containers and Closures

Components and drug product containers and closures should be handled and stored in a manner that minimizes contamination. Bagged or boxed components of drug product containers, or closures, should be stored off the floor and suitably spaced to permit cleaning and inspection. Composition of drug product containers and closures should be such that they not only protect the product from outside elements, but they do not react with the product placed inside

(i.e., a plastic container should not be used to repackage an oral liquid that is in an organic solvent as the organic solvent might leach materials out of the container and into the solution). Most drugs deteriorate as a result of being exposed to oxygen and/or moisture so using repackaging materials that can eliminate or minimize harmful external environment factors are generally preferred.

Production and Process Controls

Procedures and process controls usually exist in the form of a written document that describes how a drug product should be produced. It is critical that technicians be familiar with and follow the written procedures because it ensures that a particular drug product will have the same identity, strength, quality, and purity each time it is prepared.

Most pharmacies use repackaging control cards or production worksheets to promote consistency in the production of drug products (see Figure 8-1). Each card outlines the products, components, and procedures specific to the repackaging of a given drug dose and dosage form. A repackaging card is generally established for each dosage form of a given product (i.e., if a pharmacy repackages dexamethasone tablets in several different strengths, then a card would be needed for each strength.) Written procedures and yield checks are only two parts of an effective production and process control system, the other components are record keeping, quality control, and end product testing. The latter will be discussed later in this chapter.

Determining how much a process should produce and comparing it against the actual results is an excellent way to verify that the product was produced properly. Usually, before producing the product, a technician calculates the theoretical yield (i.e., the number of doses that can be repackaged from a bulk container of drug) and after, the pharmacist compares the predicted yield against the actual yield.

Packaging and Labeling Control

Most pharmacies do not purchase preprinted labels, but generate their own custom labels by using the pharmacy computer, typewriters, or word processing equipment. Many automated packaging machines have built-in label-printing capabilities. Written procedures should be in place explaining how label detail is ensured as

Name of Product _____
Dosage Form _____
Dosage Strength
  or Concentration _____
Amount/Packaged Unit _____
Container Type and Size _____
Drug Code Number _____

Auxiliary Label _____

Special Considerations (Storage, Stability,
Packaging Materials, Delivery Volume, etc.)
_____
_____
_____

Item No.	Date	Manufacturer's			Pharmacy Exp. Date	Units Pkg'd	Pharmacy Control No.	Pkg'd By:	Approved By:			Date Released
		Name	Lot No.	Exp. Date					Drug	Quan.	Label	
1												
2												
3												
4												
5												
6												
7												
8												
9												
10												
11												
12												

Label Format:

Label Samples
Reverse Side

Figure 8-1. Department of Pharmacy Services Repackaging Production Worksheet.

Adapted from Pesko, LJ. Repackaging Pharmaceuticals in Institutional Practice. In: Brown TR, editor. *Handbook of Institutional Pharmacy Practice*, 3rd ed. Bethesda, MD: American Society of Hospital Pharmacists, 1992.

well as how packaging materials such as glass vials are examined for cracks or paper-foil laminates are inspected for proper adhesive bond.

Labeling errors are one of the most common errors made in the repackaging process. Repackaged products can be mislabeled (i.e., misbranded) if different label lots are not kept separate from each other. Only the number of labels needed for the theoretical yield of the bulk container should be prepared plus one which is affixed to the permanent record. If extra labels are inadvertently produced, they should be defaced and discarded to prevent misbranding of other products.

When checking the final labeled product the pharmacist examines the product(s) to ensure that the information on the label (e.g., identity, strength, and expiration) is correct.

Holding and Distribution

Holding of drugs prior to distribution is sometimes required for quality control. Analysis of the final product may be deemed necessary. During this quarantine period it is imperative that these products are stored under the appropriate conditions for temperature, humidity, and light so that the identity, strength, quality, and purity of the drug products are not affected. All quarantined items should be documented and labeled as such. If conditions differ for repackaged medications, those conditions should be noted in writing.

As mentioned earlier, production should be done with the aid of "set up" trays which contain and isolate all components for each product as well as labels and production logs. Set up trays should be checked and signed off by a pharmacist before and after production.

Laboratory Controls

Most pharmacies do not maintain laboratory controls or quarantine products for any set period of time since repackaged and non-sterile compounded drug products are intended for immediate use or only short-term storage. Evaluations and expiration dating are different for these products than commercially manufactured drug products. Methods for determining stability and appropriate expiration dating will be presented later in this chapter.

Records and Reports

Keeping accurate records of the repackaging process (including equipment cleaning, maintenance, and use) is extremely important for several reasons. First, records may be needed to determine what components make up the final product in case one or more of the components is recalled. Second, repackaging records provide in-process and final-product accountability. Errors may often be detected by comparing lot numbers of individual components with the lot numbers recorded on the log sheet. Weights and measures are useful and important if the actual yield does not closely approximate theoretical yield. Third, records and reports are useful when determining the efficiency of a facility's repackaging program, as well as comparing the amount of product that was produced against the amount that was wasted, which helps the pharmacy adjust the quantities it produces.

Records should be maintained for all drug product components, containers, closures, and labeling for at least 1 year after the expiration date (or longer if so defined by local law or the institution's policy). Equipment cleaning, maintenance, and use should be included in individual equipment logs.

Batch production and control records should be prepared for each batch of drug product produced and should include complete information relating to the production and control of each batch. These records should include

- Dates of production
- Identification of each component used in the manufacturing process, supplier, lot number, and expiration date
- Identification of equipment used
- Weights and measures of the components used
- In-process and laboratory controls
- Statement of actual yield
- Complete labeling control records including samples of the labels
- Description of the drug product containers and closures
- Identification of the persons performing each step of the process
- Sample label

Good manufacturing practices should form the foundation of a repackaging program. Although not always directly applicable to the institutional personnel, good manufacturing practices do support many of the specific guidelines that have been established for institutionally based repackaging programs.

NONSTERILE COMPOUNDING

The intention of extemporaneous compounding is to individualize drug therapy for a specific patient. For example, a patient may require an oral medication with a dosage strength of one-half of the commercially available product, therefore tablets are cut in half and repackaged for the patient.

At times, it may be feasible to prepare small batches of a product because several patients have similar needs or one patient may need large amounts of a compounded product. Batch size should be small enough to ensure all products will be used prior to their expiration, but large enough to avoid preparing additional batches in the immediate future.

Equipment

Although state boards of pharmacy provide a list of equipment needed for compounding, the product and dosage form being compounded dictates what is needed. All equipment and accessories should be maintained and the maintenance should be documented. All pharmacies have torsion balances but depending upon compounding needs some may need to have equipment that offers improved accuracy or a capacity for weighing large items. At least annually, the weighing equipment should be certified and the certification documented. The equipment should be situated on level nonvibrating surfaces away from drafts where humidity is low. Guidelines for checking torsion balances can be found in pharmacy reference texts such as *Remington's Pharmaceutical Sciences*[3] or the *USP-NF*.[1] Weights should be stored in rigid boxes with labeled compartments for the weights. They should only be handled with plastic tipped forceps, because soiling by human hands will increase their weight.

The selection of graduated cylinders should match the items routinely compounded as well as satisfy regulatory requirements. For accuracy, a graduate with a capacity equal to or slightly larger than the volume to be measured should be used (i.e., 80 ml of liquid should be measured in a 100 ml graduate). A rule of thumb is to measure no less than 20% of the capacity of the graduate (i.e., the smallest amount of liquid measured in a 100 ml graduate is 20 ml, the smallest amount measured in a 5 ml graduate is 1 ml). Calibrated syringes of the proper size may be more useful than graduates at times, especially when consideration of clean up time is taken into account. It is much easier to discard a 20-cent syringe than it is to properly clean a 10 ml graduate that was used to measure a viscous (thick, dense liquid) component. The use of syringes also helps ensure total delivery of ingredients such as viscous materials. Some thick, dense liquids are more easily weighed, taking into account their specific gravities, than measured with graduates or syringes.

Mortars and pestles are used to crush, grind, and blend various medicinal ingredients. The mortar is a deep bowl and the pestle is a club shaped tool that when stamped or pounded vertically into the well of mortar causes the contents of the mortar to become pulverized. Mortars and pestles are made of different materials and come in assorted sizes. Common mortars and pestles used in pharmaceutical compounding are fabricated in smooth glass, porcelain, or the rough-surfaced Wedgewood variety. The Wedgewood mortars and pestles have rough surfaces that when rubbed together produce enough shear force to reduce hard crystals and powders down to fine powders quickly and uniformly. Porcelain mortars have a smoother finish than Wedgewood, so they are used for blending powders and pulverizing soft aggregates or crystals. Glass mortars are used for liquid preparations or for mixing components that stain or are oily. Usually glass mortars are the choice for use with chemotherapeutic drugs.

The compounding area should be stocked with bond and glassine weighing papers, disposable weighing cups, stainless steel and plastic spatulas of various sizes, ointment slabs, ointment pads, disposable and reusable suppository molds, funnels, filter paper, beakers, glass stirring rods, pH paper and appropriate personnel garb, cleaning equipment, and supplies. A heat source, refrigerator, freezer, and devices such as blenders should be available as well as a sink with hot and cold water. Cleaning of equipment is part of the overall compounding process and it is essential to the quality of the operation.

Inactive Ingredients

In addition to the active or therapeutic ingredient(s) in products, there can be a number of inactive or nontherapeutic ingredients that function as diluents, binders, colors, glidants, lubricants, flavoring, sweeteners, and suspending agents to name a few. Although the term inert is often used to describe these ingredients, there is an increasing awareness that in certain combinations these ingredients will exert their own effect and may alter the performance of the active ingredients.[3]

Commonly Compounded Products

Common types of compounding include the placing of a commercially available oral drug into an oral suspension or the compounding of an enteral nutrition formulation. Other typical compounded items are topical dermatologic ointments and creams as well as rectal and vaginal suppositories not available commercially in the desired vehicle or dosage form.

Oral Suspensions

Drugs that are available commercially only as oral solids are often needed in a liquid form because of the ease of liquid administration or the ability to individualize pediatric doses on a mg/kg basis. To make a suspension from a capsule or tablet, the following steps are usually taken:
1. Powdering of tablets with a mortar and pestle or the emptying of the contents of capsules
2. Wetting the powder to make a paste [4,5]
3. Diluting the wet powder to the desired concentration with a suspending agent
4. Adding a flavoring agent

Coatings of tablets can be removed by rubbing the tablets with gauze pads saturated with ethyl alcohol. The alcohol should be allowed to evaporate before the tablets are placed in the mortar for grinding. Sustained-release tablets should not be crushed for use in a suspension. Ready to use suspending agents are commercially available. Their ingredients should always be checked for preservatives, coloring, flavoring, and alcohol content which can cause adverse effects especially in neonates, particularly preterm infants.[4]

Enteral Nutrition Formulas

Several enteral nutrition formulas are available as ready-to-feed liquids, prepackaged in a variety of volumes and caloric densities. The primary advantages of ready-to-feed liquids are the convenience and microbiologic safety since they are closed systems similar to intravenous products. Powdered products are a useful option because the exact content and concentration of the components in a nutritional regimen can be customized to fit the patient's specific needs and generally cost less than ready-to-feed products. Customized enteral products can easily be contaminated with bacteria so institutional procedures should be strictly adhered to during preparation, storage, and administration. Steps for preparing enteral formulas are displayed in Table 8-1.[6]

Ointments and Creams

These products are usually prepared extemporaneously by mechanical incorporation of the active ingredient into commercially available ointment or cream base (petroleum jelly, Aquaphor™, cold cream, Eucerin™). The medications are often insoluble in the base, therefore it is necessary to grind them into a very fine powder using a mortar and pestle to make it easier to disperse in a uniform manner. The active ingredient is usually incorporated slowly into a small amount of base and then later added to the remainder of base. It may be necessary to use about 5% of an oil or an oil-miscible substance to help disperse the active ingredient uniformly when preparing an oleaginous ointment. Water soluble salts can be dissolved in a small volume of water before being incorporated into an ointment base.

It is important to fill an ointment jar neatly because messy jars may cause the patient to question the quality of the preparation. The surface of the ointment should be slightly lower than the top of the jar so that the ointment does not touch the inside of the lid when the lid is placed on the finished product. This is accomplished by resting the blade of a spatula on one side of the ointment jar and positioned slightly lower than the top of the jar on the other side. When the spatula is in the jar, slightly lower than the jar top, it forms a slight recession in the ointment. Before placing the lid on the container, the lip of the jar can be wiped with a clean low-lint tissue to remove ointment residue prior to the placement of the lid.[3]

Suppositories

Suppositories are made using molds that are available in various shapes and sizes as well as disposable and reusable types. The active ingredient of a suppository is dispersed or dissolved in a melted suppository base. Once the base has been prepared it is poured into a suppository mold, allowed to cool (usually under refrigeration), and removed by opening the mold.

Table 8–1

An Example of Modular Feeding Mixing Guidelines

Step 1. Determine volume of water needed for preparation.
A. Determine patient's enteral fluid requirements.
B. Subtract fluid contributed by macro- and micronutrient modules.
C. The remainder equals the fluid required for formula preparation.

Step 2. Measure water.
A. Measure total volume of sterile water required to prepare formula.
B. Set aside 50–100 ml of water for later use an an irrigant for preparation equipment.
C. Add remaining water to a large beaker with a magnetic stirring bar.
D. Place beaker on a magnetic stirring plate.
E. Initiate stirring.

Step 3. Add protein module.
A. Accurately measure protein module.
B. Add protein module to stirring water.
C. Let stir for 5–10 minutes to promote stabilization.

Step 4. Add carbohydrates, vitamins, minerals, and trace elements.
A. While protein is stirring, measure carbohydrates, vitamins, minerals, and trace elements.

B. Add carbohydrates, vitamins, minerals, and trace element modules.
C. Let stir for 2–3 minutes.

Step 5. Add fat.
A. Measure the fat while the solution is stirring.
B. Add the fat module.
C. Stir for 5–10 minutes.

Step 6. Transfer to the feeding bag or storage container.
A. Transfer the feeding to the feeding bag or storage container.
B. Irrigate the beaker used for mixing with the 50–100 ml of water set aside earlier.
C. Add the irrigated solution to the formula.

Step 7. Add dye.
A. Add adequate dye to color the feeding.

Step 8. Label feeding.
A. Immediately label feeding with label containing:
   1. Complete nutrient composition or formulate
   2. Patient identification (name and medical record number)
   3. Preparation date
   4. Expiration date

Adapted from Teasley-Strausburg, editor. *Nutrition Support Handbook*. Cinncinnati, OH: Harvey Whitney Books, 1992.

Suppositories are formulated on a weight basis so that the amount of medication that replaces a portion of the vehicle is taken into account in the formulation.[3] Suppositories can be packed in bulk by placement in labeled ointment jars or individually wrapped in foil and placed in prescription boxes. Generally, suppositories are stored under refrigeration.

Techniques for Compounding

One of the drawbacks of compounding ointments and creams in the pharmacy is the cleanup required when ingredients such Doaks Tar are used.

An alternate method to the ointment slab, ointment pad, or mortar and pestle compounding technique is the "baggie" method. Using an 8 by 14 inch amber plastic bag, mainly used to cover light sensitive intravenous products, can help eliminate the nasty cleanup of tar derivatives. To make a 2% Doaks Tar in a 1:1 mixture of ketoconazole cream and desoxymetasone 0.25% cream, one would follow these steps:

1. The plastic bag is turned "inside out" so that approximately one-half of the bag overlaps upon itself. Combine the ingredients in the bag. The creams are placed in

the bag by squeezing the contents directly from the tubes or by placement with the aid of a spatula. The required amount of Doaks is poured into the bag from a graduate (or squeezed from a calibrated dropper or expelled from a disposable syringe) directly onto the mound of creams in the bag. After all the ingredients have been placed in the bag, the portion of the bag which had overlapped upon itself is unfolded to its original position.

2. Next the bag is closed in a twisting manner similar to closing a plastic garbage bag (while doing so, excess air is expelled from the bag.) The twisted portion of the bag is then tied in a knot which provides a tightly sealed container.

3. The bag full of its contents is then "kneaded" like bread over and over causing the contents to mix well under the shear pressure.

4. After kneading the bag, scissors are used to cut one corner of the bag off (not much needs to be cut off) and the contents are squeezed into the appropriate sized ointment jar in a manner similar to the method bakers use when decorating a cake with frosting.

5. After the contents of the bag are completely expelled from the bag, the bag is discarded and the graduate is cleaned. Clean-up is easier if a graduated dropper or a disposable syringe is used.

The baggie method also works well when ingredients need to be dissolved in a vehicle before they are geometrically diluted into the base ointment or cream. After ingredients are dissolved and incorporated into a small amount of the base ointment or cream, the ingredients can be placed in the plastic bag as described above. The kneading of the bag over and over provides a very uniform mixture.

Another suggestion to help decrease compounding time of ointment and creams is to work with quantities that coincide with contents of base ointments or creams (i.e., if 45 g of a hydrocortisone cream base are requested, ask the pharmacist to change the quantity to 60 g so that contents from a commercial 60 g tube can be used rather than weighing out 45 g.) If the product is for an outpatient, the quantity can be changed and the number of refills adjusted to reflect the total quantity prescribed (i.e., 45 g with three refills can be changed to 60 g with two refills).

Expiration Dating, Labeling, and Record Keeping

General guidelines are

1. When a manufactured final-dosage-form product is used as a source of active ingredient, use no more than 25% of the manufacturer's remaining expiration dating or 6 months, whichever is less;

2. When a USP or NF chemical, not a manufactured final-dosage-form product, is used, use no more than 6 months;

3. In other cases, use the intended period of therapy or no more than 30 days, whichever is less.[2]

Always consult a pharmacist to determine arbitrary expiration dates.

Labeling

Each compounded product should be labeled with the generic or chemical name of the active ingredients (and inactive if warranted), strength or quantity, pharmacy lot number, expiration date, and any other useful information such as storage requirements. Labels should comply with local, state, and federal laws. (see chapter 4)

Documentation

Each step of the compounding process should be documented. This includes the ingredients, formula, procedure, log of compounded items, batch records sample labels, and equipment checks. The recording of the compounding procedure should be precise to ensure the consistency among all lots produced by the pharmacy. The origin of formulas should be noted with copies of published articles or page numbers of reference texts if these texts are readily available.

REPACKAGING

As pharmaceutical manufacturers prepared, packaged, and distributed more and more of the commonly prescribed medications, the role of the pharmacy changed from formulator, compounder, and packager to repackager of commercially available products. Pharmacies repackage medications from bulk containers into patient-specific containers, including unit-of-use, single-unit, or single-dose packaging.

Unit-of-Use Packaging

Unit-of-use packaging is characterized by either a vial, an envelope, or a plastic bag containing several doses of the same medication. Before dispensing, a prescription label containing the patient's name, and administration directions, is affixed to the package. Unit-of-use packaging is suitable for inpatient or outpatient dispensing. Medications are prepared this way in advance of requests.

As the benefits of unit-of-use packaging became known, further modifications gave rise to the unit-dose concept. Unit-dose packaging includes single-unit and single-dose packages.

Single-Unit Packaging

Single-unit packaging contains a single-dosage form, for example, one tablet or capsule, or one teaspoonful (5 ml) of an oral liquid.

Single-Dose Package

The single-dose package is often confused with the single-unit package. The important difference is that the single-dose package always contains one dose of the drug for a given patient. A single-dose package contains two tablets when a given patient's dose is two tablets. A single-unit package contains only one tablet. (A complete glossary of terms can be found at the end of the book).

The availability of single-unit and single-dose packages from manufacturers has reduced the need for personnel to repackage as much as they once did. However, repackaging is still performed because not all medications are available in unit-of-use, especially oral liquid medications for pediatric patients and a number of the less commonly prescribed oral solids. (Refer to appendix 8-A and 8-B for more information.)

Batch versus Extemporaneous Repackaging

Extemporaneous repackaging is repackaging of quantities of medications that will be used within a short period of time while batch repackaging is the periodic repackaging of large quantities of medications in unit-dose packages.

Extemporaneous repackaging is done on an as needed basis. The quantities repackaged are based on the anticipated immediate need. Usually these medications have limited or unknown stability or are prescribed infrequently.

Batch processing lends itself to medications that have extended stability and are prescribed frequently. Batch production is also thought to save time, materials, and money. Good manufacturing practices and end-product testing are often used with batch repackaging programs to prevent errors.

Containers and Repackaging Materials

Repackaging materials and the package itself must protect the drug from harmful external elements such as light, heat, moisture, air, and (in the case of sterile products) microbial contaminants. The material must not deteriorate during the shelf life of the drug. Packages should be lightweight and made of materials that do not interact with the dosage form. In this context, repackaging materials should not absorb, be absorbed by, or chemically interact with the drug. Materials that are recyclable or biodegradable are preferred over those that are not.

Packages should be constructed so they do not deteriorate with normal handling. They should be easy to open and use, and should not require any additional training or experience to use. Packages should allow for contents to be inspected by the person administering the medication, unless the pharmaceutical properties of the drug preclude its being exposed to light.

The *USP XXII* defines containers and closures on the basis of the degree to which the contents are protected. These degrees of protection are defined as follows:

1. *Light-resistant containers* protect the drug from the effects of incident light by virtue of specific properties of which they are composed, including any coating applied. If protection from light is required, a clear and colorless or a translucent container may be made light-resistant by means of an opaque enclosure.
2. *Well-closed containers* protect the contents from extraneous solids and from loss of the drug under ordinary handling, shipment, storage, and distribution conditions.
3. *Tightly sealed containers* protect their contents from contamination by extraneous liquids, solids, or vapors; from loss of the drug; and from effervescence, deliquescence, or evaporation under ordinary handling, shipment, storage, and distribution conditions.

4. *Hermetic containers* are impervious to air or any other gas under ordinary or customary conditions of handling, shipment, storage, and distribution.[1]

The classification set forth by *USP XXII* designates package types as class A, least amount of moisture permeation; class B, more moisture permeation; class C, more moisture than class B; and class D, highest amount of moisture permeation.

Manufacturers of repackaging materials and repackaging equipment describe their products on the basis of type of package that is achievable—class A, B, C, or D—with class A being the best and class D being the worst. It is generally accepted that class A or class B packages are needed to extend the stability of a repackaged product beyond the few days following repackaging.

REPACKAGING EQUIPMENT

Repackaging equipment can be manual, semi-automated, or fully automated. These systems are reviewed as they pertain to repackaging of oral solids, oral liquids, and injectables. The more manual the system, the more variability is introduced in the package quality and the less chance the package has of attaining a class A or class B rating. A greater number of repackaging systems are available for oral solids than for any other dosage form, because most doses dispensed in institutions are oral solids. Appendix 8-C lists manufacturers of packaging equipment and supplies.

Oral Solid Systems

Pouch and Blister Systems

Oral solids may be packaged in blister packages or in pouch packages. Blister packages are composed of an opaque and nonreflective backing that is usually used for printing or labeling. The backing should be easy to peel from the blister portion of the package and is generally composed of paper or a paper-foil laminate. Backing that is made entirely of paper may range in thickness from light (about the thickness of construction paper) to heavy (about the thickness of light cardboard).

The blister portion is composed of a dome or bubble of transparent material that is flat bottomed. The transparent material is plastic. The plastic may be either high-density or low-density polyethylene or a combination of polyethylene densities and polypropylenes. PVC has also been used as a blister package plastic.

Blister packages are more rigid than pouch packages and therefore may protect the contents of the container better, but do not lend themselves to the automated repackaging systems found in institutional practice. Automated blister packaging is generally confined to the pharmaceutical industry, but such blister packages are used with some manually operated repackaging programs in institutional practice.

Pouch packages have one or both sides composed of an opaque, nonreflective surface intended for printing. This surface is generally a paper-foil laminate. The opposite side of the pouch can be made of the same paper-foil laminate, a paper-foil-polyethylene laminate, or a transparent polyethylene-coated cellophane.

The pouch package is probably the most common for batch repackaging. The pouch package lends itself to relatively inexpensive automated machinery applications in institutional practice.

Manual Systems

Manually operated oral solid repackaging systems use either pouch packages or blister packages. Both pouch packages and blister packages use either heat sealing or adhesive sealing. As a rule, adhesive sealing systems produce class B, C, or D packages and heat sealing systems generally produce class A, B, C, or D packages.

Pouch Systems

Manual pouch repackaging systems use clear or light-resistant plastic bags (usually PVC). The tablet or capsule is dropped into the bag, and the bag opening is sealed with an adhesive. This system provides a class D package. Manual pouch systems can also be heat sealed by a hot knife blade sealing the end of the plastic bag. Although heat sealing provides a better seal than adhesive, the package is usually a class D because of the packaging material. A label is typed directly on the package before the product is added or on a regular stock label and affixed to the package after it is sealed. This system is generally reserved for extemporaneous packaging.

Blister Systems

Manual blister repackaging systems use a plastic blister package that is made of a clear PVC or a laminate of PVC and low-density polyethylene plastic. The blisters or bubbles come in various sizes, depending on the type and size of the product being repackaged. The blisters can be filled on a tabletop or placed in specially designed holders to cradle the package. The blisters are filled with the drug, and then a paper, paper-foil, or vinyl-paper-foil backing is attached to the blister by removing a protective covering from an adhesive strip on the backing material and applying pressure to the blister and backing material. Blister packages are heat sealed in a heat seal press, which resembles a waffle iron. The heat seal places heat and pressure on the backing material, while the blisters remain protected by the well-like device that holds them.[8]

The adhesive blister package can create a class B, C, or D package while the heat seal blister system can create a class A, B, C, or D package.

Automated Systems

Automated oral solid repackaging systems, or unit-dose strip packaging machines, operate in basically the same fashion as blister packing machines. They all produce a pouch package made of two polyethylene-paper-foil laminates or a polyethylene-paper-foil laminate and a polyethylene-cellulose laminate. Tablets or capsules are manually fed into a wheel that drops the dose into a pouch formed by two heated wheels, and the package is sealed. Individual packages are separated by a serrated knife blade, that perforates the strip of pouches as it passes out of the machine. The labeling information is printed on the laminate by means of a stencil-and-ink system (wet or hot stamp) or a computer-generated printing system that interfaces with the packaging machine. The printing process occurs before the dose is dropped into the pouch.

Automated repackaging machines can package from 60 to 120 doses of a single drug per minute. A device can be attached to the top of the automated strip packaging machine to eliminate the need for an operator to feed tablets and capsules into the wheel.

To prevent contamination of oral solid packaging equipment, only non-penicillin and non-oncolytic drugs should be repackaged.

Oral Liquid Systems

Manual Systems

Manual repackaging systems for oral liquids can be divided into those that use a glass or plastic vial as the reservoir for the liquid medication and those that use a glass or plastic syringe. Manual repackaging systems that require vials have three different closure systems: screw cap vials, vials with permanently affixed tops and small fill holes for medication, and vials that require the addition of a cap that must be crimped. An operator uses syringes, burettes, pipettes, or graduates to measure and transfer the liquid into the vial.

Manual systems for repackaging oral liquids into syringes use either of two methods of repackaging. The first method relies on the operator transferring the liquid to a suitable vessel (such as a beaker) and withdrawing the liquid into the syringe. An ordinary syringe can be used for this process if the number of dosage units is relatively small. Many pharmacies choose to use a reusable glass or disposable plastic Cornwall type syringe (often referred to as a magic syringe or a spring loaded syringe) to speed the filling process. The Cornwall syringe method also offers greater reliability in fill volumes, since the syringe is preset with the appropriate volume to dispense. There are systems that use a burette instead of a syringe. With the burette method, the operator attaches a specially designed cap to the bulk bottle that allows a syringe to be introduced into the bottle; the contents are then withdrawn via the syringe by inverting the bottle.[8]

Semi-automatic Systems

Semi-automated systems are manual systems that use some piece of automated equipment as part of the filling or sealing process. These semi-automated filling pumps are either volumetric or peristaltic in design and can be used with either oral syringes or vials.

Volumetric Pumps

Volumetric pumps operate on the same principle as do Cornwall syringes. The volume to be dispensed into the container is preset based on the draw-back setting and the type of reservoir selected for the pump.

Peristaltic Pumps

Peristaltic pumps get their name from the form of pumping action they employ in delivering fluid. Peristaltic action is created by a series of roller wheels being pulled across a length of tubing. As each wheel passes over the tubing, the tubing is crimped and a small volume of fluid is forced down the tubing. Peristaltic pumps offer some advantages over volumetric pumps, including a faster rate of delivery for larger volumes (10 ml and above) and ability to deliver fairly viscous liquids.

When many units are to be produced a peristaltic pump usually requires frequent recalibration. Volumetric pumps need less recalibrating than peristaltic pumps and are more accurate and reliable for delivering fluid volumes of less than 10 ml.

Like most mechanical devices, these pumps come with several convenience factors. Most of the pumps display the volume of fluid being dispensed and the number of dispensing cycles (number of units filled); fill cycle times can be set automatically with rest periods established between each fill; and alarms are available to alert the operator to an empty container. Pumps also are furnished with foot pedal actuators that allow the operator to control the delivery and rest cycle of the fill.

Automated Systems

Automated liquid repackaging machines are available that fill, seal, and label the medication. Plastic cups are used as the fluid reservoir, and the sealing system is a PVC-paper-foil overseal. The over-seal acts as the label stock, and the labeling is printed directly on the seal as the machine fills and seals the product in much the same way the automated oral solid packaging machines do. A peristaltic pump delivers a predetermined amount of fluid into each cup as the cups pass by the filling orifice. The overseal is attached by using heat and pressure until a strong bond is made between the cup and the PVC-paper-foil seal. The individual finished packages are separated when the machine cuts the overseal paper between cups. Machines are equipped with a variety of sensors that detect and signal problems associated with the fill cups, sealing foil, printing tape, and general machine failure. These machines, capable of producing 20 to 32 units per minute, are used in packaging liquids with volumes of 15 ml, 30 ml, or 45 ml. The final package produced by these machines can attain a class A rating.

COMMONLY REPACKAGED PRODUCTS

Oral Liquids

Oral liquids are usually repackaged in glass or plastic oral vials or oral syringes. Glass containers were commonly used in the past because of properties of inertness, visibility of contents, stability, and FDA acceptance.

Plastics began to be used for repackaging pharmaceuticals in the 1980s. The acceptance of plastics was slow at first because of some of the early materials used. However, they have become more and more popular because newer products are inert, cheaper to produce and ship, weigh less, and are usually unbreakable.

Glass or plastic vials are the most frequently used containers for oral liquids. They are composed of the reservoir and a closure system, generally a rubber stopper or a screw cap made of plastic or metal. The screw cap is generally lined with a paper-vinyl inner cap. The rubber stopper is frequently made of butyl rubber with an aluminum or plastic overseal to hold the stopper in place. Some plastic and glass vials use a paper-lined aluminum foil cap as a closure system; this cap is affixed to the vial by crimping the top over a lip in the vial. Other systems contain a pre-affixed rubber seal that accepts a blunt cannula for semi-automated filling. After filling, the self-sealing closure has a tamper evident seal applied to help ensure product integrity. Another oral liquid container system is a plastic vial with a unique closure system. A plastic ball fits into a small filling hole in the bottom of the vial. The ball provides a friction fit to prevent liquid from escaping from the container. The top of the vial has a paper-foil laminate pull-off tab that allows for labeling or just serves as a tear-off seal.

Oral syringes are similar to injectable syringes, except they are not sterile and a hypodermic needle cannot be connected to the syringe which prevents the injection of oral products parenterally. Oral syringes are composed of either a glass barrel and a plunger made of plastic and rubber or a plastic barrel and a plastic plunger. Many of the oral syringe systems have caps for the syringe hub to help maintain the integrity of the liquid the syringe contains. A tamper evident seal exists that can be applied over the cap and barrel of the syringe. Caution must be given to caregivers who use the oral syringe system to ensure that the syringe caps are kept out of reach of small children to prevent them from accidentally swallowing a cap. These caps should not be placed on syringes intended for outpatient use.

Respiratory Medications

Some pharmacies repackage medications that are used in respiratory treatments. The repackaging requirements of respiratory medications are similar to those of injectable medications. The container and respiratory medication should be sterile and free from pyrogens. If a respiratory medication is contained in a syringe, the syringe should not accept a needle in order to avoid the possibility of injecting the medication parenterally. This is the same premise used in the design of oral syringes, which do not accept needles. Respiratory syringes are available in clear and amber glass in 3 ml and 5 ml sizes.

Topical Medications

Topical medications in an ointment or cream vehicle can be repackaged into glass or plastic jars. Topical creams and gels that are intended for administration into the vagina may be repackaged into vaginal syringes specifically designed for this purpose. These syringes can be purchased with a tube adapter to fit almost any size tube of ointment or cream.

EXPIRATION DATING, LABELING, AND RECORD KEEPING

USP XXII establishes guidelines based on the moisture permeability of the final package for assigning expiration dates for repackaged oral solids and liquids. It does so because the type of repackaging materials and the closure system are important because they can affect the expiration date of the final product.

Labeling is the responsibility of the dispenser and should take into account the nature of the drug repackaged, the characteristics of the containers, and the storage conditions to which the article may be subjected in order to determine a suitable expiration date for the label.[1] *USP XXII* states that an expiration date cannot be later than the date of the original package. In the absence of stability data to the contrary, such date should not exceed (1) 25% of the remaining time between the date of repacking and the expiration date on the original manufacturer's bulk container, or (2) a 6-month period from the date the drug is repackaged, whichever is earlier.

Considerable technical advances have occurred in the area of labeling, partly as a result of using computers in institutional practice. In particular, the personal computer has greatly improved the quality and efficiency of the label production process. Current federal labeling requirements are described in the ASHP Technical Assistance Bulletin on Single Unit and Unit Dose Packages of Drugs (appendix 8-A).

The technical bulletin states that the control number or the lot number should appear on the package. The lot number, which is the number assigned by the repackager to the dosage form being repackaged, is often generated from the date the product is repackaged and another number or letter is added to designate the order in which the dosage form was repackaged that day. For example:

Lot Number: A111595

This was the first product repackaged on November 15, 1995. The second product repackaged on that date would be:

Lot Number: B111595

The repacking date may also be displayed backwards, as follows:

Lot Number: A951511

The lot numbering system should be simple to use. The more complicated the system, the greater the likelihood for errors to occur in assigning and interpreting the lot number.

Most labels are applied manually to the finished product, but labeling guns similar to those used in retailing for affixing price labels to goods, are available which make labeling semi-automated.

Maintaining accurate and complete records of the repackaging process is a necessity mandated by standards of practice and governmental regulation. Accurate records help in managing inventory and monitoring the efficiency of the repackaging process.[9,10] Such records can provide a focal point for a quality assurance program and maximize the technician's role in repackaging.

Like labeling systems, record keeping systems are now computerized. Although computer record keeping programs provide more flexibility in the quantity and type of information that can be gathered, hard copies of certain records such as sample labels and production sheets are still needed. The types of repackaging records that should be kept include formulation records, prepackaging records, and daily repackaging logs.

Formulation records provide pertinent information to the repackaging technician about container type, labeling information, stability, processing equipment, and hazardous materials information on a drug-by-drug basis. For example, the following information would be kept on file and referred to each time tamoxifen citrate 10 mg tablets are repackaged.

Drug: Tamoxifen citrate
    Strength: 10 mg
      Dosage form: Oral tablet
      Packaging material: Poly-foil to
        poly-foil
      Equipment: MPL strip packager

Precautions: The operator should use gloves and mask during production.

Expiration dating: Use FDA guidelines

Prepackaging records contain actual information about the drug being repackaged, for example:

Drug: Tamoxifen citrate

Strength: 10 mg

Dosage Form: Oral tablet

Date of repackaging: 11/15/95

Manufacturer's data

Name: XYZ

Lot number: 9AJB57

Expiration date: 6/97

Repackager's data

Lot number assigned: A111595-1

Expiration date assigned: 05/15/96

Expected yield:____

Quantity repackaged:____

Signatures

Person packaging: JG

Person checking: DF

Prepackaging records are organized by drug so that several batches can be entered in the same record and contain information on all the repackaging runs of the drug. See Figure 8-1 for an example of a repackaging control record form. Note that since the formulation and prepackaging records contain overlapping information, they can be combined into a single record for a given drug. Finally, the prepacking record should have a sample label affixed, for example:

Tamoxifen citrate: (XYZ)

10 mg oral tablet

Expiration date: 051596

Lot number: A111595-1

Anytown Hospital, Anycity

The production worksheet shown in Figure 8-1 lists daily repackaging activity and is used to track production records for a given shift or person and should contain the following information:

Date

Drug, strength, and form repackaged

Lot number assigned

Quality packaged

Extemporaneous or batch

Name of repackager

This record is not a necessity, but many pharmacies find it helpful in tracking productivity. It can serve an important function in recording lot numbers if lot numbers are determined by the date and order in which products are repackaged.

QUALITY CONTROL

A well defined quality control and end-product testing program is essential to ensure the continuous production of high-quality repackaged medications. Since several technicians and pharmacists may deal with many products when repackaging medications, strict adherence to the principles of good manufacturing practices is essential to quality control.

Quality control of repackaging involves in-process controls and end-product testing. In-process controls include written procedures, formal training of the operators of the system, maintenance of equipment, and checkpoints during the process.[11] End-product testing is discussed in a later section of this chapter.

Personnel Training and Competency

Formal training programs are important because they promote consistency and standardization. Over time training programs can pay for themselves by preventing the loss of medication, supplies, and personnel time associated with improper repackaging. Training can lengthen the life of equipment by teaching proper operating procedures, cleaning and maintenance, and adjustment and repair of malfunctioning machinery. Teaching aids such as programmed texts and video presentations are available through professional organizations.

Written Procedures

Technicians should be familiar with the pharmacy's procedures for repackaging. Most procedures will include what is expected regarding cleanliness; labeling format; assignment of expiration dates; container size in relation to the size or volume of the drug being repackaged; operational procedures for the setup, operation, and cleanup of equipment; the type and detail of records; and quality assurance and testing procedures. Since procedures are usually reviewed and updated annually it is a good idea to review the procedures with the staff after each update.

Maintenance of Equipment

Most equipment that is used in the repackaging process requires maintenance. Maintenance can be part of the daily operation of the equipment, or it can be done on a set schedule. Regularly scheduled preventive maintenance can extend the life of equipment, which decreases overhead in the repackaging operation. Preventive maintenance reduces equipment failures and ensures that equipment is operating to the manufacturer's specifications.

Checkpoints

Checkpoints are the steps in the repackaging process that are crucial to ensuring a high quality package. It is important to double check each step.

Check-points include the following:

1. Double checking to ensure that the drug and dosage form being repackaged are the ones that are supposed to be repackaged. It is also important to ensure that the bulk product has not expired.
2. Double checking the fill volumes to ensure that the amount of liquid delivered is proper for the dose and the container selected.
3. Double checking any calculations that may be needed for reconstituting a product to arrive at a given dosage.
4. Double checking the information (e.g., spelling) on a label, stencil, or a computer screen to ensure that the label is complete and accurate.

End-Product Testing

End-product testing is the type of quality control most industries practice. End-product testing requires sampling the final product and determining whether it meets all the standards it met before being subjected to repackaging. Examples of end-product testing include testing a sterile product for sterility and testing a package of a solid or liquid oral dosage for moisture impermeability. The uniformity and potency of a product can be tested by a number of chemical analyses. End-product testing is not generally performed for basic repackaging processes, but may be used more commonly in institutional practice to validate certain types of sterile compounding.

CONCLUSION

Personnel who are engaged in nonsterile compounding must adhere to the basic principles of good manufacturing practices. By taking advantage of the technology that is available today, pharmacies can ensure that high-quality products are produced. This technology includes computers, equipment, and end-product testing programs geared to institutional use. No effort should be spared to ensure that the repackaged medication is of the highest quality attainable.

RECOMMENDED READING

Autian J. Drug packaging in plastics, Part I,II,III. *Drug Cos Ind.* 1968;102:79.

Beck AV. Hospital unit-dose packaging. *Hosp Topics* 1968;46:49–54.

Benya TJ. Records—A control device in production. *Am J Hosp Pharm.* 1966;23:385.

Feldman MJ, Sourney PF, Kaul AF. Determining the date of manufacture of drug products for lot numbers. *Am J Hosp Pharm.* 1979;36:1545.

Gupta VD, Stewart KR, Gupta A. Stability of oral solid drugs after repackaging in single-unit containers. *Am J Hosp Pharm.* 1980;37:165–9.

Kenna FR. Strip packaged medications. *Hosp Topics* 1966;44:104.

Mandl FL, Greenburg RB. Legal implications of preparing and dispensing drugs under conditions not in a product's official labeling. *Am J Hosp Pharm.* 1976;33:814.

Miller RW. Pharmaceutical manufacturers and unit dose packaging. *Am J Hosp Pharm.* 1967;24:76.

Nold EG. Stability of drugs repackaged into unit containers. *Am J Hosp Pharm.* 1977;34:1294.

Pesko LJ. Repackaging Pharmaceutical in institutional practice. In: Brown TR, editor. *Handbook of Institutional Pharmacy Practice.* Bethesda, MD: American Society of Hospital Pharmacists. 1992.

Proceedings of seminar on drug stability as affected by environment and containers. Washington, DC: U.S. Food and Drug Administration; 1967.

Reamer JT, Grady LT. Moisture permeation of newer unit dose repackaging materials. *Am J Hosp Pharm.* 1978;35:787–93.

Reamer JT, Grady LT , Shangraw RF, *et al.* Moisture permeation of typical unit dose repackaging materials. *Am J Hosp Pharm.* 1977; 34:35–42.

Ritter FT. Panel discussions: Unit dose dispensing—Container manufacturers' viewpoint of unit dose packaging. *Bull Parent Drug Assoc* 1968;22:175.

Sacharow S. A guide to unit-dose packaging. *Drug Cos Ind* 1968;103:90–161.

Stolar MH. Expiration dates of packaged drug products. *Am J Hosp Pharm.* 1979;36:170.

Varsano J. Pharmaceuticals in plastic packaging. *Part I. Drug Cos Ind* 1969;104:72.

REFERENCES

1. USPC. *The United States Pharmacopeia,* 22nd rev., and the *National Formulary,* 17th ed. Rockville, MD: The United States Pharmacopeial Convention; 1989.
2. ASHP. ASHP technical assistance bulletin on compounding nonsterile products in pharmacies. *Am J Hosp Pharm.* 1994;51:1441–8.
3. Gennaro AR, editor. *Remington's Pharmaceutical Sciences.* 18th ed. Easton, PA: Mack Publishing; 1990. p. 1631, 1658, 1660.
4. ASHP. *Handbook on Extemporaneous Formulations.* Bethesda, MD: American Society of Hospital Pharmacists; 1987.
5. Szkutnik AJ. Extemporaneous formulations and quality assurance. In: Brown TR, editor. *Handbook of Institutional Pharmacy Practice.* 3rd ed. Bethesda, MD: American Society of Hospital Pharmacists; 1992;235–45.
6. Teasley–Strausburg KM, editor. *Nutrition Support Handbook.* Cincinnati, OH: Harvey Whitney Books; 1992.
7. USPC. *Drug Information for the Health Care Professional, Nutrition Support Handbook. Vol. I,* 14th ed. Rockville, MD: The United States Pharmacopeial Convention; 1994.
8. Stack PE. Method for the aseptic filling of unit dose syringes. *Am J Hosp Pharm.* 1974;31:762.
9. Proksch RA. Compounding and repackaging—need for complete records. *Hosp Pharm.* 1980; 15:344–55.
10. Henry B, Auberman J. Unit dose prepackaging: a guide for development of policies and procedures. *Hosp Pharm.* 1980;15:357–63.
11. Patel JA, Curtis EG, Phillips GL. Quality control guidelines for single unit packaging of parenterals in the hospital pharmacy. *Am J Hosp Pharm.* 1972;29:947–51.

SELF-ASSESSMENT QUESTIONS

1. Describe the difference in quantities produced when comparing batch repackaging and extemporaneous packaging.

2. Which type of repackaging, extemporaneous or batching, results in the most wasted product? Why?

3. How does a blister package differ from a pouch package?

4. What type of expiration dating is given to oral solids when repackaged in pouch packaging made of materials of class A or B rating?

5. Automated blister packaging equipment is commonly seen in hospital pharmacies.

   a. True   b. False

6. What are GMPs?

ANSWERS TO SELF-ASSESSMENT

1. Batch repackaging produces many unit-dose containers of medication at one time, while extemporaneous packaging usually results in a limited number of dosing units.

2. Batch repackaging results in more wasted product because it is very difficult to predict exactly how much of a product will be used over a certain period of time. With the high cost of labor, the efficiencies of mass repackaging of frequently used products and immediate dispensing without a number of manipulations usually outweigh the product waste. Product costs, labor costs, and batch sizes must be constantly monitored.

3. A blister pouch is a semirigid pouch that is generally reserved for oral solid medications. The package is composed of two parts: a backing, which is usually made up of a paper-foil material and a front or facing material, which is a small plastic blister or bubble that holds the medication. The blister portion of the package can either be clear or amber. The pouch package is flexible and is composed of two parts; a paper-foil laminate that is joined to another paper-foil laminate or to a clear cellophane type material to form a small pouch.

4. Six months from the date of repackaging or 25% of the remaining time left between the date of repackaging and the expiration of the oral solid, whichever is less.

5. b. False. Due to the cost of automated blister packaging devices, they are usually only found in pharmaceutical companies' packaging divisions.

6. GMPs are good manufacturing practices.

ASHP Technical Assistance Bulletin on Single Unit and Unit Dose Packages of Drugs

Drug packages must fulfill four basic functions:

1. Identify their contents completely and precisely.
2. Protect their contents from deleterious environmental effects (e.g., photodecomposition).
3. Protect their contents from deterioration due to handling (e.g., breakage and contamination).
4. Permit their contents to be used quickly, easily, and safely.

Modern drug distribution systems use single unit packages to a great extent and, in fact, such packages are central to the operation of unit dose systems, intravenous admixture services, and other important aspects of pharmacy practice. These guidelines have been prepared to assist pharmaceutical manufacturers and pharmacists in the development and production of single unit and unit dose packages, the use of which has been shown to have substantial benefits.

A *single unit* package is one that contains one discrete pharmaceutical dosage form, i.e., one tablet, one 2-ml volume of liquid, one 2-g mass of ointment, etc. A *unit dose* package is one that contains the particular dose of the drug ordered for the patient. A single unit package is also a *unit dose* or *single dose* package if it contains the particular dose of the drug ordered for the patient. A unit dose package could, for example, contain two tablets of a drug product.

General Considerations

Packaging Materials. Packaging materials (and the package itself) must possess the physical characteristics required to protect the contents from (as required) light, moisture, temperature, air, and handling. The material should not deteriorate during the shelf life of the contents. Packages should be of lightweight, nonbulky materials that do not produce toxic fumes when incinerated. Materials that may be recycled or are biodegradable, or both, are to be preferred over those that are not. Packaging materials should not absorb, adsorb, or otherwise deleteriously affect their contents. Information should be available to practitioners indicating the stability and compatibility of drugs with various packaging materials.

Shape and Form. Packages should be constructed so that they do not deteriorate with normal handling. They should be easy to open and use, and their use should require little or no special training or experience. Unless the package contains a drug to be added to a parenteral fluid or otherwise used in compounding a finished dosage form, it should allow the contents to be administered directly to the patient (or IPPB apparatus or fluid administration set) without any need for repackaging into another container or device (except for ampuls).

Label Copy. Current federal labeling requirements must be adhered to, with attention also given to the items at right.

The desired copy and format are as follows:

Nonproprietary Name
(and proprietary name if to be shown)
Dosage Form (if special or other than oral)
Strength
Strength of Dose and Total Contents Delivered
(e.g., number of tablets and their total dose)
Special Notes (e.g., refrigerate)
Expiration Date
Control Number

1. *Nonproprietary and proprietary names.* The nonproprietary name and the strength should be the most prominent part of the package label. It is not necessary to include the proprietary name, if any, on the package. The name of the manufacturer or distributor should appear on the package. In addition, the name of the manufacturer of the finished dosage form should be included in the product labeling. The style of type should be chosen to provide maximum legibility, contrast, and permanence.

2. *Dosage form.* Special characteristics of the dosage form should be a part of the label, e.g., extended release. Packages should be labeled as to the route of administration if other than oral, e.g., topical use. In a package containing an injection, the acceptable injectable route(s) of administration should be stated on both outer and inner packages, i.e., both on the syringe unit and carton (if any).

3. *Strength.* Strength should be stated in accordance with terminology in the *American Hospital Formulary Service*. The metric system should be used, with dosage forms formulated to provide the rounded-off figures in the *USP* table of approximate equivalents and expressed in the smallest whole number. Micrograms should be used through 999, then milligrams through 999, then grams. Thus, 300 mg, *not* 5 gr, nor 325 mg, nor 0.3 g; 60 mg, *not* 1 gr, nor 0.06 g, nor 64.5 mg, nor 65 mg; 400 mcg, *not* 1/150 gr, nor 0.4 mg, nor 0.0004 g; ml (milliliters) should be used instead of cc (cubic centimeters).

4. *Strength of dose and total contents delivered.* The total contents and total dose of the package should be indicated. Thus, a unit dose package containing a 600-mg dose as two 300-mg tablets should be labeled "600 mg (as two 300-mg tablets)." Likewise, a 500-mg dose of a drug in a liquid containing 100 mg/ml should be labeled "Delivers 500 mg (as 5 ml of 100 mg/ml)."

5. *Special notes.* Special notes such as conditions of storage (e.g., refrigerate), preparation (e.g., shake well or moisten), and administration (e.g., not to be chewed) that are not obvious from the dosage form designation are to be included on the label.

6. *Expiration date.* The expiration date should be prominently visible on the package. If the contents must be

reconstituted prior to use, the shelf life of the final product should be indicated. Unless stability data warrant otherwise, expiration dates should fall during January and July to simplify recall procedures.

7. *Control number (lot number).* The control number should appear on the package.

Product Identification Codes. The use of product identification codes, appearing directly on the dosage form, is encouraged.

Evidence of Entry. The package should be so designed that it is evident, when the package is still intact, that it has never been entered or opened.

Specific Considerations

Oral Solids

1. *Blister package.* A blister package should
   a. Have an opaque and nonreflective backing (flat upper surface of package) for printing.
   b. Have a blister (dome or bubble) of a transparent material that is, preferably, flat bottomed.
   c. Be easily peelable.
   d. If it contains a controlled substance, be numbered sequentially for accountability purposes.
2. *Pouch package.* A pouch package should
   a. Have one side opaque and nonreflective for printing.
   b. Be easily deliverable, i.e., large tablets in large pouches, small tablets in small pouches.
   c. Tear from any point or from multiple locations.
   d. If it contains a controlled substance, be numbered sequentially for accountability purposes.
3. The packages should be such that contents can be delivered directly to the patient's mouth or hand.

Oral Liquids

1. The packages should be filled to deliver the labeled contents. It is recognized that overfilling will be necessary, depending on the shape of the container, the container material, and the formulation of the dosage form.
2. The label should state the contents as follows: Delivers ____mg (or g or mcg) in ____ml.
3. If reconstitution is required, the amount of vehicle to be added should be indicated. These directions may take the form of "fill to mark on container" in lieu of stating a specific volume.
4. Syringe-type containers for oral administration should not accept a needle and should be labeled "For Oral Use Only."
5. Containers should be designed to permit administration of contents directly from the package.

Injectables

1. The device should be appropriately calibrated in milliliters and scaled from the tip to the fill line. Calibrated space may be built into the device to permit addition of other drugs. The label should state the contents as follows: Delivers ____mg (or g or mcg) in ____ml.

2. An appropriate size needle may be an integral part of the device. The needle sheath should not be the plunger. The plunger should be mechanically stable in the barrel of the syringe.
3. The device should be of such a design that it is patient ready and assembly instructions are not necessary.
4. The sheath protecting the needle should be a nonpenetrable, preferably rigid material, to protect personnel from injury. The size of the needle should be indicated.
5. The device should be of such a design that easy and visible aspiration is possible. It should be as compact as possible and of such a size that it can be easily handled.

Parenteral Solutions and Additives

1. The approximate pH and osmolarity of parenteral solutions should be stated on the label. The amount of overfill also should be noted. Electrolyte solutions should be labeled in both mEq (or millimole) and mg concentrations. Solutions commonly labeled in terms of percent concentration, e.g., dextrose, should also be labeled in w/v terms.
2. Parenteral fluid container labels should be readable when hanging and when upright or in the normal manipulative position.
3. Drugs to be mixed with parenteral infusion solutions should be packaged into convenient sizes that minimize the need for solution transfers and other manipulations.
4. Partially filled piggyback-type containers should
   a. Be recappable with a tamperproof closure.
   b. Have a hanger.
   c. Have volume markings.
   d. Be designed to minimize the potential for contamination during use.
   e. Contain a partial vacuum for ease of reconstitution.
5. If an administration set is included with the container, it should be compatible with all large volume parenteral delivery systems.

Other Dosage Forms—Ophthalmics, Suppositories, Ointments, etc. Dosage forms other than those specifically discussed above should be adequately labeled to indicate their use and route of administration and should adhere to the above and other required package labeling and design criteria.

Approved by the ASHP Board of Directors, November 14–15, 1984. Revised by the ASHP Council on Clinical Affairs. Supersedes the previous version, which was approved on March 31–April 1, 1977.

The bibliographic citation for this document is as follows: American Society of Hospital Pharmacists. ASHP technical assistance bulletin on single unit and unit dose packages of drugs. *Am J Hosp Pharm.* 1985; 42:378–9.

APPENDIX 8-B

ASHP Technical Assistance Bulletin on Repackaging Oral Solids and Liquids in Single Unit and Unit Dose Packages

To maximize the benefits of a unit dose drug distribution system, all drugs must be packaged in single unit or unit dose packages.[a] However, not all drugs are commercially available in single unit (or unit dose) packages. Therefore, the institutional pharmacist must often repackage drugs obtained in bulk containers (e.g., bottles of 500 tablets) into single unit packages so that they may be used in a unit dose system.

Certain precautions must be taken if the quality of drugs repackaged by the pharmacist is to be maintained. The guidelines presented herein will assist the pharmacist in developing procedures for repackaging drugs in a safe and acceptable manner:

1. The packaging operation should be isolated, to the extent possible, from other pharmacy activities.

2. Only one drug product at a time should be repackaged in a specific work area. No drug products other than the one being repackaged should be present in the immediate packaging area. Also, no labels other than those for the product being repackaged should be present in the area.

3. Upon completion of the packaging run, all unused stocks of drugs and all finished packages should be removed from the packaging area. The packaging machinery and related equipment should then be completely emptied, cleaned, and inspected before commencing the next packaging operation.

4. All unused labels (if separate labels are used) should be removed from the immediate packaging area. The operator should verify that none remains in the packaging machine(s). If labels are prepared as part of the packaging operation, the label plate (or analogous part of the printing apparatus) should be removed or adjusted to "blank" upon completion of the run. This will help assure that the correct label is printed during any subsequent run. There should be a procedure to reconcile the number of packages produced with the number of labels used (if any) and destroyed (if any) and the number of units or volume of drug set forth to be packaged.

5. Before beginning a packaging run, an organoleptic evaluation (color, odor, appearance, and markings) of the drug product being repackaged should be made. The bulk container should also be examined for evidence of water damage, contamination, or other deleterious effects.

6. All packaging equipment and systems should be operated and used in accordance with the manufacturer's or other established instructions. There should be valid justification and authorization by the supervisor for any deviation from those instructions on the part of the operator.

7. The pharmacist should obtain data on the characteristics of all packaging materials used. This information should include data on the chemical composition, light transmission, moisture permeability, size, thickness (alone or in laminate), recommended sealing temperature, and storage requirements.

8. Unit dose packages and labels should, to the extent possible, comply with the "ASHP Guidelines for Single Unit and Unit Dose Packages of Drugs."[1]

9. Whenever feasible, a responsible individual, other than the packaging operator, should verify that (a) the packaging system (drug, materials, and machines) is set up correctly and (b) all procedures have been performed properly. Ultimate responsibility for all packaging operations rests with the pharmacist.

10. Control records of all packaging runs must be kept. These records should include the following information: (1) complete description of the product, i.e., name, strength, dosage form, route of administration, etc.; (2) the product's manufacturer or supplier; (3) control number; (4) the pharmacy's control number if different from the manufacturer's; (5) expiration dates of the original container and the repackaged product; (6) number of units packaged and the date(s) they were packaged; (7) initials of the operator and checker (if any); (8) a sample of the label and, if feasible, a sample of the finished package, which should not be discarded until after the expiration date and which should be examined periodically for signs of deterioration; and (9) description (including lot number) of the packaging materials and equipment used.

11. It is the responsibility of the pharmacist to determine the expiration date to be placed on the package, taking into account the nature of the drug repackaged, the characteristics of the package, and the storage conditions to which the drug may be subjected. This date must not be beyond that of the original package.[b]

12. All drugs should be packaged and stored in a temperature- and humidity-controlled environment to minimize degradation caused by heat and moisture. A relative humidity of 75% at 23°C should not be exceeded. Packaging materials should be stored in accordance with the manufacturer's instructions and any applicable regulations.

13. Written procedures (both general and product specific) governing repackaging operations should be prepared and updated as required. Any deviation from these procedures should be noted and explained on the control record. Operators must understand the procedures (and operation of all packaging equipment) before commencing the run.

14. Applicable FDA and USP requirements concerning the type of package required for specific drug products must be followed.

15. Drugs and chemicals with high vapor pressures should be stored separately from other products to minimize cross contamination.

References

1. American Society of Hospital Pharmacists. ASHP guidelines for single unit and unit dose packages of drugs. *Am J Hosp Pharm.* 1977; 34:613–4.
2. Stolar MH. Expiration dates of repackaged drug products. *Am J Hosp Pharm.* 1979; 36:170. Editorial.

---

[a]A *single unit* package is one which contains one discrete pharmaceutical dosage form, e.g., one tablet or one 5-ml volume of liquid. A *unit dose* package is one which contains the particular dose of drug ordered for the patient. A *single unit* package is a *unit dose (or single dose)* package if it contains that particular dose of drug ordered for the patient.

[b]For specific recommendations on expiration date policy, see Reference 2.

Revised by the ASHP Board of Directors, November 16–17, 1978. Developed originally by a joint working group of the American Society of Hospital Pharmacists and the American Society of Consultant Pharmacists and representatives of the drug packaging industry. The original document subsequently was approved officially by the Boards of Directors of ASHP and ASCP. FDA reviewed the original document and commended ASHP and ASCP for developing the guidelines.

The bibliographic citation for this document is as follows: American Society of Hospital Pharmacists. ASHP technical assistance bulletin on repackaging oral solids and liquids in single unit and unit dose packages. *Am J Hosp Pharm.* 1983; 40:451–2.

Manufacturers of Packaging Equipment and Supplies

Containers and Closures

Abbott Laboratories
Hospital Products Division
1 Abbott Park Road
Abbott Park, IL 60064
(Empty vials)

BAXA Corporation
13760 East Arapahoe Road
Englewood, CO 80112
(Containers, closures, and filling
  systems)

Becton-Dickinson and Company
1 Becton Drive
Franklin Lakes, NJ 07417
(Syringes and syringe tips)

Burron Medical, B. Braun of America
824 - 12th Avenue
Bethlehem, PA 18018
(Containers and filling systems)

Lyphomed, Inc.
Division of Fujisawa, USA, Inc.
Parkway North Center
3 Parkway North
Deerfield, IL 60015
(Empty vials)

Medi-Dose/EPS Inc.
1671 Loretta Avenue
Feasterville, PA 19053
(Containers and closures)

Sherwood Medical
1831 Olive Street
St. Louis, MO 63103
(Syringes and closures)

Smith and Nephew
1845 Tonne Road
Elk Grove Village, IL 60007
(Containers)

3M Company
3M Center
220-8W
St. Paul, MN 55144
(Tamper-evident closures and seals)

West Company
1041 West Bridge Street
Phoenixville, PA 19460
(Containers and all closure
  components)

Wheaton Laboratories
1501 North Tenth Street
Millville, NJ 08332
(Containers and equipment)

Automated Packaging Equipment

Baxter Healthcare Corporation
1 Baxter Parkway
Deerfield, IL 60015
(ATC machine)

Econodose, Inc.
1236 Watson Avenue
Ypsilanti, MI 48917

Euclid Spiral Paper Tube Corporation
339 Mill Street, P.O. Box 458
Apple Creek, OH 44606
(Equipment and supplies)

Medical Packaging, Inc.
11-10 Ilene Court
Belle Mead, NJ 08502
(Equipment and supplies)

Odessa Packaging
202 North Bassett Street
P.O. Box 487
Clayton, DE 19938
(Equipment and supplies)

**Equipment and Supplies for
Packaging Oral Solids,
Oral Liquids, Injectables, and
Miscellaneous Products**

Phenix Box and Label Co.
P.O. Box 695
Olathe, KS 66061
(Dispensing containers, bags,
  prescription tape)

Popper and Sons, Inc.
300 Denton Avenue
New Hyde Park, NY 11040
(All types glass syringes; needles,
  pipettors)

Production Equipment, Inc.
17 Legion Place, Box 236
Rochelle Park, NJ 07662
(Prepackaging equipment for tablets
  and capsules)

Prop'r Products, Ltd.
500 South Minnesota Avenue
Sioux Falls, SD 57102
(Liquid measuring/storage devices)

Shamrock Scientific Spec. Systems
  Inc.
34 Davis Drive
Bellwood, IL 60104
(Packaging machines, unit dose
  materials, medication containers,
  bags)

Shaw-Clayton Plastics, Inc.
123 Carlos Drive
San Rafael, CA 94903
(Hinged lid plastic containers)

St. Charles Manufacturing
1611 E. Main Street
St. Charles, IL 60174
(Specialty hoods/fume hoods)

SystaModules
Division of MISSCO Corp.
P.O. Box 1059
Jackson, MS 39205
(IV preparation units with LAFH;
  general packaging and
  compounding units)

Terumo Corp.
P.O. Box 589
Elkton, MD 21921
(Insulin syringes)

U.S. Clinical Products
1900 Jay Ell Drive
P.O. Box 831667
Richardson, TX 75083-1667
(IVA seals)

Wrap Ade Machine Co., Inc.
189 Sargeant Avenue
Clifton, NJ 07103
(Strip packaging equipment/supplies)

**Equipment and Supplies for
Printing and Labeling**

Briggs Corp.
P.O. Box 1698
Des Moines, IA 50306
(Labels and auxiliary labels,supplies)

Health Care Logistics, Inc.
315 Town Street, P.O. Box 25
Circleville, OH 43113-0025
(Label/auxiliary labels, label
management system)

Mayfield Printing Co.
P.O. Box 469
Mayfield, KY 42006
(Computers labels, auxiliary labels, IV
labels)

Pharmex
207 Tuckie Road
Willimantic, CT 06226
(Labels,label systems, miscellaneous
supplies)

Phenix Box and Label Co.
P.O. Box 695
Olathe, KS 66061
(Computer labels, auxiliary labels)

Shamrock Scientific Spec. Systems
Inc.
34 Davis Drive
Bellwood, IL 60104
(Labels and labeling equipment)

Syntest Corporation
40 Locke Drive
Marlboro, MA 01752
(Label printers)

U. S. Clinical Products
1900 Jay Ell Drive
P.O. Box 831667
Richardson, TX 75083-1667
(Pressure sensitive, preprinted labels)

**Equipment and Supplies for
Packaging Oral Solids,
Oral Liquids, Injectables and
Miscellaneous Products**

Artromick International
4800 Hilton Corporate Drive
Columbus, OH 43243-4150
(Packaging systems, labels, control
drug packaging)

Associated Bag Company
400 W. Boden Street
Milwaukee, WI 53207
(Zip lock bags, biohazard bags)

Automated Prescription Sys.
P.O. Box 868
Pineville, LA 71361-0868
(Baker counting systems for oral solid
medications)

Baker Company, Inc.
P.O. Drawer E
Sanford, ME 04073
(Laminar air-flow hoods, biological
safety cabinets/supplies)

BAXA Corporation
14-C Inverness Dr. East
Englewood, CO 80112
(Oral liquid syringe and ointment;
filing equipment and supplies)

Baxter Healthcare Corporation
Pharmacy Division
1425 Lake Cook Road
Deerfield, IL 60015
(Needles, laminar air-flow hoods,
ancillary supplies)

Burron Medical Inc.
Hospital Products Division
824 Twelfth Avenue
Bethlehem, PA 18018
(Liquid packaging equipment, filter
needles and straws, vacuum
transfer devices, oral syringe
systems)

B. W. Darrah, Inc.
115 S. 4th Avenue
St. Charles, IL 60174
(Reusable security control containers)

Ertel Engineering Co.
P.O. Box 3449
Kingston, NY 12401
(Semi-automatic liquid fillers)

Forma Scientific
Mill Creek Road
P.O. Box 649
Marietta, OH 45750
(Laminar air-flow hood, safety
equipment)

Germfree Equipment Mfg. Div.
7435 N.W. 41st Street
Miami, FL 33166
(Vertical and horizontal laminar flow
hoods, fume hoods)

Health Care Logistics, Inc.
315 Town Street, P.O. Box 25
Circleville, OH 43113-0025
(Oral solid and liquid packaging
systems)

Healthtek, Inc.
870 Gold Flat Road
Nevada City, CA 95959
(Flexible admixture containers,
ambulatory infusion system, vial
venting system)

Kinematics and Controls Corp.
14 Burt Drive
Deer Park, NY 11795
(Powder and liquid filler machines)

LGS Health Products
14055 Cedar Road
South Euclid, OH 44188
(Pill splitter)

Labconco Corp.
8811 Prospect
Kansas City, MO 64132
(Vertical laminar air-flow hoods,
safety cabinets)

Lionville Systems, Inc.
Lionville, PA 19353
(Unit dose packaging equipment,
supplies)

Lunaire Environmental, Inc.
4 Quality Street, Box 3246
Willamsport, PA 11701
(Laminar air-flow equipment,
environmental rooms, incubators)

MMI of Mississippi, Inc.
232 East Georgetown Street
P.O. Box 488
Crystal Springs, MS 39059-0488
(Laminar air-flow hoods, safety
equipment, IV preparation
modules)

Markwell Medical Institute
P.O. Box 085173
Racine, WI 53405
(Button infuser for subcutaneous
   injections)

Mayfield Printing Co.
P.O. Box 469
Mayfield, KY 42006
(Bags)

Medi-Dose, Inc.
1671 Loretta Avenue
Feasterville, PA 19047
(Unit dose packaging and labeling
   system for solids, liquids,
   injections; light protection
   system; autoclavable bags; tote
   boxes and supplies)

Medipak Customer Services
P.O. Box 3248
Winchester, VA 22601
(All types of containers for various
   dose forms, UV light containers,
   quick seal equipment)

Milcare
A Herman Miller Company
8500 Byron Road
Zeeland, MI 49464
(Unit dose packaging)

National Instrument Co.
4119-27 Fordleigh Road
Baltimore, MD 21215
(Liquid filling machines, thermal
   impulse sealers)

Pak Devices, Inc.
4734 Spring Road
Brooklyn Hts., OH 44131-1098
(Strip packaging equipment, label
   printing equipment)

Pennsylvania Glass Prod.
430 N. Craig
Pittsburgh, PA 15213
(Glass droppers, dropper bottles,
   containers, applicators)

Pharmaceutical Innovators
P.O. Box 308
West Union, IA 52175
(Prepackaging equipment and
   supplies)

Miscellaneous

A & D Engineering, Inc.
2165 W. Park Court., Ste. M
Stone Mountain, GA 30087
(Analytical balances)

Alsop Engineering Company
P.O. Box 3449
Kingston, NY 12401
(Stainless steel tanks, mixers, filters
   and filtering apparatus)

American Med Industries
505 Laurel Avenue
Highland Park, IL 60035
(EZ-swallow pill crusher)

Apex Medical Corporation
P.O. Box 1235
Sioux Falls, SD 57101
(Medicating, dosing, and
   administering aids)

Artromick International
4800 Hilton Corporate Drive
Columbus, OH 43243-4150
(Needle disposal system)

Associated Bag Company
400 W. Boden Street
Milwaukee, WI 53207
(Disposable supplies)

Baxter Healthcare Corporation
Pharmacy Division
1425 Lake Cook Road
Deerfield, IL 60015
(IV filtration devices)

Bernhard Industries, Inc.
300 71st Street, S.435
Miami Beach, FL 33141
(Steam inhaler)

Briggs Corp.
P.O. Box 1698
Des Moines, IA 50306
(File trays, narcotic cabinets,
   miscellaneous supplies)

Brooklyn Thermometer Co.
Dept. 583
Farmingdale, NY 11735
(Environmental thermometers,
   thermo-regulators, hygrometers,
   hydrometers, recorders)

Burron Medical Inc.
Hospital Products Division
824 Twelfth Avenue
Bethlehem, PA 18018
(Specialty IV sets, flow control
   devices, miscellaneous IV supplies)

CHEK-MED System
423 N. 21st Street, Ste. 203
Camp Hill, PA 17011
(Patient education system, identa-
   drug system)

Contempra Furn. Div.
Fisher Scientific Corp.
922 Philadelphia Street
Indiana, PA 15701
(Complete lab furnishings,
   equipment)

Controlled Environ Equip.
3 Delta Drive
Westbrook, ME 04092
(Contamination control MATS/wipers)

Fisher Scientific Co.
1600 Parkway View Drive
Pittsburgh, PA 15205
(Protective garments, lab equipment,
   chemicals, general lab supplies)

Forma Scientific
Mill Creek Road
P.O. Box 649
Marietta, OH 45750
(Environmental rooms, incubators,
   miscellaneous products)

HEALTH-TEK, Inc.
870 Gold Flat Road
Nevada City, CA 95959
(IV filters, flexible admixture
   containers, ambulatory infusion
   system, infusion contamination
   tester)

Health Care Logistics, Inc.
315 Town Street, P.O. Box 25
Circleville, OH 43113-0025
(Tablet crushers, suppository molds,
   security seals, miscellaneous
   supplies)

Inforite Corporation
1670 S. Amphlett Boulevard, Ste. 201
San Mateo, CA 94402
(Portable data entry system)

Inter Innovation LeFebure
P.O. Box 2028
Cedar Rapids, IA 52406
(Security systems and equipment,
closed circuit TV, bullet resistive
windows and supplies, safes and
vaults)

Kole Enterprises
P.O. Box 020152
Miami, FL 33102-0152
(Shipping equipment, supplies,
containers)

Lab Line Instruments, Inc.
Lab Line Plaza
Melrose Park, IL 60160
(Furnaces, heaters, mixers, stirrers,
incubators, general lab equipment)

Lab Safety Supply Co.
P.O. Box 1368
Janesville, WI 53547-1368
(Safety equipment and supplies,
personal protection storage and
handling, hazard control)

Lifescan Inc.
2443 Wyandotte Street
Mountain View, CA 94043-2312
(Blood glucose monitoring,
management system)

MMI of Mississippi, Inc.
232 East Georgetown Street
P.O. Box 488
Crystal Springs, MS 39059-0488
(Creative design services)

Maddak, Inc.
Pequannock, NH 07440-1993
(Home health care equipment and
supplies)

Mayfield Printing Co.
P.O. Box 469
Mayfield, KY 42006
(Prescription blanks, file folders,
envelopes/statements)

Medi-Crush Company
4801 West 4th Street
Hattiesburg, MS 39402
(Medication crushing devices, plastic
lockseals, tablet cutters, needle-
syringe disposal, ambulatory med-
minders, amber IV covers)

Medi-Dose, Inc.
1671 Loretta Avenue
Feasterville, PA 19047
(Prescription supplies)

Mettler Instrument Corp.
Box 71
Hightstown, NJ 08520
(Electronic balances and accessories)

Milcare
A Herman Miller Company
8500 Bryon Road
Zeeland, MI 49464
(Administrative work environments,
modular furnishings, computer
furnishings)

Millipore Corp.
Bedford, MA 01730
(Microbiology equipment supplies,
filtration equipment/supplies,
contamination analysis
equipment)

Milton Roy
Analytical Prod. Div.
820 Linden Avenue
Rochester, NY 14625
(Spectrophotometers, refractometers)

R.C. Musson Rubber Co.
P.O. Box 7038
1320 E. Archwood
Akron, OH 44306
(Floor mats/runners/carpet mats;
anti-fatigue mats)

Novak Company, Inc.
P.O. Box 423
55 Old Field Point Road
Greenwich, CT 06836
(Rotary files, modular work stations,
administrative furnishings)

Nucleopore Corp.
7035 Commerce Circle
Pleasanton, CA 94566
(Laboratory equipment/supplies;
filtration equipment/supplies)

Omnimed, Inc.
Pine Avenue
P.O. Box 446
Maple Shade, NJ 08042-0446
(Bags, safety control seals)

Penco Products, Inc.
Brower Avenue
Oaks, PA 19456
(Office storage products)

Pharmacia Deltec, Inc.
1265 Grey Fox Road
St. Paul, MN 55112
(Infusion catheters and
devices/patient aids)

Pharmex
207 Tuckie Road
Willimantic, CT 06226
(Patient information)

Phenix Box and Label Co.
P.O. Box 695
Olathe, KS 66061
(Anti-fatigue mats)

Phonetics, Inc.
101 State Road
Media, PA 19063
(Environmental monitoring system/
security system)

PlasTies
1500 East Chestnut Avenue
Santa Ana, CA 92701
(Plastic products for packaging)

Precision Scientific Co.
3737 W. Cortlant Street
Chicago, IL 66047
(Incubators, water baths, vacuum
pumps)

Precision Systems, Inc.
16 Tech Circle
Natick, MA 01760
(Quality control equipment and
supplies, osmometers)

Pro-Tex International
P.O. Box 1038
5038 Salida Boulevard
Salida, CA 95368-0605
(Protective disposable face shields)

Pure Water, Inc.
P.O. Box 83226
Lincoln, NE 68501
(Water purification systems, distilled
water systems)

Quest Medical, Inc.
4103 Billy Mitchell
Dallas, TX 75244
(IV delivery sets, filters)

Shamrock Scientific Spec. Systems, Inc.
34 Davis Drive
Bellwood, IL 60104
(Balances, miscellaneous equipment, supplies, filing system)

R.C. Smith
801 East 79th Street
Minneapolis, MN 55420
(Modular office furnishing/casework)

Spectrex, Inc.
3580 Haven Avenue
Redwood City, CA 94063
(Laser particle counter system for fluids)

SystaModules
Division of MISSCO Corp.
P.O. Box 1059
Jackson, MS 39205
(General office furniture)

Teleautograph Corp.
8621 Bellanca Avenue
Los Angeles, CA 90047
(Omnifax, business facsimile)

Tennessee Mat Company
1400 Third Avenue South
Nashville, TN 37210-0186
(All types of floor mats and matting/cushioned/ runners/antifatigue)

U.S. Clinical Products
1900 Jay Ell Drive
P.O. Box 831667
Richardson, TX 75083-1667
(Chemo-protective gloves/garments/ prep mats/ bags; disposal system for needles)

United Pacific Industries
P.O. Box 989
Everett, WA 98206
(Latex and vinyl medical gloves)

Valleylab
5920 Longbow Drive
P.O. Box 9015
Boulder, CO 80301
(Rusable TENS Electrodes)

Vertex Industries, Inc.
23 Carol Street
P.O. Box 996
Clifton, NJ 07014-0996
(Prescription balances)

Waber Medical Specialties
Ste. 132
P.O. Box 2500
Honolulu, HI 96804
(Vacuum tube cleaner for Baker counting machines)

Adapted from *The Handbook of Institutional Pharmacy Practice*. 3rd ed. Brown TR, editor. Bethesda, MD: American Society of Hospital Pharmacists; 1992.

9 Aseptic Technique, Sterile Compounding, and Intravenous Admixture Programs

Douglas Scheckelhoff, M.S., FASHP

The purpose of this chapter is to help the technician develop a basic understanding of sterile products and the methods used to prepare them. This chapter should be mastered in sequence with the rest of the *Manual for Pharmacy Technicians*, especially chapters that have related information including calculations and measurements (chapter 3), medication orders (chapter 5), and Home Health Care (chapter 15). It is also suggested that it be used in conjunction with the ASHP videotapes *Aseptic Preparation of Parenteral Products* and *Safe Handling of Cytotoxic and Hazardous Drugs*. More detailed information is also available in the ASHP Technical Assistance Bulletin on Quality Assurance for Pharmacy-Prepared Sterile Products (appendix 9) and in the book *Principles of Sterile Product Preparation*.

The pharmacy technician can play an important role in the preparation of sterile products. Many small hospitals prepare and administer hundreds of sterile products daily while larger hospitals prepare thousands. In addition, many patients now receive intravenous drug therapy in the home. Many aspects and procedures are involved in ensuring that the process is safe and effective. For example, a structured intravenous admixture program is needed to ensure the stability, sterility, and appropriate labeling of intravenous products. Technicians and pharmacists usually work as a team in these environments, each with their own roles and expertise, to ensure that the patient receives the right drug in the right amount.

Drugs are given parenterally if patients cannot take oral medications, if a more rapid action of the drug is desired (as in an emergency situation), or if

---

Some parts of the "Aseptic Preparation of Parenteral Products " and "Chemotherapy Preparation and Handling of Cytotoxic Agents" sections were adapted from the ASHP videotapes/study guides "Aseptic Preparation of Parenteral Products" and "Safe Handling of Cytotoxic and Hazardous Drugs" respectively.

the drug is not available in a suitable oral dosage form. While the parenteral route of drug administration offers many advantages, it also has some unique preparation requirements so that patients are not harmed.

Since the drug or solution is being injected directly into the body, it bypasses the body's barriers to infection.[1] Therefore, it is extremely important that the solution be sterile, that is, free from bacteria or other living organisms. If a drug or solution that is contaminated with bacteria is inadvertently injected into a patient, the patient can suffer fatal adverse effects. Aseptic technique is the term used for all procedures and techniques performed to keep a sterile product from becoming contaminated.

Aseptic technique is the primary focus of this chapter, along with its application to different systems and dosage types. Other potential risks of parenteral therapy are addressed in the next section to emphasize the importance of using the proper techniques and appropriate caution when preparing these potentially life saving products. While nurses are often referred to as the primary caregivers involved in administering the products described in this chapter, in some hospitals or home care settings the primary caregiver may be another health care professional, the patient, or the patient's family members. Who the caregiver or caregivers are and what training and skills they have should be taken into consideration when products are prepared and dispensed and often influences the IV delivery system chosen for the patient.

LEARNING OBJECTIVES

After studying this chapter the reader will be able to
1. Describe the basics of intravenous drug therapy.
2. Describe the key elements of working in a laminar flow hood.
3. Perform basic manipulations needed to prepare a sterile product by using aseptic technique.
4. Prepare products for the systems most commonly used for IV administration of drugs and fluids.
5. Describe the risks of handling cytotoxic and hazardous drugs.
6. List the steps in drug preparation and handling that are unique to cytotoxic and hazardous drugs.
7. List the typical ingredients of a total parenteral nutrition solution.
8. Describe the manual and automated means of preparing total parenteral nutrition solutions.
9. Describe the benefits of having a formal intravenous admixture program.

PARENTERAL DRUG ADMINISTRATION

Basic aseptic technique should be used when handling parenteral dosage forms, as well as irrigations and ophthalmics (see chapter 2, Routes of Administration). Much of this chapter will address the intravenous (IV) route of administration since it is the most common route that parenteral doses are administered today. Other parenteral dosage forms include intramuscular, subcutaneous, intradermal, and epidural injections.

Basic Intravenous Therapy

In the basic setup, IV fluid is in a large-volume parenteral (LVP), usually more than 100 milliliters (ml), and hung on an IV pole or other device approximately 36 inches higher than the patient's bed. This allows the flow of IV solution to be maintained by gravity[2] (Figure 9-1). Attached to the LVP is a set of sterile tubing usually referred to as a primary IV set. The primary IV set extends down from the LVP to a catheter that has been placed in the patient's vein. Some patients' IV solution setup may differ because of the infusion device or special needs of the patient. Some of those differences are described below.

The LVP is usually a simple solution of dilute dextrose, sodium chloride or both. It may contain additives, such as potassium, if the patients clinical condition warrants it. The solution is infused continually to keep blood from clotting in the catheter and plugging it up. The fluid is also used to deliver drugs and to help prevent or reverse dehydration.

Primary IV Set—The primary IV set attached to the LVP can be any of several varieties, but most IV sets that flow by the force of gravity have several common features. The tubing has a drip chamber that is used to estimate the administration rate by counting drops as they fall through the chamber. Drip chambers are typically classified as macrodrip or minidrip based on the size

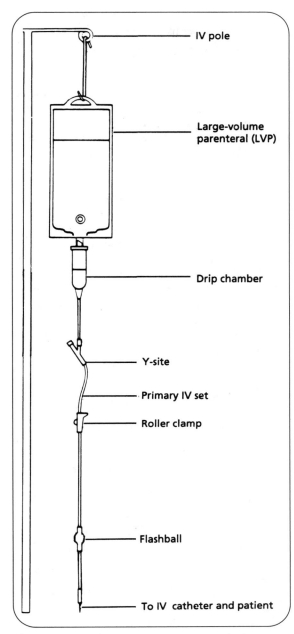

Figure 9-1. A LVP hanging on an IV pole, showing the primary IV set, including drip chamber, Y-site and flashball injection sites, and roller clamp, which can be used to control the flow of fluid.

of the drop that is formed in the drip chamber. Each set of tubing is labeled according to the number of drops it produces from one milliliter of solution. This number is used to determine how many drops should fall in a minute for the desired volume of milliliters per hour. Macro-

drip sets deliver 10 to 20 drops per milliliter, and minidrip sets deliver 60 drops per milliliter.

The rate of flow through the tubing is set by use of a roller clamp or an electronic infusion device. The roller clamp crimps the IV tubing as it is adjusted to control the flow of fluid. Electronic infusion devices, typically categorized as either pumps or controllers, are used to increase the precision and accuracy of administration. Electronic infusion devices are usually used in fluid restricted patients or when the LVP contains a drug that must be administered at a precise rate that cannot be ensured using the gravity method.

The tubing may have injection ports, either Y-sites or flashballs. Drugs or other solutions can be injected through the injection ports so they can be administered with the main solution. The systems used to give drugs through this means vary in set-up.

Secondary IV Sets—Drugs that are routinely given through the same basic IV setup are usually attached to a "secondary IV set" that is connected to the primary set (see Figure 9-14).

Catheters—Catheters are typically inserted into a peripheral vein (that is, a vein of the arm, leg, hand) or a central vein (existing in the chest near the heart). Where the catheter is inserted depends on the contents of the IV, among other things. Peripheral placement (insertion) is more common than central insertion. With peripheral catheters, there are some limitations on what can be infused and at what rate. The central catheter is more complicated and riskier to insert and maintain, but has fewer restrictions with respect to type and rate of administration.

Peripheral catheters may be any of several types. The most common is plastic, because it is flexible and can bend as the vein flexes or moves and is therefore the most comfortable for the patient. Another type is a steel needle with a short end of tubing. This type is commonly referred to as a scalp vein or butterfly because of its appearance. This type of catheter may be left in the patient's vein even without a running IV if it is periodically flushed (rinsed) with a solution to prevent it from being blocked by blood clots. It is usually used in patients that require IV therapy but are otherwise able to eat and drink, do not require supplemental fluids, and might even be ambulatory.

Central catheters can be temporary, meaning they are only used for days or weeks (such as during a hospital stay), or permanent, when used for months or years (such as with home care patients or cancer patients who require frequent infusions). Temporary central catheters are inserted by the physician via a minor surgical procedure in the patient's room. It involves a small incision and insertion of the catheter into a vein near the heart. The permanently placed central catheter also involves minor surgery, but must be done in an operating room. The central catheter gives direct access into a vein that has a high flow of blood. Therefore, solutions that might be irritating or damaging to peripheral blood vessels, which have a lower blood flow, are given centrally.

A new type of catheter that offers some of the benefits of both central and peripheral catheters is called a peripheral inserted central catheter (PICC). The PICC line, as its name implies, is inserted peripherally, but it is a long flexible catheter that travels through the vein and its tip ends near the heart where there is a high volume of blood flow.

Risks of Intravenous Therapy

Intravenous therapy offers a rapid, direct means of administering many life saving drugs and fluids. A high percentage of IV therapy is administered without any problems, but there are some risks. Many of the issues addressed in this training manual are aimed at teaching proper technique and therefore minimizing the potential for risks. Listed below are some reported complications of IV therapy that may pose risk to patients.[3]

Infection—Infections can result if a product contaminated with bacteria is infused into a patient. Bacteria can be introduced into products during preparation, administration, production, or if they are stored improperly. The rate of infection or sepsis due to a contaminated infusion has steadily decreased since health care practitioners and product manufacturers have implemented training and quality assurance programs. Despite these efforts, human touch contamination continues to be the most common source of IV related contamination.

Air embolus—The incidence of an air embolus is low, because many solutions are administered using infusion pumps equipped with an alarm that sounds when air is in the IV line. These are called air-in-line alarms. Solutions infused by gravity do not need alarms because the infusion automatically stops when there is no more fluid for gravity to push through the IV line. Even when a bag runs dry, large amounts of air are not infused. In adults it takes 150 or 200 ml of air (much less in an infant or pediatric patient) given quickly to result in harm.[3] Filters are available on some IV sets and they also stop air bubbles and add another measure of safety.

Bleeding—Bleeding may or may not be caused by intravenous therapy. When the IV catheter is removed, bleeding may occur around the catheter site. Also, if the patient has a condition that results in prolonged bleeding time, extra care and caution should be used, especially when removing the catheter.

Allergic reaction—When a patient has an allergic reaction to a substance given parenterally the reaction is usually more severe than if the same substance was given by another route (e.g., by mouth, topically, or rectally). One reason for this is that substances given parenterally cannot be retrieved like substances given by other routes. For example, substances administered topically can easily be washed off, those given orally can be retrieved by inducing vomiting or by pumping the stomach, and those substances given rectally can be flushed out using an enema. When a drug that has caused allergic reactions in a large number of patients is given intravenously, the patient should be monitored closely. If the likelihood of an allergic reaction is especially high, a test dose (a small amount of the drug) may be given to see how the patient reacts.

Incompatibilities—Some drugs are incompatible with other drugs, some types of containers, or solutions. If an incompatibility exists, the drug might precipitate, be inactivated, or adhere to the container. These outcomes are undesirable and may be difficult to detect with the naked eye. Incompatible solutions should not be administered to patients.

Extravasation—Extravasation occurs when the catheter punctures and exits the vein under the skin, causing drugs to infuse or infiltrate into the tissue. Extravasation may happen when the catheter is being inserted or after it is in place if the extremity with the IV catheter is moved or flexed too much. Using a stiff arm board to prevent excessive movement near the catheter site may help maintain regular flow and prevent extravasation and infiltration. Extravasation and infiltration can be painful and usually requires that the IV be restarted. Some drugs, such as certain chemotherapy agents, may cause severe tissue damage if they infiltrate the tissue. In some cases this tissue damage can be so severe that it requires surgery or even the loss of the limb.

Particulate Matter—Particulate matter refers to particles present in parenteral products. Particulate matter that is injected into the bloodstream can cause adverse effects to the patient. Some examples of particulate matter are microscopic glass fragments, hair, lint or cotton fibers, cardboard fragments, undissolved drug particles, and fragments of rubber stoppers. Improvements in the manufacturing processes have greatly reduced the presence of particulates in commercially available products. Similar care must be taken in the pharmacy so that particulate matter is not introduced into products; all products should be visually inspected for particulate matter before dispensing.

Pyrogens—Pyrogens, the by-products or remnants of bacteria, can cause reactions (e.g., fever and chills) if injected in large enough amounts. Since a pyrogen can be present even after a solution has been sterilized, great care must be taken to ensure that these substances are not present in quantities sufficient to harm the patient.

Phlebitis—Phlebitis, or irritation of the vein, may be caused by the IV catheter, the drug being administered (due to its chemical properties or its concentration), the location of the IV site, a fast rate of administration, or the presence of particulate matter. The patient usually feels pain or discomfort along the path of the vein (often severe), and red streaking may also occur. If phlebitis is caused by a particular drug, it may be helpful to further dilute the drug, give it more slowly, or give it via an IV catheter placed in a vein with a higher, faster-moving volume of blood.

ASEPTIC PREPARATION OF PARENTERAL PRODUCTS

As the use of parenteral therapy continues to expand, the need for well controlled admixture preparation has also grown. Recognizing this need, many pharmacy departments have devoted increased resources to programs that ensure the aseptic preparation of sterile products. The main elements these programs focus on are[4,5]

- the development and maintenance of good aseptic technique in the personnel who prepare and administer sterile products.
- development and maintenance of a sterile compounding area complete with sterilized equipment and supplies.

- development and maintenance of the skills needed to properly use a laminar flow hood (LAH).

Aseptic Technique

Aseptic technique is a means of manipulating sterile products without contaminating them. Proper use of a LAH and strict aseptic technique are the most important factors in preventing the contamination of sterile products. Thorough training in the proper use of the LAH and strict aseptic technique, followed by the development of conscientious work habits, is of utmost importance to any sterile products program.

Sterile Compounding Area

Sterile parenteral solutions must be free of living microorganisms and relatively free of particles and pyrogens. Room air typically contains thousands of suspended particles per cubic foot, most of which are too small to be seen with the naked eye, including contaminants such as dust, pollens, smoke, and bacteria. Reducing the number of particles in the air improves the environment in which sterile products are prepared. This can be done by following several practices to maintain the sterile compounding area.

A sterile compounding area should be cleaned daily and segregated from normal pharmacy operations, patient specimens, nonessential equipment, and other materials that produce particles. For example, the introduction of cardboard into the clean environment should be avoided. Traffic flow into a clean area should be minimized. Floors should be disinfected periodically, and trash should be removed frequently and regularly. Other more sophisticated aspects of clean room design include special filtration or treatment systems for incoming air, ultraviolet irradiation, air-lock entry portals, sticky mats to remove particulate from shoes, and positive room air pressure to reduce contaminant entry from adjacent rooms or hallways. These rooms are often adjoined by a room, called an anteroom, that is used for non-aseptic activities related to the clean room operation such as order processing, gowning, and stock handling.

Sterile products should be prepared in a Class 100 environment, which contains no more than 100 particles per cubic foot that are 0.5 micron or larger in size. LAHs are frequently used to achieve a Class 100 environment.

Laminar Airflow Hoods

The underlying principle of LAHs is that twice-filtered laminar layers of aseptic air continuously sweep the work area inside the hood to prevent the entry of contaminated room air. There are two common types of laminar flow hoods, horizontal flow and vertical flow.

Horizontal LAH—LAHs that sweep filtered air from the back of the hood to the front are called horizontal LAHs (Figure 9-2). Horizontal flow hoods use an electrical blower to draw contaminated room air through a prefilter. The prefilter, which is similar to a furnace filter, only removes gross contaminants and should be cleaned or replaced on a regular basis. The prefiltered air is then pressurized to ensure that a consistent distribution of air flow is presented to the final filtering apparatus. The final filter constitutes the entire back portion of the hood's work area. This "high efficiency particulate air," or HEPA, filter removes 99.97% of particles that are 0.3 micron or larger, thereby eliminating airborne microorganisms, which are usually 0.5 microns or larger.

Vertical LAH—Laminar flow hoods with a vertical flow of filtered air are also available. In vertical LAHs, HEPA filtered air emerges from the top and passes downward through the work area (Figure 9-2). Because exposure to some antineoplastic (anticancer) drugs may be harmful, they are usually prepared in vertical LAHs so that the risk of exposure to airborne drug particulates is minimized. The types of vertical LAH used for the preparation of antineoplastics contains airflow within the hood and are referred to as biological safety cabinets (BSCs). BSCs and the preparation of antineoplastics and cytotoxic dosage forms are covered later in this chapter.

The critical principle of using LAHs is that nothing interrupts the flow of air between the HEPA filter and the sterile object. The space between the HEPA filter and the sterile object is known as the critical area. The introduction of a foreign object between a sterile object and the HEPA filter increases wind turbulence in the critical area and the possibility that contaminants from the foreign object may be carried onto the sterile work surface and thereby contaminate an injection port, needle, or syringe. To maintain sterility, nothing should pass behind a sterile object in a horizontal flow hood, or above a sterile object in a vertical flow hood.

Furthermore, materials placed within the laminar flow hood disturb the patterned flow of air blowing from the HEPA filter. This "zone of tur-

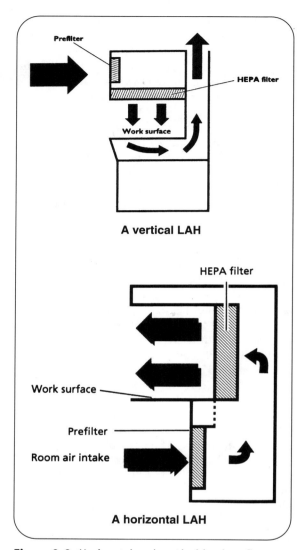

Figure 9-2. Horizontal and vertical laminar flow hoods with the basic components labeled.

bulence" created behind an object could potentially extend outside the hood, pulling or allowing contaminated room air into the aseptic working area (Figure 9-3). When laminar air flow is moving on all sides of an object, the zone of turbulence extends approximately three times the diameter of that object. When laminar air flow is not accessible to an object on all sides (for example, when placed adjacent to a vertical wall), a zone of turbulence is created that may extend six times the diameter of the object (Figure 9-3). For these reasons, it is advisable to work with objects at least six inches from the sides and front edge of the hood without blocking air vents, so that unobstructed airflow is maintained between the HEPA filter and sterile objects. Also, the hands

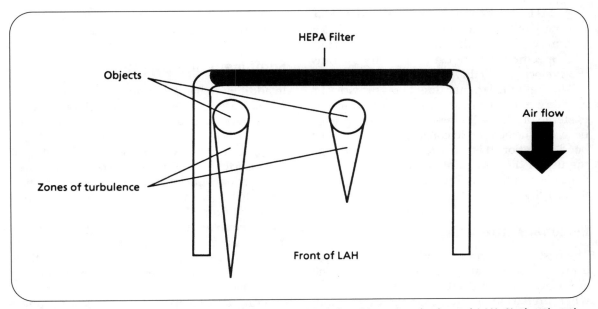

Figure 9-3. Examples of zones of turbulence created behind the objects in a horizontal LAH. Notice that the zone of turbulence of the object on the left is greater due to the object's proximity to the side of the hood, and has extended outside of the LAH. (Note: figure is not drawn to scale.)

should be positioned so that airflow in the critical area between the HEPA filter and sterile objects is not blocked.

The following are general principles for operating LAHs properly:

- A LAH should be positioned away from excess traffic, doors, air vents, or anything that could produce air currents capable of introducing contaminants into the hood.
- If it is turned off, nonfiltered, nonsterile air will occupy the LAH work area. Therefore, when it is turned back on it should be allowed to run for 15–30 minutes before it is used. This allows the LAH to blow the non-sterile air out of the LAH work area. Then the LAH can be cleaned for use.
- Before use, all interior working surfaces of the laminar flow hood should be cleaned with 70% isopropyl alcohol or other appropriate disinfecting agent and a clean, lint-free cloth. Cleaning should be performed from the HEPA filter toward the front of the LAH (in a horizontal LAH), so that contaminants are moved out of the hood. The hood should be cleaned often throughout the compounding period and when the work surface becomes dirty. Some materials are not soluble in alcohol and may initially require the use of water in order to be removed. In addition, plexiglass sides, found on some types of

laminar flow hoods should be cleaned with warm, soapy water rather than alcohol.
- Nothing should be permitted to come in contact with the HEPA filter. This includes cleaning solution, aspirate from syringes, or glass from ampules. Ampules should not be opened directly toward the filter.
- Only those objects essential to product preparation should be placed in the LAH. Do not put paper, pens, labels, or trays into the hood.
- Jewelry should not be worn on the hands or wrists when working in the LAH since it may introduce bacteria or particles into the clean work area.
- Actions such as talking and coughing should be directed away from the LAH working area, and any unnecessary motion within the hood should be avoided to minimize the turbulence of air flow.
- Smoking, eating, and drinking are prohibited in the aseptic environment.
- All aseptic manipulations should be performed at least six inches within the hood to prevent the possibility of potential contamination caused by the closeness of the worker's body and backwash contamination resulting from turbulent air patterns developing where LAH air meets room air.

- LAHs should be tested by qualified personnel every six months, whenever the hood is moved, or if filter damage is suspected. Specific tests are used to certify air flow velocity and HEPA filter integrity.

Although the laminar flow hood provides an aseptic environment, safe for the manipulation of sterile products, it is essential that strict aseptic technique be used in conjunction with proper hood operation. It is important to remember that the use of the LAH alone, without the observance of aseptic technique, cannot ensure product sterility.

Personal Attire

The first component of good aseptic technique is proper personal attire. Clean garments, which are relatively particulate free, should be worn when preparing sterile products. Clean room attire will depend on institutional policies and often are related to the type of product being prepared (appendix 9). Many facilities provide clean scrub suits or gowns for this purpose. Hair covers and shoe covers help reduce particulate or bacterial contamination, and some experts claim that the use of surgical masks and gloves is warranted as well.

Handwashing

Touching sterile products while compounding is the most common source of contamination of pharmacy-prepared sterile products. Since the fingers harbor countless bacterial contaminants, proper hand washing is extremely important. Scrub your hands, nails, wrists, and forearms thoroughly for at least 30 seconds with a brush, warm water, and appropriate bactericidal soap before performing aseptic manipulations. Wash your hands frequently and every time you re-enter the sterile compounding area. Although many institutions recommend using sterile gloves to reduce touch contamination, be careful to avoid a false sense of security. Sterile gloves are only sterile until they touch something unsterile or until they are torn and allow bacteria from the hands to enter the work area. For these reasons, always wash your bare hands thoroughly before unwrapping and putting on the gloves. Workers who have open sores on their hands or have an upper respiratory tract infection should inform their supervisor and/or consult their institution's quality assurance procedures. Often such procedures will require that they wear sterile gloves or a mask (respectively) for these conditions.

Equipment and Supplies

In addition to hand washing, another important factor in aseptic preparation of sterile products is the correct use of appropriate sterile equipment and supplies, including syringes and needles.

Syringes—Syringes are made of either glass or plastic. Most drugs are more stable in glass, so glass syringes are most often used when medication is to be stored in the syringe for an extended period of time. Disposable plastic syringes are most frequently used in preparing sterile products, because they are cheaper, durable, and are only in contact with substances for a short time. This minimizes the potential for incompatibility with the plastic itself.

Syringes are composed of a barrel and plunger (Figure 9-4). The plunger, which fits inside the barrel, has a flat disk or lip at one end and a rubber piston at the other. The top collar of the barrel prevents the syringe from slipping during manipulation; the tip is where the needle attaches. To maintain sterility of the product, do not touch the syringe tip or the plunger. Many syringes have a locking mechanism at the tip such as the Luer-lock, which secures the needle within a threaded ring. Some syringes, such as slip-tip syringes, do not have a locking mechanism. In this case, friction holds the needle on the syringe.

Syringes are available in numerous sizes ranging from 0.5 to 60 ml. Calibration marks on syringes represent different increments of capacity, depending on the size of the syringe. Usually, the larger the syringe capacity, the larger the interval between calibration lines. For example, each line on the 10 ml syringes represents 0.2 ml, but on a 30 ml syringe, each line represents 1 ml.

To maximize accuracy, the smallest syringe that can hold a desired amount of solution should be used. Syringes are accurate to one-half of the smallest increment marking on the barrel. For example, a 10 ml syringe with 0.2 ml markings is accurate to 0.1 ml and can be used to measure 3.1 ml accurately. A 30 ml syringe with 1 ml markings, however, is only accurate to 0.5 ml and should not be used to measure a volume of 3.1 ml. Ideally, the volume of solution should only take up 1/2 to 2/3 of the syringe capacity. This avoids inadvertent touch contamination caused when the syringe plunger is pulled all the way back.

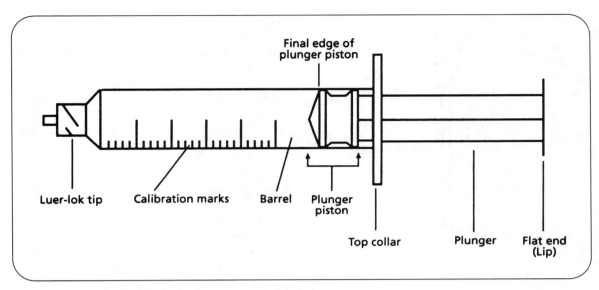

Figure 9-4. A syringe with the basic components labeled.

When measuring with a syringe, lineup the final edge (closest to the tip of the syringe) of the plunger piston, which comes in contact with the syringe barrel, to the calibration mark on the barrel which corresponds to the volume desired (Figure 9-5).

Syringes are sent from the manufacturer assembled and individually packaged in paper overwraps or plastic covers. The sterility of the contents is guaranteed as long as the outer package remains intact. Therefore, packages should be inspected, and any that are damaged should be discarded. The syringe package should be opened within the laminar flow hood in order to maintain sterility. The wrapper should be peeled apart and not ripped or torn. To minimize particulate contamination, do not lay discarded packaging on the LAH work surface.

Syringes may come from the manufacturer with a needle attached or with a protective cover over the syringe tip. The syringe tip protector should be left in place until it is time to attach the needle. For attaching needles to Luer-lock-type syringes, a quarter-turn is usually sufficient to secure the needle to the syringe.

Needles—Like syringes, needles are commercially available in many sizes. Sizes are described by two numbers, gauge and length. The gauge of the needle corresponds to the diameter of its bore, which is the diameter of the inside of the shaft. The larger the gauge the smaller the needle bore. For example, the smallest needles have a gauge of 27, while the largest needles have a gauge of 13. The length of a needle shaft is mea-

sured in inches and usually ranges from 3/8 to 3 1/2 inches.

The components of a simple needle are the shaft and the hub (Figure 9-6). The hub attaches the needle to the syringe and is often color-coded to correspond to a specific gauge. The tip of the needle shaft is slanted to form a point. The slant is called the bevel, and the point called the bevel tip. The opposite end of the slant is termed the bevel heel.

Needles are sent from the manufacturer individually packaged in paper and plastic overwraps with a protective cover over the needle shaft. This guarantees the sterility as long as the

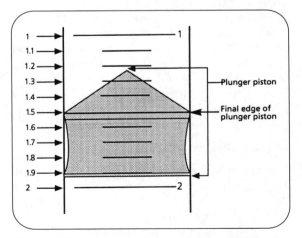

Figure 9-5. A close-up of a syringe showing how to measure 1.5 ml. Note that the final edge of the plunger piston is used to make the measurement.

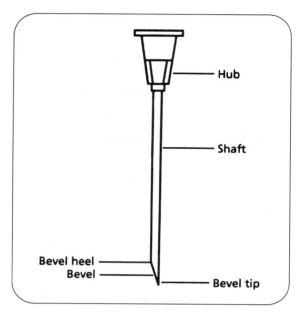

Figure 9-6. A needle with the basic components labeled.

package remains intact. Therefore, packages that are damaged should be discarded.

No part of the needle itself should be touched. Needles should be manipulated by their overwrap and protective covers only. The protective cover should be left in place until the needle and/or syringe are ready to be used. A needle shaft is usually metal and is lubricated with a sterile silicone coating so that latex vial tops can be penetrated smoothly and easily. For this reason, needles should never be swabbed with alcohol.

Some needles are designed for special purposes and therefore have unique characteristics. For example, needles designed for batch filling have built in vents to avoid the need to release pressure that might form in the vial. Another example would be needles with built in filters, meant to be used with products requiring frequent filtering such as drugs removed from a glass ampule.

Drug Additive Containers

Injectable medications are usually supplied in an ampule, vial, or prefilled syringe. Each requires a different technique to withdraw medication and place it in the final dosage form.

Ampules—Ampules are composed entirely of glass and, once broken (i.e., opened), become open-system containers. Since air or fluid may now pass freely in and out of the container, it is

not necessary to replace the volume of fluid to be withdrawn with air.

Before an ampule is opened, any solution visible in the top portion (head) should be moved to the bottom (body) by swirling the ampule in an upright position, tapping the ampule with one's finger or inverting the ampule and then quickly swinging it into an upright position (Figure 9-7).

To break an ampule properly, the head must be broken from the body of the ampule. To make the break properly, the ampule neck is cleansed with an alcohol swab and the swab should be left in place. This swab can prevent accidental cuts to the fingers as well as spraying of glass particles and aerosolized drug. The head of the ampule should be held between the thumb and index finger of one hand, and the body should be held with the thumb and index finger of the other hand. Pressure should be exerted on both thumbs, pushing away from oneself in a quick motion to snap open the ampule. Ampules should not be opened toward the HEPA filter of the laminar flow hood or toward other sterile products within the hood. Extreme pressure may result in crushing of the head between the thumb and index finger. Therefore, if the ampule does

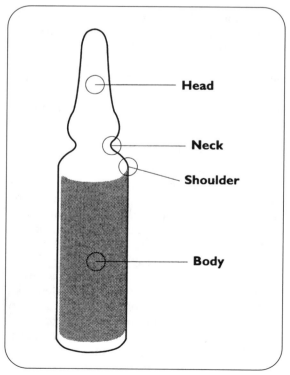

Figure 9-7. An ampule with the basic components labeled.

not open easily, it should be rotated so that pressure on the neck is at a different point.

To withdraw medication from an ampule, the ampule should be tilted and the bevel of the needle placed in the corner space (or shoulder) near the opening. Surface tension should keep the solution from spilling out of the tilted ampule. The syringe plunger is then pulled back to withdraw the solution.

The use of a filter needle (e.g., a needle with a 5-micron filter in the hub) keeps glass or paint chips that may have fallen into the solution from being drawn into the syringe. To withdraw the solution, either use a filter needle and change to a regular needle before expelling the contents, or start with a regular needle and change to a filter needle before expelling the contents. Either way, the filter needle must not be used for both withdrawing from the ampule and expelling from the syringe, because doing so would nullify the filtering effort. Usually, the medication is withdrawn from the ampule with a regular needle and then the needle is changed to a filter needle before pushing drug out of the syringe. If the syringe is used as a final container for dispensing, a filter needle should be used to withdraw the solution. Sometimes, a medication (e.g., a suspension) may need to be withdrawn from an ampule with a regular needle so that the active ingredient is not filtered out in the process.

Another device that can be used for withdrawing solutions from an ampule is the filter straw. The filter straw differs from the filter needle in that it is made out of plastic tubing rather than metal and it is longer making it easier to reach the bottom of an ampule. It also reduces the risk of needlestick during the manipulation since it does not have a sharp tip. Once the solution is withdrawn with a filter straw, however, a regular needle must be attached to the syringe to inject the solution into its final container.

Vials—A vial, unlike an ampule, is a glass or plastic container with a rubber stopper secured to its top, usually by an aluminum cover. Vials also differ from ampules in that they are used to hold powders and liquids. The rubber stopper is usually protected by a flip-top cap or aluminum cover.

Most protective covers do not guarantee sterility of the rubber stopper. Therefore, before the stopper is penetrated, it must be swabbed with 70% isopropyl alcohol and allowed to dry. The correct swabbing technique is to make several firm strokes in the same direction over the rubber closure, always using a clean swab. Swabbing helps achieve sterility in two ways: first, the alcohol acts as a disinfecting agent; and a second, the physical act of swabbing in one direction removes particles.

When piercing vials with needles, avoid coring fragments out of the rubber stopper with the needle. A core is carved out of the rubber stopper when the bevel tip and the bevel heel do not penetrate the stopper at the same point. To prevent core formation, first pierce the stopper with the bevel tip and then press downward and toward the bevel as the needle is inserted (Figure 9-8).

Vials are closed-system containers, since air or fluid cannot pass freely in or out of them. In most cases, air pressure inside the vial is similar to that of room air. In order to prevent the formation of a vacuum inside the vial (less pressure inside the vial than room air) the user should normalize pressure by first injecting into the vial a volume of air equal to the volume of fluid that is going to be withdrawn. This step should not be done with drugs that produce gas when they are reconstituted, such as ceftazidime.

If the drug within a vial is in powdered form, it has to be reconstituted. Inject the desired volume of sterile diluting solution (the diluent), such

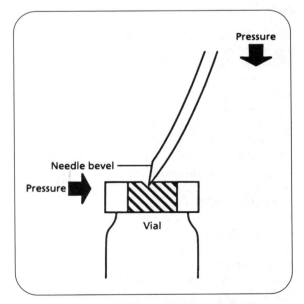

Figure 9-8. A non-coring technique of piercing a vial with a needle. Note that the needle is held on an angle—the bevel tip will pierce the vial first. As downward pressure is applied, there is a slight bend in the needle, and the bevel heel will enter through the opening made by the bevel tip.

as sterile water for injection, into the vial containing the powdered drug. An equal volume of air must be removed in order to prevent a positive pressure from developing inside the vial. Allow the air to flow into the syringe before removing the needle from the vial, or use a vented needle, which allows displaced air to escape the vial through a vent in the needle. Care must be taken to ensure that the drug is completely dissolved before proceeding. Usually gentle shaking adequately dissolves the drug contents. There are some agents that cannot be shaken as it will degrade the active ingredient (e.g., some biologic products, some investigational agents). As always, if the user is not familiar with preparation methods for the product, the package information or a supervisor should be consulted.

Vials with drugs in solution are classified as multiple-dose (also called multiple use) or single-dose. Multiple-dose vials contain a small amount of a preservative agent, added to retard the growth of bacteria or other organisms that inadvertently contaminate a product. The presence of these substances does not make the solution self-sterilizing, and the use of strict aseptic technique is still required. Preservatives are included in both "bacteriostatic water for injection" and in any multiple-dose product. Common substances used as preservatives include benzyl alcohol, parabens, phenol, and benzalkonium chloride. These substances are typically added by the manufacturer in small quantities that are not harmful when the product is dosed appropriately. Therefore, if a preparation calls for large amounts of drug solution that contain a preservative or a diluent with a preservative, the pharmacist should be consulted to verify that the total amount of preservative to be administered will not be toxic. Due to their toxicity, solutions with preservatives should not be used in preparations for pediatric or neonatal patients or for epidural or intrathecal dosage forms.

Single-dose vials have no preservative and are intended to be used one time only. Once a vial is entered with a needle, whether in a patient care area or a LAH, it should be discarded.

Prefilled Syringes—Manufacturers produce a number of products that are packaged in a ready-to-inject syringe. Drugs commonly given IM or IV are packaged this way to make them convenient for the health care provider. It is also done if the drug is commonly used in emergency situations because a prefilled syringe saves time. Prefilled syringes often have calibrations on the syringe barrel and are labeled with the concentration and total volume. These products might be used in the pharmacy to prepare a sterile product or, more likely, they are kept in patient care areas.

Preparation of Intravenous Admixtures

The usual process for preparing an admixture is that an order is received in the pharmacy and reviewed by the pharmacist. If the order is deemed reasonable and appropriate, the pharmacist will input the information into the pharmacy records (usually by entering it into a pharmacy computer system) to document the preparation and generate a label. The pharmacist then assigns the preparation of the product to support personnel. The following sequence describes the common steps technicians follow to prepare intravenous admixtures. However, keep in mind that the final IV admixture may be prepared in a variety of containers, including flexible plastic bags, glass bottles, and semirigid plastic containers.

Before compounding, assemble all materials and visually inspect vials, ampules, and IV solution containers for signs of cloudiness, particulate, matter, cracks and punctures, expiration dates, and anything else that may indicate that the product is defective. Only place materials that are necessary to prepare the product in the LAH.

Next, disinfect all injection surfaces and allow them to dry. Withdraw and measure the drug fluid from its container, using the syringe size closest to the volume to be withdrawn. To obtain as accurate a measurement as possible, remove air bubbles from the syringe by first pulling back slightly on the plunger to draw any fluid trapped in the needle into the syringe barrel, then tap the barrel and slightly depress the plunger.

Flexible Plastic Bags—Flexible plastic bags made of polyvinyl chloride (PVC) are used frequently. They are easier to store, are less breakable than glass bottles, and eliminate the need to vent the container when removing fluid.

PVC bags are available in several sizes and contain a variety of solutions. They are packaged in plastic overwraps designed to limit fluid loss. The protective overwrap should not be removed from a PVC bag until it is ready to be used. To minimize air turbulence in the critical area, position the injection port of a PVC bag, which is covered by an outside latex tip diaphragm, toward the HEPA filter when preparing an IV admixture.

To add a drug to a PVC bag, insert a needle into the injection port and inject the appropriate volume of drug fluid. Use a needle longer than 3/8 inch because the injection port of the PVC bag has two diaphragms that must be pierced (Figure 9-9). The outside diaphragm is the outside latex tip; the inside diaphragm, which is plastic, is about 3/8 inch inside the injection portal . (Note: Individual manufacturer's products may differ in appearance, but the design concept is the same.)

Glass Containers—To add a drug to a glass infusion container, first remove the protective cap from the IV bottle. Swab the rubber stopper or latex diaphragm with alcohol, let it dry, and then inject the drug fluid. To insert needles through rubber stoppers, use the previously described non-coring technique (Figure 9-8). After admixing, place a protective seal over the stopper of the glass container before removing it from the LAH.

Semirigid Containers—When using a polyolefin, semirigid container for admixture preparation, remove the protective screw cap and add drugs through the designated injection portal. Disinfecting the portal and replacing the protective cap are not necessary.

Disposal of Supplies—Syringes and uncapped needles should be discarded according to institutional policy. In some institutions they are discarded in puncture-resistant, sealable containers often called sharps containers. Other institutions use clipping devices that separate the shaft or tip of the needle from the hub, then throw the syringe away in a standard trash receptacle (needle clippings are then disposed of in sharps containers). If the pharmacist needs the syringe to verify the amount of drug added to the admixture, institutions may allow needles used in compounding to be recapped for removal and disposal. When a syringe is used to verify the amount of drug added, the plunger is drawn back to the calibration mark to indicate the amount of drug added. Then the syringe and the drug vial would be placed next to the completed and labeled product for the pharmacist to verify.

Although pharmacy technicians would probably not deal with needles except when compounding, it is important to know that compounding is one of the few situations in which recapping a needle is permitted. Most institutions have policies against recapping

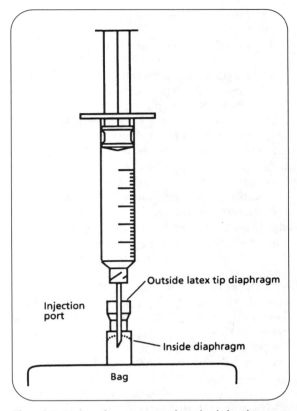

Figure 9-9. A syringe penetrating the injection port of a PVC bag. The needle must be long enough (greater than 3/8") to penetrate the inside diaphragm. (Note: figure is not drawn to scale.)

needles, since health care workers may accidently stick themselves with contaminated needles. Contaminated, uncapped needles and syringes are usually disposed of in sharps containers.

Labeling

Once an IV admixture or other sterile product is compounded, it should be properly labeled with the following information:

1. Patient name, identification number, and room number (if inpatient)
2. Bottle or bag sequence number, when appropriate
3. Name and amount of drug(s) added
4. Name and volume of admixture solution
5. Approximate final total volume of the admixture, when applicable
6. Prescribed flow rate (in milliliters per hour)
7. Date and time of scheduled administration

8. Date and time of preparation
9. Expiration date
10. Initials of person who prepared and person who checked the IV admixture
11. Auxiliary labeling—supplemental instructions and precautions. An example of a label is shown in Figure 9-10.

After it is properly labeled, perform a final inspection of the admixture for cores and particulates. All drug and IV solution containers used in preparing the admixture should be checked by the pharmacist to verify that the technician added the proper amount of the correct drug to the correct IV solution. The label and final sterile product must be validated by a registered pharmacist against the order for accuracy and completeness before dispensing it for patient use.

Each product should also include an expiration date beyond which it should not be used. This might include a time 24 hours after preparation so that unused preparations are returned for potential reuse or it might reflect the actual time that the product is considered unusable. Typically drugs are considered stable as long as they are within 10% of their labeled potency. In addition to stability, sterility concerns also factor into the assignment of expiration times. The pharmacist should assign the expiration time. Methods for assigning those times, for both standard and non-standard preparations, should be reflected in policy and procedures and substantiated by references, literature, or reasonable professional judgment.

ADMINISTRATION SYSTEMS FOR PARENTERAL PRODUCTS

As mentioned earlier in this chapter, patients receiving intravenous therapy usually have a basic IV setup that includes a LVP solution or they have catheter specifically designed for periodic injections (heparin lock, butterfly, etc.). Based on this, IV drug administration systems are typically classified as either continuous infusions or intermittent injections.

Continuous Infusions

Some drugs are administered as a continuous infusion because they are more effective and less toxic than when given intermittently. Continuous infusions include basic fluid and electrolyte therapy, blood products, and specific drugs that require tight administration control to minimize adverse effects.

Intermittent Injections

Intermittent injection systems are used to administer medications that work better when infused at defined time intervals rather than when infused continuously. The reason may be that the

---

John Doe	Adm# 565656565		Rm# 742W
Bag# 23		Hang at 12N	4/1
Cefazolin in 5% Dextrose in Water			1 g 50 mL
Infuse every 8 hours			
Infuse over 30 minutes			
Use before 12N 4/2/93		Prepared by:	
Keep refrigerated			

Figure 9-10. A sample IV label.

drug is more effective when given that way or that periodic administration reduces toxicity. Examples of drugs commonly given intermittently are antibiotics and drugs used to treat or prevent gastrointestinal ulcers.

Several types of systems are available for intermittent injections. Each system has advantages and disadvantages related to cost, flexibility, waste rates, and so on. This section addresses how to prepare products for use with each system. Institutional policies dictate specific labeling, expiration dating, and storage conditions, and so they are not addressed here.

Large Volume Parenterals

Large Volume Parenterals (LVPs) are usually defined as those IV solutions containing more than 100 ml. LVPs are usually infused as solutions of dilute dextrose and/or sodium chloride as continuous infusions with or without drug additives, but they can be used for intermittent infusions as well. These preparations may be commercially available in a ready-to-use form or may require drug additives that are added in the pharmacy.

Commercially Available

Preparations with additives are used in standard concentrations, are stable in solution for long periods of time, and are available in a variety of sizes (250 ml, 500 ml, 1000 ml) and containers (glass or plastic) depending on the product and use. Examples include lidocaine, potassium, nitroglycerin, dopamine, bretylium, and aminophylline. Ready-to-use products are advantageous because they reduce handling by the pharmacy and, therefore, the potential for contamination. In some cases these agents are used for emergency situations and may be stocked in the patient care area for immediate access.

Pharmacy Prepared

Some solutions are made in the pharmacy to meet the specific needs of patients. Solutions are prepared in different volumes (250 ml, 500 ml, or 1000 ml) and different containers (glass or plastic) depending on the drug and intended use. The preparation of LVPs in the pharmacy should follow the techniques described in the section of this chapter titled "Aseptic Preparation of Parenteral Products."

Syringe Systems

The most common drug delivery systems that use syringes are syringe pumps, volume control chambers, gravity feed, and intravenous push systems. Syringe systems require that the pharmacy fill syringes with drugs and label them. Drug stability in syringes may differ from the stability of the same drug in other dosage forms because of concentration differences.

Syringe Pumps

Syringes can be used to administer drugs by means of a specially designed syringe pump and tubing set. The pump is adjusted to administer the desired volume from the syringe over a given period of time. Pumps are either operated by a battery or a compressed spring. Pumps are also available to administer a single dose per setup or a 12- or 24-hour supply at preprogrammed intervals. Most of these setups require a special small-bore tubing set that determines the rate at which the drug is administered (as with the spring-loaded pumps). One important pharmacy implication is that doses must be sent from the pharmacy in standard syringe sizes and concentrations. This procedure allows for administering doses to patients more safely.

Volume Control Chambers (Buretrol or Volutrol)

Syringes can be used to administer drugs through a volume control, or volumetric chamber (Figure 9-11). The drug is injected through a port on top of the chamber, and solution is added from the primary LVP. With this system, minimal

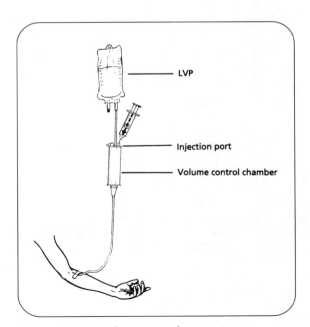

Figure 9-11. A volume control setup.

amounts of fluid can be given per dose, a method that may be beneficial in fluid-restricted or pediatric patients. This setup allows for controlled administration of fluids, since the nurse can clamp off the solution after the volume in the chamber has infused. Since multiple drugs might be in the chamber at the same time, potential for incompatibilities and unpredictable rates of administration can be problematic.

Gravity Feed

Syringes can be used to administer drugs directly by gravity if a specially designed tubing set is used (Figure 9-12). The set has an air vent through which air enters the syringe as fluid is pulled out by gravity. The syringe is prepared in the pharmacy, labeled, and sent to the nurse for administration. The system is relatively inexpensive and requires no other special equipment.

Intravenous Push

Drugs given by IV push are injected directly into the IV tubing and pushed into the patient quickly (Figure 9-13). With this method the drug is injected into an injection port, a Y-site on the IV

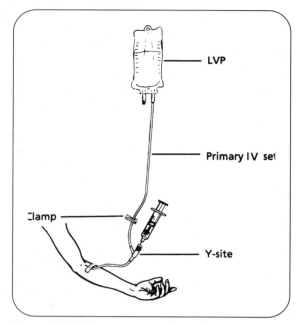

Figure 9-13. IV push setup using a Y-site.

tubing, or an injection flashball. Usually the primary IV set is clamped off just above the injection port so that the drug is delivered to the patient directly, resulting in the rapid onset of the drugs effects.

This system is used in emergencies as well as more routine situations. The disadvantage of the IV push method is it is difficult to control the rate of drug delivery with a syringe and many drugs cause the patient to experience adverse effects when given too quickly.

Small Volume Parenterals ("Piggyback" Systems)

A common method of administering drugs is adding the drug solution to a small volume parenteral or piggyback (any IV solution of less than 100 ml) and labeling it. The nurse simply attaches tubing to the piggyback and connects this secondary IV set to the primary IV set at the proximal Y-site (Figure 9-14). Piggybacking offers benefits of flexibility and ease of administration for the nurse.

The piggyback is placed higher than the primary IV (usually an LVP) so that gravity causes the drug solution to run into the patient's vein before the primary fluid. The back-check valve at the proximal Y-site closes off while the piggyback is being administered, thus preventing the piggyback solution from entering the primary IV. Once the piggyback solution has infused, the pri-

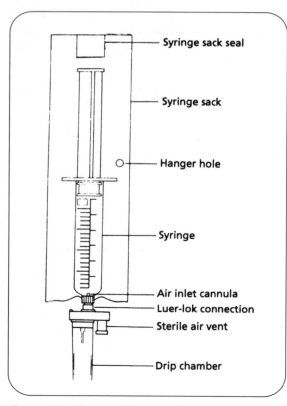

Figure 9-12. A gravity-feed syringe.

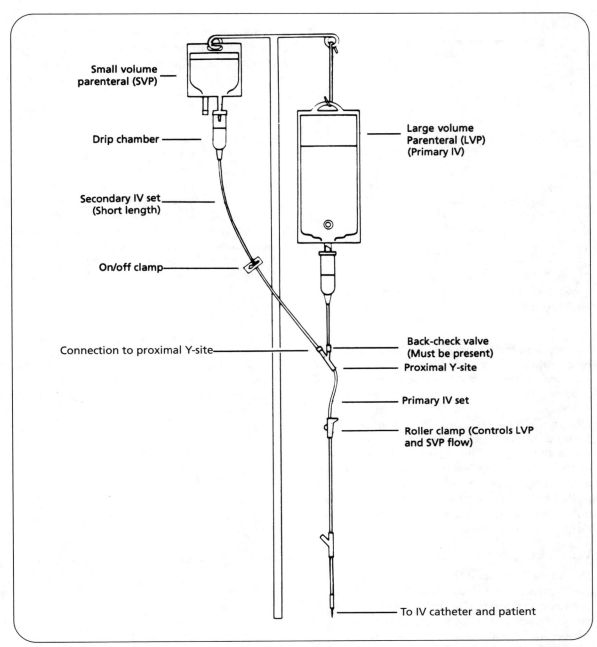

Figure 9-14. A small volume parenteral, or piggyback setup. Note that the piggyback hangs higher than the primary IV.

mary IV resumes flowing. The following systems are variations of the basic piggyback concept.

Add-Vantage®

The Add-Vantage® system (Figure 9-15) uses a specially designed bag and a vial that contains drug for reconstitution. The vial is screwed into a special receptacle on the top of the bag. To reconstitute the drug, the vial's stopper is removed by

manipulations done on the outside of the bag and the stopper remains in the bag. The IV solution then flows from the bag into the vial and dissolves and/or dilutes the drug. The bag is inverted several times to mix the drug and the IV solution. The bag is then administered to the patient in a fashion similar to the traditional piggyback setup.

The act of screwing the vial onto the bag receptacle should be performed in an LAH. The actual

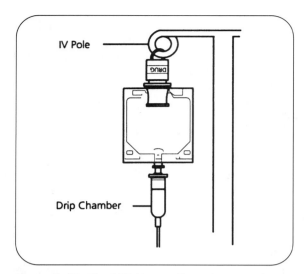

Figure 9-15. The ADD-Vantage® system setup is shown here. Note the special port at the top of the bag, which holds the medication vial.

vial top and receptacle are sterile and shielded by a protective cover until used. The pharmacy technician removes the cover at the time the vial is screwed on.

The bag's expiration date is usually 30 days after the date the vial is attached. The bag's expiration date changes to the drug expiration date when the stopper is pulled and the drug is mixed, or activated. For this reason, the stopper is usually left intact by the pharmacy and is pulled by the nurse prior to administering the dose. This way, changes in the drug order do not result in a wasted dose.

Vial Spike Systems

The Add-a-Vial® and Mini-Bag Plus® systems are similar in concept to the Add-Vantage system. The drug containing vial is attached to the bag in the pharmacy, but is not activated or mixed until just before administration. The Add-a-Vial® system uses a vial adapter. The adapter has a spike at each end; one is inserted into the drug vial and the other is inserted into the injection port of the bag. The Mini-Bag Plus® system (Figure 9-16) uses a special container that has a vial adapter and a breakaway seal. The pharmacy is responsible for attaching the drug-containing vial to the bag.

The Add-a-Vial® spike that is inserted into the bag is snapped off, or the Mini-Bag Plus® breakaway seal is broken just before administration, allowing solution from the bag to enter the drug vial and be mixed. The system does not require

special vials, because the adapters are designed to fit the commonly used vial sizes. Add-a-Vial® can be used with various manufacturers' bags. Mini-Bag Plus® requires that the manufacturer's bag be used, because the drug vial adapter is attached.

Premixed Solutions

Many drugs and doses are available in premixed form. If premixed products are not stable for long periods of time at room temperature, they are often sold frozen, and thawed by the pharmacy shortly (hours or days) before being administered. Adding drugs to these solutions is generally not recommended, and most containers do not have an injection port. These solutions are administered and handled by the nurse in the same manner as other piggyback setups.

Bags/Bottles Containing Powder for Reconstitution

Some drugs are available in powdered form in final containers of plastic or glass. This system requires that the pharmacy add to the bottle 20 to 100 ml of sterile diluting fluid such as 0.9 percent sodium chloride or sterile water for injection to

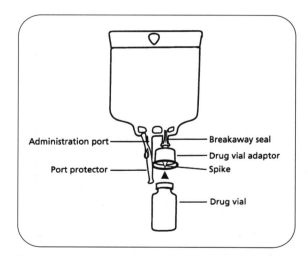

Figure 9-16. The Mini-Bag Plus® system has a special manufacturer's bag equipped with a drug vial adapter. The adapter is pushed down on the vial and snapped into place. The Add-a-Vial system operates on a similar principle except the drug vial adapter is separate from the bag and is spiked on both ends. It is attached to the drug vial first, then assembled with the bag. With both systems, the assembled product is sent to the nursing unit, where, just prior to administration, the breakaway seal is broken and the solution is mixed with the drug.

reconstitute the drug. Once reconstituted and labeled by the pharmacy, these products are administered via piggyback systems. These systems are also referred to as "drug manufacturer piggyback bottles" or DMPBs.

Controlled-release Infusion System (CRIS)®

A method of intermittent drug delivery somewhat different from syringe and piggyback types of systems is the CRIS® (Figure 9-17), which delivers the desired medication directly from the vial when it is attached to a special adapter aligned with the primary IV solution. The drug containing vial is sent from the pharmacy in ready-to-use form (powders are reconstituted before being dispensed). The nurse attaches the drug vial to the special adapter and turns a dial to direct solution flow through the drug vial and down the tubing. This system presents a labeling challenge to the pharmacy, since ready-to-use vials have limited space for patient-specific labels and expiration date stickers.

Patient Controlled Analgesia

A method of drug administration usually used with injectable pain medications is patient con-

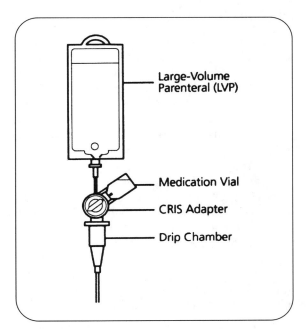

Figure 9-17. The controlled-release infusion system (CRIS®) requires a special primary IV set onto which a reconstituted vial of drug fits. The vial is spiked onto the set, and the CRIS® adapter is turned so that fluid from the primary IV enters the spiked vial to deliver drug to the patient.

Labels in figure:
Large-Volume Parenteral (LVP)
Medication Vial
CRIS Adapter
Drip Chamber

trolled analgesia or PCA, which is very effective in managing pain. Two advantages of PCAs are they eliminate the need for painful intramuscular injections and they reduce patients' anxiety about controlling their pain. The goal of PCA therapy is to relieve pain as soon as the patient recognizes a need for it. It may also reduce nursing time associated with pain medication administration.

PCA is usually administered by using either a stationary or a portable pump that infuses analgesics directly into an IV line. The pump releases a programmed amount of the pain medication into the IV tubing when the patient pushes a button. The pump is programmed to release an amount of pain medication that is specific for the patient's weight and condition. The pump is also programmed to limit how often the patient may push the button and receive pain medication. For example, the pump may be programmed to allow a patient to receive a maximum of 1 mg of morphine sulfate every 15 minutes. When the patient pushes the button, the pump injects 1 mg. If the patient pushes the button again in 10 minutes, the pump does not release drug. If the patient pushes the button at least 5 minutes later (15 minutes since the last injection), the pump again administers 1 mg. This is often referred to as a 15-minute lock-out period.

PCA preparations may be commercially available or be prepared in the pharmacy. These products involve the same techniques as other parenteral products. They differ from most other products in two regards: first, if the patient does not have other means of pain control, there might be an urgency to initiate therapy. Much of this urgency can be avoided with preplanning among the physician, the nurse, and the pharmacy. Second, these doses usually contain enough medication to last at least 8 hours and often up to 24 hours or more. The result is usually a very large amount of narcotic in one container, necessitating awareness of security issues in order to prevent diversion or theft.

Unique Infusion Devices and Containers

The delivery systems described thus far meet the needs of typical hospitalized patients. A number of new types of infusion devices and containers have been developed in the past 5 to 10 years to meet needs not met by the traditional systems. Many of these products are designed to deliver drugs through a compact system that allows the patient to receive therapy outside the hospital (e.g., at home). The system may be drug or therapy specific, such as an implanted pump with a drug reservoir for continuous low-dose chemotherapy administration. This type of system is surgically placed under the skin and the catheter is inserted in a vein. It has a built in power source and place for the drug solution, so the patient does not need to carry a pump, start a new IV periodically, or need any other supplies related to the IV therapy. The downside is that it requires surgery and can only be used for drug therapies administered in very small amounts, over long periods of time.

Another type of system uses an elastomeric infusion device that acts as its own pump, not requiring gravity or an electronic infusion device. These systems are similar in concept to a water balloon inside a plastic bottle. The balloon is filled with drug solution and the pressure of the container forces it through the tubing eliminating the need for a separate pump. These systems, whether used for hospitalized patients or home care patients, present unique challenges in filling technique, drug stability, and administration methods, among others. Those preparing drugs for use in these types of devices should become familiar with the devices themselves to prevent errors and complications.

PREPARATION AND HANDLING OF CYTOTOXIC AND HAZARDOUS DRUGS

Some medications can be hazardous to those who touch or inhale them. Because hazardous drugs initially involved drugs used in treating cancer, the terms antineoplastic and chemotherapeutic were used to describe them. The term cytotoxic, or cell killer, was later used to refer to any agent that may be genotoxic, oncogenic, mutagenic, teratogenic, or hazardous in any way. Exposure to antineoplastics, as well as immunosuppressants, antiviral agents, and biological response modifiers, may pose some of these risks. Hazardous agents require special handling procedures to minimize the potential for accidental exposure.

Contact with these drugs can cause immediate problems, such as dermatitis, dizziness, nausea, and headache.[7] Studies also suggest that repeated exposure to small amounts of the drugs may cause organ or chromosome damage, impaired fertility, and even cancer.[7]

Preparation of these agents requires special procedures for labeling, storage, and transport;

protective clothing; use of Biological Safety Cabinets (BSCs); and special handling of spills and wastage. Special techniques related to the actual administration of these products to patients are not covered in this chapter. - Additional information is available from ASHP in the form of a Technical Assistance Bulletin on Handling of Cytotoxic and Hazardous Drugs.

Protective Apparel

There is no substitute for good technique, but protective apparel is another fundamental element in protecting personnel who handle or prepare hazardous drugs. Protective garments such as disposable coveralls or gowns, gloves, and shoe and hair covers may be used to shield personnel from exposure.

Most procedures require the use of disposable coveralls or a solid front gown. These garments should be made of low-permeability, lint free fabric. They must have long sleeves and tight-fitting elastic or knit cuffs. They should not be worn outside the work area and should be changed immediately if contaminated. Shoe and hair covers may also be required, depending on the institution's policies.

Wearing gloves is essential when working with hazardous drugs. Wash hands thoroughly before putting on the gloves and after removing them. Use good quality disposable, powder-free latex gloves, such as surgical latex. These gloves are preferred because of their fit, elasticity, and tactile sensation. If only powdered gloves are available, wash powder off before beginning to work.

Depending on the procedure, one or two pairs of gloves may be required. If two pairs are needed, tuck one pair under the cuffs of the gown and place the second pair over the cuff. If an outer glove becomes contaminated, change it immediately. Change both the inner and the outer gloves immediately if the outer glove becomes torn, punctured, or heavily contaminated. If only one pair is worn, tuck the glove under or over the gown cuff so that the skin is not exposed.

Every work area in which hazardous drugs are prepared should have an eyewash fountain or sink and appropriate first aid equipment. If skin or eye contact occurs, follow established first aid procedures, obtain medical attention without delay, and document the injury.

Biological Safety Cabinets

One of the most important pieces of equipment for handling hazardous drugs safely is the Biological Safety Cabinet (BSC). A BSC is a type of vertical LAH that is designed to protect workers from exposure as well as to help maintain product sterility during preparation. BSCs must meet standards set by the National Sanitation Foundation (NSF Standard 49).

Do not use horizontal LAHs to prepare hazardous drugs. They blow contaminants directly at the preparer. If possible, prepare sterile hazardous drugs in a Class II BSC. The front air barrier of the BSC protects the handler from contact with hazardous drug dusts and aerosols that are generated in the work zone. Room air is pulled into the front intake grill and filtered through a HEPA filter. The air then passes vertically, that is, downward, through the work zone. The air that has passed through the work zone goes through front intake and rear exhaust grilles, passes through a HEPA filter, and is recirculated through the work zone or exhausted to the outside. Placing objects on or near the front intake or rear exhaust grilles may obstruct the airflow and reduce the effectiveness of the cabinet.

There are several types of Class II BSCs. Type A BSCs pump about 30% of the air back into the room after it passes through a HEPA filter (Figure 9-18). Be sure not to block airflow from the exhaust filters. Type B BSCs send air from the work zone through a HEPA filter and then to the outside of the building through an auxiliary exhaust system (Figure 9-19). Type B BSCs offer greater protection because filtered air is sent outside the building and they have a faster inward flow of air.

BSCs must be operated continuously, 24 hours per day, and they should be inspected and certified by qualified personnel every 6 months. Follow the manufacturer's recommendations for proper operation and maintenance, particularly replacement of HEPA filters.

Clean and disinfect the BSC regularly. Clean the work surface, back, and side walls with water or a cleaner recommended by the cabinet manufacturer. Do not use aerosol cleaners; they could damage the HEPA filters and cabinet, and could allow contaminants to escape.

Before performing sterile manipulations, disinfect the work surface with 70% isopropyl alcohol or another suitable disinfectant and allow it to dry. Alcohol is a disinfectant and may remove some substances in the hood that water does not. Be careful not to use excessive amounts of alcohol, because vapors may

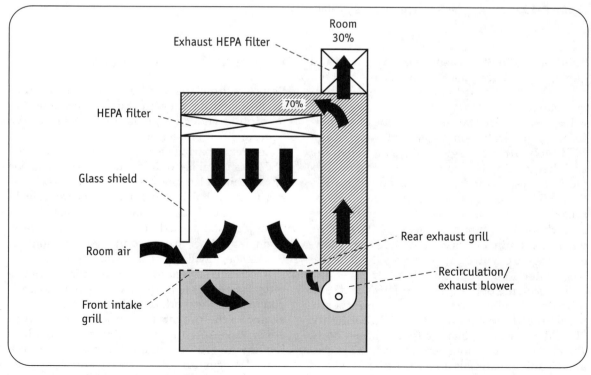

Figure 9-18. Class II Type A biological safety cabinet.

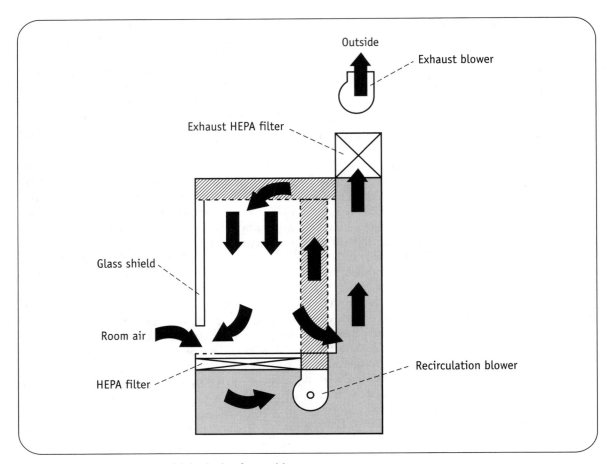

Figure 9-19. Class II Type B biological safety cabinet.

build up in the BSC. Dispose of any gauze and gloves used to clean the BSC in sealable containers with other hazardous waste; they are contaminated.

Extensive decontamination should be performed, preferably on a weekly basis and immediately after a large spill. While cleaning and disinfecting the hood, wear a gown, latex gloves, a respirator, hair cover, and eye protection, since the front shield may need to be raised. Keep the blower on and clean from the top, where contamination is least, to the bottom, where contamination is greatest. Use heavy toweling or gauze with cleaner and distilled de-ionized water. Remove the HEPA filter cover and clean inside the BSC. Lift the work tray and prop it against the back wall to clean underneath. Scrub the drain spillage trough thoroughly. Should gloves tear, change them immediately. The cleaner, water containers, protective apparel, and cleaning materials all must be handled and discarded as contaminated waste.

Preparing Hazardous Drugs

Before technicians handle a cytotoxic or other hazardous drug, they must demonstrate proper manipulative technique and use of protective equipment and materials.

Before preparing sterile hazardous drugs in a BSC, wash your hands and put on a gown and one or two pairs of latex gloves. Disinfect the work surface with alcohol. Place yourself so the front shield protects your eyes and face. Some institutions place a plastic-backed liner on the work surface. Though this liner may introduce particles into the work zone, it will absorb any small spills.

Assemble sufficient materials for the entire preparation process so you will not have to leave and re-enter the work zone. Place only items necessary to the preparation process in the work zone. Make sure that these objects do not block the downward flow of air; for example, do not hang IV bags or bottles above sterile objects. Handle sterile objects well inside the BSC so that they are not contaminated by unfiltered air at the front air barrier. Air quality is lowest at the sides of the work zone, so work at least three inches away from each side wall.

If possible, attach IV sets to containers and prime them before adding the drug. Use syringes and IV sets with locking fittings; they are less likely to separate than friction fittings. Needles are secured to these Luer-Lok fittings with a quarter turn.

When you are working with drugs in vials, pressure can build up inside the vial and cause the drug to spray out around the needle. Maintain a slight negative pressure inside the vial to prevent this. Too much negative pressure, however, can cause leakage from the needle when it is withdrawn from the vial. Another way of preventing pressure buildup is to use a chemotherapy dispensing pin. This disposable device is attached at one end to the Luer-Lok fitting of the syringe, and a pin on the opposite end is inserted into the drug vial. The device also has a venting unit that allows for constant pressure equalization, therefore eliminating any problems due to pressure imbalances.

When reconstituting a drug in a vial, use a syringe that can hold twice as much diluent as you will be drawing into the syringe barrel. This ensures that the plunger will not be pulled out of the barrel when the diluent is being drawn into the syringe. After drawing the diluent into a syringe, insert the needle into the vial top and draw the plunger back to draw air into the syringe and create a slight negative pressure inside the vial. Inject small amounts of diluent slowly and draw equal volumes of air out of the vial. Keep the needle in the vial and swirl the contents carefully until they dissolve completely. With the vial inverted, gradually withdraw the proper amount of drug solution while exchanging equal volumes of air for drug solution. Excess drug should remain in the vial. With the vial in the upright position, draw a small amount of air from the vial into the needle and hub. Then withdraw the needle from the vial.

If there is a need to transfer a hazardous drug to an IV bag, be careful not to puncture the bag. Wipe the IV port, container, and set with moist gauze and put a warning label on the IV bag. Place the IV in a sealable bag so any leakage will be contained.

When withdrawing cytotoxic or hazardous drugs from an ampule, gently tap the contents down from the neck and top portion. Spray or wipe the ampule neck with alcohol. Attach a 5-micron filter needle or filter straw to a syringe that is large enough to hold the ampule's contents. Draw the fluid through the filter needle and clear it from the needle and hub. Exchange the filter needle for a regular needle of similar gauge and length. Eject any air and excess drug into a sterile vial, leaving the desired volume in the syringe. Be careful not to create aerosols. You may then transfer the drug to an IV bag or bottle. If the dose is to be dispensed in the syringe, draw back the plunger to clear fluid from the needle and hub. Replace the needle with a locking cap. Wipe the syringe with moistened gauze and label it appropriately.

Good technique does not end with drug preparation. There are special requirements for waste disposal and cleanup. Put any glass fragments and needles in a puncture- and leak-resistant container. Do not clip the needles before disposal. Place all other materials in sealable plastic bags along with the outer pair of gloves. Seal all waste containers before removing them from the BSC, and dispose of them in designated, labeled containers. Next, remove and dispose of the gown and, last, the inner pair of gloves. When removing the gloves, be careful not to touch the fingertips of the gloves to the skin or the inside of the gloves. Finally, wash your hands.

Labeling, Storage, and Transport

Safe and effective labeling, storage, and transportation practices are essential to prevent accidental exposure to hazardous drugs. Following the appropriate guidelines with respect to these processes should begin the moment hazardous drugs enter the facility. Hazardous drugs should be identified by distinctive labels indicating that the product requires special handling (Figure 9-20). Attach the labels to drug packages and their storage shelves, bins, and areas. All the areas where hazardous drugs are stored should be marked clearly as containing hazardous drugs. Access to these areas should be limited to authorized personnel who have been trained in handling hazardous drugs.

Storage equipment should be designed to minimize breakage. For example, shelves should have front barriers and carts should have rims. Hazardous drugs should be kept at eye level or lower and stored in bins. Refrigerated hazardous drugs should be stored in bins that are separate from non-hazardous drugs.

Transporting hazardous drugs requires special precautions to prevent container leakage or

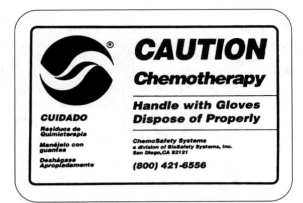

Figure 9-20. Example of a suitable warning label for cytotoxic and hazardous drugs. Other labels also may be suitable.

breakage. For example, pneumatic tube systems cause mechanical stress to containers and should not be used for transporting hazardous drugs. Carts used to transport hazardous materials should have rims to prevent the containers from falling off the cart and breaking. Hazardous drug containers must be securely capped or sealed and properly packaged to protect against leakage or breakage during transport. If leakage or breakage occurs, follow procedures described later in this section.

Waste Disposal and Spill Cleanup

Review your institution's policies and procedures for identifying, containing, collecting, segregating, and disposing of hazardous waste. Hazardous waste should be disposed of in separate containers. Regular trash should not be placed in hazardous waste containers. Handle the outside of hazardous waste containers only with uncontaminated gloves.

If you handle hazardous drugs, you should be familiar with the techniques and procedures for handling spills. In the event of a hazardous drug spill, you should use a spill kit, and the cleanup should follow established procedures. Spill kits contain all the materials needed to clean up hazardous drug spills and protect health care workers and patients. Spill kits contain protective gear: eye protection, a respirator, utility and latex gloves, a disposable gown or coveralls, and shoe covers. They also contain the equipment needed to clean up the spill: a disposable scoop and a puncture- and leak-resistant plastic container for disposing of glass fragments; absorbent spill pads; gauze and disposable toweling; absorbent

powder; and sealable, thick plastic waste disposal bags. Hazardous waste must be stored in leak-resistant containers until it is disposed of in accordance with government and institution policy.

Put up a warning sign to alert other people in the area to the hazard. Put on all of the protective equipment, including latex gloves covered by utility gloves. Put broken glass in the puncture- and leak-resistant plastic container. Absorb liquids with disposable towels or spill pads. Remove powders with dampened towels or gauze. Rinse the contaminated surface with water, wash it with detergent, and then rinse it again. Start at the outside of the spill and work toward the center. Place all the contaminated materials in sealable plastic disposal bags. In all cases it is important that the circumstances and the handling of the spill be documented in writing and kept on file.

If the area is carpeted, refer to institutional policies and procedures for handling spills in carpeted areas. Absorbent powder and "hazardous drug only" vacuum cleaners are often used to clean up spills in these areas.

If a large spill occurs in a BSC, additional steps must be taken. Use the spill kit described above and be sure to seal all contaminated materials in hazardous waste containers while the materials are still inside the BSC. Use utility gloves when handling any broken glass. Thoroughly clean the drain spillage trough and decontaminate the BSC if necessary. Transfer these containers to leak-resistant containers.

TOTAL PARENTERAL NUTRITION SOLUTIONS

Total parenteral nutrition (also known as hyperalimentation or TPN) is the IV administration of nutrients needed to sustain life: carbohydrates, protein, fats, water, electrolytes, vitamins, and trace elements.

TPN therapy is usually initiated in patients who cannot meet their nutritional needs from other sources for an extended period of time. TPN is used for patients who cannot eat (e.g., after head and neck surgery, if comatose, or before or after surgery), who will not eat (e.g., patients with chronic diseases or psychologic disorders, or geriatric patients), who should not eat (e.g., patients with esophageal obstruction or inflammatory bowel disease), or who cannot eat enough (e.g., patients with cancer, burns, or trauma).

Components of Parenteral Nutrition Solutions

TPN solutions contain base components and additives. Base components are usually mixed first and make up much of the volume of the TPN. They are composed of dextrose (carbohydrates) and amino acids (protein) and may also include fat and water. Additives are usually mixed with the base component and include life-sustaining nutrients, electrolytes, vitamins, trace elements and may also include drugs such as heparin, insulin, and H2 antagonists.

Carbohydrates are usually administered in the form of dextrose because of its low cost and easy availability. The commercially available concentrations of dextrose vary from 5 to 70%. Usually a 50 or 70% solution is used in TPN preparation, and the final dextrose concentration in the TPN is usually around 25% for solutions administered via a central vein. The dextrose concentration is significantly less for infusions intended for peripheral administration.

Protein is required for tissue synthesis and repair, transport of body nutrients and waste, and maintenance of immune function. Protein is usually given as commercially available synthetic crystalline amino acid formulations. These solutions are available in concentrated form, such as 8.5 or 10%, and diluted in the compounding process. A number of special formulations are also available for pediatric patients and patients who have kidney disease, liver disease, or are in a high stress situation (e.g., intensive care patients).

Fats (or lipids) are usually administered as fat emulsions. Administering fat emulsions not only prevents essential fatty acid deficiency, but is a source of calories. They are commercially available as 10 or 20% emulsions that are dispensed in a separate container that can be given through a peripheral IV line. Alternatively, fats can be added to the TPN solution. In this type of TPN, called a 3-in-1 solution or total nutrient admixture, the fat emulsion is considered a third base component along with dextrose and amino acids. The 3-in-1 technique offers several nutritional advantages but has certain mixing, stability, and compounding disadvantages (see the Preparation section).

Water is in all preparations and is usually derived from the components used in the preparation. Sterile water for injection may be added to obtain the desired final concentration or volume. The purpose of adding water is to offset normal bodily losses and prevent dehydration. In addition to the TPN solution, separate fluids may be given for fluid replacement.

Electrolytes are needed to meet daily metabolic needs and correct deficiencies. The electrolytes usually included are sodium, potassium, chloride, acetate, phosphate, magnesium, and calcium. Electrolytes are usually administered as a specific salt of the product. For example, sodium is frequently given as sodium chloride. Potassium can be given as potassium chloride, potassium acetate, or potassium phosphate. The patient's clinical condition and laboratory values usually determine the amount and form of electrolytes.

Vitamins are usually administered in a standard formulation of fat and water-soluble vitamins and are often abbreviated as "MVI." Commercial formulations include vitamins A, D, C, E, B_1, B_2, B_6, and B_{12}; folic acid; pantothenic acid; biotin; and niacin. When vitamin K (phytonadione) is needed it is usually given separately as an intramuscular injection. However, some clinicians add vitamin K to the TPN or use vitamin preparations that contain vitamin K.

Trace elements are required for proper enzymatic reactions and for use of energy sources in the body. Typical elements administered are copper, zinc, chromium, manganese, selenium, and iron. Commercial products are available that include combinations of trace elements and allow administration of a few milliliters to meet the daily requirements.

Orders for TPN Solutions

Procedures for ordering and dispensing TPN solutions vary and are specific to each institution. Many institutions use a standardized TPN ordering form to make the orders straighforward and consistent yet patient specific (Figure 9-21). Often a specific cutoff time for order changes or new orders is used to maximize efficiency and minimize wastage. Since setting up to make just one TPN can be wasteful, this approach saves time and money by allowing multiple bags to be prepared in a row.

TPN solutions are ordered specifically to meet a patient's metabolic and nutritional needs. These solutions are usually administered by means of a pump to maximize safety.

An order for central TPN solution might look like this:

Dextrose	250 g
Amino acids	42.5 g
Sodium chloride	60 mEq
Potassium chloride	40 mEq
Potassium phosphate	20 mEq
Calcium gluconate	1 g
Magnesium sulfate	1 g
Trace elements	2 ml
MVI-12	5 ml
Total volume	1000 ml

Infuse at 100 ml per hour.
Also give: Vitamin K 10 mg intramuscularly (IM) every week, 10% fat emulsion 500 ml intravenously 3 times per week.

Here is an example of an order for 3-in-1 central TPN solution:

Dextrose	250 g
Amino acids	85 g
Fat emulsion	50 g
Sodium chloride	80 mEq
Potassium chloride	60 mEq
Potassium phosphate	60 mEq
Trace elements	2 ml
MVI-12	5 ml
Total volume	2000 ml

Infuse over 24 hours. Give vitamin K 10 mg IM every week.

Preparation of TPN Solutions

Preparation of TPN solutions has changed considerably in the past 10 to 15 years. In the past, many of the components required preparation from nonsterile powders. Today, most TPN ingredients are available as sterile solutions, reducing the need for extemporaneous preparation. Most TPNs are made by gravity fill or by means of an automated compounding device.[8]

Gravity Fill

Gravity fill involves equipment that is normally part of an IV program. As the name implies, gravity is used to transfer the base components (dextrose and amino acids, plus IV fat emulsion in a 3-in-1 solution) into the final container. The disadvantages of this method are that it limits flexibility in the volumes of base components used, it takes longer than automated methods, and volumes cannot usually be measured accurately. There are two gravity methods of filling bags: the empty bag method and the underfill method.

The empty bag method involves starting with an empty sterile bag that will be used as the final container. Commercially available bags for this purpose have leads that can be connected to bottles or bags of the base components. The desired amounts flow into the empty bag by gravity. This method can be used for either traditional or 3-in-1 preparations.

The underfill method uses commercially available underfilled bags, which are partially filled with concentrated dextrose solution. A bottle of amino acids is connected to the underfilled bag by a tubing set and infused into the partially filled bag to make the final mixture.

With either method, other components are added by drawing each up into a syringe and injecting them through an injection port into the final container. This step is usually the final step before labeling and dispensing. Great care must be taken both in technique and accuracy, since the potential for errors is high and their ramifications are serious. Each additive must be added in the correct amount; if even one is incorrect, the entire solution for that patient must be remade, and the solution made in error is likely to be wasted. Each step must be checked by the pharmacist. To prevent waste, some institutions require that the pharmacist check the calculations and amounts of additives in syringes before they are added to the bag.

Mixing 3-in-l solutions is delicate, because the fat emulsion is actually a suspension of fat globules. Adding concentrated dextrose may "oil out," or crack, the emulsion. The proper order of mixing is to add the fats first, the amino acids second, and the dextrose last (remember the acronym "FAD," fats, amino acids, dextrose). This mixing order dilutes and buffers the fat emulsion with amino acids before the highly concentrated and acidic dextrose is added.

Automated Compounding

Automated compounding involves the use of specialized equipment to prepare the TPN solution. Three primary pieces of equipment are used, sometimes together and sometimes individually. An automated compounder prepares the base components dextrose, amino acids, and possibly fat emulsion and water; a second automated compounder adds most or all of the additives or other components; and a computer with software maintains the orders for the ingredients and controls the two compounders (Figure 9-22).

ADULT TPN/PPN PHYSICIAN ORDERS

NOTE: All TPN orders (formula and rate) must be received in the Central Pharmacy by 12 Noon to be activated the same day. Orders received after 12 Noon will be activated the following day. A bag containing 24 hours of TPN will be sent. The adult hang time is 9 p.m.

DO NOT THIN FROM CURRENT CHART

Time Processed

Clerk's Initials

1. **SELECT ONE:**

	REGULAR FORMULA	LOW K FORMULA	NO K FORMULA	LOW ACET HIGH CI	LOW Na FORMULA	PERIPHERAL FORMULA	SPECIAL FORMULA
AMINO ACIDS	6%	6%	6%	6%	6%	3%	*
DEXTROSE	☐15% ☐25%	☐15% ☐25%	☐15% ☐25%	☐15% ☐25%	☐15% ☐25%	10%	+
SODIUM -mEq/L	45	45	45	45	20	45	
POTASSIUM-mEq/L	40.5	20	0	40	40.5	40.5	
CHLORIDE -mEq/L	57.5	59	69	89	44	57.5	XXX
ACETATE -mEq/L	92.8	81.7	52.2	52.2	72.6	66.8	XXX
CALCIUM - mEq/L	5	4.5	5	5	5	5	
MAGNESIUM - mEq/L	8	5	0	8	8	8	
PHOSPHORUS -mM/L	15	7.5	0	15	15	15	

* Other Amino Acid Concentrations Available -- 3% (Renal), 4.25%   + Other Dextrose Concentration Available -- 35%

2. RATE: 25 ml/hour for 8 hours, then 50 ml/hour for 8 hours, then ____ ml/hour for 8 hours, to a final rate of____ml/hour.
   Note: All solutions containing > 3% amino acids or > 10% dextrose must be given through a central line.
3. **Vitamins** (10 ml) and **trace elements** (5 ml) are added to TPN daily, unless otherwise ordered.
4. **Vitamin K** 10 mg is added to TPN every Monday, unless otherwise ordered.
5. (optional) **Regular Insulin Human** _____ units/**liter** of TPN.
6. (optional) **Cimetidine** _____mg/**bag** of TPN.
7. **FAT EMULSION:** Infuse over 12 hours.

☐ 20% 250 ml.   ☐ Every day
☐ 20% 500 ml.   ☐ Every _____

ORDERS

1. STAT portable chest x-ray to verify central line placement, if not previously obtained. Infuse D5W at 20 cc/hr through central line until placement verified.
2. Label TPN catheter. On multi-lumen catheters, white port is designated for TPN. Do not draw blood, take CVP readings, or administer other fluid or drugs through TPN catheter/port.
3. Strict I&O's every 8 hours. Weigh ICU patients three times a week and floor patients weekly.
4. Hang fat emulsion at 0900; hang TPN at 2100. Discard unused portion of TPN.
5. Notify primary service, before hanging first bag of TPN, if blood sugar is >250 mg/dl or if phosphorus is<2.0 mM/dl.
6. Once TPN is hung, do not increase rate if blood sugar is >250 mg/dl.
7. Change TPN and fat emulsion administration sets every 24 hours.
8. Change central line dressing for TPN catheter every 96 hours or as needed per nursing policy (NS-21).
9. LABS: a. Astra-9, Magnesium, Hitachi, Ionized Ca, PT/PTT, CBC with diff with initiation of TPN, then every Monday and Thursday.
   b. Fasting triglyceride before first bottle of fat emulsion hung, then every Monday. (Draw at least 6 hours after fat emulsion infusion completed.)
   c. Obtain 24 hour urine for urea nitrogen (UNU) and creatinine (UCr) on first day of TPN, then every Monday (from 0600 - 0600).
10. Indirect Calorimetry per Nutrition Support Service
11. Finger stick for glucose every 6 hours. Follow designated sliding scale using regular insulin subcutaneously.

A. 200-249 mg% - 5 u   B. 200-249 mg% - _____ u
   250-299 mg% - 10 u **OR**   250-299 mg% - _____ u
   300-349 mg% - 15 u   300-349 mg% - _____ u
   350-399 mg% - 20 u   350-399 mg% - _____ u
   400 mg%- Call MD   400 mg% - Call MD

Supervising Physician Signature: _____

Physician Signature :_____ Physician Name Printed:_____

Beeper #:_____ Date: _____ Time: _____
WHITE-Chart   CANARY-Pharmacy   PINK-Nursing

Figure 9-21. Example of a TPN order form.

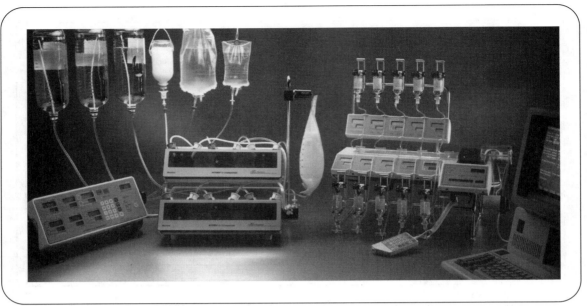

Figure 9-22. Example of the components of an automated TPN preparation device. The devices are (from L to R): The base nutrient compounder control and pump modules, micronutrient compounder, and computer for programming both compounders.

Source: Clintec Nutrition Division, Baxter Healthcare Corporation; pictured (from left): Automix® 3+3 Compounder, Micromix® Compounder, Multitask Operating System Software.

The base compounder uses special tubing that can withstand the pumping action of the machine in allocating large volumes of solutions. It accounts for the specific gravity of the solutions being used and actually weighs the amount pumped into the final container. Some compounders also weigh the original container from which solutions are pumped. It stops pumping when the selected amount has been added. The base compounder can be used with the computer, or it can be used alone. When the base compounder is used alone, the operator enters the desired volume and specific gravity of the base solution components. The device weighs the correct amounts as described above.

The additives compounder also uses special tubing that delivers exact amounts of the solutions in very small quantities. It weighs the solutions to ensure proper volumes and flushes the line between injections to avoid incompatibility problems. The additives compounder must be used with the computer and cannot be programmed alone.

The computer software controls the system and offers many safeguards. It performs many of the calculations that would otherwise be done by hand and be prone to human error, it allows the user to enter maximum safe quantities for different components, and it alerts the user to potential entry errors and inappropriate orders.

The accuracy provided by the automated compounders cannot totally substitute for all checks and balances in ensuring quality of the product. Checks and balances must be built into each step of the TPN ordering, preparation, and administration process. Calculations should be verified and double-checked, and solutions and their ingredients should be checked and double-checked, regardless of the system used. The many additives that go into a TPN solution make it complicated with respect to compatibility and stability. For example, certain concentrations of electrolytes (e.g., calcium and phosphate) will precipitate when put together and warrant that all solutions be inspected carefully before they are dispensed.

Automated compounders are used inside the LAH and must be cleaned daily according to the manufacturer's instructions. These systems require routine maintenance and calibration to ensure accurate compounding. To minimize the potential for errors, the compounders should be observed during operation. Quality control procedures may be implemented to verify final contents of the product. These systems are occasionally used for compounding other solutions. Great care should be taken to avoid compounding errors.

Administration

Most TPN solutions are made for administration through a central line (see Basic Intravenous Therapy section). This route is used because it results in immediate dilution of the solution being administered, and therefore a very concentrated solution can be administered. Administering a concentrated solution often allows the medical team to completely meet an adult patient's daily nutritional needs with 2000 to 3000 ml of TPN solution.

Occasionally, TPNs are administered through a peripheral IV line. Peripheral TPNs can contain many of the same ingredients discussed above; but to be administered peripherally they have to be diluted to lower the osmolarity. Since these solutions are more dilute they may not meet all the patient's nutritional needs. Consequently, they are often used just to supplement other caloric intake.

PEDIATRIC PARENTERAL DRUG ADMINISTRATION

Pediatric patients receive many of the same products as adults, including intermittent medications, continuous infusions, chemotherapy, TPN, and analgesics. The unique aspect of this group of patients, of course, is that their doses and solutions are much more individualized to meet their needs. Standardization of doses is not as common in pediatric patients as it is in adults. Their doses are usually calculated based on their body weight, resulting in much smaller doses than most adults receive. The volume of solution, too, is limited since their blood volume is considerably less than that of an adult.

Intermittent doses are usually given by syringe through a volume control chamber or by using a syringe pump. These systems are used to maximize accuracy of administration and minimize the amount of fluids given along with the dose of medication. Calculations should be checked and double-checked for these dilutions. An error could result in a 10-fold overdose or underdose of the drug, which could be significant in a pediatric patient.

EPIDURAL ADMINISTRATION

Epidural administration of drugs involves placing a special catheter into the epidural space of the spine. Some anesthetics and analgesics are injected into the epidural space to act on the nerve endings and provide the patient with pain relief. The placement of the catheter is a very delicate procedure and is typically performed by an anesthesiologist or a neurosurgeon. Because the drug is injected at the nerve ending, the dose needed for pain relief is greatly reduced as are many of the side effects (e.g., respiratory depression).[9]

Preparing parenterals for epidural administration requires the same aseptic technique as other parenteral products. Good technique is of utmost importance with these products, since an infection in the epidural space could be life threatening. Most epidurals must be prepared by the pharmacy and dispensed in syringes or special reservoirs designed to be used with the special pumps. All solutions given epidurally must be free of preservatives. Dosage calculations should be checked and double checked; needed doses are very small, and an error resulting in an inadvertent overdose could have severe consequences.

Epidural patient controlled —The most common use of epidural analgesia is the administration of a loading dose to initiate pain control, followed by subsequent doses as needed and administered via a PCA pump. This method is very effective in attaining the benefits of both epidural analgesia and PCA. Pump programming is similar to that for IV PCA with doses appropriate for the epidural route. Epidural doses must be prepared with drug solutions that are preservative free, meaning that they do not contain any additives to maintain sterility.

Continuous infusions—Continuous infusions of epidural analgesics are given with a device that delivers solution at a known per hour rate through the epidural catheter.

Bolus injections—Bolus epidural injections of analgesics are often used to initiate therapy or when short-term therapy is required. Bolus dosing may be sufficient to control pain without the use of a pump or continuous infusion device.

ADMIXTURE PROGRAMS

Many of the practices described in this chapter are elements of an overall pharmacy-coordinated IV admixture program. The need for such well developed programs is reinforced whenever there is a report of a patient who is harmed by an improperly prepared parenteral product. In almost all of the cases reported, the proper equipment was not used, the ingredients were not correct, personnel preparing the product where not properly trained, or some other preventable reason lead to the unfortunate outcome. Although an admixture program does not guarantee that problems will not occur, it does minimize risk to the patient by considering all factors that could potentially cause problems. The true benefit of a formal IV admixture program is that if it is well designed and managed, the whole will be greater than the sum of the parts. That is, each element alone will improve the quality of the products prepared, but with all working in concert the improvement in quality will be even greater. All of which provides the best possible outcome for the patient.

Components of a Program

The basic components of a formal IV admixture program are listed below. The need or presence of some components will depend on the scope of services provided and the type of patients served. For example, the structure of a program meeting the needs of a 100-bed hospital will differ from that of a home care pharmacy or a large teaching hospital. Each basic component is described below along with how they are superior to a system that does not utilize a formal program. Additional detail and recommended practices are also available and can be used to tailor to your own program.[10]

Policies and Procedures

Policies and procedures that are well documented and comprehensive serve as an important part of the foundation of a IV admixture program.[11,12] The policy portion of the document serves as a basis for decision making while the procedure portion serves as a description of how the task or function should be carried out.

Space

A coordinated program ideally has a space appropriate for the preparation of sterile products. Standards developed by ASHP and USP describe the desirable room layout, wall/floor/ξceiling surfaces, air quality, cleanliness, maintenance, housekeeping, and process areas needed as part of a formal program.[13] In many cases, an admixture service is operated from a room that is smaller than ideal, therefore the space must be well planned for movement of people, LAH requirements, and flow of patient orders.[4] The area should be well lighted and have as little traffic as possible. The floors, walls, and ceiling should have smooth surfaces that cannot easily harbor bacteria and can readily be cleaned and disinfected. Items like cardboard boxes can produce particulates when handled and therefore should not be brought into the IV preparation area. A room that is properly organized and structured within these guidelines will be the safest and most efficient for preparation of sterile products within the hospital.

Training

Pharmacists and technicians who work with sterile products and prepare them on a daily basis should be knowledgeable about the process.[14] Pharmacy technicians who work with these products should be trained to understand basic aseptic technique (including handling supplies, handwashing, garb, etc.), sources of contamination, how to work within a LAH, how to prepare standard types of parenteral products, and how to prepare non-standard types of preparations as needed. Technicians should demonstrate competency after learning from written training materials, videotapes, and hands-on demonstration. They should not only demonstrate proper technique but also have a sample product tested for sterility and accuracy.

Equipment

Selection and maintenance of proper equipment is important in any function, but especially important when it is relied upon to provide a clean work environment for sterile product preparation (such as with an LAH). LAHs should be cleaned before use, HEPA filters should be inspected every 6 months and have their prefilters changed regularly. Compounding equipment (such as syringe pumps used in compounding and automated TPN compounders) should be inspected and maintained according to manufacturers' recommendations. Temperature control equipment, such as refrigerators and freezers, should be monitored for temperature and be equipped with an alarm that sounds when the temperature exceeds predefined limits. All equipment (including tables, chairs, etc.) should be made of materials that are easily cleaned and disinfected (e.g., laminate or stainless steel). All equipment maintenance should be maintained on a schedule and documented.[15] Computers often are used to for a number of functions including maintaining patient profiles, generating labels, screening for incompatibilities and duplicate orders, accessing patient information (e.g., labs or diagnosis), charging, and maintaining records.[4]

Standard and Non-standard Preparations

An IV admixture program makes many different types of products, both standard (routine) and non-standard. Using the expertise of those who work in such an environment can assure that both types receive the same attention and care needed. Non-standard preparations present challenges and since they are often unusual can result in errors when made by persons not familiar with them. The use of a coordinated program, references, procedures, and general knowledge will reduce the likelihood of one of these products being prepared incorrectly. Such a program also promotes consistency in preparation and labeling.

Labeling

Countless medication errors can be attributed to poor labeling of medications. An important benefit of a IV program is that it allows for consistent, complete labeling of products prepared.[16] Usually label formats are generated by a computer and must always be clear, consistent in drug name, strength, dose, volume, and rate of administration (where applicable).

Handling

Order flow and delivery are standardized in a formal IV program. This allows for proper storage (e.g., temperature control, etc.), retrieval of unused preparations (for potential reuse) and delivery of products. This effort improves the product integrity and reduces waste by promoting use of products before they pass their expiration date.[16]

Quality Assurance

Having all sterile products prepared in one department (and often in one area) aids in the development of a coordinated, meaningful quality assurance program. Attempting to monitor and evaluate quality of sterile products that are being prepared in numerous locations throughout a hospital or other setting would be difficult and very inefficient.

Quality Assurance Program

All IV admixture programs should have a quality assurance program to ensure that products and services are of desired quality. ASHP'S Technical Assistance Bulletin on Quality Assurance for Pharmacy-Prepared Sterile Products (Appendix) provides recommendations for preparation, expiration dating, labeling, facilities, equipment, personnel education, training, evaluation, and end-product testing.

The ASHP technical assistance bulletin describes three different levels of risk for products. Products are classified into one of the three risk levels based on how they are prepared, how long they can be stored, whether they are prepared for a single patient or as part of a batch, whether they are from a sterile or non-sterile source. The characteristics of the different risk levels are listed below.

Risk Level 1

- These are sterile products without preservatives for individual patients or are batch prepared with preservatives for multiple patients.
- These are sterile products transferred into a sterile container (e.g., syringe, IV bag, or bottle).
- Storage time for these products, including administration time, should not exceed 28 hours at room temperature, 7 days under refrigeration, or 30 days if frozen.

Risk Level 2

- These products are batch-prepared without preservatives for multiple patients.
- These include products that require multiple sterile ingredients that are combined in a sterile container through a closed system transfer that are then subdivided into multiple parts.
- Storage time for these products, including administration time, can exceed 28 hours at room temperature, 7 days under refrigeration, or 30 days frozen.

Risk Level 3

- These products are compounded from non-sterile ingredients, containers or equipment or prepared from sterile or non-sterile ingredients in an open system.

The pharmacist is likely to be responsible for ensuring compliance with the guidelines and other standards of practice, but the technician's work habits and activities are likely to be affected as well. Areas of the document that affect the technician include training, policies and procedures, garb, aseptic technique, process validation, and end-product evaluation. The first four areas are covered in other sections of this chapter, but process validation and end-product evaluation require further explanation.

Process Validation

Process validation means procedures that ensure that the processes used in sterile product preparation consistently result in sterile products of acceptable quality. For most aseptic processes, validation is actually a method for evaluating the aseptic technique of personnel. Validation may be accomplished through process simulation. Process simulation is carried out just like a normal sterile product preparation process except that a microbial growth medium is substituted for the products that would normally be used. Once the sterile product is prepared, the growth medium is incubated and evaluated for microbial growth over a period of time. No microbial growth indicates that the person performing the preparation did not contaminate the product. Individuals should complete a process validation program before being allowed to prepare sterile products, and technique should be re-evaluated regularly.

End-Product Evaluation

End-product evaluation is the final inspection made by the pharmacist before the product is allowed to leave the pharmacy. It includes an inspection for leaks, cloudiness, particulate matter, color, solution volume, and container integrity. In some instances the growth medium fill procedure, described above, should be supplemented with a program of end-product sterility testing, and a method of recalling products not meeting specifications should be in place. The pharmacist also verifies compounding accuracy with respect to the correct ingredients and quantities. This check of the technician's work is an important step in ensuring that only quality products are sent for patient use.

All who work with sterile products, regardless of practice area, should be familiar with the use of the Technical Assistance Bulletin as a minimum standard.

RECOMMENDED READING

Achusim LE *et al.* Comparison of automated and manual methods of syringe filling. *Am J Hosp Pharm.* 1990;47:2492–5.

American Society of Hospital Pharmacists. Quality assurance for pharmacy-prepared sterile products. Bethesda, MD: American Society of Hospital Pharmacists; 1994. Videotape and workbook.

American Society of Hospital Pharmacists. Safe handling of cytotoxic and hazardous drugs. American Society of Hospital Pharmacists; 1990. Videotape and study guide.

Brier KL. Evaluating aseptic technique of pharmacy personnel. *Am J Hosp Pharm.* 1983;40:400–3.

Cohen MR. Proper technique for handling parenteral products. *Hosp Pharm.* 1986;21:1106.

Hasegawa GR, editor. Caring about stability and compatibility. *Am J Hosp Pharm.* 1994;51:1533–4.

Leff RD, Roberts RJ. *Practical Aspects of Intravenous Drug Administration.* 2nd ed. Bethesda, MD: American Society of Hospital Pharmacists; 1992.

McDiarmid MA. Medical surveillance for antineoplastic drug handlers. *Am J Hosp Pharm.* 1990;47:1061–6.

REFERENCES

1. Plumer AL. *Principles and Practice of Intravenous Therapy.* Boston, MA: Little, Brown and Co.; 1982.
2. Lindley CM, Deloatch KH. *Infusion Technology Manual: A self-instructional approach* and videotape. Bethesda, MD: American Society of Hospital Pharmacists; 1993.
3. Turco S, King RE. *Sterile Dosage Forms, Their Preparation and Clinical Application.* 4th ed. Philadelphia, PA: Lea & Febiger; 1994.
4. Hunt ML. *Training Manual for Intravenous Admixture Personnel.* 5th ed. Chicago, IL: Pluribus Press; 1995.
5. American Society of Health-System Pharmacists. Aseptic preparation of parenteral products. Bethesda, MD: American Society of Hospital Pharmacists, 1985. Videotape and study guide.
6. Trissel LA. *Handbook on Injectable Drugs.* 7th ed. Bethesda, MD: American Society of Hospital Pharmacists; 1992.
7. American Society of Hospital Pharmacists. Technical assistance bulletin on handling cytotoxic and hazardous drugs. *Am J Hosp Pharm.* 1990;47:1033–49.
8. Abramowitz PW, Hunt ML Jr. *Principles and Advantages of Automated Compounding: A Pharmacy Education Guide.* Deerfield, IL: Clintec Nutrition; 1992.
9. Littrell, RA: Epidural infusions. *Am J Hosp Pharm.* 1991;48:2460–74.
10. Buchanan EC, McKinnon BT, Scheckelhoff DJ, *et al. Principles of Sterile Product Preparation.* Bethesda,

MD: American Society of Health-System Pharmacists; 1995.

11. Hethcox JM. The policy and procedure manual. In: Brown TR, editor. *Handbook of Institutional Pharmacy Practice*. 3rd ed. Bethesda, MD: American Society of Hospital Pharmcists; 1992. p. 53–62.

12. Buchanan EC. Policies and procedures. In: Buchanan EC, McKinnon BT, Scheckelhoff DJ, *et al. Principles of Sterile Product Preparation*. Bethesda, MD: American Society of Health-System Pharmacists; 1995. p. 133–8.

13. Buchanan EC. Sterile compounding facilities. In: Buchanan EC, McKinnon BT, Scheckelhoff DJ, *et al. Principles of Sterile Product Preparation*. Bethesda, MD: American Society of Health-System Pharmacists; 1995. p. 25–36.

14. Buchanan EC and Schneider PJ. Personnel Education, Training and Evaluation. In: Buchanan EC, McKinnon BT, Scheckelhoff DJ, *et al. Principles of Sterile Product Preparation*. Bethesda, MD: American Society of Health-System Pharmacists; 1995. p. 9–16.

15. Schneider PJ. Equipment for sterile product preparation. In: Buchanan EC, McKinnon BT, Scheckelhoff DJ, *et al. Principles of Sterile Product Preparation*. Bethesda, MD: American Society of Health-System Pharmacists; 1995. p. 37–44.

16. McKinnon BT. Handling of sterile products within the pharmacy. In: Buchanan EC, McKinnon BT, Scheckelhoff DJ, *et al. Principles of Sterile Product Preparation*. Bethesda, MD: American Society of Health-System Pharmacists; 1995. p. 111–6.

SELF-ASSESSMENT QUESTIONS

1. Intravenous drug therapy is used
   a. when the patient is unable to take needed medications by mouth.
   b. when a drug is needed in an emergency.
   c. when a drug is not absorbed from the stomach.
   d. all of the above

2. Parenteral drug products should be
   a. free of particulate matter.
   b. sterile.
   c. free of pyrogens.
   d. all of the above

3. In the typical IV setup, an LVP is attached to a primary set that is then attached to the catheter and inserted into the patient. Drugs given intermittently are usually given
   a. through another IV line (not through the one used for the LVP).
   b. through a Y-site injection port or flashball on the primary set.
   c. by adding them to the LVP solution.

   d. none of the above

4. IV tubing used as a primary set includes which of the following?
   a. macro drip tubing (delivering 10 drops per minute)
   b. micro drip tubing (delivering 60 drops per minute)
   c. all purpose tubing (delivering 100 drops per minute)
   d. only a and b are correct

5. Large volume parenteral solution containers with potent drugs that need to be infused with a high degree of accuracy and precision are usually administered with the aid of a
   a. roller clamp.
   b. electronic infusion device.
   c. These solutions are not given IV.
   d. LAH.

6. Sterile products should be prepared in a "class 100" environment. In most pharmacies this is accomplished with the use of a
   a. room air filter.
   b. laminar Air Flow Hood (LAH).
   c. fume hood.
   d. fan cycling air 100 times per hour.
   e. none of the above

7. The space between the HEPA filter and the sterile product being prepared is referred to as the
   a. hot spot.
   b. backwash zone.
   c. zone of turbulence.
   d. critical area.
   e. none of the above

8. All manipulations inside a LAH should be performed at least _____ inches inside the hood to prevent _____.
   a. 12 inches; smoke
   b. 6 inches; backwash
   c. 10 inches; contamination
   d. 2 inches; breakage from falling on the floor.

9. Before working in the LAH
   a. interior surfaces should be wiped with 70% isopropyl alcohol.
   b. the hood should be operated for at least 15–30 minutes.
   c. hands should be washed in bacteriocidal soap.
   d. All of the above are correct.

10. Items inside a LAH should be placed away from other objects and the walls of the hood to prevent
    a. zones of turbulence.
    b. dead spaces.
    c. windows of contamination.
    d. laminar air.

11. It is permissible to touch any part of the syringe while making sterile products as long as you are wearing sterile gloves.
    a. True
    b. False

12. A 30 ml syringe with 1 ml calibrations on its barrel can be used to accurately measure 15.5 ml of a solution for injection.
    a. True
    b. False

13. To assure sterility of a new needle
    a. the user should make sure the package was intact and not damaged.
    b. wipe the needle with 70% isopropyl to disinfect it.
    c. apply additional silicone so the needle self sterilizes upon insertion into a vial.
    d. two of the above are correct.

14. To prevent core formation when entering a vial diaphragm:
    a. Only small needles should be used.
    b. Needles should be inserted quickly before a core is formed.
    c. The needle should be inserted with the bevel tip first, then pressing downward and toward the bevel so the bevel tip and heel enter at the same point.
    d. The needle should be inserted straight into the vial diaphragm.

15. Ampules differ from vials in that they
    a. are closed systems.
    b. require the use of a filter needle.
    c. can be opened without risk of breakage.
    d. ampules do not differ from vials.

16. Prior to compounding a product for parenteral administration, one should do all of the following *except:*
    a. gather all needed supplies.
    b. gather supplies anticipated for the entire shift and place them into the LAH.
    c. inspect all materials for signs they might be defective.
    d. disinfect injection sites before entry.

17. Labels for IV products
    a. should be handwritten to show personal touch.
    b. should not include anything but the drug name and the patient's name, so the patient doesn't become alarmed when reading the label.
    c. should be in a format that is consistent and easily understood.
    d. All of the above are correct.

18. Preservatives in parenteral products
    a. kill organisms and therefore eliminate the need for aseptic technique and LAHs.
    b. are harmless and non-toxic in any amount.
    c. are present in multi-dose vials.
    d. should be used in epidural dosage forms to assure sterility.

19. An IV system that uses a threaded drug vial that is screwed into a corresponding receptacle on an IV bag is called
    a. Drug-o-matic.
    b. Piggyback vial.
    c. Add-Vantage®.
    d. LVP.
    e. Cytotoxic.

20. Buretrol is a common name for a
    a. Piggyback system.
    b. Add-Vantage®.
    c. Volume Control Chamber.
    d. CRIS® system.

21. Contact with cytotoxic drugs can cause
    a. dermatitis.
    b. dizziness.
    c. nausea.
    d. possible chromosome damage, impaired fertility or cancer.
    e. all of the above

22. Cytotoxic agents are those that can be
    a. cytotoxic.
    b. oncogenic.
    c. mutagenic.
    d. teratogenic.
    e. any of the above

23. Protective apparel for those preparing cytotoxic or hazardous injections in a BSC includes
    a. a low permeability, solid front gown with tight fitting elastic cuffs.
    b. latex gloves.
    c. a self-contained respirator.

d. two of the above

24. Vertical LAHs that are Class II Biological Safety Cabinets and exhaust 100% of their air outside of the building are called
    a. Type A.
    b. Type B.
    c. horizontal LAHs.
    d. none of the above

25. After a cytotoxic agent is prepared in the pharmacy, transportation
    a. should be done immediately.
    b. should be done in a way as to minimize breakage.
    c. can be expedited with systems like pneumatic tubes.
    d. includes making the transporter aware of what they are carrying and what the procedure would be in the event of a spill.
    e. two of the above

26. Contents of a "Chemo Spill Kit" include each of the following except:
    a. gloves.
    b. goggles.
    c. a respirator.
    d. disposable gown.
    e. a loudspeaker.

27. Electrolytes are added to TPN solutions to meet metabolic needs and correct deficiencies. Examples include:
    a. amino acids.
    b. potassium chloride.
    c. vitamin D.
    d. lipid emulsions.
    e. all of the above

28. Lipid or fat emulsions are typically administered by all of the following methods *except:*
    a. as a 10% emulsion given IV through a peripheral line.
    b. as a 20% emulsion given IV through a peripheral line.
    c. as part of a 3-in-1 TPN solution.
    d. IV push.

29. Dextrose is the base component of TPN solutions most commonly given as a source of carbohydrates. Which of the following statements are true?
    a. It is available as a 5% solution that is commonly used in TPN solutions.
    b. It is available in a concentrated form (50% or more) that is diluted in the final TPN solution to approximately 25%.

c. It is available as a 70% solution that is commonly given as an separate infusion for calories and energy.
    d. All of the above are true.

30. Which of the following is FALSE concerning the gravity fill method of preparing TPN solutions?
    a. The final solution can be either the traditional formulation (amino acids and dextrose as the base) or the 3-in-1 solution (with amino acids, dextrose and fats as the base).
    b. Involves using an empty bag/bottle or using an underfilled container as the final container.
    c. Involves pumping ingredients into the final container; "gravity" really refers to the administration process for these solutions.
    d. Involves numerous checks in the system since so many additives are being measured and injected, leaving a greater potential for error.

31. Mixing of 3-in-1 solutions should be performed carefully to prevent the emulsion "oiling out." It is recommended that this be accomplished by
    a. preparing the solution in a very cold room.
    b. preparing the solution from fresh lipids.
    c. using a mixing order of fats, amino acids, and then dextrose.
    d. using a mixing order of dextrose, fats, and then amino acids.

32. Automated compounding of TPN solutions
    a. uses a compounding device to pump base ingredients into the final container.
    b. may use a device that accurately measures small quantities of electrolytes and injects them into the final container.
    c. uses a computer and software to run the compounding device.
    d. still requires the use of aseptic technique and should be done in a LAH.
    e. all of the above

33. TPN solutions are typically given through a
    a. central IV line.
    b. peripheral IV line.
    c. pump.
    d. syringe.
    e. Two of the above are correct.

34. Policies and procedures for a formal IV program typically include all of the following *except:*
    a. personnel training guidelines.
    b. quality assurance for the area.
    c. environmental monitoring procedures.
    d. names of staff working in the area.

35. Space and facilities used for sterile product preparation should
    a. be set up to meet recommendations of ASHP and USP.
    b. can be anywhere as long as it is within the pharmacy.
    c. should be carpeted to minimize noise disturbances.
    d. should have a good breeze to keep workers cool.

ANSWERS TO SELF-ASSESSMENT

1. d. Intravenous drug therapy offers some benefits in drug delivery since it provides rapid blood levels of the medication and since many drugs are not stable or absorbed in the stomach. On the other hand, there are risks associated with parenteral therapy since it is being injected directly into the body. Parenteral therapy is more expensive than oral therapy due to the need for sterility and special equipment. Therefore, the oral route should be attempted first and if not possible then the parenteral route may be used.

2. d. A basic premise required for the safe administration of any parenteral drug is that it be sterile (free of living microorganisms), free of particulate matter (undesirable particles), and pyrogens (by-products of organisms that cause fever, chills, and could lower blood pressure). Many aspects of a good IV admixture program are aimed at producing a product that meets the criteria. Products that do not meet the criteria should not be administered to the patient.

3. b. Intermittent drugs (e.g., antibiotics, anti-ulcer drugs) are often given every 6 or 8 hours through a designated location on the primary set. These locations include Y-sites (shaped like a "Y") or flashball injection sites. The only reason that another site might be required for the administration of these types of drugs would be if they were incompatible with the LVP solution, or if the LVP contained a critical drug that could not be interrupted by the intermittent drug.

4. d. Caregivers can manually control the flow rate of LVPs by counting drops in the drip chamber and adjusting the roller clamp to obtain the desired rate. The sets have a drip chamber that is calibrated to different drop sizes that allow the caregiver to visually count drops and calculate the rate of delivery. Usually the macro tubing (delivering 10 drops per minute) is used when a solution is being given at a fast rate, while the micro drip tubing (delivering 60 drops per minute) is used when a slower rate is needed.

5. b. Potent drugs that are adjusted for their effect on the patient must be controlled carefully by the caregiver. Only the use of an electronic infusion device allows this type of control. A roller clamp does control the rate of flow, but only allows the approximate rate of flow and can easily be affected by the movement of the patient.

6. b. Class 100 is defined as an environment that contains no more than 100 particles per cubic foot that are larger than 0.5 microns in size. A laminar flow hood provides a class 100 environment that can be placed in a relatively small space and is comparatively low in cost. The hood uses a blower to push air through a HEPA filter and blow it across a work surface. While some very sophisticated settings are able to filter and control air quality in an entire room and make it a class 100 environment, these are very expensive and probably more than is needed for preparation of routine sterile products.

7. d. A key principle in the use of a LAH is that nothing pass between the HEPA filter, which is blowing highly purified air, and the product being prepared. This area has been termed the "critical area" because of this important principle.

8. b. Care must be taken so that manipulations are done well inside the hood (at least six inches) to prevent backwash (i.e., unfiltered room air enters the work surface). Air movement is minimal by the time it reaches the outside of the hood and any movement or draft could allow room air to move into the hood. By working well inside the hood, this occurrence is minimized. Some users have a

tendency to work on the outside edge because it is quieter than working well within the hood, but this obviously eliminates the benefits of using the hood.

9. d. The hood should be operated for a period of time so that room air is purged from the work area. The interior surfaces of the hood should be wiped down with 70% isopropyl alcohol to disinfect them. Hands should be washed in bacteriocidal soap so that bacteria on the hands is minimized.

10. a. Materials placed within the laminar flow hood disturb the patterned flow of air blowing from the HEPA filter. This zone of turbulence created behind an object could potentially extend outside the hood, pulling or allowing contaminated room air into the aseptic working area (see Figure 9-3). When laminar air flow is moving on all sides of an object, the zone of turbulence extends approximately three times the diameter of that object. When laminar air flow is not accessible to an object on all sides (for example, when an object is placed adjacent to a vertical wall), a zone of turbulence is created that may extend six times the diameter of the object.

11. b. The barrel of the syringe can be touched and handled, but the syringe tip and plunger should never be touched. Wearing sterile gloves while preparing sterile products does not guarantee sterility since the gloves are no longer sterile once they have touched a nonsterile container or surface.

12. a. Syringes are accurate to one half of the calibrated markings. In this example that would be one half of one milliliter. Since the needed volume is at that mark it would be accurate.

13. a. Needles are sterile from the manufacturer as long as the protective overwrap is not damaged. Needles have a silicone lubricant that allows easier penetration into vials. Needles should not we wiped off since it will remove this silicone coating.

14. c. Answer c best describes the special technique that should be used to prevent a core. The other answers describe techniques that would potentially lead to a core.

15. b. Ampules are made of glass and when opened become an open system (air can pass freely); may end up with glass fragments in the solution therefore requiring the use of a filter needle; and can cut the finger of the user if not handled carefully. Vials are closed systems, do not have a risk of glass fragments and therefore do not require the use of a filter needle, and do not break on opening.

16. b. Only items needed for the preparation itself should be in the hood. Other items will introduce particulate matter unnecessarily into the work area and will create zones of turbulence disrupting the effectiveness of the LAH.

17. c. The label can play a big role in preventing medication errors. As much information as possible should be included on the label, including drug name, strength, hang time, solution, volume, patient name, room number, infusion instructions, frequency of administration, storage requirements, etc. This information should be typed or computer generated so that it is readable and should be consistent in format.

18. c. Preservatives are added to retard the growth of microorganisms in multiple dose vials. The presence of these substances should not give a false sense of security that the solution is self-sterilizing, because it is not. Strict aseptic technique is still needed. Also, if doses of drugs are significantly higher than those originally intended, larger volumes of the drug solution are given that result in larger amounts of the preservative being present which might be toxic. Therefore, if preparations involve large amounts of drug solution that contain a preservative or a diluent with a preservative, the pharmacist should be consulted to verify that the total amount of preservative to be administered to the patient will not be toxic. Solutions with preservatives should not be used in preparations for neonates, epidural, or intrathecal dosage forms due to their toxicity.

19. c. See text for description of available systems.

20. c. See text for description of available systems.

21. e. Cytotoxic agents require special handling and attention due to their potentially toxic effects. All handlers should be familiar with

these special techniques and should be aware of consequences of improper handling. All of the above are potential effects of direct exposure to one of these agents.

22. e. Handlers should be aware of what types of agents are classified as cytotoxic and therefore require special handling. Typically antineoplastics, immunosuppressants, and some antivirals are included in this category. Package inserts, material safety data sheets, or other references should be checked if a product's status is in question.

23. d. Protective apparel is doubly important with cytotoxic agents since you are not only protecting the product from contamination but also protecting the preparer from exposure. Those handling cytotoxics should wear a non-permeable gown that ties in the back and has some type of tight fitting cuffs. They should also where latex gloves that are non-powdered. If the gloves have powder on them from the manufacturer, they should be wiped clean with 70% isopropyl alcohol before use. This will prevent the powder from becoming a particulate contaminant. Use of a respirator is not needed when preparing products in a BSC since the hood filters and recycles the air.

24. b. One of the most important pieces of equipment for handling hazardous drugs safely is the BSC. A BSC is a type of vertical LAH that is designed to protect workers from exposure as well as to help maintain sterility during preparation. There are several types of Class II BSCs. Type A BSCs pump about 30% of the air back into the room after it passes through a HEPA filter. Be sure not to block airflow from the exhaust filters. Type B BSCs send air from the work zone through a HEPA filter and then to the outside of the building through an auxiliary exhaust system. Type B BSCs offer greater protection, because filtered air is sent outside the building and because they have a faster inward flow of air. Do not use horizontal LAHs to prepare hazardous drugs. They blow contaminants directly at the preparer.

25. e. Delivery of cytotoxic agents does not have to occur immediately. Once prepared, the product can receive an expiration date like any other sterile product with consideration for sterility and stability. Special handling and packaging should be used to prevent the container from breaking or leaking while in transit. Mechanical devices such as pneumatic tubes should not be used since they often jar the product, and any leakage or a spill inside a tube system would be very difficult to decontaminate.

26. e. Chemo spill kits are available commercially or can be compiled in the existing pharmacy stock. Spill kits should be assembled containing all the materials needed to clean up hazardous drug spills and protect health care workers and patients. Spill kits should contain protective gear: eye protection, a respirator, utility and latex gloves, a disposable gown or coveralls, and shoe covers. They should also contain the equipment needed to clean up the spill: a disposable scoop and a puncture- and leak-resistant plastic container for disposing of glass fragments; absorbent spill pads; gauze and disposable toweling; absorbent powder; and sealable, thick plastic waste disposal bags.

27. b. The electrolytes usually include sodium, potassium, chloride, acetate, phosphate, magnesium, and calcium. Electrolytes are usually administered (and calculated) by using a specific salt of the product. For example, sodium is frequently given as sodium chloride. Potassium can be given as potassium chloride, potassium acetate, or potassium phosphate. The patient's clinical condition and laboratory values usually determine the amount and form of electrolytes. The other components listed are commonly in TPN solutions but are not electrolytes.

28. d. Fat emulsions are administered to prevent essential fatty acid deficiency and to provide a source of calories. They are commercially available as 10 or 20% emulsion and are iso-osmolar and can be given through a peripheral IV line. Alternatively, fats can be added to the TPN solution. In this case the fat emulsion is considered a third base component along with dextrose and amino acids, and the TPN is called a 3-in-1 solution or a total nutrient admixture. The 3-in-1 technique offers several nutritional advantages but has certain mixing, stability, and compounding disadvantages.

29. b. Commercially available concentrations vary from 5 to 70%. Usually a 50% or 70%

solution is used for TPNs, and the final dextrose concentration in the TPN is usually around 25% for solutions administered via a central vein. The dextrose concentration is significantly less for infusions intended for peripheral administration.

30. c. All of the answers are true except for c. Gravity is used to transfer base solutions into the final container. This process can be slow since the dextrose is very thick in its concentrated form.

31. c. Mixing 3-in-l solutions is delicate, because the fat emulsion is actually a suspension of fat globules. Adding concentrated dextrose may oil out, or crack, the emulsion. The proper order of mixing is to add the fats first, the amino acids second, and the dextrose last (remember the acronym "FAD," fats, amino acids, dextrose). This mixing order dilutes and buffers the fat emulsion with amino acids before the highly concentrated and acidic dextrose is added.

32. e. Automated compounding involves the use of specialized equipment to prepare the TPN solution. Three primary pieces of equipment are used, sometimes together and sometimes individually: an automated compounder that prepares the base components; a second automated compounder that adds most or all of the additives or other components; and a computer with software that maintains the orders and controls the two compounders. The base compounder pumps the base components into the final container. The additives compounder also uses special tubing that delivers exact amounts of the solutions in very small quantities. It weighs the solutions to ensure proper volumes and flushes the line between injections to avoid incompatibility problems. The additives compounder must be used with the computer and cannot be programmed alone. The computer and software control the system and offer many safeguards, because they perform many of the calculations that would otherwise be done by hand and be prone to human error. They also allow the user to enter maximum safe quantities for different components and alert the user to potential entry errors and inappropriate orders. The automated compounders are used inside the LAH and must be cleaned daily according to the manufacturer's instructions.

33. e. Most TPN solutions are made for administration through a central line. This route is used because it results in immediate dilution of the solution being administered, and therefore a very concentrated solution can be administered. This route also allows the medical team to completely meet the adult patient's nutritional needs each day with 2000 to 3000 ml of TPN solution, depending on the weight and needs of the patient. Concerns over the adverse effects of a TPN solution that infuses too quickly require that a pump or other electronic infusion device be used to control its rate of administration.

34. d. Policies and procedures for IV programs typically include sections on personnel training and evaluation, acquisition, storage and handling of supplies, maintenance of the facility and equipment, personnel conduct and dress, product preparation methods, environmental monitoring, process validation, expiration dating practices, labeling guidelines, end product evaluation, housekeeping procedures, quality assurance, and documentation records. Any specific information on individuals would not fall within the purpose of these documents.

35. a. A coordinated program ideally has an appropriate space for the preparation of sterile products. Standards developed by the ASHP and USP describe the desirable room layout, wall/floor/ceiling surfaces, air quality, cleanliness, maintenance, housekeeping, and process areas needed as part of a formal program. While ideal space and facilities are still not available in some institutions, the presence of a such a program will serve to show the need for such facilities. In most hospitals, there is no better place to prepare these types of products.

APPENDIX 9

ASHP Technical Assistance Bulletin on Quality Assurance for Pharmacy-Prepared Sterile Products

Pharmacists are responsible for the correct preparation of sterile products.[a] Patient morbidity and mortality have resulted from incorrectly prepared or contaminated pharmacy-prepared products.[1-5] These ASHP recommendations are intended to help pharmacists ensure that pharmacy-prepared sterile products are of high quality.

The National Coordinating Committee on Large Volume Parenterals (NCCLVP), which ceased to exist in the 1980s, published a series of recommendations in the 1970s and early 1980s,[6-12] including an article on quality assurance (QA) for centralized intravenous admixture services in hospitals.[7] The NCCLVP recommendations, however, are somewhat dated and do not cover the variety of settings in which pharmacists practice today nor the many types of sterile preparations pharmacists compound in current practice settings.

The Joint Commission on Accreditation of Healthcare Organizations (JCAHO) publishes only general standards relating to space, equipment and supplies, and record keeping for the preparation of sterile products in hospitals.[13] The 1993 JCAHO home care standards provide somewhat more detailed, nationally recognized pharmaceutical standards for home care organizations.[14] These standards, however, also lack sufficient detail to provide pharmacists with adequate information on quality assurance activities.

The Food and Drug Administration (FDA) publishes regulations on Current Good Manufacturing Practices[15,16] that apply to sterile products made by pharmaceutical manufacturers for shipment in interstate commerce. The FDA has also published a draft guideline on the manufacture of sterile drug products by aseptic processing.[17] Both of these documents apply to the manufacture of sterile products by licensed pharmaceutical manufacturers. The Centers for Disease Control and Prevention (CDC) has published guidelines for hand washing, prevention of intravascular infections,[18] and hospital environmental control.[19] The United States Pharmacopeial Convention, Inc. (USPC) establishes drug standards for packaging and storage, labeling, identification, pH, particulate matter, heavy metals, assay, and other requirements[16]; as of this writing, there is an effort under way at USPC to develop an informational chapter on compounding sterile products intended for home use.[20]

Although the aforementioned guidelines provide assistance to pharmacists, each has certain limitations (e.g., outdated, limited scope). None of these guidelines addresses sterile product storage and administration with newer types of equipment (e.g., portable infusion devices,[21,22] indwelling medication reservoirs) or the use of automated sterile-product compounding devices.[23]

This document was developed to help pharmacists establish quality assurance procedures for the preparation of sterile products. The recommendations in this Technical Assistance Bulletin are applicable to pharmacy services in various practice settings including but not limited to hospitals, community pharmacies, nursing homes, and home health care organizations. ASHP has published a practice standard on handling cytotoxic and hazardous drugs[24];

when preparing sterile preparations involving cytotoxic or hazardous drugs, pharmacists should consider the advice in that document.

The ASHP Technical Assistance Bulletin on Quality Assurance for Pharmacy-Prepared Sterile Products *does not* apply to the *manufacture* of sterile pharmaceuticals, as defined in state and federal laws and regulations, *nor* does it apply to the preparation of medications by pharmacists, nurses, or physicians in emergency situations for immediate administration to patients. Not all recommendations may be applicable to the preparation of pharmaceuticals.

These recommendations are referenced with supporting scientific data when such data exist. In the absence of published supporting data, recommendations are based on expert opinion or generally accepted pharmacy procedures. Pharmacists are urged to use professional judgment in interpreting these recommendations and applying them in practice. It is recognized that, in certain emergency situations, a pharmacist may be requested to compound products under conditions that do not meet the recommendations. In such situations, it is incumbent upon the pharmacist to employ professional judgment in weighing the potential patient risks and benefits associated with the compounding procedure in question.

Objectives. The objectives of these recommendations are to provide

1. Information to pharmacists on quality assurance and quality control activities that may be applied to the preparation of sterile products in pharmacies; and
2. A scheme to match quality assurance and quality control activities with the potential risks to patients posed by various types of products.

Multidisciplinary Input. Pharmacists are urged to participate in the quality improvement, risk management, and infection control programs of their organizations. In so doing, pharmacists should report findings about quality assurance in sterile preparations to the appropriate staff members or committees (e.g., risk management, infection control practitioners) when procedures that may lead to patient harm are known or suspected to be in use. Pharmacists should also cooperate with managers of quality improvement, risk management, and infection control to develop optimal sterile product procedures.

Definitions. Definitions of selected terms, as used for the purposes of this document, are located in the appendix. For brevity in this document, the term *quality assurance* will be used to refer to both quality assurance and quality control (as defined in the appendix), as befits the circumstances.

Risk Level Classification

In this document, sterile products are grouped into three levels of risk to the patient, increasing from least (level 1) to greatest (level 3) potential risk and having different associated quality assurance recommendations for product integrity and patient safety. This classification system should assist pharmacists in selecting which sterile product preparation procedures to use. Compounded sterile products in risk levels 2 and 3 should meet or exceed all of the quality assurance recommendations for risk level 1. When circumstances make risk level assignment unclear, recommendations for the higher risk level should prevail. Pharmacists must exercise their own professional judgment in deciding which risk level applies to a specific compounded sterile product or situation. Consideration should be given to factors that increase potential risk to the patient, such as multiple system breaks, compounding complexities, high-risk administration sites, immunocompromised status of the patient, use of nonsterile components, microbial growth potential of the finished sterile drug product, storage conditions, and circumstances such as time between compounding and initiation of administration. The following risk assignments, based on the expertise of knowledgeable practitioners, represent one logical arrangement in which pharmacists may evaluate risk. Pharmacists may construct alternative arrangements that could be supported on the basis of scientific information and professional judgment.

Risk Level 1. Risk level 1 applies to compounded sterile products that exhibit characteristics 1, 2, *and* 3 stated below. All risk level 1 products should be prepared with sterile equipment (e.g., syringes, vials), sterile ingredients and solutions, and sterile contact surfaces for the final product. Of the three risk levels, risk level 1 necessitates the least amount of quality assurance. Risk level 1 includes the following:

1. Products
   a. Stored at room temperature (see the appendix for temperature definitions) and completely administered within 28 hours from preparation; or
   b. Stored under refrigeration for 7 days or less before complete administration to a patient over a period not to exceed 24 hours (Table 1); or
   c. Frozen for 30 days or less before complete administration to a patient over a period not to exceed 24 hours.
2. Unpreserved sterile products prepared for administration to one patient, or batch-prepared products containing suitable preservatives prepared for administration to more than one patient.
3. Products prepared by closed-system aseptic transfer of sterile, nonpyrogenic, finished pharmaceuticals obtained from licensed manufacturers into sterile final containers (e.g., syringe, minibag, portable infusion-device cassette) obtained from licensed manufacturers.

Risk Level 2. Risk level 2 sterile products exhibit characteristic 1, 2, *or* 3 stated below. All risk level 2 products should be prepared with sterile equipment, sterile ingredients and solutions, and sterile contact surfaces for the final product and by using closed-system transfer methods. Risk level 2 includes the following:

1. Products stored beyond 7 days under refrigeration, or stored beyond 30 days frozen, or administered beyond 28 hours after preparation and storage at room

temperature (Table 1).
2. Batch-prepared products without preservatives that are intended for use by more than one patient. (Note: Batch-prepared products without preservatives that

Table 1.

Assignment of Products to Risk Level 1 or 2 According to Time and Temperature Before Completion of Administration

Risk Level	Room Temperature (15 to 30 °C)	Days of Storage Refrigerator (2 to 8 °C)	Freezer (−20 to −10 °C)
1	Completely administered within 28 hr	≤ 7	≤ 30
2	Storage and administration exceeds 28 hr	> 7	> 30

will be administered to multiple patients carry a greater risk to the patients than products prepared for a single patient because of the potential effect of product contamination on the health and well-being of a larger patient group.)
3. Products compounded by combining multiple sterile ingredients, obtained from licensed manufacturers, in a sterile reservoir, obtained from a licensed manufacturer, by using closed-system aseptic transfer before subdivision into multiple units to be dispensed to patients.

Risk Level 3. Risk level 3 products exhibit either characteristic 1 *or* 2:

1. Products compounded from nonsterile ingredients or compounded with nonsterile components, containers, or equipment.
2. Products prepared by combining multiple ingredients—sterile or nonsterile—by using an open-system transfer or open reservoir before terminal sterilization or subdivision into multiple units to be dispensed.

Quality Assurance for Risk Level 1

RL 1.1: Policies and Procedures. Up-to-date policies and procedures for compounding sterile products should be written and available to all personnel involved in these activities. Policies and procedures should be reviewed at least annually by the designated pharmacist and department head and updated, as necessary, to reflect current standards of practice and quality. Additions, revisions, and deletions should be communicated to all personnel involved in sterile compounding and related activities. These policies and procedures should address personnel education and training requirements, competency evaluation, product acquisition, storage and handling of products and supplies, storage and delivery of final products, use and maintenance of facilities and equipment, appropriate garb and conduct for personnel working in the controlled area, process validation, preparation technique, labeling, documentation, and quality control.[9] Further, written policies and procedures should address personnel access and movement of materials into and near the controlled area. Policies and procedures for monitoring environmental conditions in the controlled area should take into consideration the amount of exposure of the product to the environment during compounding. Before compounding sterile products, all personnel involved should read the policies and procedures and sign to verify their understanding.

RL 1.2: Personnel Education, Training, and Evaluation. Pharmacy personnel preparing or dispensing sterile products should receive suitable didactic and experiential training and competency evaluation through demonstration, testing (written or practical), or both. Some aspects that should be included in training programs include aseptic technique; critical-area contamination factors; environmental monitoring; facilities, equipment, and supplies; sterile product calculations and terminology; sterile product compounding documentation; quality assurance procedures; aseptic preparation procedures; proper gowning and gloving technique; and general conduct in the controlled area. In addition to knowledge of chemical, pharmaceutical, and clinical properties of drugs, pharmacists should also be knowledgeable about the principles of Current Good Manufacturing Practices.[15,16] Videotapes[25] and additional information on the essential components of a training, orientation, and evaluation program are described elsewhere.[7,12,26,27] All pharmacy personnel involved in cleaning and maintenance of the controlled area should be knowledgeable about cleanroom design (if applicable), the basic concepts of aseptic compounding, and critical-area contamination factors. Non-pharmacy personnel (e.g., housekeeping staff) involved in the cleaning or maintenance of the controlled area should receive adequate training on applicable procedures.

The aseptic technique of each person preparing sterile products should be observed and evaluated as satisfactory during orientation and training and at least on an annual basis thereafter. In addition to observation, methods of evaluating the knowledge of personnel include written or practical tests and process validation.

RL 1.3: Storage and Handling. Solutions, drugs, supplies, and equipment used to prepare or administer sterile products should be stored in accordance with manufacturer or USP requirements. Temperatures in refrigerators and freezers used to store ingredients and finished sterile preparations should be monitored and documented daily to ensure that compendial storage requirements are met. Warehouse and other pharmacy storage areas where ingredients are stored should be monitored to ensure that temperature, light, moisture, and ventilation remain within manufacturer and compendial requirements. To permit adequate floor cleaning, drugs and supplies should be stored on shelving areas above the floor. Products that have exceeded their expiration dates should be removed from active storage areas. Before use, each drug, ingredient, and container should be visually inspected for damage, defects, and expiration date.

Unnecessary personnel traffic in the controlled area should be minimized. Particle-generating activities, such as removal of intravenous solutions, drugs, and supplies from cardboard boxes, should not be performed in the controlled area. Products and supplies used in preparing sterile products should be removed from shipping containers outside the controlled area before aseptic processing is begun. Packaging materials and items generating unacceptable amounts of particles (e.g., cardboard boxes, paper towels, reference books) should not be permitted in the controlled area or critical area. The removal of immediate packaging designed to retain the sterility or stability of a product (e.g., syringe packaging, light-resistant pouches) is an exception; obviously, this type of packaging should not be removed outside the controlled area. Disposal of packaging materials, used syringes, containers, and needles should be performed at least daily, and more often if needed, to enhance sanitation and avoid accumulation in the controlled area.

In the event of a product recall, there should be a mechanism for tracking and retrieving affected products from specific patients to whom the products were dispensed.

RL 1.4: Facilities and Equipment. The controlled area should be a limited-access area sufficiently separated from other pharmacy operations to minimize the potential for contamination that could result from the unnecessary flow of materials and personnel into and out of the area. Computer entry, order processing, label generation, and record keeping should be performed outside the critical area. The controlled area should be clean, well lighted, and of sufficient size to support sterile compounding activities. For hand washing, a sink with hot and cold running water should be in close proximity. Refrigeration, freezing, ventilation, and room temperature control capabilities appropriate for storage of ingredients, supplies, and pharmacy-prepared sterile products in accordance with manufacturer, USP, and state or federal requirements should exist. The controlled area should be cleaned and disinfected at regular intervals with appropriate agents, according to written policies and procedures. Disinfectants should be alternated periodically to prevent the development of resistant microorganisms. The floors of the controlled area should be nonporous and washable to enable regular disinfection. Active work surfaces in the controlled area (e.g., carts, compounding devices, counter surfaces) should be disinfected, in accordance with written procedures. Refrigerators, freezers, shelves, and other areas where pharmacy-prepared sterile products are stored should be kept clean.

Sterile products should be prepared in a Class 100 environment.[28] Such an environment exists inside a certified horizontal- or vertical-laminar-airflow hood. Facilities that meet the recommendations for risk level 3 preparation would be suitable for risk level 1 and 2 compounding. Cytotoxic and other hazardous products should be prepared in a Class II biological-safety cabinet.[24] Laminar-airflow hoods are designed to be operated continuously. If a laminar-airflow hood is turned off between aseptic processing, it should be operated long enough to allow complete purging of room air from the critical area (e.g., 15–30 minutes), then disinfected before use. The critical-area work surface and all accessible interior surfaces of the hood should be disinfected with an appropriate agent before work begins and periodically thereafter, in accordance with written policies and procedures. The exterior surfaces of the laminar-airflow hood should be cleaned periodically with a mild detergent or suitable disinfectant; 70% isopropyl alcohol may damage the hood's clear plastic surfaces. The laminar-airflow hood should be certified by a qualified contractor at least every six months or when it is relocated to ensure operational efficiency and integrity.[29] Prefilters in the laminar-airflow hood should be changed periodically, in accordance with written policies and procedures.

A method should be established to calibrate and

verify the accuracy of automated compounding devices used in aseptic processing.

RL 1.5: Garb. Procedures should generally require that personnel wear clean clothing covers that generate low amounts of particles in the controlled area. Clean gowns or closed coats with sleeves that have elastic binding at the cuff are recommended. Hand, finger, and wrist jewelry should be minimized or eliminated. Head and facial hair should be covered. Masks are recommended during aseptic preparation procedures.

Personnel preparing sterile products should scrub their hands and arms (to the elbow) with an appropriate antimicrobial skin cleanser.

RL 1.6: Aseptic Technique and Product Preparation. Sterile products should be prepared with aseptic technique in a Class 100 environment. Personnel should scrub their hands and forearms for an appropriate length of time with a suitable antimicrobial skin cleanser at the beginning of each aseptic compounding process and when re-entering the controlled area. Personnel should wear appropriate attire (see RL 1.5: Garb). Eating, drinking, and smoking should be prohibited in the controlled area. Talking should be minimized in the critical area during aseptic preparation.

Ingredients used to compound sterile products should be determined to be stable, compatible, and appropriate for the product to be prepared, according to manufacturer or USP guidelines or appropriate scientific references. The ingredients of the preparation should be predetermined to be suitable to result in a final product that meets physiological norms for solution osmolality and pH, as appropriate for the intended route of administration. Each ingredient and container should be inspected for defects, expiration date, and product integrity before use. Expired, inappropriately stored, or defective products should not be used in preparing sterile products. Defective products should be promptly reported to the FDA.[30]

Only materials essential for preparing the sterile product should be placed in the laminar-airflow hood. The surfaces of ampuls, vials, and container closures (e.g., vial stoppers) should be disinfected by swabbing or spraying with an appropriate disinfectant solution (e.g., 70% isopropyl alcohol) before placement in the hood. Materials used in aseptic preparation should be arranged in the critical area of the hood in a manner that prevents interruption of the unidirectional airflow between the high-efficiency particulate air (HEPA) filter and critical sites of needles, vials, ampuls, containers, and transfer sets. All aseptic procedures should be performed at least 6 inches inside the front edge of the laminar-airflow hood, in a clear path of unidirectional airflow between the HEPA filter and work materials (e.g., needles, stoppers). The number of personnel preparing sterile products in the hood at one time should be minimized. Overcrowding of the critical work area may interfere with unidirectional airflow and increase the potential for compounding errors. Likewise, the number of units being prepared in the hood at one time should be consistent with the amount of work space in the critical area. Automated compounding devices and other equipment placed in or adjacent to the critical area should be cleaned, disinfected, and placed to avoid contamination or disruption of the unidirectional airflow between the HEPA filter and sterile surfaces.

Aseptic technique should be used to avoid touch contamination of sterile needles, syringe parts (e.g., plunger, syringe tip), and other critical sites. Solutions from ampuls should be properly filtered to remove particles. Solutions of reconstituted powders should be mixed carefully, ensuring complete dissolution of the drug with the appropriate diluent. Needle entry into vials with rubber stoppers should be done cautiously to avoid the creation of rubber core particles. Before, during, and after the preparation of sterile products, the pharmacist should carefully check the identity and verify the amounts of the ingredients in sterile preparations against the original prescription, medication order, or other appropriate documentation (e.g., computerized patient profile, label generated from a pharmacist-verified order) before the product is released or dispensed. Additional information on aseptic technique is available elsewhere.[6,25,31]

For preparation involving automated compounding devices, data entered into the compounding device should be verified by a pharmacist before compounding begins and end-product checks should be performed to verify accuracy of ingredient delivery. These checks may include weighing and visually verifying the final product. For example, the expected weight (in grams) of the final product, based on the specific gravities of the ingredients and their respective volumes, can be documented on the compounding formula sheet, dated, and initialed by the responsible pharmacist. Once compounding is completed, each final product can be weighed and its weight compared with the expected weight. The product's actual weight should fall within a preestablished threshold for variance.[32] Visual verification may be aided by marking the beginning level of each bulk container before starting the automated mixing process and checking each container after completing the mixing process to determine whether the final levels appear reasonable in comparison with expected volumes. The operator should also periodically observe the device during the mixing process to ensure that the device is operating properly (e.g., check to see that all stations are operating).[33] If there are doubts whether a product or component has been properly prepared or stored, then the product should not be used. Refractive index measurements may also be used to verify the addition of certain ingredients.[34]

RL 1.7: Process Validation. Validation of aseptic processing procedures provides a mechanism for ensuring that processes consistently result in sterile products of acceptable quality. For most aseptic preparation procedures, process validation is actually a method of assessing the adequacy of a person's aseptic technique. It is recommended that each individual involved in the preparation of sterile products successfully complete a validation process on technique before being allowed to prepare sterile products. The validation process should follow a written procedure that includes evaluation of technique through process simulation.[35–37]

Process simulation testing is valuable for assessing the compounding process, especially aseptic fill operations.[17] It allows for the evaluation of opportunities for microbial contamination during all steps of sterile product preparation. The sterility of the final product is a cumulative function of all processes involved in its preparation and is ultimately determined by the processing step providing the lowest probability of sterility.[38] Process simulation testing is carried out in the same manner as normal production except that an appropriate microbiological growth medium is used in place of the actual products used during sterile preparation. The growth medium is processed as if it were a product being compounded for patient use; the same personnel, procedures, equipment, and materials are involved. The medium samples are then incubated and evaluated. If no microbial growth is detected, this provides evidence that adequate aseptic technique was used. If growth is detected, the entire sterile preparation process must be evaluated, corrective action taken, and the process simulation test performed again.[17,38] No products intended for patient use should be prepared by an individual until the process simulation test indicates that the individual can competently perform aseptic procedures. It is recommended that personnel competency be revalidated at least annually, whenever the quality assurance program yields an unacceptable result, and whenever unacceptable techniques are observed; this revalidation should be documented.

RL 1.8: Expiration Dating. All pharmacy-prepared sterile products should bear an appropriate expiration date. The expiration date assigned should be based on currently available drug stability information and sterility considerations. Sources of drug stability information include references (e.g., *Remington's Pharmaceutical Sciences, Handbook on Injectable Drugs*), manufacturer recommendations, and reliable, published research. When interpreting published drug stability information, the pharmacist should consider all aspects of the final sterile product being prepared (e.g., drug reservoir, drug concentration, storage conditions).[15,16] Methods used for establishing expiration dates should be documented. Appropriate inhouse (or contract service) stability testing may be used to determine expiration dates.

RL 1.9: Labeling. Sterile products should be labeled with at least the following information:

1. For patient-specific products: the patient's name and any other appropriate patient identification (e.g., location, identification number); for batch-prepared products: control or lot number;
2. All solution and ingredient names, amounts, strengths, and concentrations (when applicable);
3. Expiration date (and time, when applicable);
4. Prescribed administration regimen, when appropriate (including rate and route of administration);
5. Appropriate auxiliary labeling (including precautions);
6. Storage requirements;
7. Identification (e.g., initials) of the responsible pharmacist;
8. Device-specific instructions (when appropriate); and
9. Any additional information, in accordance with state or federal requirements.

It may also be useful to include a reference number for the prescription or medication order in the labeling; this information is usually required for products dispensed to outpatients. The label should be legible and affixed to the final container in a manner enabling it to be read while the sterile product is being administered (when possible).

RL 1.10: End-Product Evaluation. The final product should be inspected and evaluated for container leaks, container integrity, solution cloudiness, particulates in the solution, appropriate solution color, and solution volume when preparation is completed and again when the product is dispensed. The responsible pharmacist should verify that the product was compounded accurately with respect to the use of correct ingredients, quantities, containers, and reservoirs; different methods may be used for end-product verification (e.g., observation, calculation checks, documented records).

RL 1.11: Documentation. The following should be documented and maintained on file for an adequate period of time, according to organizational policies and procedures and state regulatory requirements: (1) the training and competency evaluation of employees in sterile product procedures, (2) refrigerator and freezer temperatures, and (3) certification of laminar-airflow hoods. Pharmacists should also maintain appropriate dispensing records for sterile products, in accordance with state regulatory requirements.

Quality Assurance for Risk Level 2

Because the risks associated with contamination of a sterile product are increased with long-term storage and administration, more stringent requirements are appropriate for risk level 2 preparation.

RL 2.1: Policies and Procedures. In addition to all recommendations for risk level 1, the written quality assurance program should define and identify necessary environmental monitoring devices and techniques to be used to ensure an adequate environment for risk level 2 sterile product preparation. Examples include the use of airborne particle counters, air velocity and temperature meters, viable particle samplers (e.g., slit samplers), agar plates, and swab sampling of surfaces and potential contamination sites. All aspects of risk level 2 sterile product preparation, storage, and distribution, including details such as the choice of cleaning materials and disinfectants and the monitoring of equipment accuracy, should be addressed in written policies and procedures. Limits of acceptability (threshold or action levels) for environmental monitoring and process simulation and actions to be implemented when thresholds are exceeded should be defined in written policies. For sterile batch compounding, written policies and procedures should be established for the use of master formulas and work sheets and for appropriate documentation. Policies and procedures should also address personnel attire in the controlled area, lot number determination and documentation, and any other quality assurance procedures unique to compounding risk level 2 sterile products.

RL 2.2: Personnel Education, Training, and Evaluation. All recommendations for risk level 1 should be met. In addition to recommendations for risk level 1, assessment of the competency of personnel preparing risk level 2 sterile products should include an appropriate process simulation procedure (as described in RL 1.7: Process validation). However, process simulation procedures for assessing the preparation of risk level 2 sterile products should be representative of all types of manipulations, products, and batch sizes personnel preparing risk level 2 products are likely to encounter.

RL 2.3: Storage and Handling. All storage and handling recommendations for risk level 1 should be met.

RL 2.4: Facilities and Equipment. In addition to all recommendations for risk level 1, the following are recommended for risk level 2 sterile product preparation:

1. Risk level 2 products should be prepared in a Class 100 horizontal- or vertical-laminar-airflow hood that is properly situated in a controlled area that meets Class 100,000 conditions (or better) for acceptable airborne particle levels. Class 100,000 conditions mean that no more than 100,000 particles 0.5 μm and larger may exist per cubic foot of air.[28] A positive pressure relative to adjacent pharmacy areas is recommended.

2. Cleaning materials (e.g., mops, sponges, germicidal disinfectants) for use in the controlled area or cleanroom should be carefully selected. They should be made of materials that generate a low amount of particles. If reused, cleaning materials should be cleaned and disinfected between uses.

3. The critical-area work surfaces (e.g., interior of the laminar-airflow hood) should be disinfected frequently and before and after each batch preparation process with an appropriate agent, according to written policies and procedures. Floors should be disinfected at least daily. Carpet or porous floors, porous walls, and porous ceiling tiles are not desirable in the controlled area because these surfaces cannot be properly disinfected. Exterior hood surfaces and other hard surfaces in the controlled area, such as shelves, carts, tables, and stools, should be disinfected weekly and after any unanticipated event that could increase the risk of contamination. Walls should be cleaned at least monthly.

4. To ensure that an appropriate environment is maintained for risk level 2 sterile product preparation, an effective written environmental monitoring program is recommended.[26] Sampling of air and surfaces according to a written plan and schedule is recommended.[17,26] The plan and frequency should be adequate to document that the controlled area is suitable and that the laminar-airflow hood(s) or biological-safety cabinet(s) meet the Class 100 requirements. Limits of acceptability (thresholds or action levels) and appropriate actions to be taken in the event thresholds are exceeded should be specified.

5. To help reduce the number of particles in the controlled area, an adjacent support area (e.g., anteroom) of high cleanliness, separated from the controlled area by a barrier (e.g., plastic curtain, partition, wall), is desirable. Appropriate activities for the support area include, but are not limited to, hand washing, gowning and gloving, removal of packaging and cardboard items, and cleaning and disinfecting hard-surface containers and supplies before placing these items in the controlled area.

RL 2.5: Garb. All recommendations for risk level 1 should be met. Gloves, gowns, and masks are recommended for the preparation of all risk level 2 sterile products. It must be emphasized that, even if sterile gloves are used, gloves do not remain sterile during aseptic compounding; however,

they do assist in containing bacteria, skin, and other particles that may be shed, even from scrubbed hands. Clean gowns, coveralls, or closed jackets with sleeves having elastic binding at the cuff are recommended; these garments should be made of low-shedding materials. Shoe covers may be helpful in maintaining the cleanliness of the controlled area. During sterile product preparation, gloves should be rinsed frequently with a suitable agent (e.g., 70% isopropyl alcohol) and changed when their integrity is compromised (i.e., when they are punctured or torn).

RL 2.6: Aseptic Technique and Product Preparation. All recommendations for risk level 1 sterile production preparation should be met.

A master work sheet should be developed for each batch of sterile products to be prepared. Once approved by the designated pharmacist, a verified duplicate (e.g., photocopy) of the master work sheet should be used as the preparation work sheet from which each batch is prepared and on which all documentation for that batch occurs. A separate preparation work sheet should be used for each batch prepared. The master work sheet should consist of the formula, components, compounding directions or procedures, a sample label, and evaluation and testing requirements.[39] The preparation work sheet should be used to document the following:

1. Identity of all solutions and ingredients and their corresponding amounts, concentrations, or volumes;
2. Manufacturer lot number for each component;
3. Component manufacturer or suitable identifying number;
4. Container specifications (e.g., syringe, pump cassette);
5. Lot or control number assigned to batch;
6. Expiration date of batch-prepared products;
7. Date of preparation;
8. Identity (e.g., initials, codes, signatures) of personnel involved in preparation;
9. End-product evaluation and testing specifications;
10. Storage requirements;
11. Specific equipment used during aseptic preparation (e.g., a specific automated compounding device); and
12. Comparison of actual yield to anticipated yield, when appropriate.

A policy and procedure could be developed that allows separate documentation of batch formulas, compounding instructions, and records. However documentation is done, a procedure should exist for easy retrieval of all records pertaining to a particular batch. Each group of sterile batch-prepared products should bear a unique lot number. Under no circumstances should identical lot numbers be assigned to different products or different batches of the same product. Lot numbers may be alphabetic, numeric, or alphanumeric.

The process of combining multiple sterile ingredients into a single, sterile reservoir for subdivision into multiple units for dispensing may necessitate additional quality control procedures. It is recommended that calculations associated with this process be verified by a second pharmacist, when possible; this verification should be documented. Because this process often involves making multiple entries into the intermediate sterile reservoir, the likelihood of contamination may be greater than that associated with the preparation of other risk level 2 sterile products.

RL 2.7: Process Validation. Each individual involved in the preparation of risk level 2 sterile products should successfully complete a validation process, as recommended for risk level 1. Process simulation procedures for compounding risk level 2 sterile products should be representative of all types of manipulations, products, and batch sizes that personnel preparing risk level 2 sterile products are likely to encounter.

RL 2.8: Expiration Dating. All recommendations for risk level 1 should be met.

RL 2.9: Labeling. All recommendations for risk level 1 should be met.

RL 2.10: End-Product Evaluation. All recommendations for risk level 1 should be met. Additionally, the growth media fill procedure should be supplemented with a program of end-product sterility testing, according to a formal sampling plan.[40-42] Written policies and procedures should specify measurements and methods of testing. Policies and procedures should include a statistically valid sampling plan and acceptance criteria for the sampling and testing. The criteria should be statistically adequate to reasonably ensure that the entire batch meets all specifications. Products not meeting all specifications should be rejected and discarded. There should be a mechanism for recalling all products of a specific batch if end-product testing procedures yield unacceptable results. On completion of final testing, products should be stored in a manner that ensures their identity, strength, quality, and purity. Detailed information on end-product sterility testing is published elsewhere.[7,16]

RL 2.11: Documentation. All recommendations for risk level 1 should be met. Additionally, documentation of end-product sampling and batch-preparation records should be maintained for an adequate period of time, according to organizational policies and procedures and state regulatory requirements. Documentation for sterile batch-prepared products should include the

1. Master work sheet;
2. Preparation work sheet; and
3. End-product evaluation and testing results.

Quality Assurance for Risk Level 3

General Comment on Risk Level 3. Risk level 3 addresses the preparation of products that pose the greatest potential risk to patients. The quality assurance activities described in this section are clearly more demanding—in terms of proc-esses, facilities, and final product assessment—than for risk levels 1 and 2. Ideally, the activities described for risk level 3 would be used for all high-risk products. The activities may be viewed as most important in circumstances in which the medical need for such high-risk products is *routine*. In circumstances where the medical need for such a product is immediate (and there is not a suitable alternative) or when the preparation of such a product is rare, professional judgment must be applied as to the extent to which some activities (e.g., strict facility design, quarantine and final product testing before product

dispensing) should be applied.

RL 3.1: Policies and Procedures. There should be written policies and procedures related to every aspect of preparation of risk level 3 sterile products. These policies and procedures should be detailed enough to ensure that all products have the identity, strength, quality, and purity purported for the product.[13,16] All policies and procedures should be reviewed and approved by the designated pharmacist. There should be a mechanism designed to ensure that policies and procedures are communicated, understood, and adhered to by personnel cleaning or working in the controlled area or support area. Policies and procedures should be reviewed at least annually by the designated pharmacist and department head. Written policies and procedures should define and identify the environmental monitoring activities necessary to ensure an adequate environment for risk level 3 sterile product preparation.

In addition to the policies and procedures required for risk levels 1 and 2, there should be written policies and procedures for the following:

1. Component handling and storage;
2. Any additional personnel qualifications commensurate with the preparation of risk level 3 sterile products;
3. Personnel responsibilities in the controlled area (e.g., cleaning, maintenance, access to controlled area);
4. Equipment use, maintenance, calibration, and testing;
5. Sterilization;
6. Master formula and master work sheet development and use;
7. End-product evaluation and testing;
8. Appropriate documentation for preparation of risk level 3 sterile products;
9. Use, control, and monitoring of environmentally controlled areas and calibration of monitoring equipment;
10. Validation of processes for preparing risk level 3 sterile products;
11. Quarantine of products and release from quarantine, if applicable;
12. A mechanism for recall of products from patients in the event that end-product testing procedures yield unacceptable results; and
13. Any other quality control procedures unique to the preparation of risk level 3 sterile products.

RL 3.2: Personnel Education, Training, and Evaluation. Persons preparing sterile products at risk level 3 must have specific education, training, and experience to perform all functions required for the preparation of risk level 3 sterile products. However, final responsibility should lie with the pharmacist, who should be knowledgeable in the principles of good manufacturing practices and proficient in quality assurance requirements, equipment used in the preparation of risk level 3 sterile products, and other aspects of sterile product preparation. The pharmacist should have sufficient education, training, experience, and demonstrated competency to ensure that all sterile products prepared from sterile or nonsterile components have the identity, strength, quality, and purity purported for the products.[7,13] In addition to the body of knowledge required for risk levels 1 and 2, the pharmacist should possess sufficient knowledge in the following areas:

1. Aseptic processing[17,38,43];
2. Quality control and quality assurance as related to environmental, component, and end-product testing;
3. Sterilization techniques[16]; and
4. Container, equipment, and closure system selection.

All pharmacy personnel involved in the cleaning and maintenance of the controlled area should be specially trained and thoroughly knowledgeable in the special requirements of Class 100 critical-area technology and design. There should be documented, ongoing training for all employees to enable retention of expertise.

RL 3.3: Storage and Handling. In addition to recommendations for risk levels 1 and 2, risk level 3 policies and procedures for storage and handling should include the procurement, identification, storage, handling, testing, and recall of components and finished products.

Components and finished products ready to undergo end-product testing should be stored in a manner that prevents their use before release by a pharmacist, minimizes the risk of contamination, and enables identification. There should be identifiable storage areas that can be used to quarantine products, if necessary, before they are released.[15]

RL 3.4: Facilities and Equipment. Preparation of risk level 3 sterile products should occur in a Class 100 horizontal- or vertical-laminar-airflow hood that is properly situated in a controlled area that meets Class 10,000 conditions for acceptable airborne particle levels *or* in a properly maintained and monitored Class 100 cleanroom (without the hood).[28] The controlled area should have a positive pressure differential relative to adjacent, less clean areas of at least 0.05 inch of water.[17] Solutions that are to be terminally sterilized may be prepared in a Class 100 laminar-airflow hood located inside a controlled area that meets Class 100,000 conditions.

To allow proper cleaning and disinfection, walls, floors, and ceilings in the controlled area should be nonporous. To help reduce the number of particles in the controlled area, an adjacent support area (e.g., anteroom) should be provided.

During the preparation of risk level 3 sterile products, access to the controlled area or cleanroom should be limited to those individuals who are required to be in the area and are properly attired. The environment of the main access areas directly adjacent to the controlled area (e.g., anteroom) should meet at least Federal Standard 209E Class 100,000 requirements.[28] To help maintain a Class 100 critical-area environment during compounding, the adjacent support area (e.g., anteroom) should be separated from the controlled area by a barrier (e.g., plastic curtain, partition, wall). Written policies and procedures for monitoring the environment of the controlled area and adjacent areas should be developed.[17,26]

No sterile products should be prepared in the controlled area if it fails to meet established criteria specified in the policies and procedures. A calibrated particle counter capable of measuring air particles 0.5 μm and larger should be used to monitor airborne particulate matter. Before product preparation begins, the positive-pressure air status should meet or exceed the requirements. Air samples should be taken at several places in the controlled area with the appropriate environmental monitoring devices (e.g., nutrient agar plates). Surfaces on which work actually occurs, including laminar-airflow hood surfaces and table-tops, should be monitored using surface contact plates, the swab-rinse technique, or other appropriate methods.[37,42]

Test results should be reviewed and criteria should be pre-established to determine the point at which the preparation of risk level 3 sterile products will be disallowed until corrective measures are taken. When the environment does not meet the criteria specified in the policies and procedures, sterile product processing should immediately cease and corrective action should be taken. In the event that this occurs, written policies and procedures should delineate alternative methods of sterile product preparation to enable timely fulfillment of prescription orders.

Equipment should be adequate to prevent microbiological contamination. Methods should be established for the cleaning, preparation, sterilization, calibration, and documented use of all equipment.

Critical-area work surfaces should be disinfected with an appropriate agent before the preparation of each product. Floors in the controlled area should be disinfected at least daily. Exterior hood surfaces and other hard surfaces in the controlled area, such as shelves, tables, and stools, should be disinfected weekly and after any unanticipated event that could increase the risk of contamination. Walls and ceilings in the controlled area or cleanroom should be disinfected at least weekly.

Large pieces of equipment, such as tanks, carts, and tables, used in the controlled area or cleanroom should be made of a material that can be easily cleaned and disinfected; stainless steel is recommended. Equipment that does not come in direct contact with the finished product should be properly cleaned, rinsed, and disinfected before being placed in the controlled area. All nonsterile equipment that will come in contact with the sterilized final product should be properly sterilized before introduction into the controlled area; this precaution includes such items as tubing, filters, containers, and other processing equipment. The sterilization process should be monitored and documented.[17]

RL 3.5: Garb. All recommendations for risk levels 1 and 2 should be met. Additionally, cleanroom garb should be worn inside the controlled area at all times during the preparation of risk level 3 sterile products. Attire should consist of a low-shedding coverall, head cover, face mask, and shoe covers. These garments may be either disposable or reusable. Head and facial hair should be covered. Before donning these garments over street clothes, personnel should thoroughly wash their hands and arms up to the elbows with a suitable antimicrobial skin cleanser.[19] Sterile disposable gloves should be worn and rinsed frequently with an appropriate agent (e.g., 70% isopropyl alcohol) during processing. The gloves should be changed if the integrity is compromised. If persons leave the controlled area or *support area* during processing, they should regown with clean garments before re-entering.

RL 3.6: Aseptic Technique and Product Preparation. All recommendations for risk levels 1 and 2 should be met. Methods should ensure that components and containers remain free from contamination and are easily identified as to the product, lot number, and expiration date. If components are not finished sterile pharmaceuticals obtained from licensed manufacturers, pharmacists should ensure that these components meet USP standards. Products prepared from nonsterile ingredients should be tested to ensure that they do not exceed specified endotoxin limits.[16] As each new lot of components and containers is received, the components should be quarantined until properly identified, tested, or verified by a pharmacist.

The methods for preparing sterile products and using process controls should be designed to ensure that finished products have the identity, strength, quality, and purity they are intended to have. Any deviations from established methods should be documented and appropriately justified.

A master work sheet should be developed for the preparation of each risk level 3 sterile product. Once approved by the pharmacist, a verified duplicate of the master work sheet should be used as the controlling document from which each sterile end product or batch of prepared products is compounded and on which all documentation for that product or batch occurs. The master work sheet should document all the requirements for risk level 2 plus the following:

1. Comparison of actual with anticipated yield;
2. Sterilization method(s); and
3. Quarantine specifications.

The preparation work sheet should serve as the batch record for each time a risk level 3 sterile product is prepared. Each batch of pharmacy-prepared sterile products should bear a unique lot number, as described in risk level 2.

There should be documentation on the preparation work sheet of all additions of individual components plus the signatures or initials of those individuals involved with the measuring or weighing and addition of these components.

The selection of the final packaging system (including container and closure) for the sterile product is crucial to maintaining product integrity. To the extent possible, presterilized containers obtained from licensed manufacturers should be used. If an aseptic filling operation is used, the container should be sterile at the time of the filling operation. If nonsterile containers are used, methods for sterilizing these containers should be established. Final containers selected should be capable of maintaining product integrity (i.e., identity, strength, quality, and purity) throughout the shelf life of the product.[44]

For products requiring sterilization, selection of an appropriate method of sterilization is of prime importance. Methods of product sterilization include sterile filtration, autoclaving, dry heat sterilization, chemical sterilization, and irradiation.[16,45] Selection of the sterilization technique should be based on the properties of the product being processed. The pharmacist must ensure that the sterilization method used is appropriate for the product components and does not alter the pharmaceutical properties of the final product. A method of sterilization often used by pharmacists is sterile filtration.[46] In sterile filtration, the product should be filtered into presterilized containers under aseptic conditions. Sterilizing filters of 0.22 μm or smaller porosity should be used in this process. Colloidal or viscous products may require use of a 0.45-μm filter; however, extreme caution should be exercised in these circumstances, and more stringent end-product sterility testing is essential.[26,47,48]

To ensure that a bacteria-retentive filter did not rupture during filtration of a product, an integrity test should be performed on all filters immediately after filtration. This test may be accomplished by performing a bubble point test, in which pressurized gas is applied to the upstream side of the filter with the downstream outlet immersed in water and the pressure at which a steady stream of bubbles begins to appear is noted.[46,48] The observed pressure is then compared with the manufacturer's specification for the filter. To compare the used filter with the manufacturer's specifications, which would be based on the filtration of water through the filter, it is necessary to first rinse the filter with sterile water for injection. An observed value lower than the manufacturer's specification indicates that the filter was defective or ruptured during the sterilization process. Methods should be established for handling, testing, and resterilizing any product processed with a filter that fails the integrity test.

RL 3.7: Process Validation. In addition to risk level 1 and 2 recommendations, written policies and procedures should be established to validate all processes involved in the preparation of risk level 3 sterile products (including all procedures, equipment, and techniques) from sterile or nonsterile components. In addition to evaluating personnel technique, process validation provides a mechanism for determining whether a particular process will, when performed by qualified personnel, consistently produce the intended results.

RL 3.8: Expiration Dating. In addition to risk level 2 recommendations, there should be reliable methods for establishing all expiration dates including laboratory testing of products for sterility, pyrogenicity, and chemical content, when necessary. These tests should be conducted in a manner based on appropriate statistical criteria, and the results documented.

RL 3.9: Labeling. All recommendations for risk levels 1 and 2 should be met.

RL 3.10: End-Product Evaluation. For each preparation of a sterile product or a batch of sterile products, there should be appropriate laboratory determination of conformity with established written specifications and policies. Any reproc-essed material should undergo complete final product testing. It is advisable to quarantine sterile products compounded from nonsterile components, pending the results of end-product testing. If products prepared from nonsterile components must be dispensed before satisfactory completion of end-product testing, there must be a procedure to allow for immediate recall of the products from patients to whom they were dispensed.

RL 3.11: Documentation. In addition to the recommendations for risk levels 1 and 2, documentation for risk level 3 sterile products should include

1. Preparation work sheet;
2. Sterilization records of final products (if applicable);
3. Quarantine records (if applicable); and
4. End-product evaluation and testing results.

Appendix A—Glossary

Aseptic Preparation: The technique involving procedures designed to preclude contamination (of drugs, packaging, equipment, or supplies) by microorganisms during processing.

Batch Preparation: Compounding of multiple sterile-product units, in a single discrete process, by the same individual(s), carried out during one limited time period.

Cleanroom: A room in which the concentration of airborne particles is controlled and there are one or more clean zones. (A clean zone is a defined space in which the concentration of airborne particles is controlled to meet a specified airborne-particulate cleanliness class.) Cleanrooms are classified based on the maximum number of allowable particles 0.5 μm and larger per cubic foot of air. For example, the air particle count in a Class 100 cleanroom may not exceed a total of 100 particles of 0.5 μm and larger per cubic foot of air.[28]

Closed-System Transfer: The movement of sterile products from one container to another in which the container-closure system and transfer devices remain intact throughout the entire transfer process, compromised only by the penetration of a sterile, pyrogen-free needle or cannula through a designated stopper or port to effect transfer, withdrawal, or delivery. Withdrawal of a sterile solution from an ampul in a Class 100 environment would generally be considered acceptable; however, the use of a rubber-stoppered vial, when available, would be preferable.

Compounding: For purposes of this document, compounding simply means the mixing of substances to prepare a medication for patient use. This activity would include dilution, admixture, repackaging, reconstitution, and other manipulations of sterile products.

Controlled Area: For purposes of this document, a controlled area is the area designated for preparing sterile products.

Critical Areas: Any area in the controlled area where products or containers are exposed to the environment.[37]

Critical Site: An opening providing a direct pathway between a sterile product and the environment or any surface coming in contact with the product or environment.

Critical Surface: Any surface that comes into contact with previously sterilized products or containers.[37]

Expiration Date: The date (and time, when applicable) beyond which a product should not be used (i.e., the product should be discarded beyond this date and time). NOTE: Circumstances may occur in which the expiration date and time arrive while an infusion is in progress. When this occurs, judgment should be applied in determining whether it is appropriate to discontinue that infusion and replace the product. Organizational policies on this should be clear.

HEPA Filter: A high-efficiency particulate air (HEPA) filter composed of pleats of filter medium separated by rigid sheets of corrugated paper or aluminum foil that direct the flow of air forced through the filter in a uniform parallel flow. HEPA filters remove 99.97% of all air particles 0.3 μm or larger. When HEPA filters are used as a component of a horizontal- or vertical-laminar-airflow hood, an environment can be created consistent with standards for a Class 100 cleanroom.[49]

Quality Assurance: For purposes of this document, quality assurance is the set of activities used to ensure that the processes used in the preparation of sterile drug products lead to products that meet predetermined standards of quality.

Quality Control: For purposes of this document, quality control is the set of testing activities used to determine that the ingredients, components (e.g., containers), and final sterile products prepared meet predetermined requirements with respect to identity, purity, nonpyrogenicity, and sterility.

Repackaging: The subdivision or transfer from a container or device to a different container or device, such as a syringe or ophthalmic container.

Sterilizing Filter: A filter that, when challenged with a solution containing the microorganism *Pseudomonas diminuta,* at a minimum concentration of 10^7 organisms per square centimeter of filter surface, will produce a sterile effluent.[16,17]

Temperatures (USP): Frozen means temperatures between -20 and -10 °C (-4 and 14 °F). Refrigerated means temperatures between 2 and 8 °C (36 and 46 °F). Room temperature means temperatures between 15 and 30 °C (59 and 86 °F).[16]

Validation: Documented evidence providing a high degree of assurance that a specific process will consistently produce a product meeting its predetermined specifications and quality attributes.[17]

References

1. Hughes CF, Grant AF, Leckie BD, et al. Cardioplegic solution: a contamination crisis. *J Thorac Cardiovasc Surg.* 1986; 91:296–302.

2. Associated Press. Pittsburgh woman loses eye to tainted drugs; 12 hurt. *Baltimore Sun.* 1990; Nov 9:3A.

3. Anon. ASHP gears up multistep action plan regarding sterile drug products. *Am J Hosp Pharm.* 1991; 48:386, 389–90. News.

4. Dugleaux G, Coutour XL, Hecquard C, et al. Septicemia caused by contaminated parenteral nutrition pouches: the refrigerator as an unusual cause. *J Parenter Enter Nutr.* 1991; 15:474–5.

5. Solomon SL, Khabbaz RF, Parker RH, et al. An outbreak of *Candida parapsilosis* bloodstream infections in patients receiving parenteral nutrition. *J Infect Dis.* 1984; 149:98–102.

6. National Coordinating Committee on Large Volume Parenterals. Recommended methods for compounding intravenous admixtures in hospitals. *Am J Hosp Pharm.* 1975; 32:261–70.

7. National Coordinating Committee on Large Volume Parenterals. Recommended guidelines for quality assurance in hospital centralized intravenous admixture services. *Am J Hosp Pharm.* 1980; 37:645–55.

8. National Coordinating Committee on Large Volume Parenterals. Recommendations for the labeling of large volume parenterals. *Am J Hosp Pharm.* 1978; 35:49–51.

9. National Coordinating Committee on Large Volume Parenterals. Recommended standard of practice, poli-

cies, and procedures for intravenous therapy. *Am J Hosp Pharm*. 1980; 37:660–3.

10. National Coordinating Committee on Large Volume Parenterals. Recommended procedures for in-use testing of large volume parenterals suspected of contamination or of producing a reaction in a patient. *Am J Hosp Pharm*. 1978; 35:678–82.

11. National Coordinating Committee on Large Volume Parenterals. Recommended system for surveillance and reporting of problems with large volume parenterals in hospitals. *Am J Hosp Pharm*. 1975; 34:1251–3.

12. Barker KN, ed. Recommendations of the NCCLVP for the compounding and administration of intravenous solutions. Bethesda, MD: American Society of Hospital Pharmacists; 1981.

13. Joint Commission on Accreditation of Healthcare Organizations. 1993 Accreditation manual for hospitals. Oakbrook Terrace, IL: Joint Commission on Accreditation of Healthcare Organizations; 1992.

14. Joint Commission on Accreditation of Healthcare Organizations. 1993 Accreditation manual for home care. Vol. 1. Standards. Oakbrook Terrace, IL: Joint Commission on Accreditation of Healthcare Organizations; 1993.

15. Food and Drug Administration. Title 21 Code of Federal Regulations. Part 21—current good manufacturing practice for finished pharmaceuticals, United States.

16. The United States Pharmacopeia, 22nd rev., and The National Formulary, 17th ed. Rockville, MD: The United States Pharmacopeial Convention; 1989.

17. Division of Manufacturing and Product Quality, Office of Compliance, Food and Drug Administration. Guideline on sterile drug products produced by aseptic processing. Rockville, MD: Food and Drug Administration; 1987.

18. Centers for Disease Control. Guideline for prevention of intravascular infections. *Am J Infect Control*. 1983; 11(5):183–93.

19. Centers for Disease Control. Guideline for handwashing and hospital environmental control. *Am J Infect Control*. 1986; 4(8):110–29.

20. Anon. Sterile drug products for home use. *Pharmacopeial Forum*. 1993; 19:5380–409.

21. Stiles ML, Tu Y-H, Allen LV Jr. Stability of morphine sulfate in portable pump reservoirs during storage and simulated administration. *Am J Hosp Pharm*. 1989; 46:1404–7.

22. Duafala ME, Kleinberg ML, Nacov C, et al. Stability of morphine sulfate in infusion devices and containers for intravenous administration. *Am J Hosp Pharm*. 1990; 47:143–6.

23. Seidel AM. Quality control for parenteral nutrition compounding. Paper presented at 48th ASHP Annual Meeting; San Diego, CA: 1991 Jun 6.

24. American Society of Hospital Pharmacists. ASHP technical assistance bulletin on handling cytotoxic and hazardous drugs. *Am J Hosp Pharm*. 1990; 47:1033–49.

25. American Society of Hospital Pharmacists. Aseptic preparation of parenteral products. (Videotape and study guide.) Bethesda, MD: American Society of Hospital Pharmacists; 1985.

26. Avis KE, Lachman L, Lieberman HA, eds. Pharmaceutical dosage forms: parenteral medications. Vol 2. New York: Marcel Dekker; 1992.

27. American Society of Hospital Pharmacists. ASHP technical assistance bulletin on outcome competencies and training guidelines for institutional pharmacy technician training programs. *Am J Hosp Pharm*. 1982; 39:317–20.

28. Federal Standard No. 209E. Airborne particulate cleanliness classes in cleanrooms and clean zones. Washington, DC: General Services Administration; 1992.

29. Bryan D, Marback RC. Laminar-airflow equipment certification: what the pharmacist needs to know. *Am J Hosp Pharm*. 1984; 41:1343–9.

30. Kessler DA. MedWatch: the new FDA medical products reporting program. *Am J Hosp Pharm*. 1993; 50:1921–36.

31. Hunt ML. Training manual for intravenous admixture personnel, 4th ed. Chicago: Baxter Healthcare Corporation and Pluribus Press, Inc.; 1989.

32. Murphy C. Ensuring accuracy in the use of automatic compounders. *Am J Hosp Pharm*. 1993; 50:60. Letter.

33. Brushwood DB. Hospital liable for defect in cardioplegia solution. *Am J Hosp Pharm*. 1992; 49:1174–6.

34. Meyer GE, Novielli KA, Smith JE. Use of refractive index measurement for quality assurance of pediatric parenteral nutrition solutions. *Am J Hosp Pharm*. 1987; 44:1617–20.

35. Morris BG, Avis KN, Bowles GC. Quality-control plan for intravenous admixture programs. II: validation of operator technique. *Am J Hosp Pharm*. 1980; 37:668–72.

36. Dirks I, Smith FM, Furtado D, et al. Method for testing aseptic technique of intravenous admixture personnel. *Am J Hosp Pharm*. 1982; 39:457–9.

37. Brier KL. Evaluating aseptic technique of pharmacy personnel. *Am J Hosp Pharm*. 1983; 40:400–3.

38. Validation of aseptic filling for solution drug products. Technical monograph no. 2. Philadelphia: Parenteral Drug Association, Inc.; 1980.

39. Boylan JC. Essential elements of quality control. *Am J Hosp Pharm*. 1983; 40:1936–9.

40. Choy FN, Lamy PP, Burkhart VD, et al. Sterility-testing program for antibiotics and other intravenous admixtures. *Am J Hosp Pharm*. 1982; 39:452–6.

41. Doss HL, James JD, Killough DM, et al. Microbiologic quality assurance for intravenous admixtures in a small hospital. *Am J Hosp Pharm*. 1982; 39:832–5.

42. Posey LM, Nutt RE, Thompson PD. Comparison of two methods for detecting microbial contamination in intravenous fluids. *Am J Hosp Pharm*. 1982; 28:659–62.

43. Frieben WR. Control of aseptic processing environment. *Am J Hosp Pharm*. 1983; 40:1928–35.

44. Neidich RL. Selection of containers and closure systems for injectable products. *Am J Hosp Pharm*. 1983; 40:1924–7.

45. Phillips GB, O'Neill M. Sterilization. In: Gennaro AR, ed. Remington's pharmaceutical sciences. 18th ed. Easton, PA: Mack Publishing; 1990:1470–80.

46. McKinnon BT, Avis KE. Membrane filtration of pharmaceutical solutions. *Am J Hosp Pharm*. 1993; 50:1921–36.

47. Olson W. Sterilization of small-volume parenteral and therapeutic proteins by filtration. In: Olson W,

Groves MJ, eds. Aseptic pharmaceutical manufacturing: technology for the 1990s. Prairie View, IL: Interpharm; 1987:101–49.

48. Eudailey WA. Membrane filters and membrane filtration processes for health care. *Am J Hosp Pharm.* 1983; 40:1921–3.

49. Turco S, King RE. Extemporaneous preparation. In: Turco S, King RE, eds. Sterile dosage forms. Philadelphia: Lea & Febiger; 1987:55–61.

---

[a]Unless otherwise stated in this document, the term "sterile products" refers to sterile drug or nutritional substances that are prepared (e.g., compounded or repackaged) by pharmacy personnel.

Approved by the ASHP Board of Directors, September 24, 1993. Developed by the ASHP Council on Professional Affairs.

The bibliographic citation for this document is as follows: American Society of Hospital Pharmacists. ASHP technical assistance bulletin on quality assurance for pharmacy-prepared sterile products. *Am J Hosp Pharm.* 1993; 50:2386–98.

10 | Medication Errors

Jacqueline Z. Kessler, M.S., R.Ph.
Kristin Y. Izenstark, M.S., R.Ph.

Pharmacists are responsible for the safe and appropriate use of medications in all pharmacy practice settings. As part of the multidisciplinary health care team, the role of the pharmacist is to cooperatively establish patient specific drug therapy regimens designed to achieve predefined therapeutic outcomes without subjecting the patient to undue harm.

As pharmacists become more involved in patient specific care, technicians are asked to perform tasks that have previously been restricted to pharmacists. As pharmacy technician responsibilities expand, it is important for technicians to be aware of the significance and causes of medication errors and recognize the technician's role in preventing drug errors.

Numerous terms are used to describe drug related incidents. The term drug misadventures is used to describe adverse drug reactions (unintended responses to drugs used at normal doses) and medication errors (errors related to the medication use process that may or may not result in adverse drug outcomes).[1] This chapter focuses on errors that occur during the medication use process, which includes the prescribing, dispensing, and administration phases of medication use, monitoring the patient for expected and unexpected outcomes and patient compliance.

This chapter provides insight to the incidence and significance of medication errors. It reviews common causes of medication errors and suggests measures to minimize errors. In addition, the importance of medication error reporting and monitoring is highlighted.

LEARNING OBJECTIVES

After reading this chapter, technicians should be able to
1. Describe the different types of medication errors.
2. Identify causes or factors that contribute to medication errors.
3. Describe things that can be done to prevent medication errors from occurring.
4. List examples of common errors.
5. Recognize possible consequences of actual medication errors.
6. Describe steps to be taken when an error has been identified.
7. Understand the role of quality assurance monitoring of medication errors.

TYPES OF MEDICATION ERRORS

Medication errors can occur at any point during the medication use process. They do not only occur in the pharmacy. For example, medication errors can also occur when a physician writes an order (during the prescribing process), when a nurse transcribes a medication order, when office personnel phone in a prescription to the pharmacy, or when patients do not take their medication as directed (patient compliance).

Pharmacy technicians should be aware of and concerned with all types of errors, not only those specifically occurring in the pharmacy. Sometimes a pharmacist may miss an error and a technician may be the one to notice it. According to the *ASHP Guidelines on Preventing Medication Errors in Hospitals*,[2] medication errors can be categorized into 11 different types. It is not always obvious as to which category an error belongs because of the complex nature of the medication use process. Errors may occur due to multiple factors and therefore may fit several categories.

Prescribing Errors

A prescribing error occurs at the time a drug is ordered by a prescriber for a specific patient. It may include the selection of an incorrect drug, dose, dosage form, route of administration, length of therapy, or number of doses. An inappropriate rate of administration, wrong drug concentration, or inadequate or wrong instructions for use are also considered prescribing errors. When evaluating whether a medication was prescribed in error, it is important to consider patient characteristics such as allergies, weight, age, medical indication (condition being treated), and concurrent drug therapy, among other factors. For example, a prescription for amoxicillin 250 mg PO TID may be appropriate to treat a middle ear infection in a 5-year-old child but would be too high a dose for a 12-month-old infant and thus would be considered a prescribing error. Prescriptions that are filled incorrectly due to illegible handwriting are also considered prescribing errors.

Omission Errors

Failure to administer an ordered dose to a patient in a hospital, nursing home, or other facility before the next scheduled dose would be considered an omission error. This would occur when a dose is completely omitted as opposed to one that is administered late. If a dose is ordered to be held for medical reasons, it is not considered an error. Examples of times when an omitted dose would not be an error are when the patient cannot take anything by mouth (NPO) prior to a procedure or when health care providers are waiting for drug level results to be reported. Medications that are not administered because a patient refuses to take them would not be an error.

Wrong Time Errors

Timing of administration for some medications is critical to their effectiveness. Maintaining an adequate blood level of some drugs, such as antibiotics, frequently depends on evenly spaced around-the-clock dosing. Administering doses too early or too late may affect the drug serum level and subsequently the efficacy of the drug. Nursing homes and hospitals frequently have predefined administration times to establish consistency. It could be harmful to a patient if a daily dose is administered inconsistently. It would not be realistic to expect that all morning doses be administered at exactly 0800. Therefore, an acceptable interval surrounding the scheduled time is usually established. An institution may determine that medications administered within 30 minutes of the scheduled time (30 minutes before or after) is acceptable. Medications administered outside of this window would be considered wrong time errors. Wrong time errors are occassionally unavoidable because the patient is away from the patient care area for a test or the medication may not be available at the time it is due.

Unauthorized Drug Errors

Administration of a medication to a patient without proper authorization by the prescriber is categorized as an unauthorized drug error. This might occur if a medication for one patient was mistakenly given to another patient, or if a nurse gave a medication without a physician order. Patients at home sometimes "share" prescriptions as well. Refilling a prescription that has no refills remaining without authorization from the physician would be another example of an unauthorized drug error.

Some health care facilities have guidelines or protocols established that allow flexibility in administering medications based on specific patient parameters. For example, a post-surgical protocol may allow a nurse to administer potassium chloride injection when a patient's serum potassium level falls below a specified level. The dose of potassium chloride may vary depending on how low the serum level is. Administration of medications outside of the established guidelines would be an example of an unauthorized drug error.

Improper Dose Errors

Improper dose errors occur when a patient is given a dose that is greater than or less than the prescribed dose. This type of error may occur if there is a delay in documenting (or absence of documentation) a dose that results in an additional dose being administered. Inaccurate measurement of an oral liquid would be an improper dose error. Excluded from this category would be doses that cannot be accurately measured or are not specified as in topical applications. Variances that occur from apothecary to metric conversions would be excluded as well.

Wrong Dosage Form Errors

Doses administered or dispensed in a different form from that ordered by the prescriber are classified as wrong dosage form errors. Depending on state laws and health care facility guidelines, dosage form changes may be acceptable to accommodate particular patient needs. Dispensing a liquid formulation to a patient who has difficulty swallowing tablets without a specific prescription might be an example of an acceptable dosage form change.

Wrong Drug Preparation Errors

Drugs requiring reconstitution (adding liquid to dissolve a powdered drug), dilution, or special preparation prior to dispensing or administration are subject to drug preparation errors. Examples include reconstituting a cephalexin oral suspension with an incorrect volume of water, using bacteriostatic saline for injection instead of sterile water for injection to reconstitute a lyophilized powder for injection, or not breaking the seal of a ready-to-mix heparin bag. Using a wrong base product when compounding an ointment is another example of a wrong drug preparation error.

Wrong Administration Technique Errors

Doses that are administered using an inappropriate procedure or incorrect technique are categorized as wrong administration technique errors. A subcutaneous injection that is given too deep or an intravenous (IV) drug that is allowed to infuse via gravity instead of using an IV pump are classified in this category. Eye drops instilled in the wrong eye is another example of an error in this category.

Deteriorated Drug Errors

Although sometimes cumbersome, monitoring expiration dates of products is very important. Drugs used past their expiration date may have lost potency and may no longer be effective or may be less effective. Refrigerated drugs stored at room temperature may decompose to the point that their efficacy is less than optimal. Medications that are dispensed or administered beyond their expiration date or medications that have deteriorated due to improper storage are listed as deteriorated drug errors.

Monitoring Errors

Monitoring errors result from inadequate drug therapy review. Ordering serum drug levels for a patient on phenytoin (seizure medication), but not reviewing them or not responding to a level outside of the therapeutic range would be a monitoring error. Not ordering drug levels when required or prescribing an antihypertensive agent, which lowers blood pressure, and failing to check blood pressure would be errors as well.

Compliance Errors

Medication errors are committed by patients too, when they fail to adhere to a prescribed drug regimen. These errors may be detected when a patient requests refills for prescriptions at unreasonable intervals (too long after or too soon before a refill is due) without a reasonable explanation.

Other Errors

Errors that cannot be placed into 1 of the 11 categories are grouped together in a miscellaneous category. Some of the errors as defined in the

ASHP guidelines seem to primarily apply to patients in a health care facility. These same definitions can actually be applied to home health care, clinic, or physician office, as well as the outpatient pharmacy practice settings.

INCIDENCE

Although medication errors are not uncommon, it is difficult to determine the actual numbers of medication errors. Few studies provide a complete and thorough evaluation of errors within the entire medication use process. It is hard to project data from studies on medication errors because of the different methods used to detect errors and the various definitions of errors. In addition, the focus of some studies is on just physician, nursing, or pharmacy errors, or just one component of the medication use process.

Medication errors can occur at any point in the medication use process. Millions of doses are administered daily in health care facilities and patient homes, and the volume of prescriptions filled annually in community based pharmacies is over 1.5 billion. Based on these estimates alone, it is apparent that even with a high rate of accuracy, a small percent of errors can result in a large number of medication errors.

The number of new drugs and dosage forms available continues to grow, making it difficult to keep up with new developments in pharmacy. Staying abreast of technological advances and complex medication regimens requires professional commitment. Medication error awareness and prevention must be a high priority in all health care facilities and pharmacies.

Medication Error Rates

This section describes medication error rates reported in some studies. It is intended to provide an overview of the complexity of studying medication errors due to the different monitoring, measuring, and reporting techniques used. It also reviews differences in the studies that contribute to varying medication error rates.

The Harvard Medical Study[3] that looked at the incidence of adverse events in hospitalized patients found that 19% of the adverse events that occured in hospitalized patients were related to drug complications. This study demonstrates that complications from drugs, including those caused by errors, are a signifi-

cant cause of medical management injuries in hospitalized patients.

Physician prescribing error rates in hospital and community settings have been reported to be 0.3–1.9%.[4-6] One study determined that almost one-third (28.3%) of the prescribing errors were potentially harmful if not followed up by a pharmacist.[5] Further, it has been observed that errors occurring earlier in the medication use process (prescribing phase) are more likely to be detected and corrected than those occurring later in the process (administration).[7]

Physician prescribing is only the first step in the medication use process. Other studies have evaluated medication errors occurring at various other stages as well. Error rates of pharmacist dispensing in the outpatient setting have been reported to be approximately 12%.[8,9] There is conflicting data evaluating the relationship between the number of serious errors and the number of prescriptions filled.[8-10] It has been estimated that the medication error rate in health care institutions not using a unit dose system is one error per patient per day.[11]

Medication error studies report different error rates. The pharmacy technician should recognize that the differences in error rates may be due to differences in how a study was performed, the various techniques and definitions used, and the scope of a study. Many errors are identified and corrected before medications reach the patient. Studies also show that a small percentage of errors leads to adverse events in patients.[12]

Medication Error Reporting

The rate of medication errors is often based on incident reports. Ideally, incident reports are completed by health care providers when a medication error is discovered. However, health care providers do not always submit incident reports because many personnel lack the knowledge to identify errors, the time required to document them, or they are afraid of negative consequences.

Many times errors are discovered when a pharmacist checks a prescription or medication order prior to dispensing. The error is promptly corrected before it ever reaches the patient. Often times, the error is not documented because it is not recognized as an error or the reporting process is cumbersome. For these reasons, the number of medication errors is probably higher than reported.

Reporting medication errors can sometimes be a fearful experience. Health care personnel may be afraid of disciplinary action or punitive actions, or of the backlash of reporting an error made by a coworker. They may also be concerned about liability issues should a negative outcome occur due to an error.

It is apparent that medication errors occur in all practice settings on a daily basis. Fortunately, the majority of these errors are detected and corrected before the medication ever reaches the patient. Medication errors do however reach the patient and some errors result in negative outcomes.

IMPACT OF MEDICATION ERRORS

The outcomes of medication errors range from minor discomfort to devastating long term disability or death.[13] It is often difficult to predict the outcome and significance of a medication error because so many factors are involved. Such factors include the type of medication error, the health status of the patient, pharmacologic classification of the drug involved, route of drug administration, timing of drug administration, the cost to the health care system, and the damage to the patient's trust in care providers.

Impact on the Patient

In a report of five pediatric patients who received overdoses of vincristine (a chemotherapy drug), three patients died and two recovered.[14] Of the three patients who died, two received a 10-fold overdose and the third patient was very ill with an advanced stage leukemia. The two children who recovered were in remission (their leukemia was under control) at the time and received smaller overdoses. In this situation, the health status of the patients and magnitude of the overdose helped determine the significance of the error.

Sometimes not receiving a drug or receiving it late may harm patients as well. Administration of a phenytoin (seizure medication) dose was delayed 28 hours in an elderly patient and resulted in a seizure.[15] The patient fell and fractured her jaw during the seizure, which required extensive surgery. All of these events can be attributed to one medication error—late administration of the phenytoin. Many case reports describe adverse drug events due to medication errors.

Financial Impact of Medication Errors

Not only can medication errors lead to negative patient outcomes, but they can also prolong hospital stays and increase health care expenses.[16] The treatment of adverse drug events is estimated to cost billions of dollars annually.[13,17,18] It was estimated that $1.5 million was spent in a single year to treat adverse drug events at one hospital.[17] Another study evaluated the cost of drug related morbidity and mortality in the ambulatory setting. In this study it was estimated that the United States spends $76.6 billion annually to manage those drug related occurrences, some of which were due to medication errors.[18] Not only must the cost of additional medical management be considered, but the legal fees or out-of-court settlements resulting from malpractice claims must also be considered.

In one case almost $14,000 in medical costs were incurred to treat a patient who experienced recurrent hypoglycemia (low blood sugar) due to a prescription error.[19] The pharmacist inadvertently dispensed glyburide (Diabeta®, a drug for high blood sugar) instead of diazepam (Valium®, an anti-anxiety medication).

Loss of Trust

Patients may lose trust or faith in the medical community as a result of experiencing or reading about an adverse drug event. They may choose to switch pharmacies or physicians, or maybe even hesitate to seek medical help for fear of not receiving quality care. Patients may also seek non-conventional treatments from outside the medical community. Personnel responsible for medication errors that result in significant patient injury may lose confidence in themselves as practitioners as well.

It is fortunate that most medication errors are detected and corrected before the medication is dispensed to the patient or the patient care area. However, medication errors do occur and may result in reversible or permanent negative patient outcomes. They can also be associated with a financial impact to an individual, institution, and the overall health care system.

CAUSES OF MEDICATION ERRORS AND WAYS TO PREVENT THEM

Medication errors can be attributed to a number of different causes. It would be unfair to place blame solely on an individual without considering factors that might contribute to an error. Administrators of health systems are constantly striving to decrease the presence of factors in the medication use system that contribute to medication errors. In turn, each health care provider must also strive to minimize the occurrence of medication errors. One of the best ways to do this is to become familiar with the most common causes of medication errors. Medication errors are most often attributed to one or more of the following: calculation errors, careless use of zeros and decimal points, inappropriate use of abbreviations, careless prescribing, illegible handwriting, missing information, drug product characteristics, compounding/drug preparation errors, prescription labeling, and work environment or staffing issues.

Calculation Errors

There are reports of numerous medication errors that were caused by errors in mathematical calculations. In some cases, patients have died as a result of miscalculated doses.[14,20] Calculation errors are made by prescribers, pharmacists checking doses for appropriateness or calculating doses, technicians compounding products, and nurses preparing or administering doses. Calculation errors made by health care personnel occur frequently even with the use of calculators.[21]

The pediatric population is particularly at risk since many drugs are not available in a pediatric formulations, so adult formulations must be diluted or manipulated multiple times to get the appropriate dose. One study evaluated errors in drug computations for health care personnel in a neonatal intensive care unit. Test scores were 75.6% (range of 45–95%) correct answers for nurses, 89.1% for physicians and 96% for pharmacists.[22] Many of the errors made in this study would have resulted in doses 10 times higher or lower than the dose ordered.

Personnel with multiple years of experience are just as likely to make mathematical errors as inexperienced personnel.[22-24] Calculation errors are often made by using the wrong concentration of stock solutions, misplacing a decimal point, or using wrong conversions. Personnel also neglect to double check their work, rely on their memory instead of looking up a conversion, or do not ask themselves, "Does the answer seem reasonable?"

Another way to decrease the risk of a calculation error is to ask a pharmacist or another technician to double check the calculation prior to preparing the product. The calculation should be performed independently and compared to the original answer. This system is an effective way to prevent calculation errors.

Decimal Points and Zeros

Misplacing a decimal point by one place results in errors 10-fold or possibly 100-fold greater than or less than intended. For drugs with a narrow therapeutic range (e.g., digoxin, phenytoin, lidocaine, aminoglycoside antibiotics) the consequences can be significant.

Decimal point errors can occur as a result of a miscalculation, as described above, and also when writing orders or instructions. Failure to write a leading zero in front of a number less than one (e.g., .1 mg instead of 0.1 mg) might be read as the whole number (1 mg), or writing unnecessary trailing zeros can also be confusing (e.g., 10.0 mg instead of 10 mg may be interpreted as 100 mg). Medication order sheets with lines can sometimes cause a decimal point to be overlooked on the duplicate copy that is usually sent to pharmacy. Therefore, when writing numbers, a leading zero should always be used with a decimal point for numbers less than one (0.1 mg not .1mg) and a decimal point and trailing zero should never be used for whole numbers (10 mg not 10.0 mg).

Technicians must be aware of the potential for decimal point errors due to misplaced or missing decimal points when interpreting orders. Questionable orders should be brought to the attention of the pharmacist.

Abbreviations

Medical terminology and drug names are frequently abbreviated which can lead to medication errors. Use of the abbreviation "AZT" for zidovudine (Retrovir®—an antiretroviral agent) for a patient with AIDS could be detrimental if the patient received azathioprine (Imuran®—an immunosuppressant sometimes abbreviated AZT) instead of zidovudine.

Another example of an abbreviation error is the use of "U" as an abbreviation for units. This abbreviation might result in a 10-fold error were the "U" to be read as a "zero" (e.g., 10U insulin may be read as 100 insulin). A daily order written as "QD" instead of "daily" may be troublesome since it could be read as "QID" (four times a day) or "OD" (every other day).

There are many accepted abbreviations in health care. Use of abbreviations can be efficient if everyone understands and agrees on the definitions. The Joint Commission on Accreditation of Healthcare Organizations (JCAHO) requires that institutions maintain an approved list of acceptable abbreviations and terms.[25] Not being aware of the accepted interpretation of abbreviations can lead to errors. Creating new abbreviations that are not understood by others should be avoided.[26] The American Society of Health-System Pharmacists (ASHP) recommends that an approved list be developed by the Pharmacy and Therapeutics Committee (or its equivalent).[2] Abbreviations not appearing on the approved list should be reviewed carefully before processing an order. Another recommendation from ASHP is to write out directions for medication use rather than using nonstandard or ambiguous abbreviations. The complete drug name, preferably the generic, should be used.

Technicians should become familiar with the list of abbreviations approved for their pharmacy. Such a list can be obtained from a pharmacy supervisor. Community pharmacies generally do not have a formal, approved list of abbreviations. However, posting a list of commonly accepted medical abbreviations in the pharmacy may be beneficial.

Prescribing Issues

Medication errors may result from the way a drug is prescribed. Issues associated with the prescribing component of the medication use process that may contribute to an error include verbal orders, confusion with the concentration of a product, illegible handwriting, missing information, use of the apothecary system, and writing doses based on the course of therapy as opposed to a daily dose. This section describes how these prescribing issues may lead to errors and ways to minimize potential prescribing errors.

Verbal Orders

Verbal orders can lead to medication errors when they are not transmitted clearly and the use of car phones and static connections can make verbal orders even more difficult to understand. With the number of similar sounding products available, it is easy to misunderstand a verbal order. In one case report, a verbal order was received by a nurse from a physician and then transmitted to a community pharmacy. The nurse inadvertently confused "Ismelin®" (guanethidine—potent antihypertensive agent) for "Hismanal®" (astemizole—antihistamine) and the patient received the potent antihypertensive agent for his allergy symptoms.[27]

Verbal orders should be reserved for situations when it is impossible or impractical for the prescriber to write the order or enter the order via computer. The order should be read back to the prescriber by the recipient to ensure clarity of the order. A written copy of the verbal order should be placed in the patient's medical record. Institutional pharmacies routinely require the prescriber to confirm verbal orders by signature. The use of verbal orders should be avoided in chemotherapy prescribing due to the complexity of these orders and the potentially lethal impact of mistakes with these drugs.

Although car phones, foreign terminology, accents, and poor connections can make taking a verbal order difficult, it is the responsibility of the technician to ask the other party to clarify parts of the order that are not clear. Simply asking the other party to spell the names of the drugs or other words that are unclear and repeating the order back to the other party can help ensure that the right order is received. Many states limit the acceptance of verbal medication orders to registered pharmacists. State law and pharmacy policy should be consulted to determine what role, if any, technicians play in accepting verbal orders.

Drug Concentration

Sometimes the concentration of a liquid formulation is missing from the prescription, which could result in a wrong dose being dispensed. For example, an order for amoxicillin suspension 1/2 tsp (2.5 ml) TID does not specify the concentration of the suspension causing confusion as to the actual dose ordered. It is unclear if the physician ordered 62.5 mg (1/2 tsp of 125 mg/5 ml) or 125 mg (1/2 tsp of 250 mg/5 ml).

Writing "1 amp," "1 vial," or "1 cap" can lead to errors when products come in multiple strengths, doses, or vial sizes. An "amp" of magnesium sulfate might be filled with a 2 ml amp (8 mEq), a 20 ml amp (16 mEq), or 10 ml amp of 50% concentration (40 mEq). Ambiguous doses should be clarified by a pharmacist prior to processing by the technician.

Illegible Handwriting

Physicians' poor handwriting is frequently joked about. However, illegible handwriting of any health care provider is no laughing matter when it contributes to medication errors. With the many sound-alike and look-alike drug names on the market, it is easy to understand how illegible handwriting can lead to errors. One report describes a poorly written order for Aredia® (pamidronate—a blood calcium lowering agent) 60 mg IV that was filled and administered as "Adria," a commonly spoken name for Adriamycin® (doxorubicin—a chemotherapy agent). The patient received approximately 20% of the dose before the error was noticed. The patient experienced bone marrow toxicity (decrease in blood cell counts) as a consequence.[28] Both agents are reasonable drugs for a cancer patient and are prescribed in doses of 60 mg, but the poorly written drug name led to the mix-up.

The entire order should be carefully evaluated when trying to decipher illegible handwriting. Sometimes the dose or route of administration may be helpful in determining what drug was ordered. Assistance from a pharmacist should be obtained when orders are difficult to interpret due to illegible handwriting. The prescriber should be contacted by the pharmacist to clarify orders that cannot be accurately interpreted. In some practice settings, technicians may have a role in obtaining order clarifications.

Standardized preprinted order forms for complex drug regimens are one way to minimize illegible handwriting.[2] Computerization and typewritten labeling can reduce medication errors by making the medication labels easier to read for both health care personnel and patients. The use of upper and lower case lettering also improves readability.

Missing Information

Lack of medical information about the patient, such as age, weight, height, and indication, can contribute to medication errors. Medical information is important because dose usually depends on indication and severity of the condition. Unfortunately, physicians do not routinely write the indication on prescriptions and patients do not always fully understand their conditions. In some hospital pharmacies, medical information is only available in the chart because the pharmacy computer system does not interface with the main hospital computer.

Thorough and complete medication profiles should be maintained for all patients. These profiles should include current prescription and non-prescription medications, allergies, age, height, and weight of the patient. Previous medication use is also helpful. Profiles should be kept current and referred to on a routine basis. It may be necessary to question the patient or contact the prescriber to obtain this information, because pharmacists often need it to check an order for appropriateness.

Apothecary System

The apothecary system is a system of measurement that some physicians continue to use out of habit. This can lead to errors because it is unfamiliar to many health care personnel or because it must be converted to the metric system. The fact that "1 gr" (grain) equals 60 mg or 65 mg is confusing enough, but if it is written sloppily, it could be misread as "1 gm" (for 1 gram = 1000 mg). Prescribers should be discouraged from using the apothecary system.

Apothecary conversion charts should be readily available in the pharmacy. Technicians should become familiar with commonly used apothecary symbols and their metric equivalents, which are available in chapter 3.

Course Dose vs. Daily Dose

It is common for chemotherapy drug regimens to be prescribed on a per "course" or cycle of treatment basis, as opposed to per dose basis. This practice increases the chances for medication errors because the orders are often difficult to interpret.[29] Many chemotherapy treatments require a patient to receive medication over several days and then rest (receive no drug treatment) for several days or weeks. This allows the patient time to recover from the side effects and the drugs to work in the optimal phase of the tumor cell cycle. One course of treatment may consist of several drugs given on one or more days during a specified time period.

An example of a course dose is flourouracil 4 g/m² IV on days 1, 2, 3, and 4. This order might be interpreted as 4 g/m² of flourouracil (a cytotoxic agent) daily for four days—a total of 16 g/m². One could also interpret it as 4 g/m² to be divided into four daily doses (1 g/m² daily on days 1, 2, 3, and 4). It is easy to see how course doses can be misinterpreted. Errors such as this can result in massive overdoses leading to significant morbidity or death.

Manufacturer and Drug Product Related Causes

A review of medication errors reported to the United States Pharmacopeial Convention (USP) between August 1991 and April 1993 revealed that the most common error reported was related to a problem with drug product characteristics (e.g., drug name, packaging).[30] The USP has a medication error reporting program in conjunction with the Institute for Safe Medication Practices. This program focuses on product design and characteristics. In addition to the USP program, the Food and Drug Administration (FDA) accepts reports of medication errors or potential errors via a toll-free telephone line. The FDA receives and reviews all medication error reports, whether made initially to the USP or to the FDA. Reports of potential errors can also be reported to the FDA. Among other things, the FDA uses this information to alert health care providers prior to an actual error occurring.

Characteristics of drug products that may contribute to medication errors include such things as look-alike and sound-alike drug names, the use of numbers or letters as part of the drug name, product labeling, and color coding. Drug product problems identified by USP are forwarded to pharmaceutical manufacturers. Pharmaceutical manufacturers can then address the problems by making appropriate modifications to the drug products.

Look-Alike and Sound-Alike Drug Names

There are many case reports of medications errors due to confusion surrounding drug names.[31-37] There are hundreds of examples of drug names that either sound or look like another trade or generic drug name. A list of such drug names was published in 1992. It includes pairs of similar looking or sounding drug names that have resulted in an error or could potentially lead to one.[38]

Sometimes errors occur because drug names look and sound similar, and may even be used to treat a common condition. For example, amrinone (Inocor®—a cardiac agent) was inadvertently administered to a patient instead of amiodarone (Cordarone®—an antiarrythmic agent).[32] Both drugs may be used in treating cardiovascular conditions and their generic names sound somewhat alike.

Sloppy handwriting or misspelling can contribute to drug name confusion. An order carelessly written for interferon 1 ml (an immunologic agent) was interpreted and prepared as Imferon® 1 ml (iron dextran).[31] In this case, the patient's mother questioned the dark brown coloring of the drug before it was administered and the mix-up was corrected before the patient received the wrong drug.

The likelihood of confusing two drugs with similar names is increased when the dosages of both drugs are the same. Lanoxin® (digoxin) and Levoxine® (a brand name for levothyroxine) have similar looking and sounding names and are both commonly prescribed at a dose of 0.125 mg daily.[34] Due to these similarities, the pharmaceutical manufacturer of Levoxine® changed the trade name to Levoxyl® in an effort to avoid confusion with Lanoxin®.

One report describes an error resulting from two ophthalmic ointment products having brand names that are spelled and pronounced identically.[37] One brand name, Ocu-Mycin® (gentamicin 3%), contains a hyphen and the other, Ocumycin® (bacitracin/polymixin B) does not. Given as a verbal order with vague directions such as "take as directed," one would have no way of knowing which drug was intended.

A frequently reported mix-up occurs between quinine (an anti-malarial) and quinidine (an anti-arrhythmic). The names are similar, routine doses are the same and they are frequently stocked next to one another. It is easy to see how picking one drug instead of the other could happen.

It is easy to see how sound-alike names or look-alike names can be confusing with the increasing number of drug products available. Pharmaceutical manufacturers have the responsibility to carefully select drug product names keeping patient safety in mind. Table 10-1 lists examples of drug product names that were changed to reduce the risk of prescribing errors. Health care providers can help identify potentially dangerous drug names by notifying the USP or FDA with their concerns.

Numbers or Letters as Part of the Drug Name

Manufacturers sometimes include numbers or letters as a prefix or suffix to the brand name (e.g., Tylenol #3®, Percocet-5®, Procardia-XL®). The intent may be to indicate a strength or that

Table 10-1

Examples of Drug Product Names Changed to Reduce the Risk of Prescribing Errors

Former Trade Name	Confused With	New Trade
Losec	Lasix	Prilosec
Larocin	Lanoxin	Larotid
Microx	Micro-K	MyKrox
Clonopin	Clonidine	Klonopin

needed. A patient might become extremely drowsy or confused after taking five tablets of Percocet-5®.

Letters or numbers that are omitted from brand names when writing an order can contribute to errors. The immediate release form of Procardia® may be dispensed instead of the extended release formulation in Figure 10-2 because the "XL" part of the name is left off. The extended release formulation is designed to slowly release drug over the entire day, whereas the immediate release form releases the entire dose at once. A patient might not have adequate control of his blood pressure throughout the entire day by taking the wrong formulation of Procardia®.

a product is an extended release formulation, but it can lead to errors.

Numbers in the drug name may be misinterpreted as the dose. The prescription in Figure 10-1 might be interpreted to take five tablets of "Percocet" every four hours as needed instead of one tablet of Percocet-5® every four hours as

Product Labeling

As a marketing strategy, product labels often emphasize a manufacturer's name or logo, making it difficult to readily identify the drug name and dose. Manufacturers often use the same labeling scheme including letter size, print, and background color to readily associate the prod-

Internal Medicine Consultants, Inc.
1900 West Cherry Lane
Ridge Park, MO 78993
(843) 368-7445

Edward P. Lavel, D.O.
AL2473318

Harriet Martin, M.D.
AM7739468

Name _Brian Bosly_ Age _32_

Address _2417 Hilldale Ave_ Date _12-7-97_

Rx

Percocet 5 tab PO Q 4h prn

_# 30_

Refill ☐ 1 ☐ 2 ☐ 3 ☐ 4 ☐ 5 ☑ No Refill Label ☑

☐ May Substitute _____

☐ May Not Substitute _Edward P. Lavel D.O._

Figure 10-1. Example of a drug name that contains a number as a suffix.

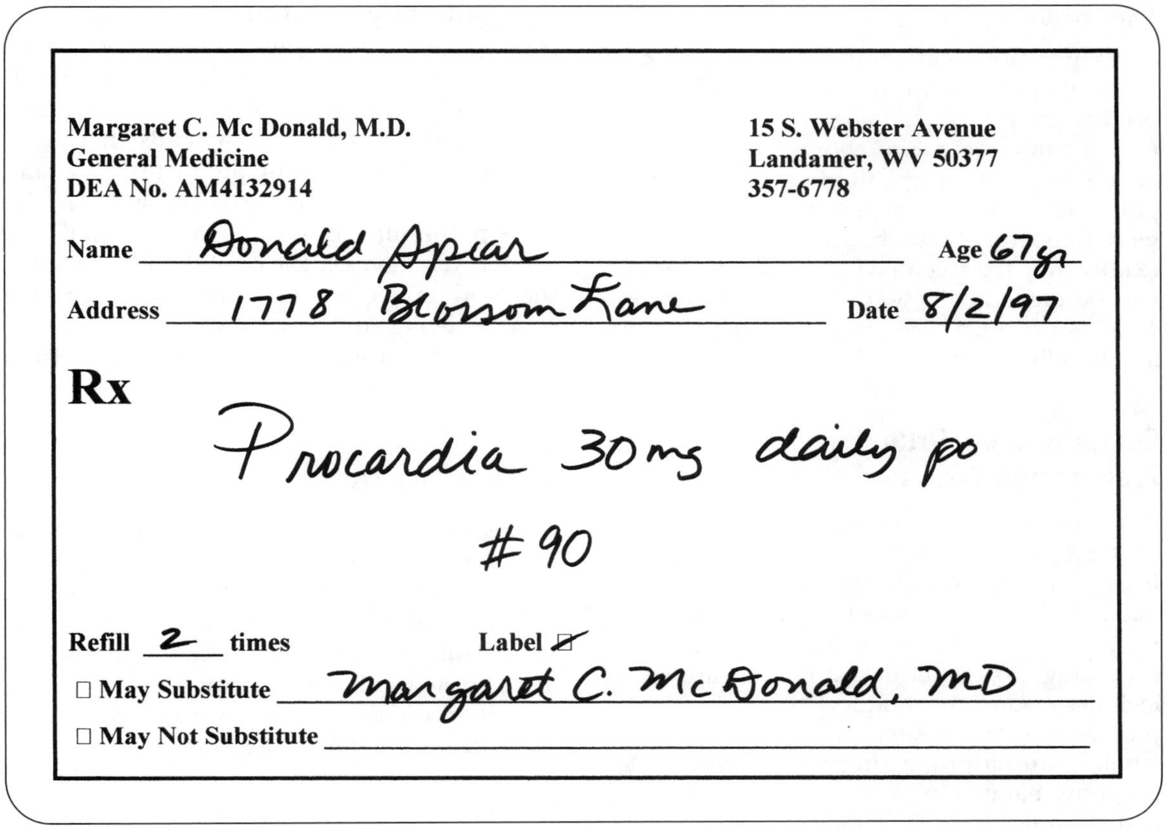

Margaret C. Mc Donald, M.D.   15 S. Webster Avenue
General Medicine   Landamer, WV 50377
DEA No. AM4132914   357-6778

Name *Donald Apiar*   Age *67yr*

Address *1778 Blossom Lane*   Date *8/2/97*

Rx

Procardia 30mg daily po

 # 90

Refill **2** times   Label ☑

☐ May Substitute *margaret C. McDonald, MD*

☐ May Not Substitute _____

Figure 10-2. Example of a drug name that should contain letters as a suffix.

uct with the manufacturer. Sometimes this strategy, which makes all labels look alike, can be detrimental.

Example 1

The dosage strength and total contents of liquid formulations are not always labeled clearly. Different vial sizes of injections may be similarly labeled with the concentration (mg/ml), but too little emphasis may be placed on the total contents of the vial. When midazolam (Versed®) first appeared on the market, it was available in a 5 mg/ml concentration in a 1 ml and 2 ml size vial. The vial size was not prominent on either label, which made it difficult to differentiate between the 10 mg (2 ml) and 5 mg (1 ml) vials.

Example 2

There have been numerous cases of a health care provider using potassium chloride (KCl) injection to flush an IV line instead of normal saline because the vial sizes and labeling of the two

products were similar. Manufacturers of potassium chloride injection are now required to use black vial caps and overseals, and prominently display a warning on the vial label that states *"must be diluted."*[39]

Color Coding

Relying on the color of product packaging is not a safe practice. Manufacturers may change their packaging color scheme at any time and color coding schemes for similar products may differ among manufacturers. Drug products with similar colors may be inadvertently misplaced in the stock areas and could easily be dispensed in error. For example both daunorubicin (Cerubidine®) 20 mg and doxorubicin 10 mg are packaged in vials that are shaped similarly and have dark blue vial caps. Plus, they are both lyophilized powders that turn into red solutions upon reconstitution. Relying on the color of the vial cap or of the diluted solution could lead to very serious errors.

Advertising

Many practices that contribute to medication errors are perpetuated through pharmaceutical product advertising. Journal advertisements may include the use of abbreviations, lack of adequate dosage strength identification, inappropriate use of decimal points, and so forth. The more frequently these things are seen, the more readily they are accepted by health care personnel and the more likely they may lead to errors. These issues must be kept in mind when reviewing drug literature.

Compounding/Drug Preparation Errors

Errors can occur during the compounding and drug preparation phase. These errors can be difficult for others to catch. Therefore, it is essential that technicians take steps to decrease the risk of making an error when compounding and preparing drug products. Such an approach includes reading the product labels carefully, not processing more than one prescription at a time, labeling prescriptions properly, storing drugs properly, maintaining a safe work environment, and keeping up with changes in the medical profession.

Reading the Label

Reading drug product labels carefully when filling an order is a step that is often neglected. This step is extremely important due to the number of product names that sound-alike or look-alike, similar product packaging, illegible handwriting, and color coding. The Institute for Safe Medication Practices recommends that pharmacy personnel read drug product labels a minimum of three times prior to processing an order to help minimize errors due to mistaking one product for another. The label should be read as the product is removed from the shelf, as the order is being prepared, and again as the finished product is set aside for the pharmacist to check, Figure 10-3.

Multiple Products

Processing more that one prescription or order at the same time can result in errors. It is easy to add a drug to the wrong IVPB diluent if several orders are being compounded simultaneously in the laminar flow hood. In this situation, it is just as easy to fill a prescription for the wrong patient or confuse the quantities to be dispensed.

Technicians should process only one prescription or common batch (all 0800 ampicillin 1 g IVPB orders) at a time. Supplies for multiple prescriptions should not be mixed together. Each prescription should be completed prior to starting the next one. Completed prescriptions waiting for a pharmacist check should be clearly separated from each other and from those that have not yet been completed.

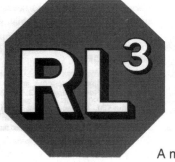

**Read Labels
Three Times**

1. When you select the drug product from a storage area or medication drawer.
2. When you prepare, label, dispense or administer the product.
3. When you return the original container or package to the storage area or discard it.

A medication error reduction tip from *HOSPITAL PHARMACY.*
Neil M. Davis, Editor-in-Chief

*Roxane Laboratories has agreed to supply free RL³ stickers. You may obtain them by: contacting your local Roxane representative, calling toll free 1-800-848-0120, extension 5000, or writing to Roxane Laboratories, Inc., P.O. Box 16532, Columbus, OH 43216-6532.

Figure 10-3. A sticker reminding personnel to read the label three times.

Source: Davis NM. A medication error reduction tip from Hospital Pharmacy. *Hospital Pharmacy,* Lippencott-Raven.

Labeling

Technicians should be familiar with the labeling requirements for prescriptions in their pharmacy as dictated by state law and pharmacy policy. If a label is handwritten, it should be done neatly and legibly. Ink cartridges and printer ribbons should be changed before the print is too faded to read, the label should be free of smudges, and the print should be aligned on the label appropriately.

Auxiliary labels provide useful information to the patient or nursing personnel. Many pharmacy computer systems are designed to identify the appropriate auxiliary labels for prescriptions. Other pharmacies use reference charts as aides. Auxiliary labels should be placed carefully on the drug container so not to cover up other pertinent information.

Deteriorated Medications

Since expired medications or improperly stored medications may have lost their potency and thus their ability to be effective, technicians should take steps to keep these medication out of the dispensing stock. In many cases it is the technician's responsibility to rotate stock. Technicians should be familiar with the pharmacy's regular system for checking for expired medications. Alhough checking expiration dates is sometimes viewed as a tedious job, it is important because it reduces the risk of making deteriorated drug errors.

When replenishing stock, always remove expired medications and place the stock with the earliest expiration date near the front to be used first. Some drugs have a short expiration date once the container has been opened. Pharmacies usually have procedures that require the date of opening or expiration date to be written on the label to help prevent use of an expired drug. Examples of drugs that usually require dating include oral suspensions and injectable drugs. Technicians should be familiar with the drugs that have short expiration dating and the procedures for indicating date of first use or expiration. It is also recommended that opened containers be marked with an "X" to readily identify the container that should be used first.

Medications that require special storage conditions, such as refrigeration or freezing should be kept in those conditions as long as possible. Drugs stored under refrigeration may only be stable for a short time out of the refrigerator.

When filling an order for a pharmacist to check, the technician must comply with the institution's policy. Some pharmacies/pharmacists require that refrigerated medications be left in the refrigerator and not on the counter, while others allow them to stay on the counter briefly.

Work Environment

Factors within the workplace may contribute to medication errors. Such things as inadequate lighting,[9] poorly designed work spaces, or inefficient workflow can make it difficult to accurately perform assigned duties. Cluttered work spaces or stock areas might increase the chances of picking up the wrong drug. The many distractions and interruptions including phone calls in a busy pharmacy can cause one to lose concentration.

Many modern pharmacies rely on specialized equipment and computers to assist in filling prescriptions. Improper maintenance of this equipment may result in unacceptable performance or necessitate the use of older, unfamiliar, or cumbersome manual systems when it breaks down. Routine maintenance schedules should be followed to prevent equipment malfunction. Technicians should be adequately trained on the proper use and maintenance of such equipment. Operating manuals should be available in the pharmacy for troubleshooting when a problem occurs.

Scheduling of staff members and the frequency of rotating shifts have shown to correlate with error rates.[40] Other factors such as staffing levels and amount of supervision may also be work environment issues to consider.

The frequency with which drug products are changed due to changes in purchasing contracts may lead to unfamiliarity of products among the staff. Significant changes should be communicated to the staff and product labels should always be read carefully.

Personnel Related Factors

Untrained, inadequately trained, or inexperienced personnel may be unfamiliar with drug names, doses, or uses of agents, which limits their ability to recognize inappropriate orders and circumstances. New technological advances make keeping up with drug use difficult even for experienced health care practitioners. The important thing is for technicians to recognize their limits and work within them, just as nurses, pharmacists, and physicians are trained to do. Relying on memory instead of checking references (dilution charts, maximum dosage ranges) or performing complicated calculations without a double check may result in errors. It is a technician's responsibility to help prevent medication errors by questioning unusual or unfamiliar orders. When situations that are abnormal or unfamiliar arise, it is always best to consult references and others before making a decision or taking action. Being aware of a potential error and not knowing what to do about it, thinking that some else will catch it, or feeling intimidated by a pharmacist or supervisor certainly increases the chances that an actual error will take place.

The lack of knowledge of medication errors and how to avoid them is another contributing factor to the occurance of medication errors. Not being familiar with common errors or medications most frequently involved in errors might cause one to think that medication errors are infrequent. The most frequently reported medication errors to the USP from August 1991 to April 1993 involved heparin, lidocaine, potassium chloride injection, and epinephrine.[30]

Deficiencies in Medication Use Systems

Medication errors cannot be attributed to human error alone. Errors are frequently due in part to defective or inadequate systems.[41] For example, stocking dangerous drugs in patient care areas (i.e., floor stock) increases the chances of an error occuring because the drugs are available to nurses without a pharmacy check. Floor stock mix-ups between potassium chloride injection and normal saline injection for flushing IV tubing, potassium chloride and furosemide injections, pre-mixed lidocaine in D5W 500 ml and plain D5W 500 ml bags and so on, can lead to serious consequences.

Pharmacy unit dose and IV admixture systems have been shown to reduce medication errors and yet many hospitals in the United States still do not have these systems in place. The unavailability of or difficulty in obtaining patient data such as current body weight, allergy information, or laboratory results contributes to medication errors.

Inefficient processes with too many or too few checks along the way or checks at inappropriate times can be considered as causes of errors. Lack of standardized procedures or outdated procedures might also lead to errors.

Being familiar with factors that may lead to medication errors and things that can be done to prevent them is the first step in reducing medication errors.

SYSTEMS DESIGNED TO PREVENT MEDICATION ERRORS

There are many ways to reduce the chance of a medication error. Institutions help minimize medication errors by fostering a well-trained and knowledgeable staff, maintaining a favorable work environment, and instituting effective policies and procedures, among other things. It is important for technicians to be familiar with the systems designed to provide additional checks in the medication use process. It is also essential that technicians ask questions when they are not familiar with the proper procedures.[4]

Well designed systems help prevent medication errors. Such systems adhere to legal requirements, and include licensed personnel, policies and procedures, multiple check systems, standardized order forms and checklists, and quality assurance activities and monitoring systems, which will be addressed later in this chapter.

Another system designed to help prevent medication errors in the outpatient setting is patient counseling. When a patient or designee drops off a prescription to be filled at the pharmacy, the pharmacist or pharmacy technician asks if the patient is allergic to any medications and asks the proper spelling of the patient's name and address among other things (see chapter 5). When the prescription is picked up, the pharmacist and the patient discuss how to take the medication, any possible side effects, and why is it important for the patient to take the medication exactly as it has been prescribed by the physician. The patient also has the opportunity to ask questions or discuss any concerns about the medication with the pharmacist. Patient counseling plays a very important role in reducing medication errors because it increases the likelihood that patients will take their medication as prescribed by the physician.

Legal Requirements

Pharmacy laws are designed to protect the public by ensuring that a knowledgeable individual double checks the results of the prescribing process and oversees the use of medications. The laws help prevent medication errors. The law requires a licensed pharmacist to be on duty during pharmacy business hours. Licensed pharmacists have to graduate from an accredited school of pharmacy, pass a licensure examination, and pass the state pharmacy law examination in order to practice pharmacy in that state.

Policies and Procedures

Another system designed to prevent medication errors is establishing policies and procedures. Policies and procedure manuals formally establish a system to prevent the occurrence of medication errors. Therefore, technicians should be familiar with the workplace's policy and procedure manual. A study of dispensing errors in an outpatient pharmacy concluded that approximately 33% of the errors discovered were due to noncompliance with company/department policies and procedures.[9]

Multiple Check Systems

Another system designed to prevent medication errors is a multiple check system. This can include the pharmacist reviewing a physician order, a pharmacy technician preparing a medication for the pharmacist to check, a nurse inspecting the dose from the pharmacy, and a patient asking questions and examining the medication before it is taken. A popular check system encourages each person to read the label three times, to remind health care professionals to spend more time reviewing medication labels carefully to prevent medication errors. A double check system is especially important when dealing with potentially lethal drugs such as cancer chemotherapeutic agents.[29]

Standardized Order Forms

Standardized preprinted orders forms have been developed to prevent medication errors by making medication orders easier to read by the prescriber, and easier for the pharmacist and nurse to interpret the orders. Figure 10-4 is an example of a standardized, preprinted order form. Preprinted forms are neatly typewritten and more legible to health care personnel. They generally make it easier for other health care personnel to double check the prescriber's order and calculations. The forms also help reduce errors primarily associated with illegible handwriting and informally educate the prescriber about which medications are on the hospital formulary.

Checklists

Checklists can be included on a standard preprinted order form. When this system is used it ensures that personnel use a systematic, thorough procedure to check medications before they are prescribed, dispensed, or administered to a patient.[29]

Education and Training

Education and training are important aspects in reducing medication errors. Technicians either receive formalized training at a community college, in organized departmental programs, or through on-the-job training. Training can include pharmacy calculations, compounding techniques, pharmacy abbreviations, preparation of intravenous medications, and computer operation skills. Health care personnel should be familiar with the classes of medications, the generic and trade names of medications, and their forms and doses. Some pharmacy technician applicants complete local community colleges before applying for a pharmacy technician position. In this situation, it is still important for the technician to complete pharmacy department training programs because they are specific for the institution and the new technician's position.

Technicians also receive training on the job. JCAHO requires organizations to prove that their personnel are competent. Ideally, on the job training will include instruction and demonstrations. After technicians have been instructed and witnessed a demonstration of a task, they are usually asked to perform the task while the educator observes. This allows the health system to document the technicians' competency.

To complement formal and on the job training, technicians should also read pharmacy literature, participate in local pharmacy organizations, and attend various continuing education lectures to improve their knowledge base. At a minimum, these programs and activities help technicians keep up with changes in formulations and recognize the differences among various medication products.[2]

Computerization and Automation

Proper use of computerization and automation are good ways to prevent medication errors. Bar coding, automatic dispensing machines, and

Cancer Chemotherapy Order Form/ADULT

Lutheran General Hospital

✚ *Advocate*

Part 1 - Chemotherapy

Orders must be received in pharmacy by 2100 for administration between 2300 and 0900

☐ Protocol # _____ 1 2 3 4 5 6 7 8 Course (Circle One)	Diagnosis	BSA M^2 ☐ Dose reduction_____ %	Height	Weight

CHEMOTHERAPY

Provide dose, select a route and designate the frequency and duration for each chemotherapy ordered.
Designate sequence, order or time in column A.   Cont. Inf. = Continuous Infusion over 24 hours

A	DRUG	DOSE	ROUTE	FREQUENCY/DURATION		
	Asparaginase	units/M^2 = U	☐ IVPB over 30 min	☐ SC ☐ IM	q	X	doses
	Bleomycin	units/M^2 = U	☐ IVP over 10 min ☐ IVPB over h	☐ Cont Inf	q	X	doses
	Carboplatin	AUC of _____ = mg/M^2 = mg	☐ IVPB over 30 min	☐ Cont Inf	q	X	doses
	Carmustine	mg/M^2 = mg	☐ IVPB over 15 min in GLASS container	☐ Cont Inf	q	X	doses
	Cisplatin	mg/M^2 = mg	☐ IVPB over 60 min ☐ IVPB over _____ h with _____ g mannitol	☐ Cont Inf	q	X	doses
	Cyclophosphamide	mg/M^2 = mg	☐ IVP over 5 - 10 min ☐ IVPB over 30 - 60 min	☐ Cont Inf	q	X	doses
	Cytarabine	mg/M^2 = mg	☐ Intrathecal ☐ IVPB over h	☐ Cont Inf	q	X	doses
	Dacarbazine	mg/M^2 = mg	☐ IVP over 1 min ☐ IVPB over 15 - 30 min	☐ Cont Inf	q	X	doses
	Daunorubicin	mg/M^2 = mg	☐ IVP over 2 - 3 min ☐ IVPB over 15 min	☐ Cont Inf	q	X	doses
	Doxorubicin	mg/M^2 = mg	☐ IVP over 10 - 15 min ☐ IVPB over 30 min	☐ Cont Inf	q	X	doses
	Etoposide	mg/M^2 = mg	☐ IVPB over 1 -2 h	☐ Cont Inf	q	X	doses
	Fluorouracil	mg/M^2 = mg	☐ IVP over 2 - 3 min ☐ IVPB over 30 - 60 min	☐ Cont Inf	q	X	doses
	Idarubicin	mg/M^2 = mg	☐ IVPB over 15 min	☐ Cont Inf	q	X	doses
	Ifosfamide	mg/M^2 = mg	☐ IVPB over 30 - 60 min	☐ Cont Inf	q	X	doses
	Mesna	mg/M^2 = mg	☐ IVPB over 15 -20 min, 30 min prior to, 4h & 8h after start of ifosfamide	☐ Mix with ifosfamide	q	X	doses
	Mesna	mg/M^2 = mg	☐ IVPB over 15 - 20 min, 4h and 8h after last ifosfamide				
	Methotrexate	mg/M^2 = mg	☐ Intrathecal ☐ IVPB over h	☐ Cont Inf	q	X	doses
	Leucovorin	mg/M^2 = mg	☐ IVP over 3 min ☐ 24 h after methotrexate ☐ Prior to fluorouracil	☐ PO	q	X	doses
	Mitoxantrone	mg/M^2 = mg	☐ IVPB over 15 min		q	X	doses
	Paclitaxel	mg/M^2 = mg	☐ IVPB over h in GLASS container	☐ Cont Inf	q	X	doses
	Vinblastine	mg/M^2 = mg	☐ IVP over 2 - 3 min	☐ Cont Inf	q	X	doses
	Vincristine	mg/M^2 = mg	☐ IVP over 2 - 3 min	☐ Cont Inf	q	X	doses
	Vinorelbine	mg/M^2 = mg	☐ IVP over 6 - 10 min		q	X	doses

Other:

Date:	Time:	Prescriber's Signature:	-Pager #:

F2736-1   © 1997 Advocate Health Care/PS LGH

Figure 10-4. Example of a preprinted chemotherapy order form.

Source: Lutheran General Hospital, Park Ridge, Illinois.

CHEMOTHERAPY FLUID/VOLUME CHART

The following table provides information for the dilution and administration of chemotherapy. This table may be utilized as a guideline when fluids, volumes and/or rates are not specified on the physicians orders.

DRUG	ROUTE	DOSE	FLUID	VOLUME	RATE
Asparaginase (Elspar)	IVPB SubQ	All[1]	D5 (or NS) -	50 ml -	30 min -
Bleomycin (Blexoxane)	IVPB SubQ	All[2]	NS -	50 ml -	1 UNIT / min -
Carboplatin (Paraplatin)	IVPB	All	D5	100 ml	30 min
Carmustine (BCNU)	Cont. Inf. IVPB	All	D5 D5	250 ml (GLASS) 250 ml (GLASS)	6 h (x4 24h) 60 min
Cisplatin (Platinol) (CDDP)	IVPB over 1h IVPB over 6h	All	NS D5.45NS	250 ml 1000 ml	1 h 6 h
Cyclophosphamide	IVPB IVPush	<= 1 gm > 1 gm All	D5 D5 -	100 ml 250 ml -	30 - 60 min 30 - 60 min 5 - 10 min
Cytarabine (Cytosar) (Ara-C)	Cont. Inf. IVPB Intrathecal	<500 mg <=1 gm > 1 gm -	D5 (or NS) D5 (or NS) D5 (or NS) NS*	250 ml 50 ml 100 ml 3 - 6 ml	24 h 30 - 60 min 30 - 60 min -
Cladribine (Leustatin) (2-CdA)	Cont. Inf.	All	NS	500 ml	24 h
Dacarbazine (DTIC)	IVPB	All	D5 (or NS)	100 ml	15 min
Dactinomycin (Cosmogen)	IVPB IVPush	All	D5 (or NS)	50 ml -	10 - 15 min 10 - 15 min
Daunorubicin (Cerubidine)	IVPB IV Push	All	NS D5 (or NS)	50 ml -	15 min 2 - 3 min
Doxorubicin (Adriamycin)	IVPB IVPush	All	D5 (or NS) -	100 ml -	30 min 10 - 15 min
Doxorubicin/Vincristine	Cont. Inf.	All	D5	500 ml	24 h
Etoposide (Vepesid) (VP-16)	IVPB	All	D5 (or NS)	<0.6, 0.4, 0.2 mg/ml	1 - 2 h
Floxuridine (FUDR)	Cont. Inf.	All	D5 (or NS)	1000 ml	24 h
Fludarabine (Fludara)	IVPB	All	D5 (or NS)	50 ml	30 min
Fluorouracil (5-FU)	Cont. Inf. IVPB IVPush	All	D5 (or NS) D5 (or NS) -	500 or 1000 ml 50 ml -	12 or 24 h 30 - 60 min 2 - 3 min
Gemcitabine (Gemzar)	IVPB	All	NS	100 ml	30 min
Idarubicin (Idamycin)	IVPB	All	D5 (or NS)	50 ml	15 min
Ifosfamide (Ifex)	IVPB	All	D5 (or NS)	250 ml	30 - 60 min
Ifosfamide/Mesna	Cont. Inf.	All	D5 (or NS)	1000 ml	24 h
Leucovorin	IVPush	All	D5 (or NS)	-	2 - 3 min
Mechlorethamine (Mustagren)	IVPB	All	D5 (or NS)	100 ml	15 min
Melphalan (Leukeran)	IVPB	All	NS	<=.45mg/ml	15 -30 min
Mesna (Mesnex)	IVPB	All	D5 (or NS)	100 ml	20 min
Methotrexate (MTX)	IVPB Intrathecal	All	D5 (or NS) NS*	250 ml 3 -6 ml	15 - 30 min
Mitomycin (Mutamycin)	IVPB	All	D5 (or NS)	50 ml	15 min
Mitoxantrone (Novantrone)	IVPB	All	D5 (or NS)	50 ml	15 min
Paclitaxel (Taxol)	Cont Inf.	All	D5 (or NS)	500 ml (GLASS)	1, 3, 24 or 96 h
Plicamycin (Mithracin)	IVPB	All	D5 (or NS)	250 ml	2 h
Teniposide (Vumon)	IVPB	All	NS	100 ml	45 - 60 min
Thiophosphoramide (Thiotepa)	IVPB	All	D5 (or NS)	50 ml	15 min
Vinblastine (Velban)	IVPush	All	-	-	2 - 3 min
Vincristine (Oncovin)	IVPush	All	-	-	2 - 3 min
Vinorelbine (Navelbine)	IVPush	All	-	-	6 - 10 min

[1] Asparaginase test dose: 2 IU (0.1ml) INTRADERMAL at least 1 hour prior to dose
[2] Bleomycin test dose: 2 units in 50 ml D5W IVPB OVER 15 - 20 min at least 1 hour prior to dose
*Preservative Free

Figure 10-4. Example of a preprinted chemotherapy order form, *continued*.

robots are used in many health care facilities to reduce medication errors. They reduce the number of health care personnel who handle the medications, which may reduce the chance for human error.[42] Pharmacy-generated medication administration records or labels are recommended to assist nurses in interpreting and documenting medication activities.[2] Packaging is getting more sophisticated; bar coded unit-dose packaging for use with an automated dispensing machine was recently introduced by one company. Bar coding also helps health care personnel avoid mistaking one patient for another. It is also recommended that there be computerized pharmacy systems in place to enable automated checking of doses, duplicate therapies, allergies, drug interactions, and other aspects of use.

Physician computer order entry is also being investigated at some institutions to decrease the number of personnel involved in the ordering process and decrease medication errors in the transcription process (where medication orders are written down by a nurse or unit clerk and sent to the pharmacy). The computer systems would also be able to alert the physician about a possible allergy problem or overdosage before the order reached the pharmacist.

THE QUALITY ASSURANCE PROCESS

What to Do When an Error Occurs

When a potential medication error occurs, for example, a pharmacy technician incorrectly fills a unit dose order and the pharmacist catches the error in the pharmacy. Usually the pharmacist will tell the technician of the error and ask the technician to correct the mistake. It is important for the technician to realize that the pharmacist's intent is to make the mistake a learning experience for the technician as well as give the technician an opportunity to ask questions. Although making a mistake is frustrating, it is important to focus on improving work habits so that the same error will not be made again.

Whatever the circumstances regarding an actual medication error, the pharmacy technician has a responsibility to inform the pharmacist about any known details. Pharmacists usually investigate the error and the severity of the consequences, and gather the details prior to contacting the nurse and the physician.

If the error is caught before the patient receives the medication, it can be corrected within the

pharmacy. If the patient has received the medication the course of action depends on the details of the error, the pharmacist may refill the medication for free and have it delivered to the patient or send a formal letter of apology to the patient. If the error has caused patient harm, the pharmacist may seek legal advice.

Documentation

When a medication error occurs, the institution's medication error reporting form should be completed according to the institution's established reporting procedures. An example of a medication error reporting form is in Figure 10-5.

The medication error reporting form should be filled out and reviewed by those involved in the error to ensure that the content is accurate and correct. Once the form is complete it is usually sent to the pharmacy supervisor and if necessary to the risk management department for review. These forms are then reviewed periodically by the institution's quality assurance committee, which consists of pharmacy, medicine, nursing, risk management, quality assurance, staff education, and legal counsel staff members.[2]

Identifying Trends

One of the roles of the quality assurance committee is to look for medication errors that occur frequently or involve high risk medications. They look for trends in the medication error process and evaluate the systems involved in the errors. Many quality assurance committees focus on the institution's systems (e.g., staff orientation and education) instead of individual staff members because in most cases medication errors are due more to poor drug distribution systems, miscommunications, faulty pharmaceutical packaging, labeling, and nomenclature, and lack of information than any one person. When there is a chance of serious errors, action is taken to improve the system and therefore minimize the possibility of errors.[43]

Making Necessary Changes

Once a trend has been identified, action must be taken to reduce the possibility of future errors. Changes may involve staff education, purchase of a more appropriately labeled medication from another company, revising department policies

Confidential Report of Occurrence
Do Not Copy (Not Part of The Medical Record)

✚ *Advocate Health Care*

☐ Bethany   ☐ Lutheran General
☐ Christ   ☐ Ravenswood
☐ Good Samaritan   ☐ South Suburban
☐ Good Shepherd   ☐ Trinity
☐ Other _____

Include Name & Medical Record No.

Name of Party Involved (print)		Age ☐ Male ☐ Female	Unit/Room No.
Street		Date of Occurrence	**Identification:** ☐ ER Patient ☐ Inpatient ☐ Out-patient ☐ Visitor ☐ Other
City State Zip Code		**Time of Occurrence** _____ Shift: ☐ Day ☐ PM ☐ Nite	**Area Incident Occurred** ☐ Operating Room ☐ Physician Office ☐ Emergency Room ☐ Bathroom ☐ Intensive Care Unit ☐ Hallway ☐ Recovery Room ☐ Facility Grounds ☐ Labor & Delivery ☐ Patient Room ☐ X-Ray ☐ Other Areas (specify) ☐ Pharmacy
Mental Status ☐ Normal/Alert ☐ Unconscious ☐ Sedated ☐ Asleep ☐ Disoriented		**Medicated Past 2 Hrs?** ☐ Yes ☐ No	
Primary Diagnosis		**Types of Medication**	**Bedrails** ☐ Up ☐ Down **Restraints On** ☐ Yes ☐ No
Attending Physician			

EVENT/OCCURRENCE   PLEASE CHECK AS MANY ITEMS AS NEEDED TO FULLY EXPLAIN OCCURRENCE

Safety / Fall Related
☐ Found on floor
☐ Fall from bed / chair / table
☐ Fall while ambulating
☐ Removed restraints
☐ Climbed over side rails
☐ Reported fall / not observed
☐ Other _____

Communication Related
☐ MD not notified / no MD response
☐ Orders / instructions carried out incorrectly
☐ Incomplete chart documentation
☐ Informed consent issue
☐ Other _____

Equipment Related (include Medical Device Reporting Form)
☐ Equipment burned patient
☐ Equipment struck patient
☐ Equipment malfunctioned / failed
☐ Equipment not available
☐ Other _____
Type: _____

Labor & Delivery Related
☐ Labor / delivery complication
☐ Forceps injury to infant
☐ Attending MD not present at delivery
☐ Other _____

Diagnosis / Testing / Treatment Related
☐ No ID band
☐ Illegible ID band
☐ Improper specimen collected
☐ Unlabeled specimen
☐ Mislabeled specimen
☐ X-Rays misread
☐ Complications of procedure
☐ Unplanned return to surgery
☐ Hematoma post procedure
☐ Catheter / tube / drain incident
☐ Delayed consult
☐ Delayed test or procedure
☐ Wasted blood product
☐ Other _____

ARREST ☐ Intubation required ☐ Resuscitated ☐ Expired

NON-MEDICAL
☐ Altercation
☐ Suicide attempt/self inflicted injury
☐ Left AMA
☐ Left without being seen

☐ Elopement
☐ Pt./family dissatisfaction
☐ Refused treatment

☐ Lost property
☐ Pt. non-compliance
☐ Other _____

MEDICATION RELATED
Medication Involved _____

☐ IV
☐ Non-IV

☐ Wrong medication or solution
☐ Wrong dose administered
☐ Wrong route of administration
☐ Wrong time (≥ 2 hrs before/after schedule)

☐ Dose omitted
☐ Prescribing concern
☐ Error discovered before administration to patient
☐ Medication reaction

☐ IV site related
☐ IV equipment related
☐ Other _____

INITIATOR'S COMMENTS: _____
_____
_____

Figure 10-5. Sample of a medication error reporting form.
Source: Lutheran General Hospital, Park Ridge, Illinois.

INITIATOR'S COMMENTS (continued)

_____
_____
_____
_____
_____

Name (print)	Signature	Date
Dept/Unit Ext.		

NATURE OF INJURY: PLEASE CHECK AS MANY ITEMS AS NEEDED TO FULLY EXPLAIN NATURE OF INJURY

☐ **No Apparent Injury**

Musculoskeletal
☐ Broken teeth/dental work
☐ Fracture/dislocation
☐ Strain/sprain
☐ Other _____
_____

Central Nervous System
☐ Cerebral vascular accident
☐ Neuro damage/deficit/loss/change
☐ Seizure
☐ Other _____

Cardiopulmonary
☐ Death
☐ Hemorrhage
☐ Other _____

Skin/Tissue/Systemic
☐ Abscess/decubitus ulcer
☐ Allergic/adverse reaction
   (non medication)
☐ Bleeding, additional
☐ Burn
☐ Contusion/abrasion
☐ Edema/swelling
☐ Hematoma
☐ Laceration/perforation
☐ Sloughing/scarring/necrosis
☐ Wound infection
☐ Other _____

Notification
☐ Attending Physician
☐ Emergency Physician
☐ Resident Physician
☐ Name _____
☐ Time called _____

Follow-up Treatment
☐ X-ray ordered/done
Result _____
_____
☐ Treatment Refused
☐ Treatment _____
_____
_____
_____

Examining Physician's Comments   ☐ No Injury   ☐ Other   ☐ Exam Refused

_____
_____
_____
_____
_____

Name (print)	Signature	Date

Supervisor Follow-up (Include Action Taken)   ☐ No Injury   ☐ Other

_____
_____
_____
_____
_____
_____
_____

Does this occurrence pertain to another department/unit?   ☐ Yes   ☐ No
If so, have you discussed this occurrence with the appropriate manager?   ☐ Yes   ☐ No

Name (print)	Signature	Date
Dept/Unit Ext.		

SEND THIS REPORT TO THE RISK MANAGEMENT DEPARTMENT

This report has been prepared at the direction of the Risk Management Department and under the authority of in-house counsel for consideration by the internal Quality Assurance Committee. This report is confidential and is subject to the Medical Studies Act.

Figure 10-5. Sample of a medication error reporting form, _continued_.

and procedures, or purchasing a piece of equipment to reduce the chance for errors.

Three ways the pharmacy department can educate its staff about actual medication errors on a continual basis are by publishing summaries of errors that have occurred in staff newsletters, conducting educational programs, and discussing medication errors as a regular agenda item at staff meetings.[2] As a technician, it is important to pay close attention to newsletters, educational programs, and discussions regarding errors to help reduce them.

If product labeling contributed to a medication error, the pharmacist usually contacts the drug company and communicates how the labeling had an impact on a specific error. The pharmacist also contacts pharmacy organizations so they can distribute the information to their members and help others to avoid making the same error.

Once a system has been identified as a contributor to medication errors, the policies and procedures are revised to eliminate or reduce the chance of future errors. The staff are inserviced or informed about the changes in procedures and why the procedures have been changed.

Monitoring the Impact of Change

If a system has been identified, the quality assurance committee makes recommendations to reduce the chance of errors in the future. After a system has been modified, the committee will continue to monitor it for medication errors to determine the impact of the changes.[43]

Technician/Pharmacist Liability Issues

Technicians and pharmacists need to be informed about how to prevent medication errors. In addition to the institution/company liability, they may be held accountable as the result of a medication error involving injury to a patient.[44]

SUMMARY

The ultimate goal of pharmacy services must be the safe use of medications by the public.[45] There are many ways medication errors can occur and there are also many ways medication errors can be prevented. Pharmacy technicians play an important role in ensuring the safe use of medications.

REFERENCES

1. Manasse HR Jr. Medication use in an imperfect world: drug misadventuring as an issue of public policy, part I. *Am J Hosp Pharm.* 1989; 46:929–44.
2. American Society of Hospital Pharmacists. ASHP guideline on preventing medication errors in hospitals. *Am J Hosp Pharm.* 1993;50:305–14.
3. Brennan TA, Leape LL, Laird NM, *et al.* Incidence of adverse events and negligence in hospitalized patients—results of the Harvard medical practice study I. *N Engl J Med.* 1991;324:370–6.
4. Lesar TS, Briceland LL, Delcoure K, *et al.* Medication prescribing errors in a teaching hospital. *JAMA* 1990; 263:2329–34.
5. Rupp MT, DeYoung M, Schondelmeyer SW. Prescribing problems and pharmacist interventions in community practice. *Medical Care* 1992;30:926–40.
6. Blum KV, Abel SR, Urbanski CJ, *et al.* Medication error prevention by pharmacists. *Am J Hosp Pharm.* 1988;45:1902–3.
7. Bates DW, Cullen DJ, Laird N, *et al.* Incidence of adverse drug events and potential adverse drug events. *JAMA* 1995;274:29–34.
8. Guernsey BG, Ingrim NB, Kokanson JA, *et al.* Pharmacists' dispensing accuracy in a high-volume outpatient pharmacy service: focus on risk management. *Drug Intell Clin Pharm.* 1993; 17:742–6.
9. Kistner UA, Keith MR, Sergeant KA, *et al.* Accuracy of dispensing in a high-volume, hospital-based outpatient pharmacy. *Am J Hosp Pharm.* 1994;51:2793–7.
10. Buchanan TL, Barker KN, Gibson JT, *et al.* Illumination and errors in dispensing. *Am J Hosp Pharm.* 1991;48:2137–45.
11. Allan EL, Barker KN. Fundamentals of medication error research. *Am J Hosp Pharm.* 1990;47:555–71.
12. Bates DW, Boyle DL, Vander Vliet MB, *et al.* Relationship between medication errors and adverse drug events. *J Gen Intern Med.* 1995; 10:199–205.
13. Leape LL. Error in medicine. *JAMA* 1994;272: 1851–7.
14. Kaufman A, Kung FH, Koenig HM, *et al.* Overdosage with vincristine. *J Pediatr.* 1976;89; 671–4.
15. Davis NM. Preventing omission errors. *Am J Nursing* 1195;95:17.
16. Classen DC, Pestotnik SL, Evans RS, *et al.* Adverse drug events in hospitalized patients. *JAMA* 1997; 277:301–6.
17. Schneider PJ, Gift MG, Lee Y, *et al.* Cost of medication-related problems at a university hospital. *Am J Health-Syst Pharm.* 1995;52:2415–8.
18. Johnson JA, Bootman JL. Drug-related morbidity and mortality. A cost of illness model. *Arch Intern Med.* 1995;155:1949–56.

19. Wou K. Costs associated with recurrent hypoglycemia caused by dispensing error. [letter] *Annals of Pharmacotherapy* 1994;28:965–6.

20. Koren G, Barzilay Z, Greenwald M. Tenfold errors in administration of drug doses: a neglected iatrogenic disease in pediatrics. *Pediatrics* 1986; 77:848–9.

21. Koren G, Barzilay Z, Modan M. Errors in computing drug doses. *Can Med Assoc J.* 1983;129:721–3.

22. Perlstein PH, Callison C, White M, *et al.* Errors in drug computations during newborn intensive care. *Am J Dis Child.* 1979;133:376–9.

23. Bindler R, Bayne T. Medication calculation ability of registered nurses. *IMAGE: J Nursing Scholarship* 1991;23:221–4.

24. Bayne T, Bindler R. Medication calculation skills of registered nurses. *J of Continuing Education in Nursing* 1988;19:258–62.

25. Joint Commission on Accreditation of Healthcare Organizations. *1996 Comprehensive Accreditation Manual for Hospitals: The Official Handbook (CAMH).* IM.3-3.2. Oakbrook Terrace, IL: Joint Commission on Accreditation of Healthcare Organizations: 1996.

26. Robertson WO. Alphabet soup: more or less? [letter] *JAMA* 1980;244:1902.

27. Cohen MR, Davis NM. Errors caused by medical office personnel. *Am Pharm.* 1993;NS33:18.

28. Davis NM. Confusion over illegible orders. *Am J Nursing* 1994;94(1);9.

29. Cohen JR, Anderson RW, Attilio RM, *et al.* Preventing medication errors in cancer chemotherapy. *Am J Health-Syst Pharm.* 1996;53:737–46.

30. Edgar RA, Lee DS, Cousins DD. Experience with a national medication error reporting program. *Am J Hosp Pharm.* 1994;51:1335–8.

31. Davis NM. A well-informed patient is a valuable asset. *Am J Nursing* 1994;94:16.

32. Cohen MR. Amrinone-amiodarone mix-up reported. *Hosp Pharm.* 1996;31:64.

33. Rodriquez G, Poretsky L. Toradol instead of tapazole. [letter] *Am J Health-Syst Pharm.* 1995;52:1098.

34. Pourmotabbed G. The naming of drugs is a difficult matter. *N Engl J Med.* 1994;331:1163.

35. Chu G, Mantin R, Shen Y, *et al.* Massive cisplatin overdose by accidental substitution for carboplatin. *Cancer* 1993;72:3707–14.

36. Malcolm KE, Hogan TT, Wyatt TL. Is the prescription really for selegiline?[letter] *Am J Hosp Pharm.* 1994;51:930

37. Cohen MR, Davis NM. Trademark similarities can cause problems. *Am Pharm.* 1993;NS33:16–7.

38. Davis NM, Cohen MR, Teplitsky B. Look-alike and sound-alike drug names: the problem and the solution. *Hosp Pharm.* 1992;27:95–110.

39. Rheinstein PH, McGinnis TJ. Medication errors. *Am Fam Physician* 1992;45:2720–22.

40. Gold DR, Rogacz S, Bock N, *et al.* Rotating shift work, sleep and accidents related to sleepiness in hospital nurses. *Am J Public Health* 1992; 82:1011–4.

41. Leape LL, Bates DW, Cullen DJ, *et al.* Systems analysis of adverse drug events. *JAMA.* 1995;274:35–43.

42. Borel JM, Rascati KL. Effect of an automated, nursing unit-based drug dispensing device on medication errors. *Am J Health-Syst Pharm.* 1995; 52:1875–9.

43. Cohen MR. Risk management of medication errors must include a careful look at the specific systems involved. *Hosp Pharm.* 1996;31:454,458,461–2.

44. Brushwood DB. Patient injury and attempted link with pharmacist's negligence. *Am J Hosp Pharm.* 1993;50:2382–5.

45. Brodie DC. The challenge to pharmacy in times of change—a report of the Commission on Pharmaceutical Services to Ambulant Patients by Hospitals and Related Facilities. Washington, DC: American Pharmaceutical Association and American Society of Hospital Pharmacists; 1966:39.

SELF-ASSESSMENT QUESTIONS

1. A medication error is defined as "an error made by a pharmacist or pharmacy technician at any time during the dispensing process."

   True or False

2. Which of the following might increase the likelihood of a medication error?
   a. reading the drug label carefully when obtaining the drug from the shelf
   b. reviewing recent medication errors at a pharmacy staff meeting
   c. asking another pharmacy technician to double check a calculation
   d. having a nurse phone in a prescription order that was communicated verbally by the doctor

3. The warning "MUST BE DILUTED" on the container cap and label must be printed by the manufacturer on which of the following products?
   a. potassium chloride inj
   b. vincristine inj
   c. digoxin liquid
   d. amoxicillin suspension

4. Manufacturers have made modifications to products in response to medication error occurrences. Which of the following changes could a manufacturer make to help prevent medication errors?
   a. Place a "hood" (stopper) on a syringe to that is designed to prevent direct injection into a vein.

b. Change the trade name of a product.
c. Decrease the size of the manufacturer's logo on the label to make it less prominent compared to the drug name.
d. all of the above

5. A prescription for diazepam (Valium®—an anti-anxiety agent) was erroneously filled with Diabeta® (glyburide—a drug that lowers blood sugar). Possible consequences resulting from this dispensing error include which of the following?
a. Patient experiences hypoglycemia (too low blood sugar) and faints.
b. Unnecessary health care expenses are incurred.
c. Patient experiences no ill effects.
d. all of the above

6. Jane Smith received the following prescription for an antibiotic to treat a respiratory tract infection on January 1:

Amoxicillin 500 mg TID × 10 days

After taking the drug for 3 days, Ms. Smith felt much better and stopped taking her medication.

On January 12, Ms. Smith presents to the pharmacy with the following prescription for another antibiotic:

Clarithromycin 500 mg PO BID × 10 days

The medication error that has occurred would be categorized as which of the following medication errors?
a. patient non-compliance
b. prescribing error
c. wrong drug dispensed
d. deteriorated drug error

7. The pharmacist asks you to prepare the following medications:

Gentamicin 1 g IVPB Q 8 hr
Cefazolin 60 mg IVPB Q 12 hr

After obtaining the necessary supplies from the shelf, you are puzzled by the number of vials needed for the gentamicin dose (13 vials). You should:
a. Prepare the doses as requested.
b. Prepare the doses as requested, but ask another technician to check your calculations.
c. Question the pharmacist about the order since you have never had to use so many vials to prepare a gentamicin dose before.

d. Prepare the doses as requested because the order has already been reviewed by a pharmacist.
e. Contact the doctor to clarify the order.

8. Katie Loden presents to your pharmacy with the prescription in Figure 10-6 and Lanoxin® (digoxin—heart medication) is dispensed. The patient calls the pharmacy several hours later and asks why her thyroid medication is a yellow round tablet instead of a light brown.

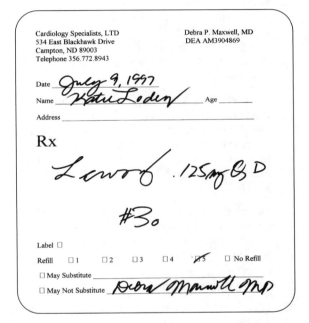

Cardiology Specialists, LTD
534 East Blackhawk Drive
Campton, ND 89003
Telephone 356.772.8943

Debra P. Maxwell, MD
DEA AM3904869

Date   July 9, 1997
Name   Katie Loden   Age _____
Address _____

Rx

Lanox   .125mg BID

#30

Label ☐
Refill   ☐1   ☐2   ☐3   ☐4   ☑5   ☐ No Refill
☐ May Substitute _____
☐ May Not Substitute Debra Maxwell MD

Figure 10-6.

This medication error would most likely be categorized as a:
a. Patient compliance error.
b. Prescribing error.
c. Wrong drug preparation error.
d. Physician error.

9. Susan Baker was in the radiology department when the nurse came to her room to administer the 0900 dose of captopril 25 mg PO three times daily (scheduled for 0900, 1600, 2200). Due to the complexity of the procedure and a number of delays in radiology, Ms. Baker did not return to her room until 1630 at which time her captopril was administered.

Which of the following is a TRUE statement regarding Ms. Baker's captopril?

a. A nursing error has been committed.
b. The medication delay resulted in a wrong time error for the 0900 dose.
c. An omission error occurred.
d. No medication error has occurred.

10. When compounding the following order, the technician inadvertently used 1 ml of the 40 mg/ml concentration solution instead of the pediatric concentration (10 mg/ml).

Gentamicin 10 mg IVPB Q 8 hr

Identify the category or categories in which this error could be classified?
a. wrong dosage form error
b. calculation error
c. improper dose error
d. wrong administration technique error
e. b and c

11. As a technician undergoing on-the-job training, you are falling behind in putting away the drug shipment that arrived earlier this morning. In an effort to save time, you fail to rotate the stock and put all the new stock in front of the containers already in the stock area.

Failure to rotate stock could lead to which of the following medication errors?
a. deteriorated drug error
b. improper dose error
c. inventory error
d. monitoring error

12. Which of the following would be considered a wrong drug preparation error?
a. using the wrong base product to compound a skin ointment
b. adding an incorrect volume of water to reconstitute a 80 ml bottle of amoxicillin oral suspension 125 mg/5 ml.
c. using the wrong diluent to reconstitute a lyophilized powder for injection
d. all of the above

13. Experienced pharmacy technicians are less likely to make calculation errors compared to technicians-in-training.

True or False

14. Which of the following may lead to a calculation error?
a. not verifying that the final answer is reasonable
b. using an inaccurate conversion
c. misplacing the decimal point
d. all of the above

15. Which of the following is least likely to lead to a wrong dose error?
a. 4 mg
b. .4 g
c. 4U
d. 4.0 units

16. Using abbreviations that have been published in reputable medical journals is acceptable since only widely accepted abbreviations are used in publications.

True or False

17. The best way to write "five thousand units of heparin" is _____.

18. Identify four things from the following order (Figure 10-7) that might contribute to a medication error.

Figure 10-7.

19. One morning you are busy preparing IVPB antibiotic orders for the 1000 delivery. The orders are:

Pat Carlson   Cefazolin 1 g IVPB Q 8 hr
Paul Cariton   Ceftazidime 1 g IVPB Q 8 hr

You decide to prepare both orders simultaneously to save time and avoid missing the delivery.

List four reasons that the chances of making an error this morning are increased.

20. Name at least five things the pharmaceutical manufacturer could do to improve labeling for this new drug product. See Figure 10-8.

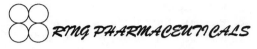

ERROMYCIN-3® INJECTION 1.0GM/mL
(errorpronemicin sulfate)

5mL vial

Figure 10-8. Drug product label.

21. Which of the following statements are TRUE regarding the practice of color coding drug product packaging and its relationship to medication errors?
    a. Color coding the vial caps red for all injectable solutions that turn red upon reconstitution would decrease the likelihood of medication errors.
    b. Developing a color coding scheme unique to a specific manufacturer would decrease the likelihood of a medication error.
    c. Color coding saves time because you do not have to read the product label.
    d. In general, color coding is an unsafe practice.

22. Which could be considered as contributing factors to medication errors?
    a. performing routine maintenance procedures on the tablet counting machine
    b. failing to read current pharmacy literature about new drug products
    c. scheduling additional staff to work during periods of heavy workload
    d. all of the above

23. Medication error rates reported in studies are probably underestimated because:
    a. only errors that result in patient injury are reported.
    b. some errors go undetected.
    c. few errors are identified and corrected during the prescribing phase.
    d. efficient anonymous reporting systems are common.

24. Which of the following statements is TRUE regarding the impact of medication errors on health care expenses?
    a. Medication errors are usually insignificant, easily corrected, and inexpensive.
    b. Medical care costs for treating negative outcomes due to medication errors are usually paid for by the health care worker responsible for the error.
    c. Health care expenses associated with medication errors costs billions of dollars each year.
    d. Malpractice claims for medication errors are usually thrown out in court.

25. Omission errors are less likely to result in negative outcomes than improper dose errors, since the patient is not receiving a harmful dose.

True or False

26. Judy Jones, a technician working in the unit dose cartfill area, notices the 25 mg and 50 mg strengths of Benadryl® are mixed together in the same storage bin. What can Judy do to correct this problem?
    a. Make no changes, since technicians are responsible to read labels carefully.
    b. Modify the stock shelf so each strength has its own section or bin.
    c. Change the label to indicate that both strengths are in the bin.
    d. Store the 25 mg strength under Benadryl® and the 50 mg strength under Diphenhydramine.

27. The technician filling a prescription for Mr. Hill notices the print on the label is faded and hard to read. What is the best way the technician could correct this problem?
    a. Hand write the patient name and directions on the label.
    b. Ask the pharmacist to change the printer ribbon before the next label is printed.
    c. Change the printer ribbon, and reprint the label for Mr. Hill's prescription.
    d. all of the above

28. Anonymous self-reporting of medication errors may be used in some institutions or companies as a means of determining the numbers/severity of medication errors.

True or False

29. A technician compounds a continuous infusion of Heparin 25,000 units in 500 ml of 5% Dextrose in Water (D5W) and places the bag on the counter for the pharmacist to check. The technician then begins to fill other medication orders. One of the orders the technician fills calls for two Heparin 5,000 unit

syringes for subcutaneous injection. The technician notices that the same patient name on the continuous infusion label and the subcutaneous injection label. What should the technician do?

a. Fill the other medication orders and assume the pharmacist will evaluate the doses.

b. Inform the pharmacist that both Heparin prescriptions have the same patient name and ask if both orders are correct.

c. Ask another technician what the standard dose of Heparin is and fill both orders.

d. Check the patient's medication profile and fill both orders for Heparin.

30. A technician fills a medication order for a 20 mg prednisone tablet with a propranolol 20 mg tablet. The pharmacy technician supervisor notices the error before the pharmacist checks all the filled medication orders. What should the technician supervisor do to prevent the wrong medication from leaving the pharmacy?

a. Tactfully call the error to the attention of the technician who made the error to correct the mistake.

b. Correct the mistake before the pharmacist also notices the error.

c. Check the stock bin to see if additional propranolol tablets were incorrectly placed in the prednisone bin.

d. Both a and c

31. A newly employed technician begins training in the pharmacy. A senior technician is training the new technician about the duties of the position. Which of the following ideas can the senior technician discuss or demonstrate that can prevent medication errors?

a. Discuss experiences the senior technicians has had with making and preventing medication errors.

b. Demonstrate the use of the credit card verification machine.

c. Demonstrate how to fill medication orders and talk on the telephone at the same time.

d. both a and c

32. A technician compounding an intravenous preparation of calcium gluconate and 5% Dextrose in Water (D5W) notices the calcium gluconate injection looks slightly cloudy before preparing the bag. What should the technician do to prevent a medication error?

a. Place the calcium gluconate vials in the refrigerator to see if the cloudiness disappears in a few minutes.

b. Place that vial of calcium gluconate back on the shelf and use another vial that looks clear.

c. Place all the calcium gluconate vials in the "shaker." The machine that helps reconstituted medications dissolve more quickly before preparation.

d. Inform the pharmacist that the calcium gluconate vials look cloudy and inspect all the calcium gluconate vials in stock.

e. Discard the vials of calcium gluconate that look cloudy.

33. The background music in the pharmacy is too loud where two technicians and a pharmacist are working. The first technician likes to work to a loud radio because he says it makes his job more fun. The second technician is having trouble hearing the phone ring. The second technician is also having trouble concentrating on his work and is worried about making a medication error because he cannot concentrate. What should the second technician do in this situation?

a. Try harder to concentrate with the music on and tell the callers on the phone to speak louder so he can hear them.

b. Tactfully ask the first technician and the pharmacist if he can turn the radio volume lower.

c. Remind himself to bring ear plugs to the pharmacy next time he is scheduled to work.

d. Wear a headset radio in the pharmacy and tell the first technician he has to answer the phone since he's the only one that can hear it ring.

34. Nancy Andrews, a pharmacy technician notices the nifedipine capsules in the automated tablet and capsule machine (ATC Machine®) are almost gone. She also notices there are no more nifedipine capsules in the pharmacy to restock the machine. What is the next action she can take to reduce the chance of a medication error?

a. Inform the technician on the next shift that the nifedipine capsules are almost gone.

b. Remind herself to order nifedipine capsules the next time she is scheduled to work.

c. Inform the pharmacist that the pharmacy is almost out of nifedipine capsules.

d. Determine the immediate needs of the patients and inform the purchasing personnel of the situation.

35. Roger Young, a pharmacy technician at Hometown Pharmacy, has the flu and has been taking antihistamines to dry his runny nose. He chose to work his scheduled shift because he knows how busy the pharmacy has been this week. However, he feels terrible and the antihistamine is making him sleepy. Roger is trying to fill prescriptions accurately but, his eyes are watery and he is having trouble reading. What should Roger do to prevent medication errors from occurring?

a. Drink a few cups of coffee to wake up.

b. Ask the pharmacist if he can go home because he is ill.

c. Drink lots of water and have chicken soup for lunch.

d. Ask the patients to read their prescriptions to him.

36. Match the medications in the first column that are commonly mistaken with the ones in the second column that result in medication errors:

Amoxicillin 250 mg capsule	Percodan® tablet
Hydroxyzine 25 mg tablet	Digitoxin 0.1 mg capsule
Potassium Chloride 20 mEq injection	Quinidine 200 mg tablet
Desipramine 25 mg tabletAmpicillin	Lidocaine 1 gm prefilled syringe
Digoxin 0.125 mg tablet	Ampicillin 250 mg capsule
Quinine 200 mg capsule	Dimenhydrinate 50 mg capsule
Epinephrine 1:1,000 injection	Hydralazine 25 mg tablet
Percocet® tablet	Furosemide 20 mg injection
Diphenhydramine 50 mg capsule	Imipramine 25 mg tablet
Lidocaine 100 mg prefilled syringe	Epinephrine 1:10,000 injection

37. The pharmacy receives a prescription for hydrocortisone 2.5% cream. The technician notices the pharmacy is out of stock in that item. The pharmacy can substitute Hydro-cortisone 2.5% ointment without calling the doctor.

True or False

38. A nurse discovers the continuous infusion being administered to Mr. Williams contains potassium chloride 40 mEq. Due to Mr. Williams kidney problems the continuous infusion prescribed for him was supposed to be without potassium chloride. After the nurse discontinues the incorrect continuous infusion and hangs the ordered continuous infusion, she is required to call the physician.

True or False

39. A pharmacy technician notices that two different looking tablets are mixed together in the ciprofloxacin 500 mg tablet bin in the automatic tablet and capsule machine (ATC-212® an automated dispensing device). The filling log indicates the machine was refilled the day before and the lot number is significantly different than the previous refill log entries. What should the technician do in this situation?

a. Remove the different looking tablets and discard them.

b. Nothing, assume the manufacturer has changed the look of the tablets.

c. Inform the pharmacist of the situation immediately.

d. Nothing, the personnel who refilled the machine rarely make mistakes.

40. A pharmacy technician supervisor notices several technicians making the same calculation error. In the next technician staff meeting, the supervisor discusses the errors with the group without mentioning who made the mistakes. The supervisor also demonstrates how to perform the calculation correctly. This practice can help prevent medication errors.

True or False

41. The purpose of a national medication error reporting program is to share experiences among health care personnel so that patient safety can be improved. It also can contribute to educational efforts to prevent future medication errors.

True or False

42. Name at least five departments or members of a quality assurance committee that are responsible for reviewing reports of medication errors.

43. Name three ways a pharmacy can educate the staff about actual medication errors on a continuous basis.

44. Technicians and pharmacists may be held legally responsible for a medication error that causes harm to a patient.

    True or False

ANSWERS TO SELF-ASSESSMENT

1. False. A medication error may occur anytime during the medication use process—prescribing, transcription, dispensing, administration (patient compliance) and by personnel other than pharmacists or pharmacy technicians.

2. d. Verbally transmitted orders can easily be misunderstood especially with the number of sound-alike drugs names on the market. In this case, the order was verbally communicated twice—from the physician to the nurse and then again to the pharmacist.

3. a. Undiluted potassium chloride injection should never be injected directly into a patient's vein due to the potential for an irregular heart beat and possibly death. The USP implemented this labeling requirement in response to the many potassium chloride injection errors reported.

4. d. All of the changes may decrease the potential of a medication error. The first one, the hood would prevent direct intravenous injection of a dangerous concentration or dose and remind health care personnel that the drug must be diluted prior to injection. Changing a drug name to one that is distinctly different from others would decrease the chance of a sound-alike or look-alike error. Ancillary information on a drug label such as a manufacturer logo should be small enough so that it does not distract from critical information (drug name, strength, concentration, route, etc.).

5. d. Outcomes of errors depend on many factors. Some patients may be more prone to ill effects due to their overall health, age, weight, or underlying diseases. Consequences may occur from taking the wrong drug (low blood sugar) and by not taking the correct medication (increased anxiety due to not taking diazepam). In some cases a patient may not experience any adverse effect from the incorrect medication.

6. a. Patients have a responsibility in the medication use process to take their medication as instructed. Not taking the entire prescription could have lead to inadequate treatment with symptoms reappearing a short time later. The new prescription for a newer, more costly agent may have been prescribed because the physician was not aware that Ms. Smith stopped taking her amoxicillin after 3 days. This may have lead the physician to believe that amoxicillin was ineffective and an alternate agent was required. It is assumed that Ms. Smith was adequately counseled by the pharmacist when the amoxicillin was dispensed.

7. c. Technicians should not feel intimidated about questioning a pharmacist about orders. Pharmacists make errors just like everyone else. Remember to be tactful when posing the question.

8. b. The error was made because Levoxyl® (levothyroxine) was sloppily written by the prescriber and misread as Lanoxin® (digoxin).

9. c. An omission error occurred because the 0900 dose was not administered until the next scheduled dose was due. The patient would likely only receive two doses that day instead of three.

10. b and c. Improper dose error is the best classification for this error. The patient would have received 40 mg instead of the 10 mg prescribed. The 40 mg/ml gentamicin could have been used to prepare the IVPB accurately by using 0.25 ml instead of 1 ml.

11. a. Failure to rotate stock may result in the use of drugs with longer expiration dates being used first. Older drugs on the back of the shelf may expire before ever getting used.

12. d. All of the answers above describe a problem in the preparation of a drug prior to administration.

13. False. Number of years of pharmacy experience does not correlate with frequency of calculation errors.

14. d. All examples may lead to calculation errors.

15. a. ".4 g" could be interpreted as 4 g and would best be written as 0.4 g or 400 mg.

Both c and d would be best written as "4 units." Abbreviations should be avoided whenever possible because the "U" in "4U" could be read as "40." Trailing zeros after the decimal point should be avoided for the same reason.

16. False. Many times authors make up abbreviation for disease states or drug names/combinations to avoid having to write out lengthy terms numerous times. This is acceptable when writing an article for publication provided the full term is spelled out the first time the abbreviation is used.
    It is not an acceptable practice for writing medication orders or prescription labels.

17. "Heparin 5000 units" or "5000 units Heparin" would both be acceptable—remember to write legibly!

18. 1. use of "dig" as an abbreviation for digoxin
    2. "QD" could be interpreted as QID, OD, QOD should be written out "daily."
    3. "1 tab" is not appropriate since digoxin is available in two strengths.
    4. sloppy handwriting

19. 1. The drug names are similar.
    2. More than one order is being prepared at the same time.
    3. The patients' names are similar.
    4. It is a "rushed" work environment.

20. 1. Make the manufacturer name/logo less prominent (smaller).
    2. Omit the trailing zero in the concentration strength.
    3. Enlarge the total contents of the vial.
    4. Enlarge the drug name.
    5. Change the trade name to something that does not sound like erythromycin or E-Mycin.
    6. Change the trade name to omit the suffix "3."
    7. Use upper and lower case lettering for the drug name.

21. d. Matching vial cap colors with solution colors would not aid drug identification. Color coding unique to a manufacturer would be confusing as manufacturers change with each new drug purchasing contract. Technicians should always read the drug product label three times.

22. b. Technicians have a responsibility to continuously learn about new drugs and therapies.

23. b. There is no way to account for errors that are not detected. Other reasons might be that errors that are corrected before the drug is administered to the patient are frequently not reported and health care personnel are afraid to report errors.

24. c. Costs of treating adverse events due to medication errors, out-of-court settlements, and legal fees add up to billions of dollars annually.

25. False. Omission errors can be just as dangerous as those that result in too high a dose being given or taken because the medical treatment for which the drug is prescribed has been overlooked.

26. b. Medications with the same generic name but, with different strengths should be stored in separate bins next to each other on the shelf. There is an increased chance of error when different strengths are stored together in the same bin.

27. c. Hard to read medication labels may contribute to a medication error. The technician should try to change the printer ribbon and redo the label first. Printer ribbons should be routinely changed as established by company/department policies and procedures. However, if this is not possible due to uncontrollable circumstances, the technician (with the pharmacist's approval) should type or legibly write the label in a manner that the patient can clearly understand.

28. True. Anonymous self-reporting may be used in some institutions.

29. b. The technician should question the pharmacist about the duplicate orders. One order may have been for another patient or maybe an order to discontinue the continuous infusion was overlooked.

30. d. The second technician should tactfully point out the error to the first technician and allow the first technician to correct the mistake. This gives the first technician a chance to learn from the mistake and may prevent similar mistakes in the future. Checking the stock bin can also prevent future mistakes.

31. a. Generally discussing previous medication errors and error correction from a senior technician's experience can help teach the new technician about medication errors. Answer c is wrong because it is important

to concentrate on correctly filling medication orders without doing two things at once. Performing one task at a time can reduce the chance of medication errors.

32. d. The technician has a responsibility to be observant and inform the pharmacist about any potential medication errors. The technician should only compound this IV admixture if the calcium gluconate is clear in appearance. The technician also has the responsibility to alert appropriate personnel so that all calcium gluconate vials in the pharmacy can be inspected for the cloudy appearance.

33. b. The work environment needs to be conducive to concentrating on the duties of the position. If the music in the pharmacy is preventing the second technician from performing his duties as a technician, he should speak up tactfully and take action to correct the situation. This can prevent medication errors by improving the ability of the second technician to concentrate, hear the telephone ring, and hear the callers on the phone.

34. d. The technician has the responsibility to make sure the pharmacy has enough nifedipine capsules in order to prevent patients from missing their scheduled doses. If the pharmacy runs out of a medication, an error of omission may occur.

35. b. Roger should ask the pharmacist if he can go home because he is not feeling well. If Roger cannot concentrate on his work and is having difficulty reading, he is more likely to make a medication error.

36. Amoxicillin—Ampicillin
Hydroxyzine—Hydralazine
Potassium Chloride—Furosemide
Desipramine—Imipramine
Digoxin—Digitoxin
Quinine—Quinidine
Epinephrine—Epinephrine
Percocet—Percodan
Diphenhydramine—Dimenhydrinate
Lidocaine—Lidocaine

37. False. The physician must be contacted and the prescription would need to be changed with physician approval before the ointment can be dispensed. Dispensing a cream instead of an ointment, or vice versa, is a common mistake. In many cases, the packaging only differs by one word (i.e., ointment or cream). Most pharmacies store the ointment in a place that is separated from the creams in hopes of preventing a mistake.

38. True. The nurse must immediately contact the physician and inform the physician about the medication error. The physician will determine.if further action is needed depending on the circumstances.

39. c. Inform the pharmacist immediately of the situation. The pharmacist can help investigate and provide direction according to established policies and procedures of how to proceed.

40. True. This practice can educate the staff about the correct way to make the calculation and prevent future medication errors.

41. True. The United States Pharmacopeial Convention, Inc. (USP) Medication Errors Reporting Program is an example of a national program.

42. The committee should have representatives from pharmacy, medicine, nursing, risk management, quality assurance, staff education, and legal counsel.

43. The pharmacy can educate staff about actual medication errors with periodic newsletters, educational programs, and by reviewing medication errors reports at staff meetings.

44. True. Technicians and pharmacists both contribute to the safe use of medications by the public. If their actions result in patient harm, they may be held legally liable for their actions along with the institution and others involved.

11 | Purchasing and Inventory Control

Stephen J. Allen, M.S., FASHP

An effective purchasing and inventory control system requires all pharmacy staff to understand and actively participate in the system, however, certain staff are responsible for managing the pharmacy inventory and purchasing system. As the primary handlers of medication in the pharmacy medication preparation system, pharmacy technicians' performance is critical to the success of the purchasing and inventory control system.

This chapter describes the basic principles of pharmaceutical purchasing and inventory control. It applies to all types of pharmacy settings, including decentralized, centralized, home infusion, and ambulatory care pharmacy operations.

For technicians interested in considering a specialized position within purchasing and inventory control, or for readers desiring more in-depth study, a reading list is included in the Additional Reading section of this chapter.

LEARNING OBJECTIVES

Upon completion of the chapter on Purchasing and Inventory Control the reader will be able to

1. Demonstrate an understanding of the formulary system and its application in a purchasing and inventory system.
2. Apply the proper principles and processes when receiving and storing pharmaceuticals.
3. Identify key techniques for reviewing packaging, labeling, and storage considerations when handling pharmaceutical products.
4. Demonstrate both an understanding and the application of appropriate processes for maintaining and managing a pharmaceutical inventory.
5. Complete the appropriate processes in the handling of pharmaceutical recalls and the disposal of pharmaceutical products.
6. Execute lending and borrowing pharmaceutical transactions between pharmacies.
7. Demonstrate an understanding of those pharmaceutical products that require special handling within the purchasing and inventory system.
8. Complete basic transactions in the billing and crediting of pharmaceutical products.

THE FORMULARY SYSTEM

Most hospitals and health care systems develop a list of medications that may be prescribed for patients in the institution or health care system. This list is usually called a formulary and serves as the cornerstone of the purchasing and inventory control system. The formulary is developed and maintained by a committee of medical and allied health staff called the Pharmacy and Therapeutics (P&T) Committee. This group of physicians, pharmacists, nurses, dietitians, and administrators collaborate to ensure that the safest, most efficacious, and least costly medications are on the formulary. The products on the formulary dictate what the pharmacy should keep in inventory.

The formulary is usually available in print or through a computer system. It is produced exclusively for all health practitioners involved in the prescribing, dispensing, and monitoring medications and is a tool to determine product availability, the appropriate therapeutic uses, and dosing of medications. Most formularies are organized alphabetically by the drug's generic name, which is typically cross-referenced with the trade name products. In most cases, the storage areas in the pharmacy are arranged alphabetically by either generic or trade name of the drug. Therefore, the formulary can help the pharmacy technician determine if a product is stocked in the pharmacy and where it would be located.

It is important for pharmacy technicians to learn how the formulary is updated, and how and when changes in the formulary are communicated to the staff. Drugs are added and deleted from the formulary on a regular basis, but the frequency at which drugs are added or deleted varies among institutions. Formularies are typically updated every 12–18 months. Loose leaf formularies and on-line computerized formularies can be continuously updated, while hard bound formularies rely on supplementary updates.

Other important information available in the formulary is the dosage form, strength, concentration, and package size specified under each listing. When selecting a product from inventory the technician must consider all product characteristics such as name, dosage form, strength, concentration, and package size (Figure 11-1). Detailed review and consideration of each listing helps ensure an error-free product selection.

CEFTAZIDIME[1]   8:12.06[2]
    (Antibiotic)[3] (Fortaz®)[4]

Note: This product is restricted to Pulmonary Medicine, Hematology/Oncology or Infectious Disease Service Approval.[5]

DOSAGE[6]

Neonates:
    Postnatal age less than 7 days: 100 mg/kg divided q 12h
    Postnatal age greater than 7 days:
        Less than 1200 g: 100 mg/kg per day divided q 12h
        Greater than 1200 g: 150 mg/kg per day divided q 8h

    Infants & children 1 month to 12 yr.: 100–150 mg/kg per day divided every 8 hours; Maximum = 6 g/day

    Adjust dosage with creatinine clearance

INJECTION, 500 mg, 1 g & 2 g vials[7]

Formulary book listings usually include: [1] generic name, [2] numeric cross reference to the American Hospital Formulary Service, [3] class of drug, [4] proprietary/trade name, [5] restricted uses within the institution, [6] dosing information, and [7] dosage form and package sizes

Figure 11-1. Formulary Listing.

Source: Adapted from a typical listing in the *Children's National Medical Center Hospital Formulary*, circa 1994.

RECEIVING AND STORING PHARMACEUTICALS

One of the most useful experiences for a pharmacy technician is to witness the receipt of pharmaceuticals by the pharmacy department. Experience is useful for a number of reasons. It helps the pharmacy technician become familiar with formulary items; it demonstrates the system used to ensure that only formulary items are put into inventory; and it helps familiarize the technician with all the areas used to store drugs.

Receiving is one of the most important parts of the pharmacy operation. A poorly organized and executed receiving system can put patients at risk and elevate health care costs. For example, if the wrong concentration of a product was received in error, it could lead to a dosing error or delays in patients' receipt of therapy. Misplaced products or products not in stock also jeopardizes the patients' care and increases health care costs. To avoid these unfavorable outcomes, pharmacy technicians should become familiar with the process for receiving and storing pharmaceuticals.

The Receiving Process

In a reliable and efficient receiving system, the receiving personnel verify that the shipment is complete and intact (i.e., check for missing and damaged items) before putting items into circulation or inventory. The receiving process begins with the verification of the boxes of pharmaceuticals delivered by the shipper. The person receiving the shipment begins the process by verifying that the name and address on the boxes and the number of boxes matches the courier's shipping manifest. Each box should also be inspected for gross damage. If there is any damage or there are any discrepancies with the shipment, they should be noted on the shipping manifest or the appropriate part of the shipment should be refused. This activity should be performed in the presence of the delivery person and documented when signing for the order. This helps protect the institution from financial responsibility for products damaged in shipment, products not ordered, and products not received. Products requiring refrigeration or freezing should be processed first.

The next step of the receiving process entails checking the newly acquired products against the receiving copy of the purchase order. This occurs after the delivery person has left. A purchase order is the document created when the order is placed. It lists the items that were ordered. A purchase order has multiple copies, including an original file copy, a receiving copy, and a copy for the supplier (Figure 11-2).

The receiving copy is used by the receiver to ensure that the products ordered have been received. The name, brand, dosage form, size of the package, concentration strength, and quantity of product must match the purchase order. Once the accuracy of the shipment is confirmed, the purchase order copy must be signed and dated by the person receiving the shipment (Figure 11-2). At this point the product's expiration date should be checked to ensure that it meets the department's minimum expiration

date requirement. Frequently, departments will require that products received have a minimum of 6 months before they expire.

If a pharmacist or pharmacy technician other than the receiving technician removes a product from a shipment before it has been properly received and cannot locate the receiving copy of the purchase order, then a written record of receipt should be created. This is done by listing the product, dosage form, concentration/strength, package size, and quantity on a blank piece of paper (Figure 11-3) or the supplier's packing slip/invoice and checking off the line item received (Figure 11-4). In both cases, the name of the person receiving the product should be included and the document should be given to the receiving technician.

The Storing Process

Once the product has been properly received it must be properly stored. Depending on the size and type of the pharmacy operation, the product may be placed in a bulk, central storage area or into the active dispensing areas of the pharmacy. In any case, the expiration date of the product should be compared with the products currently in stock. Products already in stock that have expired should be removed. Those products that will expire in the near future should be highlighted and placed in the front of the shelf/bin. The newly acquired products will generally have longer shelf lives and should be placed behind packages that will expire before them. This technique is referred to as stock rotation. Stock rotation is an important inventory management principle that encourages the use of products before they expire and helps prevent the use of expired products.

Product Handling Considerations

Pharmacy technicians usually spend more time handling and preparing medications than pharmacists. This presents pharmacy technicians with the critical responsibility of assessing and evaluating each product from both a content and labeling standpoint. It also provides the technician with an opportunity to confirm that the receiving process was performed properly.

The most important work habit for a pharmacy technician to develop when handling pharmaceuticals and medication orders is to read the label three times. Reading the label

PURCHASE ORDER
Department of Pharmacy Services
Community Hospital
1 Valley Road
Suburbia, MD 20777
(333) 555-1010

Purchase Order
No. 0849
THIS NUMBER MUST
APPEAR ON ALL INVOICES,
PACKING SLIPS, BILLS,
PACKAGES AND CARTONS

Vendor: Pharmaceutical Labs
185 Commerce Ave.
Ft. Washington, PA
1-800-555-3753
Acc# 123-12345

BY_____DIRECTOR
PHARMACY SERVICES/DESIGNEE

ORDER DATE	FOB		DATE REQUIRED IN HOSPITAL	TERMS	DEPARTMENT	SHIP VIA
4/1/97	☐ HOSPITAL	☐ SHIPPING POINT	ASAP	N/A	Pharmacy	Standard

QUANTITY RECEIVED	ORDERED	DESCRIPTION	UNIT PRICE	AMOUNT
4	5	Orimune 50 × 1	$450.00	$2,250.00
50	50	Haemophilus B Vaccine Via 4s	$ 52.92	
13	12	Piperacillin 40 g Vial each	$110.00	$2,646.00
30	30	DPT Vaccine Vial 7.5 ml each	$ 56.50	
		Quantity received as indicated / one vial of piperacillin broken in shipment.		$1,320.00
				$1,695.00
		4/15/97 Joe Johnson, Pharmacy Technician		

1. Goods not in accordance with specifications will be rejected and held at vendor's risk awaiting disposal. Vendor must pay transportation both ways on all rejected material.
2. The right is reserved to cancel all or part of this order if not delivered within the time specified.
3. No price change allowed unless authorized by this office.
4. Packing slips must accompany all shipments.
5. All shipments must be prepaid.
6. Equipment supplied under this purchase order must meet all applicable O.S.H.A.. Standards.

The quantity received is recorded in the "received" column by the person receiving the order. Damaged merchandise is noted on the purchase order, and the receiver signs and dates the receipt. This information enables the purchasing agent to confirm back orders, address mechanisms for retaining or returning overages, and determine financial accountability for damaged merchandise.

Figure 11-2. Documenting receipt on a Purchase Order.

Received to stock
4 × 50's   Oral Polio Vaccine, 0.5 ml
50 × 4's   Haemophilus B vaccine vials
13 each   Piperacillin 40 gm vials
30   DTP vials, 7.5 ml

4/15/97
One vial Piperacillin   Joe Johnson
broken in shipment.   Pharmacy Technician

Receipt on blank piece of paper must include precise detail of the amount, product description, person receiving product, and the date of receipt.

Figure 11-3. Receipt of pharmaceutical on blank piece of paper.

Invoice

Shipper
Pharmaceutical Labs
185 Commerce Avenue
Ft. Washington, PA

Buyer
Community Hospital
1 Valley Road
Suburbia, MD 20777

Invoice # 12346
Invoice Date 4/01/97

Quantity		Product #	Product Description	Unit Price	Amount
5	4 rec.	6190	Orimune 50 × 1	$450.00	$2,250.00
4	✓	7183	Haemophilus B Vaccine	$ 52.92	$2,646.00
13	12. rec.	4391	Piperacillin 40 g Vial	$110.00	$1,320.00
30	✓	2727	DPT Vaccine 7.5ml Vial	$ 56.50	$1,695.00

Quantity received as indicated,
one vial Piperacillin broken in shipment.

Received   4 × 50's   Orimune
           50   Haemophilus B Vaccine.
           13   Piperacillin 40 gm vial
           30   DTP Vaccine 7.5 ml
                      4/15/97
                      Joe Johnson
                      Pharmacy Technician

Receipt on an invoice or packing slip can be done the same way as receipt on a blank piece of paper or the quantities can be checked or modified as received.

Figure 11-4. Receipt of pharmaceutical on Packing Slip/Invoice.

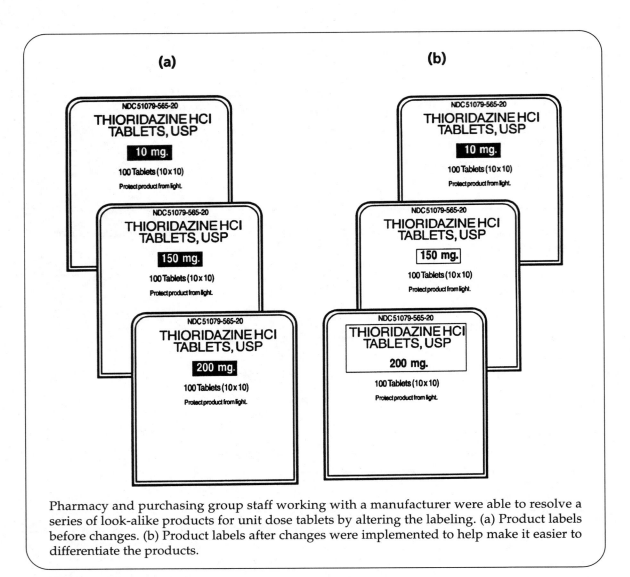

(a)   **(b)**

Pharmacy and purchasing group staff working with a manufacturer were able to resolve a series of look-alike products for unit dose tablets by altering the labeling. (a) Product labels before changes. (b) Product labels after changes were implemented to help make it easier to differentiate the products.

Figure 11-5. Look-alike product labeling.

when the product is selected, prepared, and after it has been prepared reduces the likelihood of using the wrong product, amount, or strength to prepare the medication. It is best to learn to make selection decisions based upon the written description rather than the general appearance of the product (e.g., packaging type, color, logo), since appearance often changes and may be similar to other products.

When selecting a product the expiration date of the product should also be checked. For liquids or injectable products the color and clarity of the items should be checked for consistency with the product standard. Products with visible particles, an unusual appearance, or a broken seal should be reported to the pharmacist.

Since pharmacy technicians handle so many products each day, they are in a perfect position to identify packaging and storage issues that could lead to errors. The three main issues to pay close attention to are

- *Look-alike Products.* Stocking products of similar color, shape, and size could result in error if someone fails to read the label. All staff members should be alerted to look-alike products.
- *Misleading Labels.* Sometimes the company name or logo is emphasized on the label instead of the drug name, concentration, or strength.
- *Product Storage.* Storing products that are similar in appearance adjacent to one

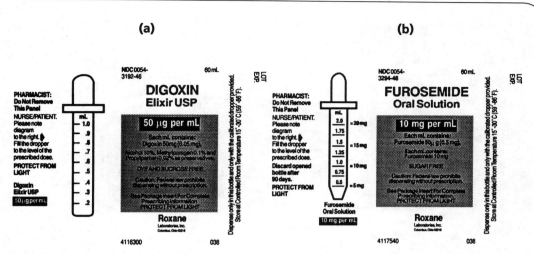

Frequently patients receive both of these medications at the same time. The two products from the same manufacturer had very similar appearances and the pharmacy staff reported their concerns for potential mix-up to the manufacturer.

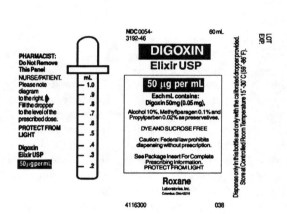

The manufacturer responded by changing the background on the digoxin label to minimize chances for mix-up. The pharmacy staff can modify storage location to further reduce the chance for error.

Figure 11-6. Product Location and Look-Alike Problem.

another can result in error if someone fails to read the label.

It is essential to alert other staff members to products that fall into one of these categories. Some pharmacies routinely discuss product handling considerations at staff meetings or in departmental newsletters, but pharmacy technicians should also discuss their concerns with co-workers and advocate changes to products with poor labeling. Examples of success stories in working with manufacturers to modify package labeling are noted in Figures 11-5 and 11-6.

MAINTAINING AND MANAGING INVENTORY

An inventory management system is an organized approach designed to maintain an adequate amount of pharmaceutical products in the pharmacy at all times. There are a variety of inventory management systems in use, such as the minimum/maximum level, the order book, and a computerized system, among others. Pharmacies often will use a combination of these systems.

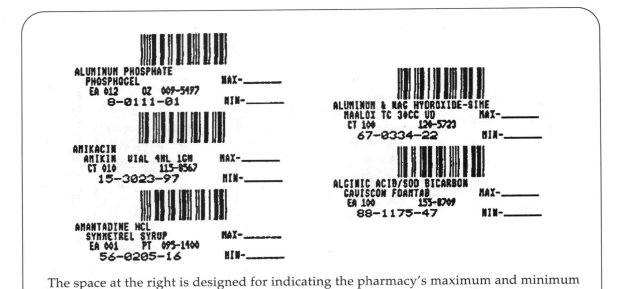

The space at the right is designed for indicating the pharmacy's maximum and minimum level of stock for the item.

Figure 11-7. Shelf labels.

The ideal system for inventory management is a computerized system. In the fully computerized inventory system each dispensing transaction is subtracted from the perpetual inventory log that is maintain in the computer, while all products received are added to the inventory log. When the quantity of a pharmaceutical product in stock reaches a predetermined point (often called "par"), a purchase order is then generated to order more of the product. This system does not depend on any one employee to monitor inventory or to reorder pharmaceuticals. The technology is available to have a computerized inventory in most pharmacies, yet interfacing a computerized inventory system with existing pharmacy computer systems designed for dispensing and patient management systems is often difficult to implement. Consequently, manual systems that require the active participation of pharmacy technicians, such as the minimum/maximum system and the order book, are frequently used.

The use of automated dispensing machines in inpatient nursing units, clinics, operating rooms, and emergency rooms has facilitated the use of computers for inventory management. These devices serve as repositories for medications that will be dispensed directly from a patient care area. There are a variety of brands of automated dispensing machines available such as Pyxis Medstation, Meditrol, Omnicell, and SureMed.

These machines are connected to the main computer terminal in the pharmacy and products are stocked in the automated dispensing machine. The machines keep track of inventory so pharmacy personnel can generate a list of what needs to be replenished. In essence, the nursing and medical personnel who use these automated dispensing machines have a computerized inventory system that the pharmacy staff manages. Medications used to restock these devices may be taken from the pharmacy's main inventory or a separate purchase order may be executed for each device on a periodic basis.

The minimum/maximum level inventory system relies on a predetermined order quantity and an order point. Shelf labels are placed on the storage bin or shelf to alert all staff to the minimum stock quantity (Figure 11-7). The pharmacy technician should always determine if the minimum stock quantity has been reached when removing a product and inform the appropriate purchasing personnel or list the item on a designated order book as described below. An assigned staff member performs a periodic inventory of the stock to identify those products that have a stock level at or below the reorder point. When the inventory is reduced to or below the order point, designated pharmacy personnel initiates a purchase order or electronically transmits a purchase order to a drug wholesaler.

Many pharmacies will use an order book system, also called a want list or want book. When pharmacists or pharmacy technicians determine that a product should be reordered, they write the item in the order book. While this approach is simple, it provides the least amount of organized control over inventory. Its success is highly dependent upon the participation of staff. Therefore, it is usually not the sole method of inventory management and is often used in conjunction with one of the other systems mentioned previously.

Whatever system is used, pharmacy technicians are vital contributors. Fluctuations in the use of pharmaceuticals will most often be identified by the pharmacy technician. Examples might include high use of asthmatic medications by the emergency room or various clinics (i.e., epinephrine, albuterol, or inhaled steroids), high doses of psychotropic medications by psychiatry patients (i.e., haloperidol and thioridazine concentrates) or high dose narcotic use by one or more oncology patients. Alerting purchasing staff to orders for unusual amounts of medications helps avoid out of stock situations and facilitates optimal inventory management. There are several more sophisticated approaches toward inventory management such as the ABC analysis and the economic order quantity. For more detailed information on these inventory methods and to learn about inventory turnover rate calculation, see the third reference in the Recommended Reading section.

Drug Recalls

Pharmaceuticals will occasionally be recalled by a manufacturer and/or the Food and Drug Administration (FDA) for reasons such as mislabeling, contamination, lack of potency, or other situations affecting the product as packaged or labeled. It is imperative that a pharmacy have a system for a rapid removal of all products affected by recalls.

Recall notices are sent in writing to pharmacies by the manufacturer of the product or by drug wholesalers. These notices indicate the reason for the recall, the name of the recalled product, the manufacturer, all affected lot numbers of the product, and instructions on how to return the product to the manufacturer. Upon receipt of the recall notice a pharmacy staff member, usually a pharmacy technician, will check the pharmacy and the institution to determine if recalled products are in stock. If none of the recalled products are in stock, a note indicating "none in stock" is written on the recall notice and filed in a recall log to document that the recall was properly addressed. If a recalled product is in stock, all products should be gathered, packaged, and returned to the manufacturer according to the instructions on the recall notice. The package should be reviewed by the pharmacist in charge prior to sending it. If patients have received a recalled product, the pharmacist in charge must take the recommended action. Upon completion of all activity regarding the product recall, a summary of actions taken should be written on the recall letter and filed in the pharmaceutical recall log. Keep in mind that it may be necessary to order more stock to compensate for those items that were recalled. In some instances, the recall may encompass all products and it will not be possible to order replacement stock.

ORDERING AND BORROWING PHARMACEUTICALS

Pharmaceutical Purchasing Groups

Most health-system pharmacies are members of a pharmaceutical purchasing group. Health systems and hospitals join together in a purchasing group to take advantage of the lower prices manufacturers offer to a large group that can guarantee a large volume of orders over long period of time (typically 1–2 years). This technique also reduces the time staff spend establishing and managing purchasing contracts. A purchasing group guarantees the price for pharmaceuticals over a contract period, which is usually one or more years. With the purchase price predetermined, the pharmacy can order the product directly from the manufacturer or from a wholesale supplier.

Direct Purchasing

Direct purchasing from a manufacturer involves the execution of a purchase order between the pharmacy and the manufacturer of the drug. The advantages of direct purchasing includes not having to pay any handling fees, the ability to order on an infrequent basis (i.e., once a month), and a less demanding system for monitoring inventory. The disadvantages include the need for a large storage capacity, dependency on the shipping firms used by the manufacturers to ship products, large amount of cash invested in inventory, and increased staff in pharmacy and accounts payable departments to prepare, process and pay purchase orders to many companies.

For most pharmacies, the disadvantages of direct ordering outweigh the advantages. As a result, the majority of health-system pharmacies primarily purchase through a drug wholesaler. There are some drugs that can only be purchased directly from the manufacturers such as some vaccines, growth hormone muromonab (OKT3®), anti-thymocyte globulin (Atgam®), and other products that require unique control or storage conditions. Consequently, most pharmacies will have a combination of direct purchases from manufacturers and drug wholesalers.

Drug Wholesaler Purchasing/ Prime Vendor Purchasing

Purchasing from a drug wholesaler permits the acquisition of drug products from different manufacturers through a single vendor. When a health-system pharmacy agrees to purchase the majority (80–95%) of its pharmaceuticals from a single wholesale company, a prime vendor arrangement is established, and customarily, a contract between the pharmacy and the drug wholesaler is developed.

Usually, the wholesaler agrees to deliver at least 95–98% of the items on schedule; offers a 24-hour emergency service; provides the pharmacy with electronic order entry devices, a computer system for ordering, bar-coded shelf stickers, and a printer for order confirmation print-outs; and a highly competitive service fee (1–5%) above cost and contract pricing. These types of services make the establishment of a prime vendor contract appealing and result in the following advantages: reducing order turnaround time, reducing time pharmacy personnel spend creating purchase orders, reducing inventory and carrying costs, reducing the amount of record keeping the pharmacy staff must do, providing computer generated utilization lists of pharmaceutical purchased, and rapid resolution of pharmaceutical ordering problems (i.e., credits and returns). Purchasing through a prime vendor customarily allows for drugs to be received shortly before use, creating a "just-in-time" ordering system. This is a highly efficient and cost effective approach toward pharmaceutical purchasing and inventory management.

Borrowing Pharmaceuticals

No matter how effective a purchasing system is, there will be times when it will be necessary to borrow drugs from other pharmacies. Most pharmacies have policies and procedures addressing this process. Borrowing or loaning drugs between pharmacies is usually restricted to emergency situations and limited to authorized staff. Borrowing is also limited to products that are commercially available, thus eliminating items such as compounded products or investigational medications. Most institutions have developed forms to document and track merchandise that is borrowed or loaned (Figure 11-8). These forms also help staff document the details imperative to error free transactions.

The department's borrow and loan policies and procedures should provide detailed directions on how to borrow and loan products, which products may be borrowed or loaned, and sources for them. Securing the borrowed item may require the use of a transport or courier service, or may include the use of the institution's security staff or other designated personnel. Knowledge of this information is vital for pharmacy technicians to understand and fulfill their responsibility when borrowing and loaning products.

PRODUCTS REQUIRING SPECIAL HANDLING

Most pharmaceuticals will be handled and processed in the inventorying and purchasing systems described above, with the exception of controlled substances, investigational drugs, compounded products, repackaged drugs, and drug samples.

Controlled Substances

Controlled substances have specific ordering, receiving, storage, dispensing, inventory, record keeping, return, waste, and disposal requirements established under the law. The *Pharmacist's Manual: An Informational Outline of the Controlled Substances Act of 1970* and the ASHP Technical Assistance Bulletin on Institutional Use of Controlled Substances provide

Community Pharmacy
555-3779

Borrowed   Lent
   From: _____   To: _____
Drug: _____
Amount: _____
              (# of vials, tablets, etc. and bulk or unit dose packaging)

Date:_____   By: _____

****

Date ordered:_____From: _____ By: _____
Date returned:_____ By: _____
Date in Loan Book:_____ By: _____
Value: $_____

Figure 11-8. Borrow/Loan form.

detailed information on the specific handling requirements for controlled substances.

There are two principles regarding controlled substances that the pharmacy technician should know: ordering and receiving schedule II controlled substances requires special order forms and additional time (1–3 days), and these substances are inventoried and tracked continuously. This type of inventory method is referred to as a perpetual inventory process. Pharmacists and, in some institutions, pharmacy technicians work with pharmacists to manage inventory, dispense, store, and control narcotics and other controlled substances.

Investigational Drugs

Investigational drugs also require special ordering, inventorying, and handling procedures. Generally, the use of investigational drugs is categorized into two distinct areas: (1) investigational drugs used in a formal protocol that was approved by the institution, and/or (2) investigational drugs used for a single patient on a one-time basis that has been authorized by the manufacturer and the Food and Drug Administration. In both cases the physician is generally responsible for the ordering and the pharmacy staff handles the inventory management of the investigational drug. Pharmacy technicians often prepare or handle investigational drugs and participate in the required perpetual inventory recordkeeping system. Again, it is important for pharmacy technicians to learn the department procedures for investigational drugs and to be

active contributors to the proper handling, storage, and inventory systems.

Compounded Products

Compounded products are another type of product handled by the pharmacy and unlike drugs ordered from an outside source, compounded products are produced in the pharmacy. These products may include oral liquids, topical preparations, or sterile products.

The use of these products requires that prescribing patterns and expiration dates be monitored closely. Compounded products typically have short expiration dates ranging from days to months. Since it is likely that pharmacy technicians will identify usage patterns and determine stock and product needs, procedures for monitoring patient use, product expiration dates, and additional stock needs must be well known and adhered to by technicians to prevent stock shortages.

Repackaged Pharmaceuticals

While most drugs are supplied by manufacturers in a prepackaged unit dose form, there are some products that the pharmacy staff is responsible for packaging. These items are generally unit-dose tablets and capsules, unit-dose oral liquids, and some bulk packages of oral solids and liquids. Each pharmacy establishes stocking mechanisms for these products and relies upon pharmacy technicians to identify and respond to production and stock needs. Generally prepackaging activities are coordinated by designated technicians, but some pharmacies may integrate repackaging with other pharmacy technician responsibilities. Knowledge of the department's procedures for repackaging is required in order to prevent disruptions in dispensing activities.

Nonformulary Items

Nonformulary items also require special handling. No matter how much planning is devoted to formulary management, there will be patients who need medications not routinely stocked in the pharmacy. It is usually the pharmacist who determines when a nonformulary medication should be ordered into stock. However, the pharmacy technician is often in the best position to monitor the supply and determine when and if additional quantities should be ordered. Since nonformulary medications do not have a set storage location in the pharmacy, they fall outside normal inventorying mechanisms. Consequently, manual tracking mechanisms and computer system queries of active nonformulary orders are the two most common techniques used to monitor and order these products.

Medication Samples

The last products requiring special handling are medication samples. Traditional inventory management and handling practices do not work well with medication samples for two reasons. First, medication samples are not ordered by the pharmacy. They are usually provided to physicians by the drug manufacturer free of charge, oftentimes without the pharmacy's knowledge. Second, samples are not usually dispensed by the pharmacy. These factors make it difficult to know who to contact if a medication sample is recalled and to ensure that medication samples are not sold. Due to difficulties in controlling samples, most institutions allow samples to be stored and dispensed in ambulatory clinics only after being registered with the pharmacy for tracking purposes. These difficult logistical and control factors have led many institutions to adopt policies that do not allow medication samples at all.

If your institution does allow samples, they will probably be stored outside the pharmacy and require that pharmacy personnel register and inspect the stock of medication samples. Pharmacy technicians are sometimes involved in inspecting medication sample storage units. These technicians are often responsible for deter-

mining if a sample is registered with the pharmacy, stored in acceptable quantities, labeled with an expiration date that has not been exceeded, and generally stored under acceptable conditions. Review your department's policies and procedures regarding medication samples to learn the role of the pharmacy technician.

PROPER DISPOSAL AND RETURN OF PHARMACEUTICALS

Expired Pharmaceuticals

The most common reason drugs are returned to the manufacturer is because they are expired. The process for returning drugs in the original manufacturer packaging is straight forward and not particularly time consuming if done routinely. Returning expired products to the manufacturer or wholesaler prevents the use of these products, while enabling the department to receive either full or partial credit for them. To return products, pharmacy personnel must complete the paperwork required by the manufacturer/wholesaler and package the product so that it may be shipped. Technicians often perform these duties under the supervision of a pharmacist. Some pharmacies contract with an outside vendor that completes the paperwork and coordinates the return of these products for an agreed upon fee. In this case, the pharmacy technician need only assist the returned goods vendor with the location and packaging of expired pharmaceuticals.

Pharmaceuticals compounded or repackaged by the pharmacy department cannot be returned and must be disposed of after they have expired. It is important to dispose of these products for safety reasons. Proper disposal prevents the use of subpotent products or products where sterility can no longer be guaranteed. The precise procedure for disposal is dependent upon the type and content of the product. Some products such as expired repackaged solids can be disposed via the general trash removal system, while others such as expired compounded cytotoxic products must be disposed of according to hazardous waste removal procedures. Each institution has detailed procedures for hazardous waste removal and the pharmacy technician should be familiar with these procedures. Disposal of expired compounded or repackaged pharmaceuticals by the pharmacy technician should be completed under the supervision of the pharmacist.

Another type of product requiring disposal rather than return is chemicals. Most pharmacies will stock a supply of chemical grade products for compounding external or oral pharmaceutical products. Examples of chemical products include sodium benzoate or sodium citrate (preservatives), lactose or talc (exipients), and active ingredients such as hydrocortisone, triamcinolone, neomycin, or lidocaine powders. When such products expire, they should be disposed of in accordance with the institution's hazardous waste procedures.

Expired controlled substances are disposed of via a unique process. These products may not be returned to the manufacturer or wholesaler for credit. They must be destroyed and the destruction must be documented to the satisfaction of the Drug Enforcement Administration (DEA). The DEA provides a specific form, entitled "Registrant's Inventory of Drugs Surrendered" (Form 41), for recording the disposal of expired controlled substances (Figure 11-9). The actual disposal of expired controlled substances should be completed by a company sanctioned by the DEA or by a representative of the state board of pharmacy. The DEA disposal of controlled substances form should be completed properly and submitted to the DEA immediately after the disposal has occurred. A copy of the record of disposal form will be signed by a DEA representative and returned to the pharmacy where it is kept on file. Previously, the DEA allowed for shipment of expired controlled substances and the completed disposal form to the regional DEA office, but this practice is no longer permitted.

The usage and disposition of investigational drugs must also be documented carefully. Expired investigational drugs should be returned to the manufacturer or sponsor of an investigational drug study according to the instructions they provide. The pharmacy technician may be responsible, under the supervision of the pharmacist, for the completion of paperwork, packaging, and shipment of the expired investigational agents. Investigational drug products that expire due to product instability or sterility issues should never be discarded. These doses should be retained with the investigational drug stock and be clearly marked as expired drug products since the investigational study sponsor will need to review and account for all expired investigational drug products.

Pharmaceuticals that need to be returned due to an ordering error require authorization from the original supplier and the appropriate forms.

The Prescription Drug Marketing Act mandates that the authorization and retention of records of returned pharmaceuticals be maintained by pharmacies in order to prevent potential diversion of pharmaceuticals. The pharmacy technician must be familiar with pharmacy department procedures for returning medications to a supplier. Typically, a pharmacy will have a process for returning mis-ordered medications to the prime drug wholesaler on a routine basis. This prevents the need for storage of overstocked or misordered products in the pharmacy. The pharmacy technician may be responsible for the completion and filing of paperwork and the packaging of returned products under the supervision of the pharmacist.

BILLING AND CREDITING PHARMACEUTICALS

The use of computers in institutional pharmacy has reduced the amount of time pharmacy personnel devote to dispensing and billing functions. Most institutional pharmacies have a computer system that manages both dispensing and billing functions. In a computerized charge-on-dispense system, billing functions occur on-line when the prescription is dispensed or when a list of all the medication that will be dispensed that day (called a fill list) is generated. Therefore, manual accounting actions are not required by the pharmacist or pharmacy technician; but what is required is an understanding of how the computer system charges for pharmaceuticals. Inaccurate order entry or changes to a patient's therapy may require that the patient receive a credit. All pharmacy technicians must learn how to credit a patient's record correctly.

In pharmacies with on-line billing functions, pharmacy technicians may be responsible for completing routine credit functions. With a charge-on-dispense system, pharmaceuticals are credited when unused doses are returned from patients' supplies. This may be associated with the discontinuation of a medication, discharge of a patient, or with unused p.r.n. medications. Generally, crediting functions are completed in conjunction with the daily exchange of unit dose cassettes or IV additive deliveries. Returned drugs are recorded on the proper patient record (e.g., medication fill list or IV admixture list) and then entered into the computer system. Patient name, account number, medical record number, pharmaceutical name and item number, units to

292 | Manual for Pharmacy Technicians

Figure 211-9. Registrants Inventory of Drugs Surrendered, (DEA Form 41).

Source: Drug Enforcement Administration.

Community Hospital
Suburbia, MD 20777

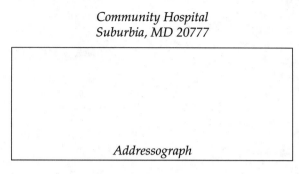

Addressograph

Instructions

After using medication, place patient information in area marked "Addressograph." Return completed form to PHARMACY to receive a resupply of medication. This form is necessary to make an exchange.

Operating Room Reservoir Stock Drug Tray		
Acetylcholine intraocular 20 mg	6017	
Atropine opth sol 1% 1 ml	6124	
Balanced salt sol 15 ml	6168	
Betamethasone inj 6 mg/ml 5 ml	6149	
Blephamide opth oint 3.5 g	7737	
Chymotrypsin opth sol 750 units	6261	
Cyclogyl opth sol 1% 2 ml	6318	
Cyclogyl opth sol 2% 2 ml	6320	
Erythromycin opth oint 3.5 mg	6998	
Fluorescein inj 10% 5 ml	6757	
Gentamicin opth oint 3.5 mg	6781	
Glycerine ann. opth sol 7.5 ml	6790	
Homatropin opth sol 5% 1 ml	6828	
Maxitrol opth oint 3.5 g	6469	
Methylene Blue inj 1% 10 ml	6624	
Methylprednisolone inj 40 mg/ml (respository)	6640	
Microfibrillar collagen hemostat	6661	

A sample manual charge ticket utilized for floor stock, emergency drug tray, or other stock medications that must be key punched into a computer system.

Figure 11-10. Stock Replacement form.

be credited, and reasons for credit are information fields that may require completion upon computer order entry. Therefore, use of a patient fill list or IV admixture fill list minimizes the need to search for this information and facilitates the efficiency of the crediting process. Pharmacy technicians should review departmental crediting procedures so they can help avoid incorrect patient charges and can maintain the accuracy of inventory.

Some pharmacies will issue or dispense medications and supplies to an inpatient unit or clinic for their stock. In this situation a manual charging system may be used in conjunction with the computer system. When a nurse or physician uses a medication or supply item from stock for a patient, the manual record is completed. The manual record is then sent to the pharmacy and a pharmacy technician, billing clerk, or office personnel charges the patient in the computer system. In this system the accuracy of the billing is dependant on how complete the form is because the data (i.e., name, account number, etc.) required to initiate the charge must be filled in by the staff member submitting the record. To improve the completeness of the form, many pharmacies provide preprinted order forms (Figure 11-10).

The use of automated dispensing machines, as mentioned earlier in the chapter, has eliminated much of the manual billing and crediting for stock medications. These machines interface with the pharmacy dispensing and billing system, and thereby eliminate most of the manual paperwork.

Finally, the non-computerized pharmacy may use handwritten records to create a system for both billing and crediting. In this situation, patient medication profiles or dispensing records have a section that details all the pharmaceuticals dispensed and credited. The medication profile/dispensing record is then used by a designated technician or clerical staff to enter into a computerized or manual billing system.

SUMMARY

The movement of pharmaceuticals into and out of the pharmacy requires an organized, systematic, and cooperative approach. The pharmacy technician plays a vital role in maintaining the functionality of these systems. Pharmacy technicians' familiarity with product conditions and uses puts them in a position to identify quality and care issues that can strengthen the purchasing and inventory control system.

RECOMMENDED READING

American Society of Hospital Pharmacists. ASHP statement on the formulary system. *Am J Hosp Pharm.* 1983;40:1384–5.

Wetrich JG. Group purchasing: an overview. *Am J Hosp Pharm.* 1987;44: 158–92.

Bicket WJ, Gagnon JP. Purchasing and inventory control for hospital pharmacies. *Top Hosp Pharm Manage.* 1987;7(2):59–74.

Yost RD, Flowers DM. New roles for wholesalers in hospital drug distribution. *Top Hosp Pharm Manage.* 1987;7(2):84–90.

Roffe BD, Powell MF. Quality assurance aspects of purchasing and inventory control. *Top Hosp Pharm Manage.* 1983; 3(3):62–74.

Soares DP. Quality assurance standards for purchasing and inventory control. *Am J Hosp Pharm.* 1985;42:610–20.

Kroll DJ. The pharmacy technician as a purchasing agent. *J Pharm Tech.* 1985; 1(1):29–31.

U.S. Department of Justice Drug Enforcement Administration. *Pharmacist's manual: an informational outline of the Controlled Substances Act of 1970.* 5th ed. Washington, DC; Apr 1986.

American Society of Hospital Pharmacists. ASHP technical assistance bulletin on institutional use of controlled substances. *Am J Hosp Pharm.* 1987;44: 580–9.

Hughes TW. Automating the purchasing and inventory control functions. *Am J Hosp Pharm.* 1985;42: 1101–7.

American Society of Hospital Pharmacists. ASHP technical assistance bulletin on use of controlled substances in organized health-care settings. *Am J Hosp Pharm.* 1993;50:489–501.

SELF-ASSESSMENT QUESTIONS

1. Which of the following methods of maintaining a formulary is more convenient and yields the most current product information in a purchasing and inventory system?
   a. formulary book
   b. computerized formulary

2. The formulary contains important information to assist the pharmacy technician in which of the following areas of product information?
   a. identification of trade names of products
   b. identification of product concentration
   c identification of package size
   d all of the above

3. Receiving and storing pharmaceuticals is a simple process that should be reserved solely for trainees and other inexperienced staff.
   a. True
   b. False

4. When receiving a shipment of pharmaceuticals the packaging slip should be used to check in the order.
   a. True
   b. False

5. Reviewing the product's expiration date is not a part of the receiving process.
   a. True
   b. False

6. When documenting the receipt of pharmaceuticals for which the purchase order or manufacturer's invoice cannot be located, which of the following information should be recorded?
   a. product name and amount
   b. product name, strength, and amount
   c. date of receipt, product name, and amount
   d. date of receipt, name of receiver, product name, strength, dosage form, and amount

7. A receiving copy of a purchase order is not required to check in an order if a manufacturer's invoice is available.
   a. True
   b. False

8. Reading a pharmaceutical product label three times is a legal requirement for pharmacists and is a practice pharmacy technicians are not encouraged to use.
   a. True
   b. False

9. Describe three product handling issues that a pharmacy technician should monitor to maintain and improve the quality of the inventory management system.

10. A want book ordering system is necessary when a minimum-maximum level system is used in a pharmacy purchasing system.
    a. True
    b. False

11. Describe three patient care situations that might require adjustment of the pharmacy's inventory level on a short-term basis.

12. The most important consideration in processing a manufacturer's recall notice is
    a. timely response in checking the inventory.
    b. timely response in removing affected products from the inventory.
    c. receiving proper credit from the manufacturer.
    d. a and b

13. Describe the primary benefits of being a member of a pharmaceutical purchasing group.

14. List two advantages of purchasing pharmaceuticals directly from the manufacturer.

15. List four disadvantages of purchasing pharmaceuticals directly from the manufacturer.

16. List three advantages of a prime vendor arrangement.

17. Effective purchasing and inventory systems make the need for a borrow and loan system obsolete.
    a. True
    b. False

18. Schedule II medications can be ordered in the same manner as all other pharmaceuticals.
    a. True
    b. False

19. Describe a few situations in which investigational drugs are used in patient care and identify who is customarily responsible for ordering investigational drug products.

20. Medication samples are routinely ordered by the pharmacy and dispensed directly to patients as ordered by the physician.
    a. True
    b. False

21. List the necessary data elements to credit a patient for pharmaceuticals.

22. List two situations that create a need to credit a patient for pharmaceuticals.

23. Schedule II controlled substances that have expired cannot be returned to a manufacturer for credit.
    a. True
    b. False

24. Investigational drug products that have expired should be discarded by pharmacy staff because there is no credit issued for expired investigational drugs.
    a. True
    b. False

ANSWERS TO SELF-ASSESSMENT

1. b. An on-line computerized formulary is generally more current than printed formularies and it can be searched more rapidly.

2. d. The formulary serves as a valuable reference in determining all aspects of product information required in a pharmaceutical purchasing system.

3. b. Receiving and storing of pharmaceuticals is an important process that should be performed routinely by experienced pharmacy staff. However, it is important for trainees and inexperienced staff to learn the receiving and storing process.

4. b. The receiving copy of the purchase order should be used to check in a pharmaceutical order because it documents precisely what was ordered. The packing slip documents the products the supplier shipped and, if shipped in error, may be different than the products ordered.

5. b. Review of the expiration date for all pharmaceuticals received is an important process that prevents short-dated or expired products from entering the pharmaceutical inventory.

6. d. It is important to document essential information about the product, the receiver, and the date of receipt.

7. b. If shipped in error, the manufacturer's invoice may be different than the purchase order. A copy of the purchase order should be available to check in a shipment of pharmaceuticals.

8. b. It is an important practice for pharmacy technicians to read a label three times to prevent selection and preparation errors.

9. A pharmacy technician may contribute positively in the handling of pharmaceuticals by:
   • identifying look-alike pharmaceutical packaging,
   • identifying unclear or misleading labels on pharmaceutical products,
   • suggesting storage locations for products that will minimize selection errors.

10. a. A want book is necessary in a minimum-maximum order system to facilitate timely identification of products that need to be ordered.

11. A pharmacy technician may be able to identify:
    • increasing inventory requirement for seasonal products, such as asthma medications;
    • increasing inventory requirements of a particular patient requiring high doses of a pain medication;
    • decreasing inventory requirements following a period of high use of a particular product by one or more patients.

12. d. The most critical processes in responding to a manufacturer's recall is a review of the inventory for affected products and removal from the hospital's inventory.

13. The primary benefits of belonging to a pharmaceutical purchasing group include:
    • obtaining preferential pricing,
    • reduction of pharmacy staff time devoted to contract matters,
    • assurance of preferred pricing over a period of 1 year or more.

14. The primary advantages of purchasing pharmaceuticals on a direct basis include:
    • no handling fees,
    • ordering is required only on a periodic basis.

15. The major disadvantages of a direct purchasing program for pharmaceuticals include:
    • need for large storage capacity,
    • reliance on independent shipping firms,
    • large amount of money invested in the pharmaceutical inventory.

16. The major advantages of a prime vendor arrangement for the purchase of pharmaceuticals include:
    - reduced order turnaround time,
    - lower inventory and carrying costs,
    - readily available drug utilization data,
    - singular system for processing credits and returns.

17. b. Even highly effective purchasing and inventory systems do not eliminate the occasional borrowing or lending of pharmaceuticals.

18. b. Schedule II medications require the use of a specific order form and require a longer turnaround time for receipt of product.

19. Investigational drugs are used in patient care on a one-time only basis or as part of an ongoing study to treat multiple patients. The physician or primary investigator is customarily responsible for ordering investigational drugs.

20. b. Medication samples are not routinely ordered by the pharmacy and require a separate system for the pharmacy to monitor drug use and storage.

21. The essential data needed to credit a patient for a pharmaceutical include:
    - patient name,
    - patient account number or medical record,
    - pharmaceutical name or item number,
    - number of units to be credited,
    - reason for the credit.

22. Two situations that create a need to credit a patient for a pharmaceutical include:
    - incorrect order entry of a pharmaceutical product,
    - return of an unused tamper proof product.

23. a. Schedule II controlled substances must be destroyed and documented according to the requirements of the DEA.

24. Expired investigational products should never be discarded and should always be returned to the study sponsor.

12 | Computer Technology

Connie Larson, Pharm.D.

Computer technology is advancing rapidly. Although computers have become more advanced and complex, they have also become easier to use. Computers are used to generate our pay checks, pump gas into our cars, process our utility bills, keep track of our credit history, and assist in the administration of health care.

LEARNING OBJECTIVES

After reading this chapter the reader will be able to
1. Describe the differences between mainframe and personal computer systems.
2. Understand basic computer terminology.
3. Describe how automation impacts the drug distribution process.
4. List the types of computer-generated work lists pharmacies use.
5. Describe the difference between the automation needs for institutional and ambulatory care (AC) pharmacies.
6. List the different types of reports that management and staff can utilize.
7. Describe how technology is used to monitor the clinical status of patients.
8. Describe the advantages of using automation for inventory control.
9. Describe the features of an automated narcotic control system.
10. List three applications for bar coding in health care.
11. List the disadvantages of touch screen technology.
12. List the advantages of light pen technology.
13. Describe the future of voice recognition technology.
14. Describe the difference between decentralized and centralized automated dispensing systems.
15. Describe the limitations of automated dispensing systems.
16. List applications for process control devices.
17. Describe the advantages of paperless charting.

PHARMACY COMPUTER SYSTEMS

If your work place is not using computers, they probably will be implemented in the near future. Although computers are expensive investments for businesses and improper use can result in damage to the equipment as well as loss of crucial information, they generally improve the efficiency, productivity, and accuracy of our work, and reduce the cost associated with common tasks.

In order to capitalize on the investment and avoid the loss of information and damage of equipment, many institutions designate a knowledgeable person to manage the computer system and serve as a resource to staff. Designated personnel also ensure that safeguards are built to avoid accidental access to functions that could jeopardize the system. Pharmacy technicians should know who their staff resource person is and how to contact computer support personnel when they need assistance.

Mainframe versus Personal Computer-Based Systems

Working with computer systems requires a basic knowledge as well as some specific training for the system used in a technician's work place. There are different types of computers, and their unique characteristics make each suitable for different situations. Mainframe computers are large, expensive, powerful computers, designed to process large amounts of data that are shared by numerous people. Because they generate a lot of heat, mainframe computers need to be stored in large, temperature-controlled rooms. Institutional pharmacies use mainframe systems to access patient information (e.g., room number, age, sex, weight, and laboratory data). Ambulatory care pharmacies use mainframes to record patient prescriptions and access insurance and billing information.

Dummy terminals are an inexpensive way for a large number of users to access information from a central computer's memory. Dummy terminals are useless unless they are connected to a mainframe system. Dummy terminals allow pharmacies to access patient information, such as patient medication profiles and allergy information.

Minicomputers are smaller scaled mainframe computers. They are commonly used by several people within a small organization or by a department within a large organization. Minicomputers are used to form Local Area Networks (LAN). LANs are also commonly used by small groups of people.

Pharmacy personnel use minicomputers to access patient information just as they would use a mainframe.

Microcomputers or personal computers (PC) are stand-alone systems that run software pro-

grams and manage data accessed from a larger source such as a mainframe. PCs have traditionally been used for word processing, spreadsheets, database management, desktop publishing and telecommunication programs. With the advent of larger PCs that can be used as central file servers, many PCs can be interconnected in a LAN. This allows PC users to share information as needed, such as with a pharmacy order entry system. In the client/server model, LANs can be interconnected with other PCs, other LANs, minicomputers, and mainframes. In this scenario, information can be shared among the various systems. Today, PCs are as powerful as early mainframes and are available in desktop models, portable laptops, and hand-held models.

Interfaces are connections between two or more computer systems that enable data to be transferred. The interface can be uni-directional, allowing one-way information to be entered or removed, or bi-directional, which allows data to be sent back and forth from system to system. Building interfaces can be very complicated and expensive. The interface limits the amount of information you can receive from other departments that have their own system, such as the hospital laboratory. For example, interface applications provide patient laboratory data and input of pharmacy medication charges for institutional pharmacies and allow retrieval of patient insurance information and payment processing in ambulatory care pharmacies.

The number of pharmacy departments that use computer systems has increased from 63.9% in 1990 to 75% in 1992, based on two ASHP surveys. A computerized pharmacy system was defined in the surveys as a system that at a minimum maintains patient medication profiles and generates prescription or dispensing fill lists. In the 1992 survey 86% of the pharmacy departments had at least one microcomputer.[1]

As the practice of pharmaceutical care grows and pharmacists' responsibilities become more and more patient focused, the opportunity for technician involvement with computers will increase. Many of the tasks traditionally performed manually by technicians, such as cart filling, floor stock replacement, IV admixing and prepackaging, are now being modified so that some of the work can be done by computers.

Microcomputers are used for pharmacy activities such as quality assurance, drug information, drug utilization evaluations, adverse drug reaction reporting, nonformulary drug use and workload statistics computing. An on-line policy and procedure manual and drug formulary allows frequent updating. Technicians also play a larger role in the collection, input, and organization of such data into microcomputer systems.

The type of computers an organization or department may require depends on the users' needs, financial resources, and the systems already available within the organization. Pharmacy systems can be part of an institution's mainframe system or purchased separately as stand-alone systems. Several computer companies offer mainframe systems with pharmacy components and others offer stand-alone pharmacy systems (e.g., Digimedics, Cerner, HBO). If the basic system is not comprehensive, additional software can be purchased to help the pharmacy department meet its operational and informational needs.

Institutional Distribution Functions

Results of a 1992 ASHP survey noted that complete unit-dose drug distribution services were offered by 90% of the responding community hospital pharmacies.[1] Automation can have a significant impact in this area.

The type of computer system the pharmacy uses determines the type of information available to the pharmacy. Data that is input into a stand-alone pharmacy system can be entered manually or transferred into the system via an interface with the hospital's mainframe system. Depending on the complexity of the interface, the information the pharmacy receives through the interface could be simple demographic information or complete medication orders, lab results, and procedures. When an interface involves demographics only, then the pharmacy must input the patients' medication orders manually.

Databases

The pharmacy department or an institutional technology service specialist is responsible for building the system's database during the installation of the system. In order to enter patient medication orders or prescription information, a database must be in place to accommodate all the information that is unique to the institution or pharmacy such as room numbers, patient care areas, formulary medications, inventory, insurance and billing information. Tools that assist drug therapy monitoring by screening patient profiles for drug-drug, drug-food, drug-disease and drug-lab interactions, and also maximum dose, dose range and duplicate therapy checking, are often included with a system. However, maximum dose and dose range checking may require modifications.

System Security

Access to the pharmacy computer system is controlled by the use of sign-on passwords or numbers. These access codes identify the individuals using the system. Users should sign off the system so no one can enter patient orders under another's sign-on code. Different security levels can be programmed so that only pharmacists can verify medication orders and only authorized individuals can access databases.

Medication Order Entry

A patient record will have sections for demographic information and a medication profile. Medication orders are entered into the system by using predefined commands or menu options to select the type of medication order. Usually, the type of medication order (IV piggybacks (IVPB), syringe medications, large volume parenterals (LVP), and unit-dose products) determines the data input requirements and type of label that will be printed. For example, label requirements are different for IVPB, syringe medications, LVPs, and unit-dose products. Once you are in a medication section of the entry screen(s), short codes or mnemonics can be used for the medication (name, strength, and dosage form), medication and schedule or groups of medications specific to a medical service or physician. Medication order entry can be time consuming but short codes speed up the order-entry process by minimizing the number of keystrokes needed. Medications can also be searched for by entering the first few letters of a drug name, though this approach takes longer than the short code approach.

Other information that needs to be entered manually or automatically includes the medication administration schedule, the medication's start and stop date and time, charging information, label quantity, and any precautions or instructions that may be necessary for a label (e.g., protect from light).

After the medication order is entered, the pharmacy technician should make sure the right medication, dosing schedule, and dose was entered into the correct patient's profile. Medication orders entered by technicians must be verified by a pharmacist before they can be active. Institutions use a variety of methods to identify the orders that are awaiting verification. Some computer systems highlight or make unverified orders flash. Pharmacy technicians should familiarize themselves with the system used at their institution.

Patient Medication Profiles

Patient medication profiles are usually organized by medication type and/or by order of input. Active medication orders should be listed first and they should be separated from the discontinued medications. Discontinued medications should only be available for review upon entering an appropriate command or at the end of the profile.

If profiles are arranged by medication type the first section of the medication profile may list all scheduled unit-dose and bulk medications. The second section may list all scheduled IVPBs and syringe admixtures. The third section may list all prn medications. The fourth section may list all LVPs. Discontinued medication orders would be last and grouped as above. Medication orders within a medication-type might be listed alphabetically or from newest to oldest order. Also, certain medication orders should be readily identifiable on the patient's profile because of their type, examples include investigational drugs, restricted drugs, nonformulary drugs, and controlled substances (CS). Identification could be by a variety of means such as the use of a heading or asterisks. An example of this profile structure is depicted in Figure 12-1.

Work Lists

The organization of the profile dictates the types of work lists that can be generated. The typical pharmacy work list is used for unit-dose cart fill. The cart-fill work list extracts medication information from the patient profile to be used for dispensing medications for a patient. Work lists are also used for cart-fill updates, IV pick, IV fill, IV fill updates, and labels. Work lists contain patient-specific information with the exception of pick lists. Pick lists contain the quantity of each medication needed to provide multiple patients with a supply of medications for a specified time period (e.g., 12 or 24 hours), including the quantity of IV solutions and additives/medications to meet the needs for small and large volume parenterals. Work lists can be printed on a daily basis or as often as necessary depending on the computer system and the

pharmacy's requirements. A 24-hour cart fill is common, but often times IV admixtures are produced in batches (e.g., one batch per shift), to decrease waste. Other reports the pharmacy needs are admission, discharge, and transfer (ADT) notices to ensure that patient medications are delivered to the right place. Pharmacy systems also generate medication administration records (MAR) that are primarily used by the nursing staff.

Patient Record

ID #: 11111111   **Room #:**437 West   **Unit:** CCU

Name: Example, XYZ   **Doctor:**ABC

Allergy: penicillin

Sex: Male   **Age:**37   **Ht:**72 inches   **Wt:**84 kg

Admit Date: 5/3/98   **DRG:**127

Diagnosis/problem list: Congestive Heart Failure

Comments: PCN allergy—Ceftizoxime OK; received previously with no problems.

MEDICATION PROFILE
Scheduled Medications

5/4	Nitroglycerin oint	Dose: 2" top	q6hr
5/3	Digoxin tab 0.25 mg	Dose: 1 po	qAM
5/3	Aspirin EC tab 325 mg	Dose: 1 po	BID
5/3	Amiodarone tab 200 mg	Dose: 2 po	BID
5/3	Erythromycin 500 mg inj	IVPBq6hr	Stop date: 5/14/98
5/3	Ceftizoxime 1gm inj	IVPBq8hr	Stop date: 5/14/98

Prn Medications

5/4 Triazolam 0.125 mg tab Dose: 1 po qhs prn sleep

5/3 Acetaminophen
      325 mg tab   Dose: 2 po q4hr prn pain

IVs

5/3 Dobutamine 1000 mg in D5W 250 ml

Conc: 4 mg/ml

Infuse 5 mcg/kg per min

Note: send infusion sheet; patient wt. 84 kg

5/3 NaCl 0.9% 1000 ml

Infuse 125 ml/hr

Discontinued Meds

None

Figure 12-1. Profile structure.

Ambulatory Care Prescription Functions

Like institutional pharmacies, ambulatory care (AC) pharmacies want to streamline work flow, reduce costs, increase efficiency and productivity, and decrease errors. Computers have been useful to help realize these goals.

Generally, pharmacists lack the time to provide the needed level of clinical services such as patient counseling. Computers allow pharmacists to spend more time providing clinical services (pharmaceutical care). The type of information ambulatory care pharmacies manage is similar to the inpatient pharmacy (e.g., patient drug profile, inventory management). Computer functions important to an ambulatory care pharmacy operations are shown in Table 12-1.

An important distinction between an ambulatory care pharmacy and an institutional pharmacy is that ambulatory care pharmacies are responsible for billing and collecting payment for their products while institutional pharmacies may be responsible for billing, but not collecting payment. Ambulatory care pharmacies need payer and insurance carrier information and third-party billing functions as part of the computer database. These features allow the processing of insurance claims while the patient's prescription is being filled. Because health plans vary with regard to medications covered, co-payment, and generic substitution requirements, computers are instrumental in preventing pharmacies from dispensing prescriptions that are not in accordance with the payers insurance information.

In some cases an ambulatory care pharmacy may have access to inpatient records of its affiliated organization and vice versa. The sharing of information among practice settings promotes continuity of care because pharmacists in both settings can access their patient's drug profile to see what medications the patient was on as an inpatient or outpatient. However, care must be taken when a patient is admitted to the hospital because patients often receive their medications from more than one pharmacy. In such a case, the affiliated pharmacy's patient record may be incomplete.

Management Functions

Pharmacy departments are responsible for managing their resources effectively and controlling costs. Computers allow management and staff to

Table 12-1

Ambulatory Care Computer Functions

Database Maintenance
1. Drug file (medications and IV solutions)
   a. Mnemonics
   b. Brand and generic name
   c. Price structure
2. Physician file
   a. Phone number
   b. Address
   c. Drug Enforcement Administration (DEA) number
3. Clinical monitoring
   a. Drug-drug, drug-food, drug-disease, drug-lab interactions
   b. Dose range checking
4. Payer and insurance information

INTERFACES

Patient Information

1. Demographic information (age, address, phone, sex)
2. Allergies, weight, height, diagnosis
3. Insurance

Prescription Processing

1. Patient identification by:
   a. Name
   b. Patient number
   c. Prescription number
2. Prescription information
   a. Medication name, dose, route, frequency, duration, and expiration date
   b. Quantity of medication and refills if allowed
   c. Comments and special instructions
   d. Patient education material
   e. Receipts
3. Pharmacist verification of orders entered by technicians
4. Label generation
5. Price inquiry

Management Functions

1. Distribution reports
   a. Narcotic utilization records
2. Financial reports
   a. Billing information
3. Workload data
4. File maintenance

generate reports that can help evaluate and improve work flow and medication use. Printed reports give management the opportunity to analyze and interpret data more thoroughly. Some common and valuable reports used by management include monitoring nonformulary drug use, drug usage patterns, drug costs, productivity, work load, and pharmacist interventions. Intervention data can be useful for justifying clinical pharmacist positions or additional resources. The most useful report details the type of intervention (e.g., prevention of medication error), time spent, dollar impact, and significance of the intervention (e.g., life threatening situation). Unfortunately most systems do not have built-in reports so they must be "written" by the pharmacy department.

Patient-Monitoring Functions

Basic Patient-Monitoring Functions

Most computers automatically perform some patient-monitoring functions (i.e., clinical activities) such as checking for therapeutic duplications, drug-drug, drug-food, drug-disease, and drug-lab interactions and IV compatibility.

Therapeutic duplication checking detects patients on drugs in the same American Hospital Formulary Service (AHFS) pharmacologic-therapeutic classification or if there is more than one order for the same medication.

Drug-drug interaction checking identifies drugs in a patient's profile that may cause problems when taken concomitantly. For example, when terfenadine and ketoconazole are used together they can cause arrhythmias and death. The medication formulary database sets the level of significance related to the interaction. Some drug combinations have the potential to cause only minor problems, and the benefit of the combination may outweigh the risks.

Drug-food interaction checking informs the user that the patient has been prescribed a drug that has the potential to cause problems with certain foods. Often times, certain foods will decrease the efficacy of a drug or increase the likelihood of an adverse reaction. This interaction notification serves as a prompt for the pharmacists and other health care professionals to provide patient counseling in order to minimize problems.

Drug-disease interaction checking identifies drugs that may cause problems with the patient's medical condition. For example, aspirin can increase the risk of bleeding and is generally contraindicated for patients with hemophilia.

Drug-lab interaction checking detects medication orders that might interfere with certain laboratory tests.

IV compatibility programs check medication orders for potential problems with physical incompatibilities (e.g., precipitation of ingredients or color changes) and stability of components (e.g., greater than 10% decomposition of one or more components in an admixture in 24 hours or less).

If a problem is detected, the user will receive an alert message. As noted, when alerting the user most computer systems divide interactions into levels of significance and allow the pharmacist to document an action on the patient's profile when overriding the alert. The ability to print the interaction information and view or print a monograph related to the alert information is also available on most systems.

Be aware that these patient-monitoring functions are intended to assist the pharmacy staff in providing quality patient care, but oftentimes, can be a nuisance. For example, IV incompatibility information programs may alert inappropriately or not provide suitable information. Therapeutic duplication checks often alert for appropriate drug therapy combinations. Sometimes manipulation of the database settings in the medication formulary can decrease nuisance alerts. If not, turning off certain patient monitoring functions may be necessary. As time progresses, the quality of these monitoring functions should improve as feedback is given to computer software suppliers.

Additional Patient-Monitoring Functions

Other on-line patient-monitoring features include screening doses to make sure they don't exceed maximum dose or dosage range recommendations and screening for drugs that are contraindicated in patients who are pregnant or lactating. Institutions that use uncommon doses as part of protocols can customize dosing guidelines to suit specific populations (e.g., geriatrics, pediatrics, and neonatology). Pharmacokinetic monitoring programs are also common. These programs use patient specific data to generate dose and frequency recommendations.

An important patient monitoring tool that has grown in popularity in the provision of pharmaceutical care is on-line intervention documentation. Newer pharmacy systems are incorporating pharmacists' interventions as part of the order entry process. These systems guide the pharmacist through the pharmaceutical care model. Online documentation promotes continuity of care by improving communication among staff members. This function may be part of a pharmacy stand-alone system or a mainframe system. The information can then be downloaded to a PC and incorporated into a spreadsheet or database program for analysis.

Inventory and Narcotic Control

Pharmacy technicians typically play an active role in the areas of inventory and narcotic control. Computerization of inventory functions is useful in tracking costs, purchases and usage, wastage, discarded or outdated inventory, and items loaned to or borrowed from other pharmacies. The ability to generate purchase orders when a preset medication-specific reorder point is reached ensures adequate stock. Vendor computer files are useful for keeping records of purchase agreements for minimum order quantity, price, price payment policy, and return goods policy.

Narcotic control features commonly used are reports for daily controlled substance (CS) use by patients, quantities dispensed to nursing units or pharmacy areas, and error and discrepancy records. Most systems provide separate controls for schedule II drugs.

Computerized inventory records allow pharmacies to update their inventory upon receipt and dispersal, record and maintain records on all purchases of CS, and maintain records of expired CS. Appropriate security clearance is important for narcotic control records and should be limited to the technicians and pharmacists involved with record keeping. Automated dispensing systems (described later) can offer greater control of CS over traditional lock and key systems. Systems that dispense by dose offer the greatest control.

CURRENT TECHNOLOGY

Before available technologies are implemented, their contribution to the effective operation of the pharmacy and the benefits to be realized by the department must be weighed. These technologies require informed, educated operators who understand how technology can be used. The goal should be to increase quality and reduce errors in the most cost-effective manner. Automation can allow departments to maintain or increase the level of service without significant changes in staffing. The use of technology is much more likely to change the scope of a technician's responsibilities than result in job elimination. Current computer technology used in health care includes bar coding, touch screens, light pens, voice recognition, medication packagers and unit-dose apportionment systems, automated dispensing systems, process control devices, and paperless charting.

Bar Coding

Bar codes are a unique arrangement of lines (thick and thin) used to identify the item on which they are printed. The bar code identifies the drug name, strength, dosage form, lot number, and expiration date of a particular drug product. In order to translate the bar code, a hand held or fixed position scanner is needed. Some pharmacies, community and institutional, use bar codes to save time and promote accuracy when performing tasks such as ordering, distributing, returning inventory, billing patients for drugs dispensed, crediting patients for drugs returned, and filling and checking unit-dose carts.

Bar codes have helped health care teams ensure that the right patient receives the correct drug, dose, dosage form, via the correct route, and at the correct time. To do so in an institutional setting, bar codes are assigned to each nurse, medication, and patient.[2] Before the nurse gives a dose to a patient, the nurse scans her or his bar code, the patient's bar code, and the medication bar code. The system then verifies that the patient, medication, and time are correct. If an error exists, such as a contraindication (e.g., allergy) or incorrect medication or patient, the system notifies the nurse. If the system doesn't identify any problems, the nurse administers the medication, and the system charts it as given.

Bar codes are also used in the ambulatory care setting to verify the accuracy of filled prescriptions. In this situation, the stock medication bottle and the prescription and the prescription label are bar coded. The bar codes are then scanned to ensure that they match. If they don't, the pharmacist or technician is notified and the error is corrected.

Basically, bar codes present information in a manner that allows a computer to read it. Although bar coding systems accurately identify medications and patients, pharmacists and technicians should not rely on such systems completely. It is still important for pharmacists and technicians to check their work to ensure accuracy and appropriateness.

Touch Screens and Light Pens

Touch screen technology senses the location of your finger as it nears or touches a screen. Touch technology is limited because it has poor resolution and large fingers tend to be inaccurate. Light pen technology is similar to touch screen technology. A hand-held pen that contains a light-sensitive tip is used instead of your finger. This allows for better accuracy. Physician order entry systems often use light pen technology.

Voice Recognition

Voice recognition technology will eventually replace the need to use a keyboard to enter data. The goal of voice-input systems is for the system to recognize any person speaking and not just a particular voice. Currently most applications only recognize a particular voice and a limited number of words. Voice recognition technology is primarily used by physicians to transcribe patient discharge summaries. Some PC software packages use this technology for verbal interactions and it could be useful for documenting pharmacists' interventions or patient education in medical records.

Automated Packaging and Unit-dose Apportionment Systems

Computerization has improved the unit-dose packaging process tremendously. Prior to computers, unit-dose packaging was efficient but the manual preparation of template labels was very time consuming. Time is saved with computers because both steps occur simultaneously. In addition, most computer systems used for packaging can produce labels with bar codes and keep records to be used for quality assurance.

Automated Dispensing Systems

Traditional unit-dose drug distribution systems are very labor-intensive. The use of automation in this area is an important issue for hospital pharmacy departments. Automated dispensing systems save time and allow better control and tracking of inventory. An automated dispensing system is a storage, dispensing, and charging device for medications. The different systems vary with regard to storage capacity, amount of space needed for the device(s), functionality, cost, and the ability to store refrigerated medications.[3] There are two broad applications for these systems: decentralized (e.g., Pyxis MedStation, Baxter SureMed, Owen HealthCare Meditrol) and centralized (e.g., Baxter ATC-212, Automated Healthcare Automated Pharmacy Station [APS]).

Decentralized Systems

Decentralized systems are located in the patient care unit and usually contain floor stock medication and supplies, and controlled substances. The systems are designed to solve medication management problems such as lost billing charges, pilferage, narcotic diversion, and poor record keeping.[4] Health care professionals use automated dispensing systems to dispense medications, return medications, record medication waste, and generate reports among other things. For these reasons, they could replace current unit-dose systems and the need for satellite pharmacies to dispense.

System Access

To access the system, a code must be entered by the employee, which dictates the level of security. The menu of options available to each employee can be controlled to provide the desired level of security. Options, security, and codes for levels for pharmacy employees are usually assigned by the pharmacy computer system administrator. All functions are performed on a patient-specific basis and can be traced to an individual transaction. The actual dispensing of medications may be by single-dose or the system may allow access to limited quantities. Single-dose dispensing devices are less error-prone than systems that allow access to multiple drugs.

Technician Roles

Usually, technicians assume most of the responsibilities for the operation and stocking of the decentralized devices, which allows the pharmacist to spend more time on clinical activities.

Centralized Systems

Centralized systems are located in the central pharmacy and they are used to improve the manual unit-dose cart fill process. Currently, these systems cannot accommodate all dosage forms because of size or the need for refrigeration, so manual cart-fill systems must supplement these systems.

The Baxter ATC-212 is a device that packages patient-specific doses of oral solid medications. This system uses bulk medications that are unit-dosed at the time of dispensing. The system will print a pick list for items not stocked in the device. The system requires manual entry of patient medication orders unless it is interfaced with another system. Technicians are primarily responsible for stocking the device.

Advantages. Advantages of the systems like the ATC-212 include cost savings associated with purchases of bulk medications and the ability to alert the technician when medication canisters need to be refilled.

Disadvantages. Systems like the ATC-212 system do not stock unit-dose injectable medications and can only generate general pick lists (not patient-specific) when manually requested to do so.

Robotic Cart Fill

The Automated Pharmacy Station (APS) is another type of centralized system that combines bar code technology, a network system of micro-computers, a conveyor system, and a robot to pick drugs and place them into patient medication drawers. The APS cart fill process has a high degree of accuracy. The system is capable of generating bar coded labels for patient identification (ID) and medication drawer location. The system knows the patient's location and generates an alert if the patient has moved. It then prints a new bar code-printed name label if appropriate. The system will check the patient's profile and request that the drawer be placed on the conveyor if the patient has medications to be refilled. The APS system scans the patient ID bar code and then the robotic arm delivers the appropriate medications to the drawer. A manual fill list is generated for items not in the APS system's inventory. Return medications can be credited to a patient by scanning the medication and the patient bar code under the credit function.

Advantages. The strength of the APS system is the accuracy associated with the use of bar coding to identify patient drawers, and medications. Medications are returned to stock in their pre-assigned location by the robotic arm. Other important advantages of this system include good inventory control, removal of expired drugs from stock before they can be dispensed, and cart fill process suitable for having pharmacists check only manually picked medications. State laws will have to be reviewed to better determine what pharmacists must check when an automated system is in place. This technology is also used in the ambulatory care setting to fill patient-specific prescriptions.

Disadvantages. The disadvantage of the APS system is the requirement of proprietary cassettes, and special packaging materials and equipment to work with the system. Also, the time required to repackage unit-dose tablets is a distinct disadvantage of this system. However, an increasing number of wholesale companies are repackaging medications so they are ready for use in the machine.

Technicians are typically responsible for complete operation of this APS system, including packaging, stocking, inventory control, cart fill, manual fill, and troubleshooting.

Process Control Devices

Computerized pumps are often used in the IV admixture area of institutional pharmacies. Such computerized pumps are used to prepare adult and neonatal total parenteral nutrition (TPN). These prepare the base solution and add electrolytes and micronutrients. Other computerized pumps are available to fill batches of syringes.

Technicians are usually involved in the operation of these devices. Some common responsibilities include entering patient orders into the system, setting up the correct medication solutions, setting up log sheets for quality assurance purposes, and operating the device.

Paperless Charting

Paperless charting involves computerized patient medical records. Documentation consumes an excessive amount of nursing time and automation of the process should provide the nurse with more time for patient care. Many hospitals have installed bedside terminals for nursing documentation. An advantage of the system would be the on-line availability of the patient's record to any number of people simultaneously. There would be access to the patient's history from the moment of admission without having to wait for access to the patient's chart. On-line medical records would be ideal for audits, drug use evaluations, and retrospective studies.

CONCLUSION

Computers are everywhere. Students are learning how to use them in the classroom and use computers for their school work. Computer knowledge is a valuable resource to have for any job and computer courses are available at most community colleges, which often have convenient campus locations. Some large organizations may offer computer courses for their employees at no cost. In addition to the more traditional responsibilities that technicians perform, they play an important role in managing computerized systems so pharmacists have more time for direct patient care activities.

Computers can handle a wide variety of functions. Every year technology will expand to include more applications for pharmacy. Technicians can expect to see their roles change as new technologies are developed in health care.

RECOMMENDED READING

Blissmer RH. *Introducing Computers—Concepts, Systems, and Applications.* New York: John Wiley & Sons, Inc.; 1992–1993 edition.

Kinkoph, S, *et al. Computers—A Visual Encyclopedia.* Indianapolis, IN: Alpha Books; 1994.

REFERENCES

1. Crawford SY, Myers CE. ASHP national survey of hospital-based pharmaceutical services—1992. *Am J Hosp Pharm.* 1993;50:1371–404.
2. Hynniman CE. Drug product distribution systems and departmental operations. *Am J Hosp Pharm.* 1991;48:S24–35.
3. Perini VJ, Vermeulen LC. Comparison of automated medication-management systems. *Am J Hosp Pharm.* 1994;51:1883–91.
4. Lee LW, Wellman GS, Birdwell SW, Sherrin TP. Use of an automated medication storage and distribution system. *Am J Hosp Pharm.* 1992;49:851–5.

SELF-ASSESSMENT QUESTIONS

1. Mainframe computers are:
   a. large.
   b. expensive.
   c. powerful.
   d. all the above

2. Dummy terminals have the following characteristics *except*:
   a. inexpensive
   b. function as personal computers on their own
   c. useful for a large number of people to access the system
   d. can be hooked up to mainframe systems

3. Personal computers have the following characteristics *except*:
   a. can be used as a stand-alone system
   b. useful for wordprocessing
   c. cannot run software programs
   d. can manage data from a mainframe

4. An interface is not:
   a. a connection between two or more computer systems.
   b. necessary for the transfer of data between systems.
   c. uni-directional only.
   d. valuable for receiving information from other systems.

5. Responsibilities of technicians that can be enhanced by automation include:
   a. cart filling.
   b. floor stock replacement.
   c. IV admixing and prepackaging.
   d. all the above

6. Which of the following statements is true?
   a. Technicians can gather data for quality assurance (QA) activities and use computers to organize and input data.
   b. Only pharmacists can gather data for QA activities and use computers to input data.
   c. Technicians can be responsible for data collection only.
   d. Technicians cannot collect data but can use computers to input data for report generation.

7. Which of the following statements is not true?
   a. Pharmacy stand-alone systems must have an interface to the hospital mainframe to display patient demographic information.
   b. Pharmacy systems require a database to input patient data.
   c. Interfaces can supply laboratory results to the pharmacy system.
   d. Manual data input is simplified with the use of mnemonics.

8. Which of the following statements regarding medication entries to a patient profile is not true?
   a. Short codes and mnemonics speed up the order-entry process.
   b. There are separate pathways to enter different medication types.

c. Medications can be searched for by typing in part of the drug name.
d. The use of mnemonics prevents the wrong medication from being entered on a patient's profile.

9. Information needed on the patient's medication profile includes the follow *except*:
a. start date of the medication.
b. name and strength of the medication.
c. social history.
d. route of administration for each medication order.

10. The following statements regarding technician-entered medication orders are false *except*:
a. Technicians are not allowed to enter medication orders.
b. Technician-entered medications orders are active immediately.
c. Highlighting or flashing is used to identify technician-entered medication orders.
d. Once a medication order has been entered by a technician a pharmacist can not modify it.

11. Which of the following statements concerning sign-on or access codes is true?
a. Everyone uses the same code.
b. Sign-ons identify the individual using the system.
c. All pharmacy staff has the same level of security assigned to their access code.
d. A technician should not sign off before someone else uses the same terminal.

12. Common work lists that can be computer generated are:
a. cart fill
b. IV fill
c. cart fill pick
d. all the above

13. Goals for automation in the ambulatory care setting include all of the following *except*:
a. streamline work flow
b. increase productivity
c. increase efficiency
d. increase costs

14. Information needs of an ambulatory care pharmacy include the following *except*:
a. third-party billing database
b. price inquiry
c. co-payment amounts
d. patient room number

15. Which of the following statements regarding management reports is *not* true?
a. Intervention reports can be used to help justify pharmacist positions.
b. Report features are built into the systems.
c. Data generated from a report could be used to redesign work flow.
d. Commercially available software is available to simplify the report generation process.

16. Automation provides on-line clinical monitoring for:
a. drug-drug, drug-food, drug-disease, and drug-lab interactions.
b. IV incompatibilities.
c. therapeutic duplication.
d. all the above

17. The following statements regarding on-line intervention documentation are true *except*:
a. Provides continuity of care.
b. Allows information to be downloaded for report generation.
c. Provides a communication tool for other pharmacy staff.
d. Is only available on mainframe systems.

18. Inventory control system advantages include the following *except*:
a. tracks purchases
b. tracks medication usage
c. tracks inventory costs
d. tracks personnel expenditures

19. The following statements concerning narcotic control are true *except*:
a. A separate control system for CII drugs is not desirable.
b. Access to records should be restricted.
c. Record maintenance of narcotic purchases is desirable.
d. Automated dispensing systems are frequently used for narcotic control.

20. The following statements regarding the use of automation are true *except*:
a. Automation can change the scope of a technician's responsibilities.
b. Automation requires informed, educated operators.
c. Automation increases the potential for errors.
d. Automation can increase quality.

21. The following statements regarding the use of bar coding are false *except*:

a. Requires the use of a scanner to "read" the bar code information.
b. Bar codes can identify products only.
c. Scanners must be in a fixed position.
d. Bar coding is not useful for inventory control.

22. Touch screen technology has all of the following characteristics *except:*
a. The technology senses the location of a finger as it nears or touches the screen.
b. Touch screens are difficult for large fingers.
c. Touch screen technology has a high resolution.
d. Light pen systems are more accurate than finger systems.

23. Characteristics of voice recognition technology include all of the following *except:*
a. Most systems accommodate a particular voice only.
b. The technology recognizes a limited vocabulary.
c. Voice recognition could eventually replace manual entry of data.
d. Such technology has no application in health care.

24. Advantages of newer automated packagers are
a. computer-generated labels.
b. programming sets up packaging and labeling.
c. automated labeling can be bar coded.
d. all the above

25. Characteristics of automated dispensing systems include the following *except:*
a. Automated dispensing systems are storage, dispensing, and charging devices.
b. Decentralized automated dispensing systems are not useful for tracking inventory.
c. All functions are performed on a patient-specific basis.
d. The system requires entry of patient medication orders unless obtained from an interface.

26. Disadvantages of a central automated dispensing system using robotics include all of the following *except:*
a. Expired drugs must be manually removed from the system.
b. Special medication cassettes are required.
c. A special packager is required.
d. Special packages are required.

27. Automated dispensing systems using robotics require bar coding for all of the following *except:*
a. patient location label.
b. medications.
c. system operator.
d. patient ID label.

28. Advantages of automated dispensing systems using robotics include all of the following *except:*
a. Pharmacist checking of medication cassettes is quick using the bar code scanner.
b. Returned medications can be easily credited by scanning the patient ID label and the medication.
c. High degree of accuracy for filled medications can be achieved.
d. The system restocks itself.

29. Process control devices can
a. prepare base solutions for TPNs.
b. add electrolytes and micronutrients to TPNs.
c. batch fill syringes.
d. all the above

30. Features of paperless charting include the following *except:*
a. potential to decrease the amount of time the nurse can provide patient care.
b. on-line availability of the patient medical record.
c. ideal for obtaining data for audits.
d. bedside terminals keep the nurse by the patient.

ANSWERS TO SELF-ASSESSMENT

1. d. Mainframe computers are large, expensive, powerful computers, designed to process large amounts of data.

2. b. Dummy terminals are useless on their own.

3. c. Personal computers are stand-alone systems that can run software programs and manage data accessed from a larger source.

4. c. An interface can be uni- or bi-directional. Uni-directional interfaces send data to another system but can not receive input back. Bi-directional interfaces can send data back and forth.

5. d. Technicians' roles include cart filling, floor stock replacement, IV admixing, and pre-

packing, all of which are enhanced by the use of automation.

6. a. Increasingly technicians perform a variety of QA activities, which frees pharmacists for clinical activities.

7. a. An interface is not necessary to display this information. However, if an interface is not present, this information must be entered manually.

8. d. The only thing that will prevent the wrong medication from being entered on a patient's medication profile is careful entering and checking by technicians and pharmacists.

9. c. Patients' medication profiles contain medication information such as, name and strength, start date, and the route of the medication. Social history (e.g., married, single) is included in the patient's medical record.

10. c. Technician-entered medications orders must be identifiable by the pharmacist, and such orders are often identified by highlighting or flashing.

11. b. It is important that you sign-off immediately when you are finished so that no one else uses your code.

12. d. Work lists such as, cart fill, IV fill, and cart fill pick, are used by technicians to identify tasks to be completed.

13. d. Increased costs is not a goal in the use of automation. However, decreasing cost is one of the goals.

14. d. Patient room numbers are used in institutional pharmacies, not ambulatory care pharmacies.

15. b. Reports usually must be developed by the pharmacy.

16. d. Computers are capable of screening medication orders at the time of order entry for drug-drug, drug-food, drug-disease, and drug-lab interactions; IV incompatibilities and therapeutic duplication.

17. d. Intervention programs can be on mainframes interfaced to PCs or could be on a pharmacy stand-alone system without an interface.

18. d. Inventory control programs track issues related to medications not personnel.

19. a. A separate control system for CII is advisable because of the record keeping required for CIIs.

20. c. While there can be errors with any system manual or automated, automating a system is likely to decrease the potential for errors.

21. a. Scanners are needed to read bar codes and may be hand held or in a fixed position, such as, mounted into a table top, and items are waved over the top of the scanner to be read.

22. c. Poor resolution is one of the disadvantages.

23. d. Voice recognition technology has very important applications for health care. In the future, technology will be so advanced that a system will be able to recognize any voice input and convert it to the printed word. Health care professionals are likely to use this technology to document information in a patient's medical record.

24. d. Labels were previously prepared manually. Computer can be used to set up packaging and labeling, with provisions for bar coding labels if desired.

25. b. Automated dispensing systems are very useful for tracking inventory. The systems track dispensed medications, returned medications, wasted medications, and individual transactions.

26. a. Expired drugs are automatically removed when the robotic arm reads the medication's bar code.

27. c. During the cart fill process, bar coding of the medication, patient ID label, and patient location allow the robot to pick the right medication, for the right patient in the right location.

28. a. The bar code check of the filled cassette is very time consuming. Because of the system's high degree of accuracy it may be possible soon to eliminate the pharmacist check of machine-filled medications. Manual picks would still require a pharmacist's check.

29. d. Process control devices are computerized pumps that assist in the preparation of IV admixtures.

30. a. Increasing nursing time for patient care is a major advantage.

13 | Institutional Pharmacy Practice

Steven Lundquist, Pharm.D.

Institutional settings are facilities where patients receive health care in a structured manner, such as hospitals and nursing homes. Pharmacy plays an important role in institutional settings. The primary responsibility of the pharmacy department is to provide medications and services that help ensure safe and effective use of medications. However, the scope of responsibilities for pharmacy is ever changing and expanding to meet the challenges of rising health care costs, reduced health care resources, and advances in technology.

Institutional pharmacy practice centers around products and patient care services. Traditional product-focused services include procurement, storage, preparation, administration, and distribution of drugs and supplies to patients. Technicians are an integral part of the pharmacy team that provides these services. However, as the pharmacy profession continues to expand its realm of activities toward direct patient care, the responsibilities and opportunities for technicians also expand. This chapter provides a general overview of institutional pharmacy practice, discusses the current roles and responsibilities of pharmacy technicians, and identifies the potential impact the changing health care environment has for the pharmacy technicians. Although this chapter concentrates on institutional pharmacy practice, it does not describe all aspects. Refer to Recommended Reading for further detail.

LEARNING OBJECTIVES

After completing the chapter the reader will be able to

1. Describe the forces causing changes in health care practices in institutions.
2. Understand the differences between centralized and decentralized pharmacy services. Understand the roles and responsibilities of technicians in each of these different settings.
3. Understand and define a unit-dose system.
4. Be able to define pharmaceutical care and how it relates to the technician's new roles.
5. Be able to explain how quality control and quality improvement are used in institutional pharmacy practice.

HISTORICAL OVERVIEW AND CURRENT PRACTICES

Pharmacy services have existed in institutional settings in one form or another for many years. Pharmacy services 30 years ago usually consisted of a central pharmacy located in the basement of the hospital, which was very limited in its responsibilities and number of personnel. The focus was medication products including compounding, repackaging, and relabeling multi-dose supplies to be used by nurses for patient care. Bulk supplies of medications were often kept on the nursing station as floor stock. When a patient needed a medication, the nurse would obtain the medication from the floor stock, perform all calculations, and prepare the product. The nurse would also prepare all intravenous (IV) medications directly on the patient care floor without the use of a laminar flow hood.

Fortunately, the practice of institutional pharmacy has made tremendous advances over the last 30 years. Pharmacy has moved from a profession focused primarily on medication preparation and distribution to that of providing services to help get the best outcome from the drug therapy. This evolution has occurred as a result of many internal and external forces. Two major forces are the impact of new technology and the enormous burden placed on health care by rising costs and diminishing resources.

Technology and Pharmacy

Technology has impacted our normal daily living. We are able to obtain information and communicate easier and quicker with the use of cellular phones, satellites, fax machines, and computer networks. Technology has helped industries improve the speed and quality and increase the quantity of the goods they produce. These technological advances have certainly found their way into the health care system. Drug companies can now manufacturer mass quantities of medications in a ready to use unit-dose (which will be discussed later in this chapter). This has made a significant impact on pharmacy because it is not burdened with extemporaneous preparation of medications and the errors, waste, and cost associated with the process.

Another significant technological advance is automation. Automation technologies have replaced many of the manual tasks within pharmacy. Automation allows pharmacy technicians and pharmacists to devote more time and resources to patient-focused activities. Examples of automation in institutional practices are the micromix and automix machines and drug dispensing machines. The micromix and automix are used to prepare hyperalimentation solutions (see chapter 9). Automated drug dispensing machines (e.g., Pyxis®, Meditrol®, SureMed®, etc.) can be placed in a patient care area to allow health care providers to obtain medications at the point of use. These machines keep track of which medication was removed and to whom the medication is to be administered, as well as who removed the medication. A more detailed description and example of automation appears in chapter 12.

Computers are commonly used to streamline the medication use process and reduce the chance of making an error. For example, physicians are now entering medication orders directly into an institution's computer system. On-line entry of medication orders eliminates the need to transcribe, manipulate, or re-enter medication orders, and it generates a typed label that is affixed to the final product. Physician order entry significantly reduces the number of steps in the medication use process and can reduce interpretation and transcription errors and the time it takes to get medications to patients.

These are just a few examples of how technological advances reduce the time pharmacy personnel spend performing tedious tasks, increase productivity, and improve the quality of pharmacy services. Although automation has replaced certain tasks performed by technicians, it has also created new opportunities. Technicians are often given the responsibility of operating and maintaining these forms of automation. In addition, the time saved on traditional product-focused tasks can now be used to assist the pharmacist with patient-focused tasks. For example, technicians may be asked to obtain lab results for pharmacists to use when evaluating the appropriateness of certain drug regimens.[1]

Financial Implications

The financial burden on health care systems continues to have huge ramifications for patients and institutions. There are many reasons for increased health care costs: one example may be the Medicare and Medicaid legislation that allowed institutions to receive full reimbursement for fees determined by the physicians. This removed the incentive for institutions to control their costs and did not promote competition, which meant institutions were not stimulated to provide the best services at the lowest cost. Today, institutions and payers are trying to reduce costs and improve the quality of care by developing alternative practice settings, establishing reimbursement guidelines, and implementing changes to streamline patient care services.

Health care maintenance organizations (HMOs) are an example of an alternative practice setting. Employers may use an HMO to provide health benefits for their employees. The HMO centralizes the delivery of care to improve efficiency and reduce waste and cost. The reimbursement HMOs receive from the employer are capitated. This means that the HMO receives a fixed amount of money for each employee enrolled in the plan, regardless of the care the patient receives. Thus it is best for the HMOs if they provide cost-effective care with the focus on preventive care and wellness. Examples of other alternative practice settings include home health care, mail order prescription services, and managed care companies.

ORGANIZATIONAL STRUCTURE OF INSTITUTIONS

Health care institutions are usually organized into several levels of management. Managers at the top of an organization are primarily involved in setting a direction and vision for the hospital. As you move down the organizational structure, the responsibilities become more defined and are targeted to meet the goals of the hospital. Each level of management is designed to allow a diverse range of activities to be performed in an organized manner. Without clear levels of responsibility and a chain of command, the activities of employees would be unorganized, inefficient, and unproductive. Figure 13-1 is an example of a typical organizational structure.

At the top of an organization is the chief executive officer (CEO), president, or hospital director. The CEO helps set a direction for the hospital by creating a vision and mission for the institution. The CEO reports to the hospital's board of directors and is responsible for ensuring that necessary budget, personnel, and operations are in place to help achieve the mission of the hospital. The medical staff and the second level of management report directly to the CEO.

Hospitals usually have a chief operating officer (COO), or vice president, representing a second level of management. The COO is responsible for the daily operations of the hospital. Another second-level manager is a chief financial officer (CFO). The CFO is responsible for the financial management of the hospital. Because of the large number of personnel represented by nursing, another second level of management may be referred to as an associate director or vice president of nursing. The number of additional levels of management is a factor of the size and scope of services provided by the health care institution.

The individual departments within an organization are routinely grouped by either patient care (e.g., nursing, pharmacy, radiology), ancillary (e.g., materials management, environmental services), or support services (e.g., medical records information systems). Variations of this organizational structure are being used to improve quality of patient care, improve efficiency, and reduce cost. One example is the patient-focused care model (explained later in this chapter). Managers are given responsibility for all employees and activities provided to specific patient types (i.e. surgery, pediatric, or medicine patients). The philosophy is for the employees to function as a team with everyone having a role in providing patient care, regardless of discipline or the tasks performed.

PHARMACY DEPARTMENT STRUCTURE

The director or chief of pharmacy services is at the top of the pharmacy department hierarchy. The number and levels of management below the director of pharmacy depend on the department's size and scope of services. For example, a hospital affiliated with a university may need a manager to coordinate the residency program and another manager to coordinate pharmacy students, staff development, and all clinical pharmacy services. However, pharmacy department structure is most often based on the types of operations provided by the institution, such as centralized or decentralized pharmacy services.

Centralized Pharmacy Services

Centralized pharmacy services, as the name implies, handle pharmacy personnel, resources, and functions from a central location. Central

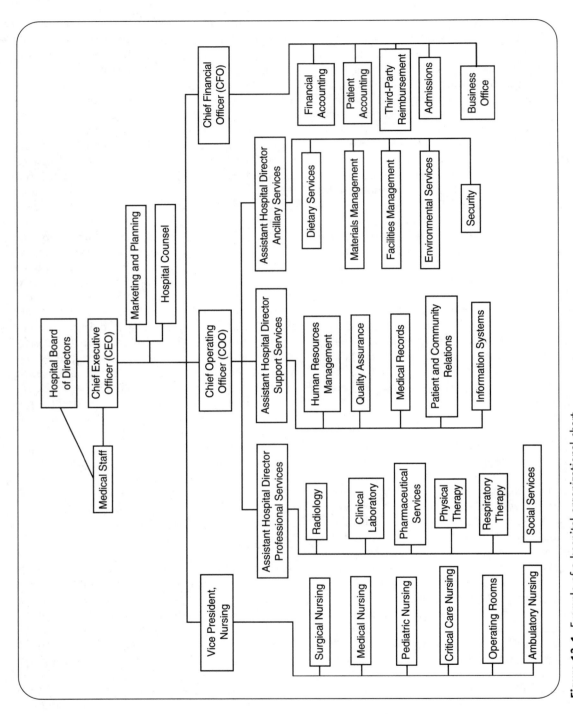

Figure 13-1. Example of a hospital organizational chart.

Source: Brown TR, editor. *Handbook of Institutional Pharmacy Practice*, 3rd ed. Bethesda, MD: ASHP; 1992.

pharmacies are often located in the basement of hospitals. A typical centralized pharmacy may contain an area for the preparation of intravenous medications (i.e., antibiotic piggybacks, large-volume parenterals with additives, total parenteral nutrition, chemotherapeutic agents), a medication cart filling area, an outpatient prescription counter, and a storage area for medications and supplies. Central pharmacy services are often used when resources (personnel, equipment, and space) are limited. The advantage of centralized services is that less staff is needed to control, store, inspect, prepare, and dispense medications for the entire institution.

The main disadvantages are the lack of face to face interactions with patients and other health care providers and the time it takes to deliver medications. Centralized pharmacies make it difficult for pharmacists to have access to the information needed to make appropriate therapeutic assessments of medication orders. The time to deliver medication orders to all areas of the institution from a central location may be slow.

The technician responsibilities in a central pharmacy may involve the preparation of IVs, hyperalimentation and chemotherapeutic agents, filling patient medication carts, delivering narcotics, extemporaneous compounding (i.e., products not available from a manufacturer), functions related to quality control and quality improvement, billing, and miscellaneous paperwork.

Decentralized Pharmacy Services

Decentralized pharmacy services do not replace centralized pharmacy services but are used in conjunction with a central pharmacy. Decentralized pharmacy services are provided from within a patient care area. The most common form of decentralized pharmacy is a pharmacy satellite. A pharmacy satellite is a designated area where drugs are stored, prepared, and dispensed for patients. Pharmacy satellites are often staffed by one or more pharmacist(s) and technician(s). The proximity of the pharmacy satellite to the patients and other health care providers gives the pharmacist more opportunities to interact with patients for the purpose of obtaining pertinent information, monitoring and assessing their response to drug therapy, and disseminating patient education materials. The pharmacist also has more opportunities to discuss the plan of care, answer drug information questions, and make appropriate drug therapy recommendations face to face with other health care providers.

The disadvantage of decentralized pharmacies is that it requires additional resources. Additional resources include personnel to staff a decentralized satellite, equipment (e.g., laminar flow hood, computers, printers), references, and a second inventory of medications and supplies.

The technician's role in decentralized pharmacies varies from institution to institution. The technician's role in the satellite is a major factor in the ability of the pharmacist to provide pharmaceutical care. Some responsibilities of satellite technicians are maintaining appropriate inventory (e.g., medications and supplies), keeping the inventory free of expired medications, cleaning and maintaining laminar flow hoods, and preparing all unit-dose and intravenous medication orders in a timely fashion. Experienced technicians may also answer some questions from nurses and make judgments on when to refer a question to the pharmacist. Thus, some technicians are responsible for all aspects of running the satellite under the supervision of a pharmacist.

Use of Clinical Practitioners

Pharmacy departments may also be structured by nonproduct services. An example may include services referred to as patient-focused care that requires the use of clinical pharmacy skills. A clinical practitioner is a pharmacist who provides patient-focused care. Clinical practitioners are involved in all aspects of drug therapy to ensure appropriate, safe, and cost effective care. Patient-focused care is accomplished by ensuring all patient-specific problems requiring drug therapy are being treated, that the medication selected is appropriate for the indication, that the dose ordered is correct, and that the dosage form and administration technique meet the patient's needs. After the medication has been administered, clinical practitioners will monitor the effects of the medication through laboratory results (e.g., drug levels, culture and sensitivity results, or serum creatine) as well as patient-specific parameters (e.g., heart rate, temperature, or respiration rate). Clinical practitioners also have a significant role in the education of patients and other health care providers regarding the use of medications. A clinical practitioner spends most of the time directly with patients and in the patient care area.

PRODUCT-FOCUSED SERVICES

Pharmacy services are changing and expanding. However, pharmacy is still responsible for the provision of medications directly to patients or other health care providers who care for patients. Fulfilling the responsibility efficiently requires that several processes, such as ordering, storing, preparing, delivering, administering, documenting, and monitoring are integrated properly.

As an example, in order for a patient to receive one acetaminophen tablet the following steps must have occurred. First, the drug has to be in the inventory. This means it was ordered from the manufacturer, received, inspected, stored, inventoried, and periodically reviewed to ensure that it has not expired. Next the medication order must be received and processed by the pharmacy so the drug can be dispensed and delivered to the nursing station. Once at the nursing station the drug is administered to the patient, and the dose is documented. In the past, compounding and repackaging was part of this process. However, the advent of a unit-dose drug distribution system eliminated this time-consuming process for most of the solid dosage forms dispensed.

Investigational drug services, if provided by the institution, represent another form of product-focused service in which the technician can play an important role. The technician may be involved in the record keeping, inventory control, preparation, and dispensing of investigational drugs. This is an important responsibility because the validity of the results and conclusions of every drug study depend on the accuracy of the dispensing records.

Unit-dose System

Unit-dose drug distribution systems prepare medications in a single unit package. In other words, the package contains a single dose that is ready to be administered to a patient. Understanding a unit-dose system is essential because technicians spend a significant part of their time obtaining, preparing, and labeling medications in a unit-dose form.

Unit-dose drug distribution systems allow a limited number of doses (usually a 12- or 24-hour supply) to be dispensed in unit-dose medication carts or via automated floor stock systems. The advantages of using a unit-dose system are listed below:[2]

1. A reduction in the incidence of medication errors.
2. A decrease in the total cost of medication-related activities.
3. A more efficient use of pharmacy and nursing personnel, allowing for more direct patient-care involvement by pharmacists and nurses.
4. Improved overall drug control and drug use monitoring.
5. More accurate patient billings for drugs.
6. The minimization of drug credits.
7. Greater control by the pharmacist over pharmacy workload patterns and staff scheduling.
8. A reduction in the size of drug inventories located in patient-care areas.
9. Greater adaptability to computerized and automated procedures.

Most medications are commercially available in unit-dose form, but some medications still must be packaged as a unit-dose medication by pharmacy personnel (see chapter 8). Intravenous medications are the best examples of those prepared in a unit-dose form by pharmacy personnel. Many IV medications are not stable in solution, and must be mixed by a technician just prior to administration.

Patient-specific characteristics are often a reason to extemporaneously prepare medications in a unit-dose form. Pediatric patients, for example, require very small doses that may not be available from the manufacturer in a unit-dose form. Some doses required for pediatric patients (especially neonates) are so small that they can not be measured accurately from commercially available products. The following scenario is an example of how a pediatric dose might be prepared in a unit-dose form.

Example: The doctor writes for an intravenous 3-mg dose of clindamycin for a patient in the neonatal intensive care unit. Clindamycin is available in a concentration of 150 mg/ml vial. The final volume for a 3-mg dose at 150 mg/ml would be 0.02 mls. Since this volume is too small to measure accurately, the technician will have to prepare a dilution. An appropriate dilution would be a 1:25 dilution, which would result in a final concentration of 6 mg/ml. The final volume for a 3-mg dose of the new concentration would be 0.5 ml. (refer to chapter 3). The technician can now, under the supervision of a pharmacist, measure, label, and dispense this medication.

Solid dosage forms may also need to be diluted. A technician may need to crush tablets, add a filler ingredient such as lactose, measure each dose using a calibrated balance, and then fold each powdered dose using a paper (referred to as powder paper) into single unit-dose packages.

PATIENT-FOCUSED SERVICES

Approximately 30 years ago pharmacists began to provide patient-focused services, called clinical pharmacy services, in addition to product services. These clinical services included pharmacokinetics dosing services, drug information services, and nutritional support services. It was realized by the profession that in order to achieve optimal outcomes and improve patient satisfaction pharmacy had to be accountable for the patient's medication-related needs.

Clinical services were eventually incorporated into the model of pharmaceutical care. Pharmaceutical care is defined as "the responsible provision of drug therapy to achieve definite outcomes intended to improve a patient's quality of life."[3] The pharmacist becomes an advocate for the patient. Not only are all medication therapy decisions made for the patient's benefit, but the patient has input into the decision-making process.

This approach also incorporates new roles for the technician. For example, one institution reported the use of technicians to record laboratory results in the pharmacist's patient database.[1] At another institution, one of the pharmacy satellites uses the technician to record the serum creatinine level for patients receiving certain medications. The pharmacist uses the serum creatinine value to assess kidney function and make appropriate recommendations for dosing the medications. Technicians also obtain other laboratory test results for the pharmacist, such as culture and sensitivities and electrolytes (e.g., potassium and sodium). Technicians can screen medication orders for nonformulary and restricted medications and notify the pharmacist when there is a need to take action on those orders. Technicians can also review and collect missing information for a patient's database such as allergies, height, and weight.

The ultimate goal of pharmaceutical care is to improve patient outcomes, enhance quality of care, heighten patient satisfaction, and decrease costs. Because of the fierce competition for health care dollars, quality care at the lowest cost may be the key to an institution's financial survival. W. Edwards Deming is known for his work in quality improvement techniques and philosophies. Deming often used the following chain reaction to illustrate the effects of quality improvement,[4] Figure 13-2.

QUALITY CONTROL AND QUALITY IMPROVEMENT PROGRAMS

Whether the pharmacy department is providing product- or patient-focused services, these need to be provided in a manner that guarantees a high level of quality. Quality has been a popular topic not only for pharmacy but for any organization providing a product or service. Quality itself is difficult to describe because the term implies a positive connotation but denotes nothing measurable. Quality may be identified when a product or service meets predetermined standards, such as a health care institution that has been accredited or certified. Quality may also be defined by what customers perceive. The pharmacy's customers can be patients, nurses, other pharmacists, or even accrediting agencies (e.g., Joint Commission on Accreditation of Healthcare Organizations [JCAHO]). Ensuring quality can be approached by two methods or concepts—quality control and quality improvement. Each is important and has a specific role in pharmacy.

Quality Control

Quality control is a process of checks and balances (or procedures) followed during the manufacturing of a product or provision of a service to ensure that the end products or services meet or exceed specified standards (e.g., zero errors, zero problems). The start of any quality control program requires complete written procedures and training for all staff involved in that procedure. Checks and balances usually occur at critical points in the process. For example, a quality control system for the preparation of Cefazolin 1-gm IVPB may start with the technician pulling the Cefazolin vial from stock and checking to make sure it is the right drug and strength, calculating the correct volume to withdraw, drawing up the correct volume of drug, injecting it into the bag, checking for any particulate matter or leaks, and checking the label for accurate and complete information (i.e., correct patient's name, drug, dose, route, diluent). Quality control is necessary to prevent defective products from reaching the patient. It is especially desirable when IV products are being prepared. An error or defect in an IV medication may cause significant morbidity and even death.

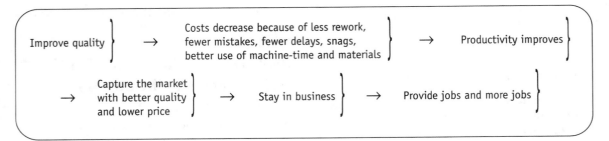

Figure 13-2. The Deming Chain Reaction.

Reprinted from *Out of the Crisis* by W. Edwards Deming by permission of MIT and The W. Edwards Deming Institute. Published by MIT, Center for Advanced Educational Services, Cambridge, MA 02139. Copyright 1986 by The W. Edwards Deming Institute.

A disadvantage of quality control is the time and resources it adds to the process. Although quality control identifies and prevents errors or defects, the underlying cause is not always identified or corrected. As a result, the underlying problem still exists, and defects will continue. Quality improvement, an alternative method, is one approach that reduces the problems and improves the product or service.

Quality Improvement

Quality improvement, also known as continuous quality improvement (CQI), is a scientific and systematic process involving monitoring, evaluating, and identifying problems and developing and measuring the impact of the improvement strategies. CQI concentrates on problems within a system, not on the person. It requires that decisions be based on fact (data) and not on a hunch or opinion. Various tools have been used to identify problems, assist in the data collection, and analyze the data. The use of these tools requires an understanding of when, how, and why a tool is used. For example, brainstorming is an excellent method of generating ideas and breaking down barriers between individuals or departments, because everyone in the group is given an opportunity to express an opinion. Another tool is a flow diagram, which is a visual display of a given procedure. Everyone participates in a workflow diagram because each individual may have a unique role in the process not known to others in the CQI group. Through a workflow diagram, everyone has the same understanding of the process. An example of a tool involving statistics is a run chart which tracks patterns and trends over a period of time. The temperature of a medication refrigerator can be plotted each day on a run chart, allowing immediate action before medications are affected if the temperature becomes too high or low.

CQI requires that everyone participate. All employees are encouraged to offer ideas in the CQI cycle. An example of a CQI program used by many health care institutions is the FOCUS-PDCA® cycle, which in fact was developed by a health care organization, Hospital Corporation of America (HCA).

Quality control and quality improvement programs are required by many of the accrediting agencies, such as JCAHO or the Health Care Financing Administration. The technician can be a valuable resource in the preparation for surveys or inspections by these agencies. For example, the technician may be responsible for ensuring that refrigerator logs are completed, medication units are inspected, and IV hoods are inspected on a routine basis and documented accordingly. The technician may also assist in the database management for other pharmacy quality improvement services, such as adverse drug reaction (ADR) reports, medication occurrence reports, and drug use evaluations.

THE FUTURE

The trend is for hospitals to become more involved in critically ill and intensive care patients. In critical care settings, the technicians are already valuable assets because they can accurately prepare emergency intravenous drips. Automation and technology continue to change trends in health care. The role of technicians is already integral to automation. The growing use of micromix and automated dispensing machines will increase opportunity for technicians.

The role of the pharmacy technician has and will continue to change as health care systems change. The pharmacy technician must continue to be flexible, adaptable, and knowledgeable about new technologies and services. Thus, the technician is encouraged to attend any educational sessions or inservices on new skills, automation, and technology. The technician should volunteer and participate in any available programs such as continuous quality improvement or data collection for upcoming JCAHO inspections. Following these guidelines, the technician can stay one step ahead of change.

RECOMMENDED READING

Brown TR. *Handbook of Institutional Pharmacy Practice.* 3rd ed. Bethesda, MD. American Society of Hospital Pharmacists; 1992.

REFERENCES

1. Hudkins JE, Crane VS. Role of pharmacy technicians in hospital formulary maintenance. *J Pharm Technol.* 1988;4(Jul/Aug):144–56.
2. American Society of Health-System Pharmacists. *Practice Standards of ASHP 1995–1996.* Bethesda, MD: ASHP; 1995. p.11
3. Hepler CD, Strand LM. Opportunities and responsibilities in pharmaceutical care. *Am J Hosp Pharm.* 1990;47:533–43.
4. Walton M. *The Deming Management Method.* New York: Putnam Publishing Co; 1986, p. 25.

SELF-ASSESSMENT QUESTIONS

1. Which of the following have had a role in rising health care costs?

   a. Medicare
   b. Medicaid
   c. JCAHO
   d. a and b
   e. none of the above

2. Which of the following are forms of technology used by pharmacy technicians in an institutional pharmacy?

   a. Micromix®, Automix®
   b. Pyxis®, Meditrol™, SureMed®
   c. computers
   d. all of the above
   e. none of the above

3. Which of the following health care settings have been developed to reduce cost and/or increase patient satisfaction?

   a. managed care companies
   b. home health care companies
   c. mail order prescription companies
   d. health maintenance organizations
   e. all of the above

4. Which of the following statements regarding shrinking health care dollars is false?

   a. Technicians now have less responsibility.
   b. Hospitals are now looking for the most cost-effective means of providing services.
   c. Alternative practice settings such as HMOs are more common.
   d. The use of automation to streamline services is increasing.

5. Which of the following is an/are advantage(s) to a centralized pharmacy?

   a. easy to control medications
   b. reduces inventory compared with a decentralized pharmacy
   c. reduces the number of personnel required to operate a pharmacy
   d. all of the above

6. Which of the following are advantages of a decentralized pharmacy?

   a. Pharmacy services are closer to the patient.
   b. Requires fewer resources.
   c. The technician can assist the pharmacist in the providing pharmaceutical care.
   d. a and c
   e. all of the above

7. Indicate which functions the technician can perform from a decentralized pharmacy.

   a. Prepare doses in a unit-dose form.
   b. Perform pharmacokinetic calculations for gentamicin dosing regimen.
   c. Collect patient laboratory results for the pharmacist.
   d. Screen questions in the satellite.
   e. a, c, and d
   f. a and d

8. Which of the following statements regarding pharmaceutical care is false?

   a. Pharmaceutical care is the responsible provision of drug therapy to achieve definite outcomes intended to improve a patient's quality of life.
   b. Pharmaceutical care only affects the activities of the pharmacist.

c. Pharmaceutical care allows the patients to have input into decisions regarding their drug therapy.

d. none of the above

9. In which of the following activities can a technician assist in the provision of pharmaceutical care?

a. obtaining laboratory results
b. providing counseling for a patient
c. screening orders for nonformulary/restricted drugs
d. pharmacokinetic dosing of a medication
e. a and c

10. Which of the following are disadvantages of a centralized pharmacy?

a. Lack face to face interaction with other health care providers
b. Difficult to access information kept in the patient's medical chart
c. Increased time to deliver medications
d. a and b
e. all of the above

11. Which of the following best defines a unit-dose system?

a. All medications are kept on the nursing station in bulk quantities.
b. All medications are packaged in a single dose that is ready to be administered to a patient.
c. A unit-dose system increases the number of errors compared with a system where bulk supplies of medications are dispensed.
d. none of the above

12. Which of the following statements is true regarding ready-to-use systems?

a. increase waste
b. increase errors
c. increase cost
d. all of the above
e. none of the above

13. Which of the following statements regarding pharmacy directors are false?

a. Pharmacy directors are typically at the top of the pharmacy department hierarchy.
b. Pharmacy directors are responsible for all the activities of the department.
c. Directors often report to one of the hospital administrators (COO, or one of the vice presidents).

d. Pharmacy directors can operate all activities independent of other departments or managers.

14. Which of the following statements regarding organizational structures are false?

a. A typical organizational structure will have a CEO at the top of the hierarchy.
b. All health care institutions have the same organizational structure.
c. Organizational structures are important to maintain clear levels of responsibility and chain of command.
d. All of the above are false.
e. All of the above are true.

15. Which of the following is a true statement regarding unit-dose systems?

a. Unit-dose systems are helpful in preparing medications for specialty patients like pediatric patients.
b. Unit-dose systems increase the chance of errors.
c. Unit-dose systems increase workload for nurses.
d. Unit-dose systems decrease the level of drug control.

16. Which of the following statements regarding quality are false?

a. Quality control is a process of checks and balances.
b. Quality may be defined by what customers perceive.
c. Because quality is something that can not be directly measured, it is more important to focus on the quantity of products made.
d. none of the above

17. The following are true about quality improvement *except*:

a. Quality improvement falls under the total responsibility of the pharmacy director.
b. Quality improvement is an important part of preparing for a JCAHO survey.
c. Quality improvement concentrates on problems within a system, rather than on individuals.
d. all of the above

18. Which of the following statements on technology are false?

a. Technology will continue to be used to help improve the efficiency of pharmacy services.

b. Technology in pharmacy has provided new opportunities for pharmacy technicians.

c. Technology and automation continue to interfere with pharmacy in the provision of patient focused pharmaceutical care.

d. a and c

e. All of the above are true.

19. Which of the following regarding quality control are false?

a. Quality control is a method used only after a medication has been prepared.

b. Quality control is a process of checks and balances.

c. The checks and balances often occur at critical points in the process.

d. Although quality control prevents errors or defects from occurring, the underlying cause may not be identified or corrected.

e. none of the above

20. The following are true about CQI *except:*

a. CQI focuses on people problems.

b. CQI is a scientific/systematic approach to quality.

c. CQI allows decisions to be made by objective data alone.

d. c and d

e. a and b

21. Which of the following statements is correct?

a. Computers have frequently been used with success by pharmacy departments. However, physicians using computers for medication order entry have increased errors and added several steps to the medication use process.

b. Physician order entry can decrease the number of steps in the system and reduce the potential for errors.

c. Physician order entry will eliminate the role of pharmacists in the review of appropriate medication therapy.

d. all of the above

22. Which of the following statements are false?

a. The CEO of the hospital is the individual to whom the board of directors reports.

b. CFO stands for Chief Financial Officer and is responsible for the financial management of the hospital.

c. COO stands for Chief Operating Officer and is responsible for the daily operation of the hospital.

d. The CEO helps set a direction for the hospital by creating a vision and mission for the institution.

e. b and c

23. Which of the following statements is true about a pharmacy satellite?

a. A pharmacy satellite is a decentralized form of pharmacy services.

b. Pharmacy services from a satellite pharmacy are performed in or near the patient care area.

c. Pharmacy satellites are located in the central pharmacy.

d. Pharmacy satellites eliminate the need for pharmacy technicians.

e. a and b

f. a, b, and d

24. Which of the following are strategies to cut the costs of a health care institution?

a. Cut personnel.

b. Reduce the length of time that patients spend in the hospital.

c. Shift patient care to the ambulatory care setting.

d. Improve efficiency of existing services.

e. All of the above are examples to cut costs.

25. The following statements are true about Quality Control (QC) *except:*

a. QC builds checks and balances throughout the process.

b. Training is important for a QC program.

c. Written policy and procedures are not needed if you have a QC program.

d. QC is extremely useful for IV products because of the potential for morbidity and mortality.

e. all of the above

ANSWERS TO SELF-ASSESSMENT

1. d. Medicare and Medicaid have contributed to the rising health care costs.

2. d. Micromix®, Automix®, Pyxis®, Meditrol™, and SureMed® computers are all examples of technology used by technicians in pharmacies.

3. e. All have been developed to reduce health care cost and increase patient satisfaction.

4. a. Technicians are being used for more activities. Technicians are now responsible for

many activities formerly reserved for pharmacists (e.g., managing investigational drug programs, using automated technology).

5. d. All are advantages to a centralized pharmacy. A centralized pharmacy allows for efficient control, storage, inspection, preparation, and dispensing of medications with fewer personnel.

6. d. A decentralized pharmacy allows pharmacy services to be closer to the patients, expands the role of the pharmacy technician, but increases the need for resources (i.e., equipment, references, inventory, etc.)

7. e. The technician can perform many tasks from a decentralized pharmacy including, but not limited to preparing unit-dose products, collecting laboratory results, and screening questions for the pharmacist. The application of pharmacokinetics is a clinical skill that pharmacists are trained to provide.

8. b. Technicians participate in the provision of pharmaceutical care by gathering patient specific laboratory results that are used to assess drug therapy.

9. e. Obtaining laboratory results and screening orders for nonformulary/restricted drugs are activities the technician can perform to assist the pharmacist in the provision of pharmaceutical care.

10. e. All are disadvantages to a centralized pharmacy. These disadvantages are based primarily on the location of the pharmacy.

11. b. A unit-dose system prepares each dose in ready to use form. The advantages to a unit-dose system can be reviewed in this chapter under "Unit-dose System."

12. e. None of the above are true about unit-dose systems. The reader is again referred to the "Unit-dose System" section of this chapter.

13. d. Pharmacy directors must collaborate with many departments to provide the best services for patients.

14. b. Many organizational structures may exist, depending on the size, type of institution (i.e., teaching vs. community) and other factors.

15. a. Unit-dose systems are particularly valuable in specialty practices like pediatrics.

16. c. Quality should always be more important than quantity.

17. a. Quality improvement requires the participation of all individuals involved, not just a few.

18. c. Technology may change the focus of pharmacy's responsibilities, but these changes offer new opportunities and responsibilities.

19. a. Quality control consists of checks and balances built in throughout the process.

20. a. CQI looks at the entire system. CQI is based on the principle that most problems are system related, not people related.

21. b. Although computers can not eliminate errors, they have reduced errors related to transcription and manipulation of orders. In addition, computer order entry reduces the number of steps in a medication use process.

22. a. The CEO is at the top of the organizational structure and stands for Chief Executive Officer, but the CEO reports to the board of directors.

23. e. A pharmacy satellite is a decentralized form of pharmacy services and is located on or near the patient care area. The pharmacy technician has many opportunities to work in a pharmacy satellite. Please refer to the section "Decentralized Pharmacy Services" for a more detailed description of the technician's role in the pharmacy satellite.

24. e. All are examples of methods for cutting costs. All of these strategies may affect the technician. These strategies offer opportunities for the technician to obtain new responsibility and knowledge about pharmacy services.

25. c. Written procedures are very important in QC. Without written procedures, the potential for deviating from the production process may introduce errors and defects into the product.

14 | Ambulatory Care Pharmacy Practice

Richard K. Lewis, Pharm.D., MBA

This chapter describes those characteristics of pharmacy practice that are unique to ambulatory care and the important role pharmacy technicians play in providing pharmacy services in this setting. Specifically, this chapter will offer a review of ambulatory care pharmacy history and current practices; compare and contrast different types of ambulatory care practices; and describe the activities performed by pharmacy technicians in this environment. The importance of customer service and communication skills will be emphasized. Third-party payer programs, claims processing, and formularies as components of pharmacy workflow will also be discussed.

Many of the issues important to an ambulatory care setting have been covered in other chapters. In particular, it may be useful to review the chapters on law, calculations, and interpreting medication orders.

LEARNING OBJECTIVES

After reading this chapter, the technician should be able to
1. Discuss the history and current practices of pharmacy in ambulatory care.
2. List the similarities and differences between the variety of ambulatory care practice sites (i.e., chain, independent, clinic, managed care, and mail order).
3. Explain the importance of exceptional customer service and communication skills in the outpatient pharmacy environment.
4. Explain the typical prescription distribution process in an ambulatory care pharmacy.
5. Describe the role of the technician in ambulatory care pharmacy.
6. Describe how third-party payment programs affect prescription processing in ambulatory care.

HISTORICAL OVERVIEW AND CURRENT PRACTICES

The majority of pharmacy practice takes place in an ambulatory care setting, and it is this setting that has been the basis of the public's perception of pharmacy for hundreds of years. Over time, pharmacy practice in ambulatory care has changed significantly. Historically, the pharmacist (or apothecary) compounded medications in the corner drug store and was often consulted by patients to help treat their common ailments. In fact, prior to the enactment of the 1951 Durham-Humphrey Amendment to the Food, Drug and Cosmetic Act, there was no definition of prescription drugs, allowing pharmacists to dispense medications without a physician's order. Of course, now pharmacists can only dispense prescription drugs upon receipt of a valid prescription.

The mass production of pharmaceuticals by large drug companies began in the 1950s and resulted in several changes. The need for pharmacists to compound prescriptions decreased and many community pharmacies became more focused on selling a large variety of retail items. As this trend continued, pharmacists spent less time talking to patients about their medications. In fact, in the 1960s, many professional pharmacy organizations encouraged pharmacists to refrain from discussing medication issues with patients and many pharmacy schools taught students that such activity would interfere with the physician-patient relationship.

During the 1970s, some pharmacists began practicing "clinical pharmacy." Clinical pharmacists, who primarily practiced in hospitals, were monitoring specific drugs, rounding with the medical team, and filling an important role in hospital patient care. One of the reasons this occurred in the hospital was because of the pharmacists' ability to reduce costs. In addition, pharmacy organizations and pharmacy schools began encouraging patient-pharmacist interaction. During this same time, pharmacists practicing in ambulatory care settings continued to focus on prescription dispensing and there was an expansion in chain pharmacies. Unlike the hospital setting, there was little financial pressure to reduce unnecessary prescription use in the ambulatory care setting because most patients still paid cash for their prescriptions.

In the 1980s, the cost of health care became a significant public policy issue and managed care began to grow. With managed care came restructuring of health care reimbursement and the movement to minimize the amount of time patients spend in hospitals. In ambulatory care, pharmacist-patient communication was emphasized and the role of pharmacy technician was expanded to include more prescription filling activities.

In the early 1990s, health care reform became a major item on political agendas. While health care reform continues to be debated on the legislative level, major payers are forcing market changes by demanding lower costs for health care. With respect to pharmacy, there was a great deal of debate about the cost of pharmaceuticals. Attempts to manage the cost of pharmacy services and products resulted in the expansion of managed care and mail order pharmacy operations, and the advent of pharmacy benefit management firms (PBMs). One of the most significant changes during this time period was the enactment of the Omnibus Budget Reconciliation Act of 1990 (OBRA 90), which required states to implement drug use review (DUR) programs within their Medicaid system. A major component of the DUR program is the requirement that pharmacists review a patient's prescriptions for drug-related problems and, at least, offer counseling on prescription medications at the time of dispensing. It should be noted that many states added the DUR/counseling requirement to their pharmacy practice acts to include all patients, not just Medicaid patients.

PRACTICE SITES IN AMBULATORY CARE

Traditionally, the ambulatory care practice site has been the community pharmacy. However, in recent years, the number and type of ambulatory care practice sites have grown to include hospital-based clinic pharmacies (general and specialty), mail order pharmacies, pharmacies in physician office buildings and nondispensing practices such as pharmacist-managed clinics, office practices, and PBMs. The roles and responsibilities of technicians in most of the dispensing operations are very similar.

Community Pharmacies

Community pharmacies are often stand-alone businesses that fill prescriptions, sell a variety of nonprescription products (e.g., cough and cold preparations, toiletries) and counsel patients about proper use of their medications. Most community pharmacies employ pharmacists and technicians. There are two distinct types of community pharmacies, independent and chain.

Independent Community Pharmacies

Independent pharmacies are likely to be recognized as "the corner drugstore." The services offered by independent pharmacies vary, depending on the pharmacist, location, and patient population served. The owner of an independent pharmacy is most likely the pharmacist-in-charge. Many independent pharmacies specialize in areas such as durable medical equipment (DME) or medical supplies and compounding. Some independent pharmacies also serve nursing homes.

Chain Pharmacies

A corporate-owned group of pharmacies is generally recognized as a chain pharmacy. These pharmacies are usually large business entities with common policies and procedures. Pharmacists as well as technicians are employees of the corporation. Chain pharmacies often offer discount prescription filling services, accept a large number of insurance plans, and offer the convenience of multiple locations. Some chains (as well as some independents) also offer cholesterol screening, flu shots, and blood pressure monitoring services.

There are also some pharmacies that are considered "small chains" or "independent chains." These are often independent pharmacies that have grown to add new locations in a community. These small chains usually consist of three to seven pharmacies.

Clinic Pharmacies

Clinic pharmacies and pharmacies in physician office buildings usually offer the same scope of services as many community pharmacies but may have less focus on selling retail products other than medications. Because of the proximity of these pharmacies to the prescribers, there is generally greater access to patient information.

Clinic pharmacies and physician office building pharmacies may differ in ownership and licensure. Clinic pharmacies associated with a hospital are likely to be owned by the hospital and operated under the direction of the hospital pharmacy department. Because of this relationship, the hospital-owned pharmacy may receive contract pricing from a buying group, through the manufacturer, or through disproportionate share pricing (hospitals and clinics serving a disproportionate share of indigent patients are eli-

gible to buy pharmaceuticals at government rates). In these instances, the pharmacies are not allowed to dispense prescriptions to non-hospital patients because their pricing may give them an unfair advantage over community pharmacies. In other words, if a patient entered a hospital-owned pharmacy receiving contract prices with a prescription from the physician's office down the street, the pharmacy may not be able to legally fill the prescription.

In the private physician office building, pharmacy services are more likely to be a contracted service with a local independent or chain pharmacy. In this case, the pharmacy operates just like any other community pharmacy. It should be noted however, that clinics associated with a hospital may also hire an outside vendor to provide pharmacy services.

Specialty Clinic Pharmacies

Because of the specific needs of some specialty clinics, pharmacies will occasionally be located in these areas. For example, oncology clinics often have their own pharmacies. These pharmacies usually specialize in the preparation of chemotherapeutic agents for on-site administration.

Managed Care Pharmacies

Some managed care organizations own and operate physician office buildings or clinic practices and may also operate pharmacies in these buildings. These pharmacies operate much like community or other ambulatory care pharmacies but may only carry those drugs on the organization's formulary and may only serve the patients enrolled in the managed care plan.

Mail Order Pharmacies

Mail order pharmacies are mostly large-scale operations that mail maintenance medications (i.e., medications that patients take on a regular basis) to the patients' homes. Mail order pharmacies have become increasingly popular with insurance companies and some patients because they are convenient and are often thought to have lower prices. These pharmacies can process thousands of prescriptions in a 24-hour period. Many mail order pharmacies now partner with PBMs to offer distribution and DUR services. The role of the technician in these pharmacies is usually the same as in other ambulatory care sites, except there is no face-to-face patient contact. Instead, most communication with patients occurs over the telephone. Therefore, good telephone communication skills are essential.

TECHNICIAN RESPONSIBILITIES IN AMBULATORY CARE

The role of pharmacy technicians in ambulatory care practice is essential to an efficient and effective operation. Generally, it is the responsibility of technicians to maintain and operate all aspects of the drug distribution process under the supervision of pharmacists. This includes receipt of the prescription order, computer order entry, claims processing, prescription filling and labeling, compounding, inventory maintenance, and other activities as directed by the pharmacist. The demands on the pharmacist to assess the patient and prescription for drug-related problems and to appropriately counsel the patient requires technician support that is timely, complete, and accurate.

Customer Service and Communication Skills

Possibly the most important qualifications of those who serve the public is the ability to provide good customer service and practice good communication skills. This is especially true in the health care setting where the patient is the customer. Patients are often not feeling well and have a low tolerance for inconveniences and perceived rudeness of employees. Technicians should always approach patients in a positive, polite, and caring manner. In addition to being a good business practice, a positive interaction with the technician helps prepare the patient for an open and productive interaction with the pharmacist. Technicians must also respect and be considerate of the patient's confidentiality and maintain a sense of privacy when discussing medications.

Technicians must be prepared to handle demanding patients appropriately. Sometimes demanding patients will create difficult situations and the technician should work closely with the pharmacist to develop a game plan for handling such situations. For example, a patient may demand a quickly filled prescription or argue over the price of a co-pay. In such situations, always clarify that you understand the issue (perhaps it is a simple misunderstanding),

and never escalate an argument by raising your voice or by challenging the knowledge of the patient. Part of the game plan should include when to defer the situation to a pharmacist.

The use of the telephone in community pharmacy also requires proper communication skills. Physicians, patients, and other pharmacies may be calling, so it is important to identify yourself as the pharmacy technician. This may prevent the caller from taking the time to ask a lengthy question just to be put on hold and then have to ask the pharmacist the question again.

Third-Party Payment Programs

One of the most unique and time consuming activities in the ambulatory care pharmacy setting is dealing with third-party payment programs. Third-party programs are insurance or entitlement programs that reimburse the pharmacy for products delivered and services rendered. Although there are hundreds of third-party programs administered by organizations ranging from large insurance companies to small employer or union sponsored employee benefit programs, there are only two major mechanisms for pharmacy reimbursement, fee-for-service and capitation.

Fee-for-service

In a fee-for-service system, the pharmacy bills the third party each time an eligible product is dispensed or services rendered. The third party then reimburses the pharmacy. The amount charged and amount reimbursed varies depending on the cost and time involved.

Capitation

Capitation is popular with managed care programs. Under a capitated payment program, a pharmacy receives a set amount of money for a defined group of patients, regardless of the number of prescriptions or amount of services received. The dollar amount is usually in terms of per patient per month. For example, the third-party payer may agree to pay the pharmacy $2 per member per month. Therefore, if the program has 100 patients, the pharmacy receives $200 each month. Even if one of the patients does not use the pharmacy, the pharmacy still receives the $2 for that patient. Likewise, if a patient receives multiple medications and uses the pharmacy 10 times per month, the pharmacy also receives only $2 for that patient.

Eligibility Verification

Because of the variety of third-party programs, there are a variety of methods of ensuring eligibility. Most programs offer membership cards to their patients. These cards often carry the basic information such as name and identification number. However, the technician may have to collect additional information from the patient, such as date of birth and address. Most third-party programs are on-line through the pharmacy computer and will notify the pharmacist or pharmacy technician if there is a problem with eligibility. Another situation to be aware of is that some third parties will cover family members, but the membership card will only list the primary beneficiary.

Formularies

A formulary is a list of drugs approved by a third party for reimbursement. Formularies are developed to help control cost and improve the quality of the drug therapy their patients receive (e.g., cost-effective therapy). However, formulary drugs will vary between third parties because of differences in contract prices and rebate agreements with the manufacturers, among other reasons. If a patient presents a prescription for a drug that is not on the third party's formulary, the pharmacist should be alerted to the problem so that he or she can take appropriate action.

Co-payments/Deductibles/ Spend-downs

Many third parties require the patient to pay a co-payment (or deductible) each time a prescription is received. There are three basic co-payment arrangements designated by third parties: flat rate, variable rate, and straight percentage. A flat rate requires a specific co-pay regardless of the drug received and cost of the drug. A variable rate may require a different co-pay if the patient insists on a brand name product over a generic. A percentage co-pay requires the patient to pay a percentage of the total cost of the medication. The amount paid by the patient would then increase as the cost of the prescription increased.

A spend-down (also known as a front-end deductible) differs from a co-pay or deductible in that it is assessed over a defined period of time and not on a per prescription basis. A spend-down requires a patient to spend a defined amount of out-of-pocket dollars on prescriptions within a year before the third party pays anything. For example, a patient may have a spend-down of $500 over a period of one year. This patient will have to buy $500 worth of prescription drugs (out-of-pocket) first, and then the third party will pay for the remaining prescriptions during the rest of the year.

PRESCRIPTION PROCESSING AND WORKFLOW

The objective of this section is to highlight the unique components of prescription processing in the ambulatory care setting. The specific role of a technician in a pharmacy will vary depending on the preference of the pharmacist or the policies of the employer.

Prescription Reception

The patient will bring his or her prescription(s) to the prescription reception area (or "In Window") of the pharmacy. This is often the first contact the patient has with the pharmacy, so good customer service is essential. Because it is the first contact, it is also important to gather accurate data about the patient and verify that the prescription is complete (see chapter 5 for a list of items needed for a complete prescription). The typical data that should be collected include
- Correct spelling of name
- Address and phone number
- Allergies
- Patient's birthdate
- Weight for children and infants
- Payment information
- Desire for generic substitution

If the patient is hesitant to provide this information, explain the purpose of collecting it (i.e., for insurance reimbursement, recall notices, dosage calculations).

If the patient has previously experienced an allergic reaction to a medication, the technician should document the reaction and alert the pharmacist. The technician's role is only to document the reaction. The assessment of the reaction and discussion with the patient should be left to the pharmacist. The pharmacist will need to evaluate the type of allergic reaction experienced by the patient, determine if it may be a potential problem with the patient's current prescription, and make recommendations as appropriate.

Many pharmacies accept a large number of insurance plans, and it is important for the technician to be familiar with the requirements of each plan or at least know where to find the information.

The laws and regulations regarding generic substitution vary from state to state, but usually there must be agreement among the prescriber, patient, and pharmacist before a generic product is dispensed over a brand name product. If the prescription is written generically (e.g., furosemide), then the generic can usually be dispensed. However, if the prescription is written for the brand name product (e.g., Lasix) and marked "may substitute," the patient should be asked if he or she prefers the generic or brand name product. Since all drugs are not available as generics, the technician should be familiar with which generics are available. When unsure of availability, the technician should ask if the patient prefers the generic product if one is available. In certain cases, it will be important to inform the patient that some insurance plans will not cover brand name products when a generic is available or that the insurance plan may require a higher co-pay for brand name products.

The last question the patient should be asked at the reception area is if he or she plans to wait or return later for the prescription. From a customer service perspective, it is important to prioritize the prescription-filling process and efficiently adjust workflow as necessary to provide a timely service and accommodate the customer's needs.

Prescription Computer Entry

After the prescription has been received, the next step is to enter the prescription into the pharmacy computer system. There are hundreds of pharmacy software vendors and some pharmacies develop their own software, so the details of the prescription entry process will differ between sites. However, the basic process of keying in the patient and prescription information and generating a label should be the same. Additionally, most insurance plans are on-line, which allows for virtually immediate responses to the pharmacy's insurance claims.

As the patient and prescription information is entered into the computer, the software and/or the on-line third party will verify the patient's eligibility for payment, as well as formulary and therapeutic problems. The technician should be prepared to handle payment problems, however,

therapeutic problems should be referred to the pharmacist. When a problem does occur, the computer generates an alert message for the pharmacy. Common error messages are reviewed below.

Refill Too Soon

This message deals specifically with refill prescriptions and the time period between filling prescriptions. Typically, third parties allow patients to receive a 30-day supply of medications. If the patient attempts to refill that prescription within a significantly shorter time period (e.g., 15 days after the last prescription), the prescription cannot be processed without prior approval from the third-party payer.

Missing/Invalid Patient ID

This or a similar message would indicate that the patient who is entered into the pharmacy computer does not appear to be enrolled in the insurance program. Upon receiving this message, the patient information entered should be examined for mistakes. Perhaps the name was misspelled, identification number mistyped, or other required information left out. Because some insurance plans will use a PBM to manage their pharmacy services, the prescription may need to be processed under the name of the PBM instead of the name of the third-party payer.

Drug-Drug or Drug-Allergy Interaction

Most pharmacy software will screen the patient profile for drug and allergy information. If interactions are detected, the program will alert the user. Some software will not only identify an interaction but indicate the potential severity of the reaction. When receiving this message, the technician should alert the pharmacist to the problem.

Nonformulary/Not Covered

Many third-party payers have formularies (a list of covered drugs). If a nonformulary drug is entered into the pharmacy computer, the message received will indicate that the drug is not covered, and payment will not be made for that drug. When receiving this message, the technician should alert the pharmacist.

Patient Profile Maintenance

The patient profile is a list of the prescriptions received by a patient and all corresponding prescription information (i.e., original date, refill dates, prescribing physician). The patient profile assists the pharmacist in evaluating the appropriateness and efficacy of the patient's drug therapy. One use of the patient profile in ambulatory care that is unique in comparison with the inpatient environment is for assessment of patient compliance. For example, if a patient received a 30-day supply of medication but did not return to the pharmacy for a refill until 45 days later, the pharmacist will likely investigate the discrepancy to determine if a problem has occurred, if the patient is noncompliant, or if the prescribed therapy has been changed. The patient profile contains private and confidential information; therefore, this information should never be discussed with anyone other than the patient and the pharmacist.

Prescription Filling and Labeling

The actual filling and labeling of prescriptions is one of the most common pharmacy technician activities in ambulatory care (some states restrict labeling to the pharmacist only). This process must be completed in a timely and accurate manner. Any mistakes in the process are not only dangerous but time consuming and obstructive to the workflow. Pharmacy technicians should be cautious to ensure that all prescriptions meet the five rights: (1) the right drug, (2) in the right dose, (3) in the right dosage form, (4) with the right label, and (5) for the right patient. Any error discovered by the pharmacist will often be returned to the technician for correction.

Automation

The use of automated devices to fill and label prescriptions in ambulatory care is increasing and is likely to grow rapidly over the next several years. Such automation will increase the productivity of the pharmacy and the pharmacy technician. With the increase in automation comes an increase in the technician's responsibility for maintaining and filling such devices; however, the final check still remains with the pharmacist. Technicians should strictly follow the policies, procedures, and standards developed within the pharmacy in filling automated devices. An error in filling could result in a large number of misfilled prescriptions if not caught by a pharmacist.

Compounding

One of the valuable services provided by ambulatory care pharmacy is compounding prescriptions. The majority of compounding in this setting involves making suspensions for pediatric patients who need a smaller dose than what is commercially available or for patients who cannot swallow tablets or capsules. In addition, many combination topical products are prepared in ambulatory care settings. (Refer to chapter 8 for more detailed information on compounding.)

Most pharmacies keep a "recipe book" that contains a step by step guide on how to prepare compounds that are routinely ordered. It serves as a reference on what ingredients to use, how to prepare the compound, and stability information (e.g., refrigeration requirements and expiration dates). The technician's role is to compound the prescription following the appropriate recipe, document all necessary information, and label the product appropriately for the pharmacist to complete the final check.

Dispensing

The last step in the prescription-processing function is dispensing. Technicians can assist pharmacists in the dispensing process by making sure all the medications that belong to a patient are ready to be dispensed and by collecting payment from the patient when appropriate.

A large and important component of the dispensing function is patient counseling. OBRA 90 requires pharmacists to offer counseling to patients (refer to chapter 4, for detailed information on OBRA 90). Many potential drug-related health problems and prescription errors can be prevented through effective communication between the patient and the pharmacist.

Transferring Prescriptions

The laws regarding the transfer of prescriptions between pharmacies vary among states and among different classes of drugs. However, the pharmacist is always ultimately responsible for the information transferred. The transfer of a prescription to another pharmacy is usually initiated by a phone call from the pharmacy needing a transferred prescription. A technician may pull the original prescription from files and/or pull up the data on the computer, but the actual transfer of information is usually the responsibility of the pharmacist.

The same is true for prescriptions being transferred into the pharmacy. In this case, the process begins when a patient requests to transfer the prescription from another location. At that point, it is important for the technician to obtain as much information as possible from the patient about the prescription. At a minimum, the pharmacist needs the patient's name and the name of the pharmacy currently holding the prescription. If a patient brings in his or her old bottle, it may be useful to troubleshoot the labels. For example, if the label indicates there are no refills, the physician will have to be called to authorize the refill.

NONPRESCRIPTION MEDICATIONS

Nonprescription medications, or over-the-counter (OTC) drugs, can be purchased without a prescription. Because of the availability to the consumer and relatively low out-of-pocket expense, some third-party payers will not include OTCs on their formulary or will require that a provider has written a prescription for the OTC before covering it under the benefit. Some of the common OTC products available include drugs for cough and cold, antacids, laxatives, pain medications, topical preparations, anti-diarrheal products, diabetic care products, weight control products, ophthalmic products (eye preparations), otic products (ear preparations), and nutritional supplements. In addition, a variety of home health care supplies such as ostomy bags, crutches, and wheel chairs are available.

In recent years, consumers have been increasingly interested in taking care of their health through self-education, exercise, and proper diet. In addition, more and more patients are choosing self-treatment for their acute illnesses (i.e., coughs, colds, heartburn). The increasing cost of health care, lack of medical insurance, inaccessibility of medical care, availability of more diverse and sophisticated self-care products, and increasing number of prescription drugs being switched to nonprescription status are some of the reasons patients are getting more involved in their own health care. These trends present tremendous opportunities for the pharmacy profession to provide patients with the guidance and information they need to use OTC products effectively.

Pharmacy technicians are usually the first to encounter patients when they approach the pharmacy; therefore, the technicians should familiarize themselves with the location of the OTCs and be able to direct patients to specific products. However, it is very important for tech-

nicians to know when to answer a patient's question and when to refer the patient to the pharmacist. For example, if a patient asks a technician to help with returning a crutch the patient rented for a sprained ankle, the technician can usually take care of the patient. On the other hand, if the patient also asks if he or she can take aspirin for the pain, the technician should refer the patient to a pharmacist.

REFERRING PATIENTS TO A PHARMACIST

There are three reasons that technicians should always refer patients with drug (prescription or OTC) or health-related questions to a pharmacist: drug-drug interactions, drug-disease state interaction, and need for physician referral.

Drug-Drug Interactions

The patient may be taking prescription or other nonprescription drugs that may interact with OTC drugs. For example, drugs for use in heartburn and acid indigestion that were previously available by prescription have only recently entered the OTC market. Some of these drugs interact with prescription drugs such as medications used for heart disease, blood pressure, seizure disorders, etc. They may also interact with other OTC drugs. Therefore, while these drugs may be appropriate for some patients, they may not be appropriate for others.

Drug-Disease State Interaction

Some OTC drugs may adversely affect the patient's existing disease state by making the condition worse or precipitating a disease that is in remission. Pharmacists are trained to know the effect of drugs on disease states and can make appropriate recommendations.

Need for Physician Referral

Often, patients may come to the pharmacy with seemingly simple problems while in reality the problem is complex. For example, a patient may ask for an OTC drug recommendation for a headache. The technician may feel pressured to give a recommendation based on her/his own experience or what she/he heard a pharmacist recommend previously. However, the appropriate response from the technician is to refer the patient to a pharmacist. Pharmacists are trained to interview patients and determine if a patient's complaint is an indication of a more serious medical condition that requires further evaluation.

Another common question a technician may receive concerning nonprescription medications is whether or not insurance companies pay for OTC products. In general, many insurance companies do not pay for OTC products. But, there are a few exceptions to the rule, and therefore it is best to check the insurance plan before giving a patient a yes or no answer.

SUMMARY

This chapter has provided an overview of ambulatory care pharmacy practice. As more and more health care is provided in the outpatient setting and as the complexity and breadth of OTC and prescription drugs continue to increase, the role of pharmacists in counseling and monitoring patients becomes increasingly critical to the safe and effective use of medications. The role of pharmacy technicians in maintaining an effective and efficient drug distribution process is critical to the success of ambulatory care pharmacies. Technicians must be knowledgeable and proficient in the use of automation and pharmacy computer systems and efficient in filling prescriptions. Technicians must also maintain a working knowledge of third-party payers and their prescription policies. Finally, technicians must provide excellent customer service through friendly and caring interactions with patients.

RECOMMENDED READING

Cooke C, Wilson M. Managed care organizations, today and tomorrow. *Am Drug*. 1994; Nov:67–74.

Abramowitz PW, Mansur JM. Moving toward the provision of comprehensive ambulatory care pharmaceutical services. *Am J Hosp Pharm*. 1987;44:1155–63.

Fincham JE, Wertheimer AI, editors. *Pharmacy and the U.S. Health Care System*. Binghamton, NY: Pharmceuticals Products Press; 1991.

SELF-ASSESSMENT QUESTIONS

1. The Durham-Humphrey amendment:
   a. defined "prescription" drugs.
   b. required pharmacists to offer patients counseling on their medication.
   c. allowed pharmacists to dispense any drug without a prescription.
   d. none of the above

2. True or False: Managed care outpatient pharmacies operate very similarly to community or other ambulatory care pharmacies but may maintain a smaller variety of drugs because of restrictive formularies.

3. An important aspect of an ambulatory care pharmacy technician's job is:
   a. counseling patients about drug interactions.
   b. good customer service and communication skills.
   c. educating physicians about pharmacology.
   d. none of the above

4. True or False: Technicians should always identify themselves as pharmacy technicians when answering the phone.

5. True or False: One question that should be asked when a patient drops off a prescription is whether the patient plans to wait or return later to pick up the prescription.

6. True or False: Typically, third-party plans with formularies will not pay for drugs that are nonformulary unless prior approval is obtained.

7. True or False: The sole purpose of the patient profile is to maintain the patient's insurance information.

8. True or False: Technicians can assist the pharmacist in the dispensing process by counseling the patient on their medication.

9. True or False: In the ambulatory care setting, a list of drugs approved by a third party for reimbursement is a formulary.

ANSWERS TO SELF-ASSESSMENT

1. a. The 1951 Durham-Humphrey Amendment to the Food, Drug and Cosmetic Act gave a definition to "prescription" drugs and prohibited pharmacists from dispensing these drugs without a valid medication order. The OBRA 90 regulations required pharmacists to offer counseling to Medicaid patients. Many state practice acts quickly expanded the OBRA 90 guidelines to all patients.

2. True. The functions performed by technicians and pharmacists are usually the same throughout all ambulatory care pharmacies. However, since managed care pharmacies usually only care for their own patients, they

will keep inventory to a minimum by limiting the items they stock.

3. b. Good customer service and communication skills are essential in ambulatory care practice (for both the technician and the pharmacist). Some patients will not be feeling well and may be less tolerant of delays in receiving their prescriptions or perceived rudeness of employees. A friendly and caring interaction between the technician and the patient sets the stage for a productive patient interaction with the pharmacist.

4. True. If mistaken as the pharmacist, the caller (physician, patient, etc.) may ask a therapeutic question that would need to be referred to the pharmacist. This would tie up the phone line for additional time and create an inefficient workflow.

5. True. The technician must prioritize activities within the prescription filling process. If a patient is returning at a later time (perhaps the next day), other prescriptions for waiting patients may take precedence.

6. True. A formulary is a list of drugs that are covered under a particular third-party plan.

Occasionally, a nonformulary drug is needed for a patient. In these cases, the pharmacist or physician can ask for prior approval and provide the third party the details of why the nonformulary drug is needed for the patient.

7. False. The patient profile has multiple purposes, including the storage of the patient's insurance information. It also serves as a tool for the pharmacist in assessing potential drug interactions, allergy contraindications, and patient compliance.

8. False. The technician's role is to ensure an efficient drug distribution process so that the pharmacist has time to counsel the patient.

9. True. The formulary is usually used by the third party to promote cost-effective use of drugs. If a patient presents a prescription for a nonformulary drug, the technician can assist the pharmacist by determining what alternatives are available within the same drug class, but the pharmacist will need to evaluate the drug and patient variables to make appropriate recommendations.

15 Home Care Pharmacy Practice

Mary Ann Kliethermes, B.S., Pharm.D.
Karen E. Bertch, Pharm.D.

Home health care is defined as the provision of health care services in the patient's home, versus the institutional setting or provider's office.[1] Home care pharmacy is part of home health care practice. The majority of pharmaceuticals in non-institutional settings are provided through the community pharmacy system. The niche of home care pharmacy is to provide intravenous medications and high technology services in the home. Much of the material covered in chapter 9, Aseptic Technique, Sterile Compounding, and Intravenous Admixture Systems, complements this chapter. Technicians planning to practice in a home care setting should review both chapters thoroughly.

LEARNING OBJECTIVES

After reading this chapter the reader should be able to

1. Identify the historical reason for establishing home care services and the impetus for the growth of the home care industry.
2. Cite the seven goals of home care therapy.
3. Identify the members of the home care team and describe their primary roles in the home care process.
4. Identify five diseases or conditions commonly treated with home care services.
5. Identify the top drug classes used in home infusion therapy. List one or two parameters for these drugs that affect how they are used in the home environment.
6. Group sterile products based on the level of risk to a patient.
7. Compare the advantages and disadvantages of the four different infusion systems available for use in a patient's home.
8. Describe the mechanisms of operation for four infusion systems available to patients at home.
9. List the labeling requirements for sterile products that are to be used in a patient's home.
10. Outline the factors that are important to consider when determining expiration dates for sterile products used in the home care setting.

11. Discuss the characteristics and indications of the various venous access devices available for use by home care patients.

HISTORICAL OVERVIEW AND CURRENT PRACTICES

Patients first began receiving infusion therapy in the home, rather than in an institutional setting, in the late 1970s. The driving force for sending patients home was twofold. The cost of keeping patients in the hospital to receive long term intravenous antibiotic therapy or parenteral nutrition was becoming too expensive. It also was a hardship for patients and their families to "live" in the hospital for the duration of their treatment. These patients often required minimal intensive medical care, only needing the care associated with their infusion therapy. The search for alternatives to hospitalization led to the development of programs to treat long-term infusion patients at home and the birth of the home infusion industry. In the past 20 years we have seen home care, and in particular home infusion, become one of the fastest growing segments of health care. Currently, approximately 5 billion dollars are spent on home infusion services in the United States.[2]

There are several reasons for the rapid growth of home infusion. A number of studies have shown that administration of long-term intravenous therapy in the home is safe, effective, and less expensive. This helped physicians and insurance companies overcome any fear or reluctance they may have had in sending their patients to home health care agencies. In addition, the explosion of technology has supported the movement of patients to the home care setting. New developments brought infusion pumps that are portable, small, and easily programmable for a wide range of therapies, and in some cases disposable. This has made it easier to teach non-professionals, such as patients and their families, to administer complicated therapies at home. Although consumers have demanded home care, citing their improved quality of life, ability to return to work, and greater independence, the strongest impetus came from the dramatic changes in our health care system. Escalating health care costs forced hospitals to decrease the length of time patients spent in the hospital. As a result, patients are discharged earlier in the course of treatment and often need additional care when they get home. The need for more intensive med-

ical care and support in the home provided the opportunities for the home health care industry.

Home infusion services are provided by a number of organizations including hospitals, community pharmacies, home health nursing companies, integrated health care systems, and independent home infusion companies. After the tremendous expansion of home health care organizations, we are now seeing a consolidation, with mergers of companies and shifting of dominance among the providers of home infusion services.

SUMMARY OF HOME CARE PRACTICE

Purpose and Goals of Home Infusion Therapy

The purpose of home care pharmacy practice is to provide high technology therapy, which is usually provided in an institutional setting, at home. The intentions of these services are summarized in Table 15-1. Overall, the major goal is to provide safe and effective infusion therapy in the home. However this therapy must also be cost effective.

The Home Care Process

A patient enters the home care process a number of ways. Usually a physician will recom-

Table 15-1

Goals of Home Care

- Allow patients to leave the hospital earlier
- Allow patients to receive therapy without being hospitalized
- Allow patients to return to work or normal activities sooner
- Allow patients to recuperate in the comfort of the home environment
- Decrease health care costs
- Provide safe and effective therapy and care
- Achieve a smooth non-stressful transition of therapy between the hospital and the patient's home

mend that a patient completes therapy at home. In some instances the patient and the patient's family push for home therapy. Other times the patient's insurance company may dictate where therapy will be provided. Sometimes this is mediated by an insurer's agent called a case manager. This person works to manage the cost of medical care for the patient and may be very influential in steering a patient to home care. The hospital may also initiate the process as it tries to control its costs by reducing patients' length of stay.

Once the decision to send a patient home has been made, a social worker or a discharge planner contacts the home care agency and initiates the process. In many hospitals the discharge planner is a registered nurse with home care experience. The discharge planner will begin preparing the patient for home therapy.

An intake coordinator at the home care company receives the patient referral. This person is responsible for retrieving the patient's demographics (address, phone number, etc.), diagnosis, requested home care therapy, pertinent medical data, and insurance information. The intake coordinator is often a nurse, but can also be a technician specially trained for the job.

When all the necessary data has been obtained, the home care team decides to accept or refuse the referral. This determination is based on the ability and willingness of the patient and/or the caregivers to perform the tasks required to administer therapy at home, the appropriateness and feasibility of the therapeutic plan, and the assurance that home care therapy will not place undue financial burden on the patient or the home infusion company.

Once the patient is accepted, the home care team begins providing services. This includes determining the necessary medical supplies (e.g., tubing, dressing, needles and syringes); selecting an appropriate infusion device (gravity system, pump, etc.); preparing the drug in a sterile environment; assembling the appropriate patient educational materials and home care paperwork; and negotiating charges with the insurer. When all materials and supplies are ready, a delivery is made to the patient's home. The pharmacy technician may be involved in gathering supplies, educational material, and paperwork and arranging delivery. The technician is always involved in preparation of the drugs.

The initial patient visit is made by a registered nurse trained in home infusion. Once the patient has been informed of his/her rights and responsibilities as a home care patient, the nurse begins to teach the patient about the supplies and drugs, and how to care for the catheter so the patient can eventually administer the medications. If a patient cannot administer the medications, a caregiver learns, or on rare occasions, a nurse will administer the medications. Several nursing visits are often required to ensure the patient has been taught properly.

The initial referral process usually extends over 24- to 48-hours, it occasionally must be performed in just a few hours. Empathy is essential in this process. Many times home infusion of medications overwhelms the patients and their caregivers. What may be routine for the home care professional is often very foreign to the patient. Therefore, crucial members of the team (i.e., home care nurse, pharmacist) must be available (usually by pager) to the patient 24 hours a day, 7 days a week.

After the initial visit, the home care team develops a care plan for the patient. The care plan includes how the home care team will monitor the patient's therapy and watch for complications of therapy, as well as signs that the therapy is effective. The patients are visited or contacted by home care team members on a regular basis to assess their status, inventory their supplies, and make interventions when necessary. Generally, supplies and drug are prepared and delivered weekly. The home care team maintains records of the patient's home care course. This is the patient's home care chart and includes documentation of all communications concerning the patient, physician orders and prescriptions, records of drugs and supplies sent to the patient, and laboratory results. The goal of the home care process is for the patient to experience a successful course of therapy without any adverse events. Once home care therapy is completed the patient is discharged from the home care service.

THE HOME CARE TEAM AND SPECIFIC ROLES

The members of the home care team are listed in Table 15-2. The primary team members are actively involved in the care of the majority of home infusion patients. Secondary members are involved only when a particular patient requires their services.

Table 15–2

Members of the Home Health Care Team

Primary Members
- Physician
- Registered Nurse with infusion skills
- Registered Pharmacist
- Pharmacy Technician
- Reimbursement Specialist
- Delivery Representative
- Patient Service Representative
- Patient and/or Caregiver

Secondary Members
- Registered Dietitian
- Respiratory Therapist
- Social Worker
- Physical Therapist
- Occupational Therapist
- Certified Nursing Assistant (CNA)

Physician

The physician is the leader of the team and ultimately responsible for the care of the patient. The physician provides the direction of care. Any major changes in therapy requires the physician's approval. To ensure the physician remains in charge of the patient's care, the physician reviews and signs the Certificate of Medical Necessity and Plan of Treatment. Physician drug orders (prescriptions) are usually received by the pharmacist over the phone, similar to the community pharmacy setting. Written and signed physician orders received via facsimile machine, however, are becoming more common. In the home care environment the physician does not see the patient on a daily or even weekly basis. The physician often relies on the nurse and/or pharmacist to evaluate and report the patient's clinical condition.

Nurse and Pharmacist

The infusion nurse and pharmacist are key members of the team. They work together to coordinate patient supplies, develop a plan of care, monitor and document the patient's status, communicate with the physician, coordinate physician orders, and make appropriate interventions. The nurse and pharmacist not only select the infusion device, but both should be proficient in programming and troubleshooting the devices. Both disciplines are intensely involved in assessing and educating home care patients. The disciplines work jointly to perform the organization's clinical quality assurance activities such as measuring and documenting catheter infections, re-hospitalizations, adverse events (including adverse drug reactions), and outcomes of the plan of care. Together, the nurse and pharmacist are responsible for communicating and coordinating all patient care activities.

Nurse

The nurse is the primary educator of the patient, responsible for teaching all aspects of home care therapy. When visiting the patient, the nurse assesses the patient's physical status, adherence to treatment plan, condition of the catheter, and psychosocial issues the patient may be facing. Maintenance of all intravenous catheters is the sole responsibility of the nurse. Home care infusion nurses are skilled in placement of peripheral catheters and many are skilled in the insertion of peripheral long term catheters or the PICC catheter (discussed later in this chapter). Nurses also schedule and perform all blood work that is ordered.

Pharmacist

The pharmacist is solely responsible for the proper acquisition, compounding, dispensing, and storage of drugs. The pharmacist is also an educator, responsible for instructing the patient and the nurse on the drugs being administered. The pharmacist regularly assesses the home care patient with a focus on monitoring the laboratory data, the patients symptoms, and compliance with drug therapy. Important additional clinical pharmacy roles are pharmacokinetic dosing of vancomycin and aminoglycosides, nutritional support services, as well as input in selection of the most appropriate drug for the home care patient. The pharmacist is the drug information source for all other team members.

Pharmacy Technician

Pharmacy technicians support the pharmacist by performing the majority of the technical pharmacy functions. These consist of generating medication labels; compounding, preparing, and labeling medications; and maintaining the compounding room and drug storage areas. The technician is the coordinator of the IV room, working with the pharmacist to arrange the mixing schedule, ordering and maintaining drug and mixing supplies, and performing quality assurance on compounding activities. Other functions the technician may be responsible for are managing the warehouse and inventory of non-drug supplies, accounts receivable, picking and packaging of supplies for shipment to patients, and delivery of supplies to the patient. In smaller companies, the pharmacy technician may wear many of these hats. In larger companies, an individual is hired (who may be a pharmacy technician) to perform each of these latter functions. For example, some technicians may be experienced drivers and only make patient deliveries.

Reimbursement Specialist

Although not active in direct patient care, the reimbursement specialist is a key to the economic viability of the company. The reimbursement department is the interface between the insurer, and the home infusion company and patient. The primary responsibility of this department is to coordinate all the billing and collection for services provided. To fulfill this responsibility, reimbursement specialists brief staff regarding the services and drugs that are paid for by the insurers, negotiate the price of services with insurers, and brief the insurers regarding the status of the patient and the therapeutic plan. The timeliness of this function is crucial to the financial survival of the organization.

Patient Service Representative

Many companies employ a patient service representative. This person's job is to contact the patient or caregiver weekly. The representative is responsible for controlling the patient's inventory of supplies and screening for problems. Occasionally a pharmacy technician may be responsible for this job.

Patient and/or Caregiver

Not to be forgotten as team members are the patient and/or the caregivers. In home care much of the burden falls on their shoulders. They must be involved in the decision making and the development of the care plan. The patient's right to be involved is clearly stated in the rights and responsibilities document that is presented on the initial visit.

TYPES OF HOME CARE THERAPIES

Antibiotic Therapy

The administration of antibiotic therapy is the leading home infusion service offered, comprising 40 to 70% of the current home infusion business.[3,4] There are four classes of antibiotics that constitute over 80% of home infusion antibiotic therapy (Table 15-3).[4] Since antibiotics have been discussed in chapter 6, this discussion will just focus on the intricacies of these drugs in home infusion.

Cephalosporins, such as ceftriaxone, cefazolin, cefotetan, and cefoperazone, comprise 33% of intravenous antibiotic courses in the home.[4] Cephalosporins are very easy drugs to use in home care because they have a low incidence of adverse reactions[4] and require minimal monitoring. Ceftriaxone is often prescribed because it can be given once daily, which decreases the costs of supplies and requires less work for the patient and/or caregiver. Most cephalosporins are stable for 10 days, ideal for weekly deliveries. The only exceptions are cefotetan and cefoperazone, which are stable for 4 and 5 days respectively.

Penicillins comprise 23% of intravenous antibiotic courses in the home.[4] The top four drugs in this class are ampicillin/sulbactam (Unasyn), ticarcillin/clavulanate (Timentin), nafcillin or oxacillin, and penicillin G. Penicillins are more

Table 15–3

Most Common Antibiotics Used in Home Care

- Cephalosporins
- Penicillins
- Vancomycin
- Therapy for AIDS related infections:
  Ganciclovir
  Foscarnet
  Acyclovir
  Amphotericin B
  Pentamidine

difficult to use in the home because they need to be given so frequently (every 4 to 6 hours). These types of dosing regimens are difficult for some patients to adhere to because of the time it takes out of their day. Portable pumps, called ambulatory pumps, that can automatically give intermittent doses throughout the day are often required for penicillin therapy. Stability is another problem with this class. Ampicillin has short stability and must be mixed in the home prior to infusion. The availability of the ADD-Vantage® system (see chapter 9) has made mixing in the home much easier and safer. Most of the other penicillins have just 7-day stability. Pushing penicillins to their stability limit is of concern because they may break down as they expire, and the break down products are associated with an increased risk of allergic reactions. The most common adverse effect in this class is allergic reaction, such as rash. Penicillins are also very irritating to veins, frequently causing phlebitis (redness and inflammation of the vein). It is highly recommended that patients receiving penicillins at home have a central catheter.

Vancomycin is the third most frequently prescribed drug in home care, accounting for 21% of the orders.[4] Vancomycin should be infused at a rate of 1 gm over 60 minutes to prevent Red Man Syndrome (discussed in chapter 6). This can be accomplished by using a pump or infusion control device, or by placing vancomycin in larger amounts of fluid (e.g., 150 to 250 mls). Individualized patient dosing of vancomycin may be done by the pharmacist using pharmacokinetics and the results of vancomycin blood levels. Vancomycin is irritating to the veins, and in the home setting is best given through a central catheter. If a peripheral catheter is used, vancomycin should be placed in 150 to 250 mls of solution to avoid vein irritation.

Intravenous Antibiotic Therapy

Most available intravenous antibiotics can be used in the home environment. However, relatively few infectious diseases require long term infusion therapy. Five of the more common infectious diseases seen in home care patients are listed in Table 15-4.

Osteomyelitis

Osteomyelitis is an infection that occurs when bacteria invades bone. Bacteria can enter bones via the blood (e.g., in patients with bacteria in the blood), via nearby tissues such as muscle and skin (e.g., when infections of the skin pass from infected tissue to adjacent bone) or via the external environment (e.g., due to a penetrating wound or a fracture where the bone breaks through the skin). The most common bacteria causing osteomyelitis is *Staphylococcus aureus*. This is a gram positive organism that is commonly found on skin. Becoming more common, is osteomyelitis due to other types of bacteria such as gram negatives and anaerobes.

The main symptoms of osteomyelitis are fever, and pain and tenderness near the affected bone(s). The diagnosis is usually based on X-rays and a blood value called erythrocyte sedimentation rate (ESR). The ESR is abnormally high in patients with osteomyelitis. The antibiotic chosen to treat the infection is based on bone cultures when available, or on the organism most likely to cause osteomyelitis. Treatment usually depends on how the patient got the infection. The duration of therapy is usually 4 to 6 weeks, but may be longer. Patients' symptoms and ESR are monitored. With treatment of the infection, the ESR should return to normal.

Septic Arthritis

Septic arthritis is an infection of the tissue that lines the joints, which is called the synovium. The synovium has an extensive blood supply that allows bacteria present in blood to easily enter the joint space. People with trauma to a joint, artificial joints, and arthroscopy are more susceptible to this infection. Patients with diabetes, arthritis, and cancer are also at higher risk for septic arthritis. Therapy consists of surgical drainage of pus from the joint followed by 2 to 3 weeks of intravenous antibiotic therapy. Antibiotics are chosen based on cultures of the drainage. If the causative bacterium is *Staphylococcus*, treatment is recommended for 4 weeks.

Table 15–4

Common Infectious Diseases In Home Care Patients

- osteomyelitis
- septic arthritis
- cellulitis
- endocarditis
- AIDS related infections

When patients with artificial joints develop septic arthritis, it is an extremely painful and costly experience. These patients often require surgical removal of the joint, followed by 6 weeks of intravenous antibiotic therapy, and then the joint is replaced with a new artificial joint.

Cellulitis

Cellulitis is an acute inflammatory infection of the skin that often extends deep into the subcutaneous tissue (tissue under the skin). Cellulitis is often secondary to events such as puncture wounds, ulcers, bites and illicit drug injections. *Streptococcus* and *Staphylococcus* bacteria, found on the skin, are the most common causes of cellulitis. Usually cellulitis can be treated with 14 days of oral antibiotics. However serious infections such as diabetic foot ulcers and human or animal bites may require intravenous therapy.

Endocarditis

Endocarditis is an infection of the heart valves or heart tissue. Patients who get endocarditis usually have an underlying heart defect such as congenital heart disease (born with heart defect), rheumatic heart disease (result of an infection), an artificial heart valve, or a history of illicit drug abuse. Endocarditis can be difficult to diagnose because the symptoms, such as fevers, night sweats, fatigue, weakness, and malaise can be caused by several different medical conditions. The diagnosis of endocarditis is based on blood cultures and ultrasound images of the heart. Endocarditis is treated with 4 weeks of intravenous antibiotics. Antibiotics are chosen based on the organism identified in the blood cultures. Depending on the causative bacteria, combination therapy with two drugs may be required for the first 2 weeks of the 4-week course.

Infections in Acquired Immunodeficiency Syndrome Patients

Patients with acquired immunodeficiency syndrome (AIDS) often contract a number of different infections. The virus that causes AIDS, the human immunodeficiency virus (HIV), suppresses the patients' immune systems and makes them more susceptible to infections. *Pneumocystis carinii* pneumonia (PCP) is the most common opportunistic infection in AIDS patients. The symptoms are a dry cough, and labored or difficult breathing. Therapy begins with 3 weeks of intravenous pentamidine or trimethoprim/sulfamethoxazole. Chronic maintenance therapy with oral antibiotics usually follows. Both of these drugs have the potential for serious toxicity in AIDS patient. Pentamidine can cause severe hypotension if infused too fast. It can also cause acute and severe drops in blood glucose due to a direct toxic effect on the pancreas. In the home setting, pentamidine should be placed on a pump to control infusion rate. Many home care protocols require the immediate availability of normal saline infusion and a syringe of 50% dextrose so these side effects may be treated. Trimethoprim/sulfamethoxazole can cause a high number of allergic reactions in patients with AIDS.

Fungal Infections

Infections with fungi, such as *Candida albicans, Histoplasmosis, Coccidiomycoisis*, are also common in patients without a competent immune system. Amphotericin B is the primary treatment for these infections. Patients may need to receive amphotericin B infusions for 1 to 2 months. AIDS patients require maintenance therapy following their treatment courses, which is often accomplished with the oral anti-fungal agent, fluconazole. Many patients experience fever, chills, and shakes from amphotericin infusions. This reaction often requires pre-medication with oral acetaminophen and diphenydramine. Some patients have such severe reactions that IV meperidine and hydrocortisone are given. The home care infusion pharmacy usually supplies these pre-medications. Infusions of amphotericin should always be given with an infusion pump. Normal saline, commonly used to flush the catheter before and after infusion of medication, is incompatible with amphotericin B. Mixing the two results in precipitate. Therefore, dextrose 5% syringes for flushing of the catheter are compounded by the pharmacy when amphotericin is used in the home.

Immunosuppressed patients are susceptible to *Mycobacterium avium intracellulare* (MAI), part of the tuberculosis family. This infection is very difficult to treat, often requiring a patient to take up to five different medications concurrently. Therapy options include the oral agents: clarithromycin, ethambutol, rifabutin or rifampin, ciprofloxacin, and clofazine. Amikacin is the only intravenous agent for treating MAI. The duration of therapy is indefinite. However most patients cannot remain on amikacin more than several months due to side effects.

Cytomegalovirus is a common viral infection in AIDS patients. The infection manifests itself primarily as retinitis (infection of the retina or back portion of the eye) with blurred vision, or enteritis (infection of the intestines) with diarrhea. The infection is treated with 3 weeks of intravenous ganciclovir or 2 weeks of foscarnet followed by daily maintenance therapy. Ganciclovir almost always causes bone marrow toxicity in AIDS patients. Filgrastim (Neupogen®) therapy is often added to offset the bone marrow toxicity. Foscarnet can cause kidney damage if the patient does not drink plenty of fluids or the drug is infused too fast. To help prevent this, foscarnet is compounded in 500 to 1000 ml of fluid and infused with a pump, or 500 to 1000 ml of normal saline is given prior to each infusion.

Parenteral Nutrition

Patients with Crohn's disease (inflammatory disease of the small and large intestines) and bowel loss or dysfunction are the major recipients of parenteral nutrition. Malnutrition associated with cancer and AIDS is another indication for parenteral nutrition. Patients that absorb some nutrients from the food they eat, but not enough to completely sustain them, may also require supplementation with parenteral nutrition. These patients differ in that they require smaller volumes of parenteral nutrition and may not need daily infusions.

Patients receiving parenteral nutrition often require other intravenous medications. Many of these medication are not compatible with parenteral nutrition. This creates a difficult situation to manage in the home. The patient must learn to stop and start the parenteral nutrition, and adequately flush the catheter in order to administer other medications. One solution is for these patients to have a central catheter with at least two separate lumens. Another solution is for the parenteral nutrition to be cycled to infuse over 8 to 12 hours at night instead of continuously over 24 hours.

Common parenteral nutrition 3-in-1 solutions (contain lipids) are stable for 9 days and bags without lipids are stable for 14 days. However, a number of ingredients in parenteral nutrition are stable for only 24 hours. These drugs are called patient adds and must be injected into the bag prior to infusion by the patient or caregiver in the home. Examples of drugs that the patient must add are insulin, heparin, vitamins, and H2-antagonists (cimetidine, ranitidine). It is advisable to limit what a patient must add to a parenteral nutrition bag to those which are absolutely indicated. This is not only for sterility reasons, but also for the sake of compliance, and patient stress. Drugs a patient needs to add should never be sent in ampule form.

Parenteral nutrition patients require intensive monitoring. This includes weekly laboratory tests (chemistry and CBC), glucose and fluid status monitoring, and patient weights. Monitoring progress toward the therapeutic goals of increasing the patient's weight and improving his/her nutritional status, as well as screening for complications such as liver toxicity and bone break down, is a continual process. Before a week's supply of solution is mixed, the pharmacist must review these parameters, as well as others. If these values are abnormal, the pharmacist must make recommendations to the physician, followed by appropriate changes in the parenteral nutrition formula (e.g., electrolyte content; volume; or the amount of glucose, lipid, or protein in the solution). To avoid making parenteral nutrition bags that cannot be used, mixing of a patient's parenteral nutrition should be coordinated by the technician to follow scheduled laboratory blood draws and pharmacist and nursing assessments and visits. Changes to parenteral nutrition formulas are common, especially the first few months of therapy. Patients on long term parenteral nutrition tend to stabilize after several months and require less monitoring.

Chemotherapy

Most chemotherapy is given in a clinic setting, but a number of chemotherapy agents have been given in the home environment. Chemotherapy regimens reserved for home are those requiring prolonged infusion, usually greater than 24 hours. The agents that tend to be used in this manner are 5-fluorouracil, cyclophosphamide, adriamycin, vincristine, vinblastine, and taxol.

5-Fluorouracil is the most common agent that is administered in the home care environment. Continuous infusions of 5-flourouracil are used in treatment protocols for gastrointestinal (stomach, intestine, colon) and liver cancers. A central line is highly recommended for patients receiving chemotherapy at home to avoid the risk of extravasation (leaking of chemotherapy into the skin resulting in severe damage to the skin). Side effects, primarily bone marrow toxicity and stomatitis (sores in the mouth), are frequent with this class of drugs. Many patients require the addition of filgrastim therapy to counteract the chemotherapy induced drop in white blood cells.

Some oncology clinics and offices have home infusion pharmacies mix chemotherapy for their patients. The chemotherapy is compounded usually for IV push or short IV infusion administration in the clinic or office. When the home infusion company assumes this role, the home care team does not routinely monitor the patients.

Pain Management

The term pain management identifies infusion therapy for patients with chronic pain and pain associated with terminal illnesses. Intravenous medications are used when oral, rectal, or transdermal alternatives are not effective. Ninety percent of home care narcotic orders are for morphine.[4] When morphine is not acceptable, other drugs used for pain control are hydromorphone, meperidine, fentanyl, or fentanyl with bupivacaine. Usually one bag or cassette with enough narcotic to last the patient a week is dispensed at a time. In order to accomplish this, morphine solution is usually provided in concentrations of 5 to 50 mg per ml.

In the home environment, narcotics can be given subcutaneously, intravenously, epidurally, or intrathecally. When the patient has an intravenous catheter, pain management is given via this route. The subcutaneous route is often used in patients without intravenous access. Intrathecal and epidural routes are saved for those patients who cannot achieve adequate pain control with intravenous therapy. Infusion of narcotics is accomplished using patient controlled analgesia (PCA) pumps (see chapter 9 for a complete description). Attainment of adequate pain control, such that the patient has a decent quality of life, is the goal of the home care team. Assessment of the patient's pain by team members is done on a continual basis.

Enteral Therapy

Some home infusion pharmacies may also provide enteral therapy. Enteral nutrition is the administration of specialized formulas, high in required nutrients, through the stomach to meet a patient's nutritional needs. Those patients who can eat, drink the enteral formula. Other patients who cannot eat (e.g., are comatose) but have a working stomach, receive the formula through tubes placed through their nose down into their stomach, or surgically to their stomachs. Home infusion companies become involved when enteral nutrition is being administered continu-

ously via a feeding tube with or without a pump. When this technology is used, it often requires the expertise of the home health care team. Patients who can drink their enteral formulas, can usually get their therapy much cheaper through a community pharmacy system and do not require home care services. Monitoring of enteral patients includes detecting drug-nutrition interactions and monitoring their nutritional status.

Biological Response Modifiers

The biological response modifiers include filgrastim (Neupogen®), erythropoietin (Epogen®), interferons, and growth hormone. These agents are called high technology drugs because they are produced through genetic engineering. These drugs are fairly easy to administer through conventional subcutaneous and intravenous routes.

Filgrastim is used for treatment of chemotherapy and AIDS induced neutropenia (low white cell count). Erythropoietin is used to treat anemia. Interferons have roles in the treatment of multiple sclerosis, chronic hepatitis, cancer, and certain rare diseases. Growth hormone is used in children less than 14 years old who are short in stature due to deficiency in the hormone. All these agents are proteins that should not be shaken and require refrigeration for stability.

Other Therapies

Numerous other therapies are becoming more common in the home health care setting. In some cases patients with congestive heart failure, women with premature labor, patients with the genetic disorder alpha-1 antitrypsin deficiency, and simple dehydration are being treated at home with drugs that were previously infused in institutional settings.

COMPOUNDING IN THE HOME CARE SETTING

Pharmacy technicians, under the supervision of pharmacists, are responsible for the correct preparation of sterile products. It is important that the pharmacy technician become familiar with appropriate procedures to ensure that pharmacy-prepared sterile products are of high quality.

Clean Rooms

A clean room is an enclosed space, containing one or more clean zones, where the concentration of airborne particles is controlled. Most home infusion companies either have a clean room or sterile compounding area. The major difference between the two is the designated specifications for control of potential microbial contamination. In a clean room, the whole room environment is controlled for microorganisms within designated specifications. In the sterile compounding area, the sterile product preparation room only needs to be functionally separate from nonsterile product preparation and constructed to minimize particulate and microbial contamination. Although it would seem like a clean room is the best option, new technology and products allow companies to prepare products safely in sterile compounding rooms. A few state boards of pharmacy have mandated the use of clean rooms, but generally the home infusion company decides which type of room to use.

Clean rooms minimize the accumulation of particulates and microbial growth by using smooth, seamless, nonporous, and nonshedding building materials; temperature and relative humidity controls; and air filtration devices.[5] These rooms coupled with policies that prohibit shedding materials (e.g., cardboard boxes) and porous and nonsterile materials from entering the room, and require personnel to be properly trained and dressed in sterile garments establish the cleanest compounding environment possible.

Clean rooms are classified based on the number of particles in the room. A room with no more than 1 particle of 0.5 micron size per cubic foot of space is a Class 1 clean room. A room with no more than 100,000 particles of 0.5 micron size per cubic foot of space is a Class 100,000 clean room. At a minimum clean rooms must be certified by a qualified contractor every 6 months or when the room is relocated.

Sterile compounding areas are less formal in design and do not require formal certification.[5] The number of particles per cubic foot of space in a sterile compounding area can increase the chances of contaminating a product during preparation. However, when products are prepared in a sterile compounding area different techniques and approaches to preparing sterile products are employed to reduce the risk of contamination.

Most infusion providers look to voluntary practice standards for guidance on quality assurance issues. Two professional pharmacy organizations have provided guidelines intended to help pharmacy personnel ensure that pharmacy-prepared IV admixtures are of high quality. The American Society of Health-System Pharmacists (ASHP) published the "ASHP Technical Assistance Bulletin on Quality Assurance for Pharmacy-Prepared Sterile Products."[6] The United States Pharmacopeial Convention issued an informational chapter on "Sterile drug products for home use."[7] In the ASHP technical bulletin, sterile products are grouped into three levels of risk to the patient. These categories depend on how much time elapses between when the drug is compounded and when it is administered; in other words, the expiration dating. These levels increase from least (level 1) to greatest (level 3) potential risk and have different quality assurance recommendations for product integrity and patient safety[6] (Table 15-5).

The rationale behind the risk level approach is that the greater the chance of contamination or the greater the risk of microbial growth in the product, the more careful providers should be to safeguard the sterility of the IV admixture. In this case, a parenteral nutrition solution prepared by gravity transfer from manufacturers' bottles or bags, refrigerated for 7 days or less before administration, and given to a patient over a period not exceeding 24 hours would be an example of a relatively low risk product in level 1. The highest risk of contamination would entail batch preparation of parenteral nutrition solutions with investigational L-glutamine prepared from nonsterile powdered glutamine in an open reservoir. Most products prepared for use by home care patients fall into risk level 2 because they are stored for more than 7 days.

Methods to access an individual's aseptic techniques and environmental monitoring programs are often used to identify potential sources of contamination. Once a source is identified, steps can be taken to improve the environment. In addition, pharmacy technicians can play a major role in preserving clean environments by maintaining them properly. Chapter 9 reviews the principles relating to sterile compounding and maintaining clean environments.

High Technology Systems

The home infusion therapy industry's need for technology to improve the patient's quality of life and save the infusion companies money has resulted in a number of products that allow med-

Table 15–5

Sterile Product Risk Levels

Risk Level	Storage Conditions*			Products	Quality Assurance Level
	Room Temperature	Refrigerator	Freezer		
1	completely administered within 28 hrs	</= 7 days	</= 30 days	unpreserved sterile products for 1 patient; batch-prepared products with preservatives;closed system aseptic transfer of pharmaceutical obtained from licensed manufacturer into sterile final container	least
2	storage and administration exceeds 28 hrs	> 7 days	> 30 days	batch-prepared products without preservatives; closed system aseptic transfer of combined multiple sterile ingredients obtained from licensed manufacturer in a sterile reservoir before subdivision into multiple units	more
3				compounded from nonsterile ingredients or compounded with nonsterile components, containers, or equipment; use of open-system transfer or open reservoir for sterile or nonsterile combined multiple ingredients before terminal sterilization or subdivision into multiple units	most

*Storage Conditions: Room Temperature (15 to 30°C), refrigerator (2 to 8°C), freezer (–20 to –10°C).
Adapted from: ASHP technical assistance bulletin on quality assurance for pharmacy-prepared sterile products. *Am J Hosp Pharm.* 1993;50:2386–98.

ications to be delivered to patients at home. In most cases the device chosen by the home care provider dictates the type of bag the medication or solution will be dispensed in and to a greater extent the type of supplies (e.g., tubing, needles) the technician will have to assemble for the patient. Technicians should become familiar with the infusion products and the supplies the home infusion company uses to care for its patient population.

There are four types of infusion systems available for patients to use at home: the minibag infusion via gravity system, syringe infusion via syringe device, rate-restricted IV administration set systems, and ambulatory electronic infusion pumps. Home care providers select the most appropriate infusion device based on several factors, the most important being the patient's needs (Table 15-6). In addition to the patient's needs, cost and reimbursement are also important factors that home care providers consider when selecting a system.[8,9] A range of issues to consider when selecting an infusion system are listed in Table 15-7. All of these factors have an impact on the cost-effectiveness and appropriate selection of infusion devices. Unfortunately,

Table 15–6

Patient Needs Assessment for Selecting Infusion Systems

- Age
- Diagnosis
- Clinical condition
- Manual dexterity
- Ambulatory status
- Working status
- Number of therapies
- Training ability for self-administration
- Caregiver presence in the home
- Nursing support requirements
- Travel time from home infusion provider

Adapted from: Saladow J. Ambulatory systems for i.v. antibiotic therapy: making sense of the options. *Infusion* 1995; April:17–29.

Table 15–7

Cost Issues Associated with Infusion System Selection

- Product design
- Product efficacy
- Product reliability
- Product availability
- Ease of staff training
- Ease of patient/caregiver training
- Nursing interaction time
- Pharmacy handling time
- Pharmacy filling time
- Ability of device to minimize complications
- Ability of device to minimize waste
- Storage space needed at provider's facility
- Storage space needed in patient's home
- Manufacturer and/or distributor support
- Ease of product disposal
- Down-time and repair cost
- Inventory costs

Adapted from: Saladow J. Ambulatory systems for i.v. antibiotic therapy: making sense of the options. *Infusion* 1995; April:17–29.

the industry has yet to firmly quantify and analyze this impact. Selection is also complicated by the vast array of products that are marketed as the most economical method for therapy delivery.

Minibag Infusion via Gravity System

The minibag infusion via gravity system can be one of the most cost-effective methods to deliver medications. In fact, it is the standard intravenous administration set used for hospitalized patients in the United States. However, in the home care setting this system may be more expensive than in the institutional setting due to the cost associated with nurses teaching patients and caregivers, and troubleshooting problems.[8] Other limitations of the system are the expectation that patients or caregivers will manually connect the bag to the infusion tubing, and set and maintain the infusion rate; the increased risk for touch contamination; and the problems the cumbersome IV pole (on which the bag hangs) causes patients who are ambulatory or trying to work.

The AddVantage® and Add-a-Vial® systems are special types of minibags used for drugs with short stability. With both systems, the patient/caregiver activates the vial just before administration so that the drug mixes with the diluent in the minibag. This is more expensive than the traditional minibag system mentioned above because of the specially designed minibags that both systems use and the special drug vials used with the AddVantage® system. Both of these systems have the same limitations as the traditional minibag system. See chapter 9 for a more detailed description of special types of minibags.

Syringe Infusion System

The syringe infusion system is another very cost-effective system. Syringes are also easier to prepare and store than the containers used with other systems. The limitations of the syringe systems are the small volume of fluid that can be stored in one syringe. The volume limitations result in requiring the preparation of concentrated dilutions, the potential for increased time spent educating patients and caregivers, potential for malfunctions of the electrical devices used to push the solution from the syringe, and restrictions it imposes on those ambulatory or working patients.[8] Syringe infusion systems that are currently available are the Bard/Baxter Mini-Infuser, Becton Dickinson/McGaw Infuser, Baxa

Dual Rate Infuser, Excelsior ESP Infusion System, and Medex 2001 and 2010 models. These devices are commonly used for administration of IV antibiotics to the home care patient. The 3M Medifuse® syringe system is unique in that it uses a mechanical rather than electronic syringe driver along with a series of proprietary infusion sets that control the medication rate.

Rate-restricted IV Administration Systems

Rate-restricted IV administration sets are used with proprietary fluid reservoirs that are designed specifically for use in the home care setting. The tubing used with this system is designed to infuse the solution at a set rate. The only way to change the rate of infusion is to change the tubing. There are three general types of proprietary fluid reservoirs that can be used in this system, the elastomeric balloon, mechanical, and electronic controlled pressure and chemical release systems.

Elastomeric Balloons

Elastomeric balloon systems were first used for delivering antibiotics and chemotherapy agents to patients outside of the hospital. Infusion Systems developed the first device of this type, now called the Baxter Intermate® Elastomeric Infusion System. As the home care industry grew, so did the number of other elastomeric balloon infusion systems. These reservoirs consist of multiple layers of elastomeric (i.e., stretchy, elastic-like) membranes that are contained within a hard or soft shell. When the device is filled with diluent and drug, the elastomeric material expands like a balloon filling up with air. When tubing is attached to the device and the patient's catheter the elastic balloon forces the solution through the tubing and into the patient. The tubing controls the rate of the infusion, which can range from 0.5 to 200 ml/hour.[8] These devices do not have alarms and safety features, thus they may not be suitable for medications that require a critical infusion rate (i.e., dobutamine) or cause tissue damage if extravasation occurs.[9] However, advantages of elastomeric balloons are that they are small and lightweight, thus convenient for use in ambulatory or working patients, and they are easy to use which makes patient training simple.

A few of the elastomeric balloon systems that are currently available are Block Medical Homepump® and Homepump Eclipse®, McGaw Ready Med®, and Secure Medical MedFlo II®. Baxter Healthcare's Infusor System and Block Medical's

Extended Use Homepump® are designed specifically for administering chemotherapy and other long-term continuous infusions. Elastomeric balloon reservoirs can be filled with syringes manually, via an automated filling pump, or by using a pump designed specifically for filling the elastomeric system. It is important that the technician or pharmacist prime the tubing to remove air before sending the elastomeric balloon device to a patient. Manipulation of these devices versus other systems may take more pharmacy technician time due to the need to add diluent and drug. However, automated filling pumps can reduce the preparation time.

Mechanical Systems

Several mechanical systems that rely on positive pressure similar to elastomeric balloons have been developed. The I-Flow SideKick® infusion system was introduced in 1992. It consists of a round pump housing that unscrews and opens in two halves, a round disposable plastic bag that holds either 50 ml or 100 ml of fluid and an IV flow control set. Once the two halves are screwed together, a spring-loaded pressure plate in the upper half of the pump housing applies positive pressure to the lower half containing the diluent and drug. As the clamp on the attached IV set is opened, the positive pressure forces fluid out of the bag at a rate controlled by the tubing. Infusion sets are available as disposable, pre-attached, or as a separate set that is detached from the disposable bag and reused for future doses. This reusable set offers the advantage of lowering the overall cost per dose.[8] I-Flow also developed two additional devices similar in design and concept, the Paragon® and Paragon Elite®. The Paragon® is like the SideKick® except it holds 110 ml of fluid and its spring mechanism is designed for more accurate delivery and slower infusion rates. It was designed to give longer-term continuous infusions like chemotherapy. The Paragon Elite® has the additional feature of a built-in battery, which can provide a series of alarm conditions. The disposables for all three of these I-Flow devices are available only from Solopak Pharmaceuticals. All of these devices are manually filled with a syringe or a pharmacy-automated filling pump.

Electronic Controlled Pressure and Chemical Release Systems

In early 1994, an electronic controlled pressure device, the Maxx®100 by Medication Delivery Devices, was introduced. This system consists of a rectangular shaped housing and a series of disposable reservoir bags with pre-attached IV flow control sets.[8] Detachable IV sets may be used and reused for multiple doses, again reducing the cost of each dose delivered. A proprietary plastic bag is placed inside the device housing on top of a bladder, which expands with air and applies pressure to the bag when the device is closed and turned on. The IV tubing controls the drug administration rate once the clamp on it is opened. It differs from the previously discussed rate-restricted systems in that it provides controlled pressure pumping via an electronic system rather than by positive pressure. It also has audible and visual alarms. The Maxx®250 infusion system, a 250 ml version of the Maxx®100 system was recently released. Proprietary minibags or standard Abbott or Baxter minibags prefilled with diluent may be used in this device.

The SmartDose® by River Medical provides positive pressure by a combination of a chemical reaction and mechanical pressure. It incorporates a hard plastic outer infusion container, administration set, and drug vial adaptor. The infusion container houses two flexible multi-layered membranes. This device is manually filled with diluent using a syringe or automated filling pump. Recently, this device container became available with pre-filled diluent. The drug is then added by syringe or by attaching the drug vial adaptor to the fill port of the SmartDose® container. An advantage of this system is that the actual mixing of the drug can occur in the patient's home just prior to infusion.[8] When ready for a dose, the patient attaches an IV set to the container, connects it to the catheter, and depresses a round start button at the top of the container. This releases CO_2 gas that exerts a constant pressure forcing fluid out of the container. It requires proprietary reusable IV administration sets that are attached prior to infusing. These devices take minimal pharmacy technician time to assemble due to the availability of pre-filled diluent bags designed specifically for the devices. In many cases, only a prescription label need be attached to the finished product.[8]

The rate-restricted IV administration systems described offer significant advantages in the delivery of antibiotics and other medications to home care patients. Unfortunately, many of them still require addition of diluent to the reservoirs. When more are available with pre-filled diluents, these systems will be more convenient, reduce pharmacy admixture time, increase flexibility use, and be more cost-effective.

Ambulatory Electronic Infusion Pumps

A number of ambulatory electronic infusion pumps on the market are designed to deliver various therapies to home care patients. Many of these devices integrate infusion and computer technologies. Some of these devices are designed to administer a single therapy such as parenteral nutrition while others can accommodate multiple types of therapies utilized in the home.[8,9] Today there are more than 25 ambulatory electronic infusion devices available.

Ambulatory electronic infusion pumps are small, lightweight, and can be worn by the patient during infusions. They offer a wide range of infusion rate settings and volumes. These features are controlled by the electronic components of the individual device. Moreover, these pumps can infuse out of standard IV containers or proprietary reservoirs. Selection of an ambulatory device depends on patient-, therapy-, and infusion service-related factors. Table 15-8 reviews these factors. The device selected for a patient on home infusion therapy may ultimately determine how the patient views the home care experience.[10,11]

Ambulatory infusion devices are typically divided into two broad categories, therapy-specific and multiple therapy devices.[12] Therapy-specific devices are designed to provide single therapies such as pain management or TPN. Operation of these devices is fairly straightforward, and can be done by clinicians and patients. Common therapy-specific devices include the Abbott Provider® products and the SIMS Deltec CADD® infusion pumps. Other therapy-specific devices are found in Table 15-9. The CADD® pumps are the most widely used ambulatory infusion devices in the United States. All of these devices are therapy-specific and relatively simple to program.[14] The CADD-TPN®, CADD-PCA®, and CADD-Plus® are designed specifically for TPN infusions, pain medications, and antibiotics, respectively. The CADD-TPN® has two proprietary sets that connect to standard TPN containers, one containing a 0.22 micron filter for non-lipid-containing TPN solutions and one containing a 1.2 micron filter for lipid-containing TPN solutions. The CADD-PCA® and CADD-Plus® devices use proprietary 50 ml or 100 ml cassettes with attached tubing that contain the diluent and/or drug. They are manually filled with a luer-lock syringe. In addition, other IV containers can be used with these two devices by attaching a bypass spike adaptor with tub-

Table 15–8

Factors Influencing Selection of Ambulatory Infusion Device[10,11]

Patient-related Factors	Therapy-related	Infusion Service-related
• Age	• Number of Drugs	• Distance from Home Care Office
• IV Access	• Drug Stability and Compatibility	• Reimbursement Issues
• Ambulatory Status	• Duration of Infusion	• Nursing Support Requirements
• Level or Presence of Caregiver Assistance	• Dosing Schedule or Pattern	
• Environment	• Volume of Infusate	
	• Patient Controlled Dose Needs	
	• Accuracy of Small Volume Delivery	
	• Life of Battery	

ing. Filling of the cassettes or containers requires the technician to remove air from them because the pumps do not contain air-eliminating filters.

Multiple therapy devices allow providers to carry a single device that may be used for any patient with different therapies. Inventory can be consolidated, capital equipment costs can be overcome more quickly, and clinical staff training is simplified. These devices can infuse continuously or intermittently and may be used to infuse TPN solutions, antibiotics, antineoplastic agents, and pain medications. Most are single-channel, allowing infusion of only one medication at a time. Others are multiple-channel, capable of infusing up to four different drugs at different rates.[10,12] Table 15-10 lists the multiple-channel devices. Furthermore, newer devices offer telemedicine capabilities whereby information can be transmitted over standard telephone lines via the use of modems, from the patient's

Table 15–9

Therapy-Specific Ambulatory Infusion Devices[12]

Device	Manufacturer	Primary Therapy
Provider One	Abbott Laboratories	Parenteral nutrition
Provider 5500	Abbott Laboratories	Patient-controlled analgesia
Provider 6000	Abbott Laboratories	Continuous and intermittent infusions, patient-controlled analgesia
Pain Management Provider	Abbott Laboratories	Patient-controlled analgesia
EZ-Flow 80-2	Creative Medical Development	Antibiotics, antivirals
H-Tron V 100	Disetronic Medical Systems	Insulin
Panomat Series	Disetronic Medical Systems	Micro-infusions (terbutaline)
WalkMed 350	Medex Inc.	Low-dose continuous infusions
WalkMed PCA	Medex Inc.	Patient-controlled analgesia
MiniMed 506	MiniMed Technologies	Insulin
MiniMed 404-SP	MiniMed Technologies	Micro-infusions (terbutaline)
CADD-1	SIMS Deltec Inc.	Chemotherapy
CADD-PCA	SIMS Deltec Inc.	Patient-controlled analgesia
CADD-Plus	SIMS Deltec Inc.	Antibiotics, chemotherapy, dobutamine
CADD-TPN	SIMS Deltec Inc.	Parenteral nutrition
CADD-Micro	SIMS Deltec Inc.	Micro-infusions (insulin, terbutaline)

Table 15–10

Multiple Channel (Therapy) Ambulatory Infusion Devices[12]

Device*	Manufacturer
AIM Infusion System	Abbott Laboratories
Verifuse**	Block Medical Inc.
EZ-Flow 480**	Creative Medical Development
VIVUS 2000**	I-Flow Corporation
VIVUS 4000**	I-Flow Corporation
Vector MTI**	Infusion Technologies
MedMate 1100	Patient Solutions
Sabratek 6060 Homerun**	Sabratek

*Able to infuse all of the following therapies: antibiotics, chemotherapy, continuous therapies, patient-controlled analgesia, parenteral nutrition.
**Denotes devices with telecommunications capabilities.

home to the health care provider's office. Providers can change infusion rates, correct alarm conditions, track patient compliance, and view or print infusion status reports without making a home visit.

New ambulatory infusion devices continue to be developed. Disposable devices that infuse large volumes of fluid using disposable batteries are on the horizon. It is important for home infusion providers to keep up with the latest infusion device technology so they can provide the high quality of care that patients and third-party payers expect. Furthermore, pharmacy technicians must become familiar with the different ambulatory infusion devices available. This knowledge will allow technicians to choose the appropriate supplies when preparing products and sending supplies patients need to use the devices.

Automated Compounding Devices

Automated compounding devices are based on peristaltic pump principles similar to infusion pumps. Patient-specific parenteral nutrition formulations and the benefits of providing 24-hour, single-container TPN and hydration bags have driven the need for automated compounding devices. The need is especially prevalent in home care practice, since the patient usually gets a 1- to 2-week supply of TPN or fluids. Automated compounding devices are also used to prepare complex multicomponent sterile products such as nutrition formulations and cardioplegia solutions, as well as batch preparations of other solutions.

Several automated compounding systems are currently marketed including Nutrimix® (Abbott Laboratories), MicroMacro Compounder® (Baxa), Automix® and Micromix® (Clintec Nutrition), and Hyper-Former® (McGaw). The advantages of these devices over manual compounding are increased efficiency and accuracy, automatic calculations (software-driven systems), potential reduction in labor, reduction in materials, and demonstrated cost-effectiveness.[13,14] Disadvantages of a completely automated system are the potential for equipment malfunction and power outages. Automated compounding devices are available with proprietary tubing that attach to the device. Proprietary or other manufacturers' containers are then connected to the tubing. It is important that the device operator removes air from the filled container prior to sending it to the patient. Removing air avoids ambulatory infusion device alarms and eliminates other problems.

Special considerations are taken when using automated compounding devices. Home infusion companies use a compounding sequence or manufacturing practice that minimizes the potential for gross or subtle incompatibilities, especially when mixing total nutrient admixtures (TNAs). It is essential that technicians recognize the importance of these sequences and practices, because technicians often play a major role in, or are completely responsible for following the sequence. The order of mixing of components as well as their final concentrations is important for TPN solution stability. Many manufacturers of automated compounding devices have predetermined additive sequences available for use by operators of these devices.[15] The development of dual-chamber bags in which the lipid is contained in the upper portion of the bag, while the other TPN components are in the lower portion of the bag, also may improve the safety of TNA formulations. These bags extend stability (up to 30 days). The patient or caregiver activates the bag by removing a white strip and gray bar just prior to infusing. These bags can be filled using an automated compounding device. To ensure stability throughout the administration period some medications, such as multivitamins and insulin, are added by the patient just prior to infusion.

Labeling and Expiration Dating

Labeling in home care practice is similar to that in institutions. However, there are some unique requirements. The product is considered an outpatient prescription, thus it must meet state board of pharmacy requirements (see chapter 4). The label should be written so lay people (nonmedically trained people such as patients and caregivers) can interpret and understand the directions.

The information required by law for a home care product label includes the patient's name, prescription number, prescribing physician, and date (Figure 15-1). The patient's address is optional, however, it may simplify delivery procedures. Directions for use should state the rate and frequency of administration, and any special handling or storage requirements. The name and amount of drug contained in one dose and the appropriate volume for that amount should be listed. Then, the name and volume of admixture solution equivalent to one dose of drug is indicated. The actual expiration date established for the product is noted. The individual(s) who prepared and checked the admixture must initial the label. Finally, auxiliary labeling should include federal transfer labeling and optionally, specific precautionary labels or storage instruction labels can be applied to the product. The bottle or bag sequence may be listed as well to help track the specific number of

doses ordered and/or the total number of doses administered.[6]

Expiration dating has important implications in home care practice, as it may dictate whether the pharmacy can prepare batches, reduce waste, and decrease the frequency of deliveries to the patient. Expiration dates for admixtures are based on stability and sterility data.[6,7] Most home care pharmacists have references that list expiration dates for products or their components. The most common reference is the *Handbook on Injectable Drugs*, but many pharmacists keep files containing published research articles on stability. Technicians need to be aware of expiration dates on products they use to make sterile admixtures. When a product expires in a particular month of a year, it can be used through the last day of the month listed.

A product can quickly change or deteriorate as a result of changes in pH, temperature, and drug structure that may cause solubility problems; drug adsorption to and absorption within product containers; and chemical degradation due to hydrolysis, oxidation, reduction, or photolysis. The method of delivery, either the system or technique, and environment of the drug administration can also affect stability.[6,7] Home care practice demands that the pharmacist assign a maximum expiration date that is still within appropriate stability limits. A common problem is the use of drugs with limited stability at room temperature. For drugs to be given via an ambulatory infusion device, at least 24-hour stability at room temperature or warmer is required.[10] For drugs that have limited room temperature stability, the patient or caregiver may be taught how to prepare the drug immediately before administration. Although a product may be stable for an extended period, its sterility and potential for bacterial growth must also be a factor in assigning an expiration date. Sterile products not intended for prompt use should be stored at no higher than 4°C to inhibit microbial growth, unless room temperature storage is warranted.[7]

Packaging and Transport

Temperature control during transportation of sterile products to a patient's home is critical. Appropriate packaging must be used to keep the temperature near the midpoint of the product's specified range.[7] Technicians should be familiar with the pharmacy's procedures for packaging products so they can abide by them. Most admixtures are placed in a ziplock bag to prevent a

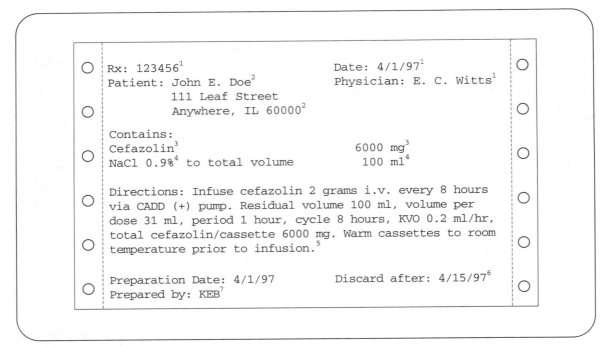

Figure 15-1. Sample home care label.

KEY: Required Labeling

1 - Prescription number, date, and prescribing physician—Is typically required by state boards of pharmacy. Used by dispensing pharmacist to verify original order.

2 - Patient name and address—The patient's name should be printed as part of the label.

3 - Name and amount of drug added—The name of the drug, preferably generic, should be stated. The amount of drug per dose or per unit dispensed (e.g.,in this case, the total amount of drug in the cassette) should be listed.

4 - Name and volume of admixture solution—The amount of admixture solution per dose should be stated. In the case of a container housing more than one dose, the volume listed should be equivalent to the total volume in the container.

5 - Directions for use—These should be easy to understand. They should include rate and frequency of administration. Any special handling or storage requirements should be stated.

6 - Expiration date—The date is usually the actual expiration date established for the product.

7 - Initials of persons who prepare and check IV admixture—State boards of pharmacy often require that this information appear on the label. In addition, this information is helpful when questions arise about product preparation.

Adapted from: Scheckelhoff DJ. Labeling of sterile products. In: *Principles of Sterile Product Preparation*. Bethesda, MD: ASHP; 1995.

problem if leakage occurs. Hazardous substances should be double bagged to protect the shipper, patient, and caregiver if leakage occurs. These individuals should be trained how to deal with a spill in case it occurs. Certain product containers such as prefilled syringes should be packaged in hard plastic or cardboard tubes, or within bubble packs to prevent movement during transit. Refrigerated items should be transported in coolers and postdelivery temperature checks should be taken to ensure that an adequate temperature was maintained. Delivery personnel should be familiar with the shipping requirements for each package. In some cases, technicians may make deliveries and should therefore be sure they understand the delivery requirements.

Supplies for the Home Care Patient

Technicians should become familiar with the supplies used by home care patients so they can communicate about supply issues with the patient and other health care professionals. This entails being aware of the various venous access devices (catheters that reside in the patient's vein through which medication or solution flows) as well as specific supplies that the patient or caregiver uses to set up an infusion, such as tubing and needles.

Venous Access Devices

Peripheral access (e.g., infusing drugs in through a needle placed in the veins of an arm) is one of the most common ways patients receive infusions in the hospital, but it does not always work well in the home care environment. Peripheral access is better for short courses of therapy than long courses of therapy. Peripheral veins often collapse or rupture, so a new vein must be used and in some cases, there are not any usable peripheral veins left. To avoid this scenario other types of venous access devices are used for patients who need long term access. Consequently, a number of extended venous access devices (that can be used for weeks to months, even years) have been developed for patients who require repeated venipuncture (the puncture of a vein for any therapeutic purpose) or who have suboptimal peripheral venous access due to advanced age, obesity, or previous irritating drug therapy. These devices are classified as tunneled central venous catheters, subcutaneous vascular access ports, and peripherally inserted central venous catheters.[10] It is important for technicians to gain a general understanding of the venous access devices commonly used. This knowledge assists technicians in selecting patient supplies more accurately and efficiently.

Two examples of commonly used tunneled central venous catheters are Broviac and Hickman catheters. These catheters were introduced in the 1970s and were made of barium-impregnated silicone rubber (Silastic®). They facilitate long-term vascular access with minimal complications. These catheters are surgically inserted into a central venous site and passed through the vein until the tip of the catheter stops at the entrance of the heart's right atrium. After insertion, the catheter is tunneled subcutaneously for a short distance to establish a barrier between the skin exit site and vascular entrance site. An external dressing or bandage is applied to the site. Available tunneled models are distinguished by the catheter material (silicone or polyurethane), number of lumens (single, double, or triple), catheter diameter (French size 3 = pediatric to 12.5 or 13.0 = double or triple lumen), lumen diameter (0.2 to 2.0 mm), and type of catheter tip.[10,16] Manufacturers of these catheters include Arrow International, Inc., Bard, Cook Critical Care, Harbor Medical Devices, and Quinton. The lumens (access ports on the catheters) are separate within the catheter, so incompatible solutions can be administered at the same time. To prevent the formation of blood clots when the catheter is not in use, a heparin solution of 100 units/ml should be locked into each lumen at least daily. The Groshung®

catheter is unique in that it has a pressure-sensitive, distal-tip slit valve (a valve at the end of the catheter with a slit in the rubber). Infusing or withdrawing fluid causes pressure that opens the valve. When the valve is closed, blood cannot flow back into the catheter. This eliminates the need for heparin locking and also decreases the risk of air embolism. These catheters are flushed with 5 to 10 ml of saline after each use and weekly when the catheter is not in use. Infections are the most common complications of tunneled venous access devices. Other complications include catheter occlusion (clogging), dislodgement (moving out of the vein), incorrect catheter positioning, and venous thrombosis (blood clots).

The subcutaneous vascular access port consists of a small volume reservoir with a self-sealing septum that is connected to a central venous catheter. This system is placed subcutaneously (under the skin) by a surgeon, usually in the chest wall, and is hardly noticeable. A dressing or bandage is unnecessary. The device is accessed by inserting a specially designed, noncoring needle called a Huber needle through the skin and port septum.[10] Single- and double-lumen devices are available. Several different products are currently on the market, including Port-a-Cath®, Infusaport®, Mediport®, and Davol®. These devices are suitable for intermittent or prolonged continuous infusions. Between infusions, the port is flushed and locked with heparin 100 units/ml, 5 ml at monthly intervals. Complications are similar to those of tunneled catheters and include infections, occlusion, and thromboses. Needle dislodgement from the septum may occur as well as pocket (the opening under the skin where the device resides) infections.

The use of peripherally inserted central venous catheters (PICC) is increasing because of their unique features. PICCs can be inserted at the bedside or at home by specially trained nurses. They are inserted through a vein in the arm, threaded through other veins in the arm, and end up with the tip resting in the superior vena cava.[10,17] PICCs may remain in place for weeks to months. An X-ray is used to confirm placement before infusing solutions that are very hypertonic such as TPN. PICC lines, also known as long-arm or long-line catheters are made of silicone (Silastic®) or flexible polyurethane and are available in single- and multilumen designs. They require daily flushing with heparin and dressing changes. Complications include phlebitis at the insertion site or along the vein, infection, cellulitis, occlusion, catheter tip migration, and thrombosis.[10,17]

Peripheral catheters are available in a number of gauges and lengths, commonly between 18 to 24 gauge and three-quarters to one inch in length. These catheters are desirable for short-term therapies. Most home care providers' protocols call for changing peripheral catheters every 72 hours.

Midline catheters are peripheral catheters but have the advantage of being 6 inches in length and may remain in place on average 7 to 10 days but even up to months. A Landmark® catheter is a common midline catheter inserted in home care patients.

Other Supplies

Patients on home infusion therapy require a number of other supplies. Many home care providers have standard supplies that are sent to most patients whether they have a peripheral or central venous catheter. In general, these supplies include alcohol pads, injection caps (caps that go onto the end of the catheters), nonsterile gloves, a sharps container, medical waste bag, and tubing. Additional supplies depend on the type of venous access and therapy, the physician, or account specifications. For drugs or fluids requiring filtration, an appropriate filter should be included.

If a patient has a peripheral line, an IV start kit will be needed, while a CVC (central venous catheter) kit is required for midline or central lines. These kits are self-contained packets of supplies required to insert IV lines or change the dressing at the line insertion site. Several catheters should be available in the home for patients with peripheral lines so that the nurse has one when the catheter is scheduled to be changed. The only centrally placed catheters that are inserted in the home are PICC lines. Other central venous access devices are placed in the hospital.

For patients requiring an ambulatory infusion device, the appropriate tubing should be sent. Thus it is important to keep a record of which device a patient is using. Batteries are required for devices that are battery-operated. Patients receiving their therapy via minibag or using a non-ambulatory infusion device may need an IV pole. These are available in portable, collapsible designs or the standard, rugged type seen in hospitals.

Heparin is supplied in different concentrations depending upon the type of venous access device. Generally, heparin 10 units/ml is used for peripheral catheters while 100 units/ml is used for central venous catheters. Many home infusion companies or institutions have specific protocols that are followed for heparin flushes. Technicians should be familiar with these protocols so that the appropriate flushing materials accompany the patient's supply order. If flush materials are sent in vial form or if drugs will need to be drawn from vials, the appropriate syringe(s) and needles should be included.

Patients on a needleless system should receive the proper materials including injection caps, vial adaptors, syringes, and syringe cannulas. Interlink® and Burron are two needleless system products currently available. Home care personnel should determine the appropriate supply use based on anticipated delivery frequency and send supplies accordingly. In many cases, patients are taught to take inventory of their supplies and review it with the appropriate personnel each time a delivery is anticipated. This minimizes over- or undersupply and helps to reduce costs.

INFECTION CONTROL AND SAFETY

All patients in the home care setting should be treated as if they are potentially infectious. As such, home care personnel must follow "universal precautions." Nurses should wear sterile gloves when manipulating catheters to maintain their integrity and nonsterile gloves when drawing blood to protect themselves. Delivery personnel should also wear nonsterile gloves or rugged work gloves when picking up medical waste and unused supplies, to prevent needlestick injuries or contact with contaminated materials that were spilled.

Patients and/or their caregivers are taught to use appropriate sterile technique when preparing their medications or fluids and when manipulating the catheter. Occasionally, there may be a break in technique that could lead to a catheter infection or sepsis. In many cases these infections can be treated with intravenous antibiotics, but some cases require antibiotics and removal of the catheter.

Collection and Disposal of Medical Waste

Most state boards of pharmacy prohibit reuse of repackaged or compounded items, including sterile products. Thus, products returned from the home environment are not recycled. Supplies returned to the home infusion company from a patient should be dealt with as described by the company's disposal policies and procedures.

In the 1980s improper disposal of medical waste was a national issue. Since then, disposal methods and recycling of waste are more regulated. All home care patients and their caregivers should be taught to dispose of hazardous and non-hazardous wastes properly.[7] Needles and other sharp materials should be placed in a hard plastic or cardboard sharps container to prevent injury. An isolated area in the home should be identified for storage of medical waste. In addition, a schedule for waste removal should be clearly developed and agreed on by the patient and the home care provider. If patients notice that their sharps container will be full before their next scheduled delivery, they should contact their home care provider as soon as possible.

CONCLUSION

Home infusion pharmacy offers a unique and challenging opportunity for the pharmacy technician. The role of the home care pharmacy technician involves substantial responsibility and the role in the maintenance of the mixing room, inventory control, and product preparation continues to expand. Home care technicians have an opportunity to learn skills not found in other types of practice sites such as dealing with high technology, infusion supplies, and venous access systems. Often there is opportunity for patient contact as well. Home infusion pharmacy is a growing field that depends on skilled pharmacy technicians to help the team provide pharmaceutical care to its patients.

REFERENCES

1. Anon. Home Health Care *Ann Int Med.* 1986;105:454–460.
2. American Society of Hospital Pharmacists. Increase in market for home infusion products and services predicted. *Am J Hosp Pharm.* 1990; 47:958
3. Anon. Report provides profile of home infusion services patients. *Am J Hosp Pharm.* 1993;50:846–9.
4. Kliethermes MA. Adverse drug reactions in home care: Report of five year data collection. Presented at HomeCare 95 Meeting of ASHP, Boston, MA. August 1995.
5. Kaplan LK. How clean is clean enough? *Infusion* 1995;August:11–8.
6. ASHP Council on Professional Affairs. ASHP technical assistance bulletin on quality assurance for pharmacy-prepared sterile products. *Am J Hosp Pharm.* 1993;50:2386–90.
7. Sterile drug products for home use. In: *United States Pharmacopeia, 23rd rev./National Formulary,* 18th ed. Rockville, MD: United States Pharmacopeial Convention; 1994. p. 1963–75.
8. Saladow J. Ambulatory systems for i.v. antibiotic therapy: making sense of the options. *Infusion* 1995; April:17–29.
9. Kwan JW. High-technology i.v. infusion devices. *Am J Hosp Pharm.* 1991;48(Suppl 1):S36–51.
10. Finley RS. Drug-delivery systems: infusion and access devices. *Highlights on Antineoplastic Drugs.* 1995;13:15–20,23–9.
11. Bowles C, McKinnon BT. Selecting infusion devices. *Am J Hosp Pharm.* 1993;50:228–30.
12. Saladow J. Ambulatory electronic infusion systems. Making sense of the options. *Infusion* 1995; July:9–21.
13. Dickson LB, Somani SM, Herrmann G, Abramowitz PW. Automated compounder for adding ingredients to parenteral nutrient base solutions. *Am J Hosp Pharm.* 1993;50:678–82.
14. Seidel AM, Woller TW, Somani S, Abramowitz PW. Effect of computer software on time required to prepare parenteral nutrient solutions. *Am J Hosp Pharm.* 1991;48:270–5.
15. Driscoll DF. Total nutrient admixtures: theory and practice. *Nutr Clin Pract.* 1995;10:114–9.
16. Viall CD. Your complete guide to central venous catheters. *Nursing 90* 1990;20:34–41.
17. Masoorii S, Angeles T. Picc lines: the latest home care challenge. *RN* 1990;44–51.

SELF-ASSESSMENT QUESTIONS

Case 1

Tom is a 54-year-old male with a 10 year history of diabetes. Tom stepped on a tack while working in the garage. He did not notice the tack in his shoe until he took off his shoes and socks that evening. The tack had cut his right foot behind the big toe and caused it to bleed. He cleaned the wound. Three weeks later, the patient began experiencing severe pain and tenderness in his right foot. He went to his doctor who noted a swollen and red right foot with a 2 cm wide and 4 cm deep ulcer behind the big toe. The patient was hospitalized for surgery to drain the wound. Cultures of bone were obtained during surgery. A diagnosis of osteomyelitis of the right foot with *Staphylococcus aureus* was made.

Tom supports a family of six. Three of his children are in college. Since there have been recent layoffs at his place of employment, he is concerned about his illness causing him to lose time at work. The patient is also concerned about the financial drain this illness will cause his family, since his HMO requires him to pay 20% of all health care expenditures.

1. Tom's diagnosis is often treated in the home health care environment.
   a. True   b. False

2. Which of the following would be home care goals for this patient?
   a. Allow the patient to leave hospital earlier.
   b. Allow the patient to return to work sooner.
   c. Decrease the health care costs associated with his therapy.
   d. all of the above

Tom's physician started nafcillin 2 gms IV every 6 hours to treat his infection and gave orders to arrange home care services for the patient. Tom is very nervous about going home. He is not sure he will be able to do what the nurses have been doing for him in the hospital. Although he knows going home will be cheaper, he is still concerned about how much this is going to cost.

3. Which of the following hospital employees coordinates Tom's transfer into the home care system?
   a. pharmacy technician
   b. reimbursement specialist
   c. discharge planner
   d. intake coordinator

4. The most appropriate team member for Tom to discuss the cost of therapy with is the:
   a. pharmacy technician.
   b. reimbursement specialist.
   c. home care nurse.
   d. home care pharmacist.

5. The pharmacist and nurse decide to use an ambulatory pump to administer Tom's nafcillin so he can return to work. The temporary technician is complaining about mixing the nafcillin for the pump, because it is so much harder than minibags. You explain to the technician that the pump is used because
   a. the company will make more money.
   b. the ambulatory pump will automatically infuse his drug every 6 hours, allowing the patient the time to work.
   c. nafcillin is more stable in ambulatory pumps.

   d. none of the above

6. Which team member would be the most appropriate to teach Tom how to use the system chosen to administer his medication?
   a. home care nurse
   b. physician
   c. pharmacy technician
   d. delivery personnel

The day has come for Tom to go home. Besides the prescription, orders are written for a PICC catheter to be inserted at home and for a CBC and erythrocyte sedimentation rate to be done weekly.

7. Which home care team member is responsible for giving the above orders?
   a. home care nurse
   b. home care pharmacist
   c. physician
   d. discharge planner

8. Which team member will insert the PICC catheter?
   a. nurse
   b. physician
   c. pharmacist
   d. none of the above

9. As the pharmacy technician you need to order enough nafcillin to provide Tom with the appropriate course of therapy. You note his diagnosis is osteomyelitis. Based on this you know his therapy will last
   a. 5 days.
   b. 4 to 6 weeks.
   c. 1 week.
   d. 3 months.

10. You are entering the orders for Tom into the computer system at your organization. You come to the CBC and erythrocyte sedimentation rate orders. You recognize these as
    a. orders nursing will need to schedule blood draws.
    b. orders the pharmacist will need to set up a monitoring plan.
    c. orders that will require the patient to have blood draw supplies in the home.
    d. all of the above

Tom has now received 5 weeks of therapy without complications. At the weekly patient rounds, the nurse reports Tom's right foot looks great. There is no more swelling or redness, and the ulcer has completely healed.

11. The patient service representative comes and tells you the patient needs seven more cassettes of nafcillin. She is a little concerned

because Tom has not been feeling "quite right" the last few days. He thinks he may have prickly heat because he has red bumps all over his chest. You take the following action

a. Tell the pharmacist about the patient service representative's concerns and wait to make the nafcillin until the pharmacist has evaluated the situation.

b. Mix 7-days worth of nafcillin, because a rash to nafcillin is common.

c. Arrange to return the nafcillin to the drug supplier because you will not be using it any more.

d. all of the above

Case II

Ken is a 35-year-old male who was diagnosed with AIDS 2 years ago. He was recently started on ganciclovir for CMV retinitis. Over the past 6 months, Ken lost 60 pounds and now he feels very weak. Ken and his physician have decided to treat his malnutrition with parenteral nutrition.

12. Parenteral nutrition is used to treat malnutrition associated with AIDS.
    a. True   b. False

13. Parenteral nutrition is a very complicated therapy, and needs to be administered in an institutional setting. Ken will have to be admitted to a hospital or long-term care facility.
    a. True   b. False

14. Ken would like to continue his job as an accountant, and wishes to start his parenteral nutrition at home. His physician and insurance case manager approves this plan because home care therapy
    a. allows patients to receive therapy without being hospitalized.
    b. allows patient to return to work or normal activities sooner.
    c. decreases health care costs.
    d. all of the above

15. The pharmacist recommends the following formula for Ken:

Dextrose 50%	1000 ml
Amino Acids 10%	1000 ml
Lipids 20%	500 ml
Multiple Electrolyte vial	40 ml
Sodium Phosphate	30 mMol
Trace Metals	5 ml
Multi-Vitamins	10 ml

You are preparing to compound Ken's parenteral nutrition solutions, which of the following will you not add to the solution?

a.	Lipids 20%	500 ml
b.	Trace Metals	5 ml
c.	Sodium Phosphate	30 mMol
d.	Multi-Vitamins	10 ml

After 2 weeks on parenteral nutrition, it becomes clear that Ken is not tolerating the high dextrose load. His physician orders Regular Human Insulin. The stress of Ken's disease causes stomach pain, and his physician orders ranitidine, an H2 antagonist, 100 mg IV daily, to be added to his parenteral nutrition.

16. Ranitidine and insulin are incompatible with his TPN formula and therefore cannot be given when the TPN is infusing.
    a. True   b. False

17. The nurse plans to draw Ken's weekly labs and change his central line dressings on Tuesdays. You should plan to mix his TPN on which day?
    a. Monday
    b. Tuesday
    c. Wednesday
    d. Sunday

18. Ken is planning to take a 2-week vacation to Hawaii. Is this a possible, given his TPN therapy?
    a. Sure, but he would not be able to infuse his TPN during the 2 weeks.
    b. Absolutely not, it would be too dangerous. He cannot go on vacation while receiving this therapy.
    c. A 9-day supply could be sent with him, but due to limited stability, the remainder would have to be shipped.
    d. none of the above

19. The pharmacist tells you that the electrolytes on Ken's most recent labs are all normal but his liver enzymes are elevated.
    a. You go ahead and mix his TPN because the electrolytes are good.
    b. You hold the mix of TPN because the elevated liver enzymes may be TPN induced and result in a change in formula.
    c. You hold the mix because the elevated liver enzymes are due to the ganciclovir.
    d. none of the above

20. As you are preparing Ken's ganciclovir, you make yourself a mental note to check on how much stock you have in the refrigera-

tor for a drug that is often given to patients on ganciclovir, just in case Ken may need it. Which drug would you check for?
a. filgrastim (Neupogen)
b. insulin
c. ranitidine
d. none of the above

21. Which of the following groups was responsible for establishing three levels of risk to patients when receiving a sterile product?
a. American Society of Health-System Pharmacists
b. Food and Drug Administration
c. United States Pharmacopeial Convention
d. National Institutes of Health

22. A pharmacy technician is preparing a 1-week supply of TPN for a patient at home, using an automated compounding device. Investigational L-glutamine is being added at the end of the mixing process. Which risk level of compounding describes this situation?
a. risk level 1
b. risk level 2
c. risk level 3
d. no risk level

23. The disadvantage(s) of minibags is/are
a. the need for an IV pole.
b. increased risk for touch contamination.
c. requirement for more nursing interaction.
d. all of the above

24. Advantages to delivering medications via syringe infusion include which of the following?
a. syringes are easy to batch fill
b. syringes require less storage space
c. the drugs stored in syringes are stable for longer
d. a and b

25. Which of the following systems is considered an elastomeric balloon device?
a. SideKick®
b. Homepump®
c. Paragon®
d. Maxx®100

26. Which of the following rate-restricted systems provides controlled pressure pumping via an electronic system rather than by positive pressure?
a. ReadyMed®
b. Paragon Elite®
c. Maxx®100
d. SmartDose®

27. Which of the following manufacturers offers a different therapy-specific device designed specifically for infusion of TPN, pain medication, antibiotics, and insulin?
a. Medex, Inc.
b. SIMS Deltec, Inc.
c. MiniMed Technologies
d. Block Medical

28. A patient will be receiving TPN and pain management at home through a home infusion therapy provider. The patient is very debilitated and his wife does not feel very comfortable with programming an infusion pump. Which of the following devices would be most suitable for use in this patient?
a. EZ-Flow 80-2®
b. MedMate 1100®
c. VIVUS 2000®
d. Provider One®

29. Required labeling information for a product going to a home care patient includes which of the following?
a. patient name, address, prescribing physician
b. prescription number, date, prescribing physician
c. precautionary labels, patient name, date of dispensing
d. bag sequence, patient address, federal transfer label

30. Selecting an appropriate expiration date for sterile products used in home care practice is important because it dictates:
a. whether the product can be prepared in batches.
b. how much will be wasted.
c. the frequency of deliveries to the patient.
d. all of the above

31. Which of the following statements is true regarding expiration dating for sterile products used in the home care setting?
a. A 24-hour stability at room temperature is required for drugs to be given via an ambulatory infusion device.
b. Changes in pH and drug structure do not affect extended stability for sterile products.
c. Sterile products not intended for prompt use should be stored at no more than 25°C to inhibit microbial growth.

d. Physical degradation due to hydrolysis, oxidation, and reduction can deteriorate a product.

32. Tunneled central venous catheter models are distinguished by which of the following features?
    a. surgery vs. bedside placement
    b. likelihood that it will become occluded
    c. flushing protocol
    d. number of lumens

33. Which of the following are true about peripherally inserted central venous catheters (PICC)?
    a. They are also called midlines.
    b. They do not require flushing with heparin.
    c. They may be inserted in the hospital or at home.
    d. Their complication rate is less than any other catheter.

ANSWERS TO SELF-ASSESSMENT

1. True. Osteomyelitis is one of the most common diseases seen in the home care environment, primarily because it requires long term intravenous antibiotic therapy.

2. d. All the goals listed are primary goals of home care and are personal goals for the patient as well.

3. c. The discharge planner or a social worker coordinates the discharge of a patient to home care from the hospital.

4. b. The reimbursement specialist is the most knowledgeable about the cost of home care therapy and insurance coverage.

5. b. Ambulatory infusion pumps can be used to automatically infuse doses throughout the day. They are ideal for patients who may have a problem adhering to an infusion schedule that requires frequent dosing.

6. a. The nurse is the primary educator of the patient at home.

7. c. Only the physician can give orders that alter the therapeutic plan.

8. a. The home care nurse has primary responsibility for intravenous catheters. Many home care nurses are trained in the insertion and maintenence of PICC catheters.

9. b. Osteomyelitis is usually treated for 4 to 6 weeks.

10. d. The nurse is responsible for scheduling and drawing blood for laboratory tests on the patient. The pharmacist is responsible for evaluating laboratory results as part of their patient assessment and monitoring function. The home care company is usually the source for all the patient's medical supplies.

11. a. A rash developing well into therapy with nafcillin is a common occurrence in the home care environment. However, it is best to find out how the rest of the home care team wants to deal with the rash before mixing or returning the nafcillin. That way you will not have wasted the nafcillin.

12. True. Parenteral nutrition, may be used to treat malnutrition associated with AIDS. AIDS patients, due to chronic diarrhea, often cannot absorb enough nutrients from the food they eat to sustain adequate nutrition.

13. False. This may have been the thought 30 years ago, however, long term infusion therapy, such as parenteral nutrition, has been shown to be safe, effective, and cheaper in the home care environment.

14. d. The answer is all of the above, as all three goals listed are part of the seven goals of home care therapy.

15. d. Multi-Vitamins are the only components of Ken's formula that has limited stability (24 hours) and must be added by the patient in the home prior to infusion. The remainder of ingredients, lipids, electrolytes, sodium phosphate, and trace metals are stable in solution for 9 days.

16. False. Both these drugs are compatible with Ken's TPN but have short term stability, therefore should be added by the patient prior to infusion.

17. c. Wednesday would be the optimal day to mix, because lab results would be available that day and the nurse would have made a patient assessment for any problem or complications on Tuesday. Any changes in the formula could be made then prior to mixing a 7-day supply of TPN.

18. c. Ken could take up to nine bags (9-day supply) with him, or more, depending on how long his formula is stable. Other arrange-

ments would have to be made for the remainder of his therapy. Often a company will ship the medication overnight to the vacation spot.

19. b. Since elevated liver enzymes are a long-term complication of parenteral nutrition, the TPN order may be changed to avoid further complications. It is best to wait until a decision has been made regarding the composition of the TPN, rather than mix the wrong TPN and waste material, time, and money.

20. a. Ganciclovir commonly causes bone marrow toxicity and resulting neutropenia (low white blood cell count) in AIDS patients. Filgrastim is frequently used as therapy for this side effect.

21. a. The American Society of Health-System Pharmacists (ASHP) published the "ASHP Technical Assistance Bulletin on Quality Assurance for Pharmacy-prepared Sterile Products." The United States Pharmacopeial Convention issued an informational chapter on "Sterile Drug Products for Home Use." In the ASHP technical bulletin, sterile products are grouped into three levels of risk to the patient. These categories depend on how much time elapses between when the drug is compounded and when it is administered, in other words, the expiration dating. These levels increase from least (level 1) to greatest (level 3) potential risk and have different quality assurance recommendations for product integrity and patient safety.

22. c. The rationale behind the risk level approach is that the greater the chance of contamination or the greater the risk of microbial growth in the product, the more careful providers should be to safeguard the sterility of the IV admixture. The product being prepared by the pharmacy technician falls into risk level 3 because of the preparation of investigational L-glutamine from a powder (a nonsterile component) in a open reservoir. Indeed, the TPN solutions are being prepared using an automated compounder which alone renders them to be classified as risk level 2. However, because of the L-glutamine, risk level 2 is superceded by risk level 3.

23. d. Minibags are considered one of the most cost-effective methods to deliver medica-

tions from an acquisition standpoint. Their limitations in home care practice include: the need for an IV pole; patient or caregiver needs to manually set and maintain the infusion rate; patient or caregiver needs to connect the set and the bag in the home, increasing the risk of touch contamination; and the requirement for more nursing interaction with the patient than other systems. Use of minibags for drugs that are given frequently can pose a problem for patients who are ambulatory and/or working because of the cumbersome IV pole.

24. d. A revived interest has surged in the delivery of medications via syringe infusion due to attempts to reduce cost. As drug containers, syringes are the least expensive. In addition, syringes are easy to batch fill and require less storage space.

25. b. Elastomeric balloon systems currently available are Block Medical Homepump® and Homepump Eclipse®, McGaw Ready Med®, and Secure Medical MedFlo II®. Baxter Healthcare's Infusor System and Block Medical's Extended Use Homepump® are designed specifically for administering chemotherapy and other long-term continuous infusions.

26. c. In early 1994, an electronic controlled pressure device, the Maxx®100 by Medication Delivery Devices was introduced. This system consists of a rectangular shaped housing and a series of disposable reservoir bags with pre-attached IV flow control sets. A proprietary plastic bag is placed inside the device housing on top of a bladder, that expands with air and applies pressure to the bag when the device is closed and turned on. The IV tubing controls the drug administration rate once the clamp on it is opened. It differs from other rate-restricted systems in that it provides controlled pressure pumping via an electronic system rather than by positive pressure.

27. b. Therapy-specific devices are designed to provide single therapies such as pain management or TPN. Operation of these devices is fairly straightforward, and can be readily done by clinicians and patients. Common therapy-specific devices include the Abbott Provider® products and the SIMS Deltec CADD® infusion pumps. The CADD® pumps are the most widely used ambulatory

infusion devices in the United States. All of these devices are therapy-specific and relatively simple to program. The CADD-TPN®, CADD-PCA®, and CADD-Plus® are designed specifically for infusion of TPN, pain medications, and antibiotics, respectively.

28. c. The VIVUS 2000 pump will allow infusion of two medications simultaneously which would be ideal for this patient receiving two therapies. In addition, it offers telecommunications capabilities that would be pertinent in this case because of the inability of caregivers to operate the device. It can be programmed by the home care provider over the phone via a modem. The other devices do not have telecommunications capabilities nor the ability to infuse two medications through the same device.

29. b. Required labeling information includes prescription number, date, and prescribing physician, usually required by state boards of pharmacy and useful to the dispensing pharmacy to verify an original order. The patient's name is mandatory but the address is optional, however, it may simplify delivery procedures. Directions for use should be simple and easy to understand. The name and amount of drug contained in one dose and the appropriate volume for that amount should be listed. Then, the name and volume of admixture solution equivalent to one dose of drug is indicated. The actual expiration date established for the product is noted. The individual who prepared and checked the admixture must initial the label. Finally, auxiliary labeling should include federal transfer labeling and as an option, specific precautionary labels or storage instruction labels can be applied to the product. The bottle or bag sequence may be listed as well to help track the specific number of doses ordered and/or the total number of doses administered.

30. d. Expiration dating has important implications in home care practice, as it may mean the ability for batch preparation in the pharmacy, a reduction in waste, and less frequent deliveries to the patient. Expiration dates for admixtures must be based on stability and sterility considerations.

31. a. Expiration dates for admixtures must be based on stability and sterility considerations. Physical and chemical breakdowns are possible. Changes in pH, temperature, and drug structure may cause solubility problems. Chemical degradation due to hydrolysis, oxidation, reduction, or photolysis can quickly deteriorate a product. Home care practice demands that the pharmacist assign a maximum expiration date that is still within appropriate stability limits. A common problem is the use of drugs with limited room temperature stability. For drugs to be given via an ambulatory infusion device, at least 24-hour stability at room temperature or warmer is required. For drugs that have limited room temperature stability, the patient or caregiver may be taught how to prepare the drug immediately before administration. Although a product may be stable for an extended period, its sterility must also be a factor in assigning an expiration date. The potential for bacterial growth must be considered. Sterile products not intended for prompt use should be stored at no more than 4°C to inhibit microbial growth, unless room temperature storage is warranted.

32. d. Available tunneled central venous catheter models are distinguished by the catheter material (silicone or polyurethane), number of lumens (single, double, or triple), catheter diameter (French size 3 = pediatric to 12.5 or 13.0 = double or triple lumen), lumen diameter (0.2 to 2.0 mm), and type of catheter tip.

33. c. The use of peripherally inserted central venous catheters (PICC) is increasing because of their unique features. PICCs can be inserted at the bedside or at home by specially trained nurses. These lines may remain in place for weeks to months. PICC lines, also known as long-arm or long-line catheters are made of silicone (Silastic®) or flexible polyurethane and are available in single- and multilumen designs. They require daily flushing with heparin and dressing changes. Complications include phlebitis at the insertion site or along the vein, infection, cellulitis, occlusion, catheter tip migration, and thrombosis.

Glossary

Absorption Base—see Anhydrous Base.

Accreditation—the process of granting recognition or vouching for conformance with a standard (usually applies to an institution).

Addressograph—a raised letter registration card similar to a credit card, that is used to imprint patient identification information on medical record documents.

Admixture—the combination of one or more sterile products and a parenteral solution.

Adsorbent—a substance with the property of attaching other substances to its surface.

Adverse Drug Event—a harmful or potentially harmful patient outcome caused by the administration or omission of a drug.

Adverse Drug Reaction—any unexpected, undesirable effect of a drug that occurred at normal doses. This includes allergic and immunologic reactions.

Aerosol—a suspension of very fine liquid or solid particles distributed in a gas and packaged under pressure. Medication is released from the container as a spray, foam, or solid. Aerosols may be inhaled internally or applied topically (externally).

Air Embolism—a phenomenon that results from air entering the body's circulation. The air creates an air lock that obstructs the outflow of blood from the right ventricle of the heart. Air may enter the circulation as a result of injury, surgery, or intravenous infusions.

Alcoholic Solution—a nonaqueous solution that employs alcohol, rather than water, as its solvent and/or vehicle.

Analgesic—a compound that relieves pain by altering one's perception of painful stimuli.

Angina Pectoris—severe constricting pain in the chest, often radiating to the left shoulder and down the arm, due to lack of oxygen to the heart muscle.

Anhydrous Base—an ointment base that contains no water but is able to absorb water, also known as an absorption base.

Anteroom—a room outside the clean room in which activities such as hand washing, gowning and gloving, removal of packaging, and sanitizing of hard-surface containers and supplies are performed to prepare for admittance to the clean room.

Anticholinergic Effects—symptoms (usually adverse effects of drugs) related to blocking of the cholinergic nervous system. Symptoms include dry mouth, constipation, rapid heart rate, blurred vision, confusion, impairment of ejaculation, and urinary retention.

Anticoagulant—an agent that prevents blood from forming a clot (coagulation).

Antiemetic—a remedy that prevents or controls nausea and vomiting.

Antihistamine—drugs used to treat allergy symptoms. They antagonize the actions of histamine, which cause many of the symptoms associated with allergies.

Antiperistaltic—an agent that impedes or arrests the waves of alternate circular contraction and relaxation of the intestines. This peristaltic action is what propels substances through the intestines. In some cases, there may be too much peristaltic activity (i.e., hypermotility) and drugs are used to decrease the hyperperistaltic state.

Antipyretic—an agent that reduces fever.

Antitussive—an agent that relieves cough.

Apothecary System—units of measure used by pharmacists primarily in the past.

Aqueous Solution—a solution that employs purified water as its vehicle. Such solutions may be ingested orally, applied topically to the skin, or injected into the bloodstream.

Arrhythmia—an irregular heartbeat.

Aseptic Technique—a set of methodologies, procedures, and techniques practiced to keep a sterile product from becoming contaminated.

Asthma—a condition of the lungs characterized by narrowing of airways that results in "shortness of breath." The condition varies over short periods of time and is caused, more specifically, by varying degrees of smooth muscle spasms, edema of the lining of the airways, and mucus in the airways.

Atherosclerosis—a condition characterized by irregularly distributed fat deposits in the vessel walls of large and medium-sized blood vessels. Atherosclerosis is a risk factor for heart disease.

Automated Compounding Devices—devices based on peristaltic pump principles that are similar to infusion pumps. They are used to prepare complex multicomponent sterile products such as nutrition formulations and cardioplegia solutions, as well as batches of other products.

Auxiliary Label—additional labels that are affixed to prescription containers to provide information beyond that which appears on the prescription label itself. Examples include "Keep in the Refrigerator" or "For External Use Only."

Bacteria—one-celled microorganisms that often cause infections and are targeted by antibiotic therapy.

Batch Repackaging—the repackaging of many unit-dose containers of medication at a time prior to receipt of prescriptions. The amount of medication packaged depends on the expected demand and the expiration date of the repackaged medication.

Benign Prostatic Hyperplasia—a noncancerous enlargement of the prostate gland that sometimes obstructs the flow of urine or causes irritation.

Biological Safety Cabinet (BSC)—a special hood designed to create a front air barrier, or "curtain," between the handler and the work zone. It is intended to protect personnel from contamination by hazardous drug dusts and aerosols that are generated in the drug preparation area.

Bipolar Disorder—a mood disorder characterized by alternating periods of euphoria (mania) and depression.

Blister Package—a semirigid package that is generally reserved for oral solid medications. The package is composed of two parts; a backing, which is usually made up of a paper-foil material, and a front or facing material, which is a small plastic blister or bubble that holds the medication. The blister portion of the package can be either clear or amber in color.

Board Certified Pharmacotherapy Specialist (BCPS)—a pharmacist who has been certified through an examination process and has demonstrated a defined level of knowledge, experience, and skill in the management of drug therapy.

Bolus—injection of an intravenous dose of medication over seconds to minutes. Also known as "IV push" where the medication is pushed into the body by means of a syringe.

Bronchodilator—an agent that increases the diameter of the bronchi and bronchioli (airways in the lungs) to improve the airflow to the lungs, primarily used to treat asthma.

Buccal Route of Medication Administration— introduces medication into the bloodstream through the lining of the cheek. Usually, a buccal medication is absorbed after being placed in the patient's mouth.

Buccal Tablet—a tablet that is placed inside the cheek where it slowly dissolves and is gradually absorbed into the bloodstream through the cheek lining (i.e., buccal route of administration).

Capitation—a type of third-party reimbursement in which the pharmacy receives a set amount of money for a defined group of patients, regardless of the number of prescriptions or services each patient receives. The dollar amount is usually in terms of per patient per month.

Capsule—a solid medication dosage form in which the drug, with or without inactive or inert ingredients, is contained within a gelatin shell.

Cathartic—a medication used to promote rapid evacuation of the bowels.

Catheter Dislodgement—movement of the catheter out of the vein.

Catheter Occlusion—clogging of the catheter occurs when blood clots form in the catheter's lumen and prevents the flow of fluids through the catheter.

Certification—the process by which a non-governmental agency or association grants recognition to an individual who has met qualifications that are predetermined by that agency or association.

Chemotherapy—one option to treat disease by means of administering specific chemical substances or drugs. Chemotherapy is most commonly used in the treatment of cancer.

Chewable Tablet—a pleasantly flavored tablet that may or should be chewed before swallowing. Chewable tablet form is most often used for pediatric medications.

Chronic Bronchitis—a condition of the lungs characterized by cough, oversecretion of mucus, and expectoration of sputum over a long period of time. People with this ailment often have frequent bronchial infections.

Chronic Obstructive Pulmonary Disease (COPD)—a group of diseases that interferes with ventilation by limiting expiration rates, includes emphysema, asthma, and chronic bronchitis.

Clean Room—an enclosed space, containing one or more clean zones, where the concentration of airborne particles is controlled. The purpose of a clean room is to minimize the potential for parenteral products to become contaminated.

Collodion—an alcoholic solution that is a liquid preparation of pyroxylin (a component of cotton fibers) dissolved in ethyl ether and ethanol. After application to the skin, the ether and ethanol evaporate and leave a pyroxylin film.

Community-acquired Infection—an infection in which the infecting organisms came from the patient's home environment or surrounding community. Organisms associated with community-acquired infections are often easier to treat than hospital-acquired infections. Infections acquired in nursing homes usually involve organisms that are more similar to hospital-acquired infections than to community-acquired infections.

Compact Disk Read-Only Memory (CD-ROM)—media on which computer software and data are often stored. People access the material saved on the CD-ROM via a computer, but they cannot save additional material on the disk.

Compressed Tablet—a tablet formed by die-punch compression of powdered, crystalline, or granular substances. The tablet may also include binders, disintegrators, lubricants, diluents, and/or colorants.

Conjunctivitis—inflammation of the mucous membrane that covers the outside surface of the eyeball and the inside surface of the eyelid (conjunctiva).

Continuous Phase—see External Phase.

Contraceptive—an agent used to prevent pregnancy.

Co-payment (deductible)—a portion of the costs of each prescription that is paid by the patient; a common copayment is 20%. May also be called a deductible. The third-party payer pays the balance.

Cream—semisolid oil-in-water or water-in-oil emulsion that may or may not contain medication. It differs from an ointment in that it is easily worked into the skin and has a lighter feel.

Credentialing—the process of formally recognizing professional or technical competence.

Cross-sensitivity—a term used to identify similar effects caused by two different agents. The term is often applied to a drug to which a patient may be allergic, if the patient is allergic to certain other drugs.

Cytotoxic—an agent or substance that is detrimental or destructive to cells. Many of the drugs used to treat cancer are cytotoxic agents.

Cytotoxic Drugs—agents that are toxic to cells and can be hazardous to those handling them if there is exposure through touch or inhalation.

Decongestant—an agent that decreases congestion. These agents are usually used to reduce congestion or swelling of the nasal lining in those who have allergic rhinitis, a cold, or the flu.

Deductible—a portion of total prescription costs for a given time period that must be paid by the patient before the third-party payer will begin paying for prescriptions in that time period. In some cases, the deductible applies to each prescription. Also called a co-payment or a "spend-down."

Default Value—the value for a field in a computer record that appears if no other information is entered.

Depression—a syndrome that is characterized by the inability to experience pleasure and by mood variations, sleep disturbances, and lack of reactivity to one's environment.

Dermatitis—inflammation of the skin.

Diabetes Mellitus—a disease of metabolism in which the ability to utilize carbohydrates is reduced and the ability to use proteins and fats is enhanced. It is caused by an absolute or relative deficiency of insulin.

Dispense As Written—an indication by the prescriber of a medication that the generic product cannot be substituted for the brand name product. May be abbreviated as "DAW."

Distal-tip Slit Valve—a valve at the end of a catheter with a slit in the rubber. It allows fluids to pass when pressure is applied, but does not allow fluid to flow backwards. It is intended to prevent catheters from becoming occluded.

Douche—an aqueous solution that is directed into a body cavity or against a part of the body to clean or disinfect.

Drug Level—slang for serum drug concentration, which reports the amount of drug present in a patient's bloodstream.

Drug Misadventures—hazards or incidents that result from risk associated with the therapeutic use of medications. This term includes adverse drug reactions and medication errors.

Drug Related Incident—any occurrence involving a drug that is not supposed to happen, or occurs inappropriately.

Dummy Terminals—computer terminals that are an inexpensive way for a large number of users to access information from a central computer. Dummy terminals are only useful when they are connected to a mainframe system.

Effervescent Tablet—a tablet containing ingredients that bubble and release medication when placed in a liquid. Once in a liquid, the tablet quickly disintegrates and dissolves before it is administered to the patient.

Electronic Charting—a computerized mechanism of documenting patient care. This method of charting bypasses the steps of writing the information on paper and then entering it into a computer system. Electronic charting may eliminate errors caused in part by illegible handwriting and transcription errors.

Electronic Mail (e-mail)—is a computer-based communication tool. Basic functions include sending and receiving messages within an organization, or with outside organizations. The system can be set up to send the same message to multiple users.

Elixir—a clear, sweet, flavored hydroalcoholic solution intended for oral ingestion.

Emollient—a substance or medication that softens or soothes irritation of the skin or mucous membranes

Emphysema—a condition of the lung characterized by destructive changes and a decrease in number of air sacs, which are necessary for the body to exchange waste gases. Symptoms include shortness of breath on exertion, and a thin and barrel-chested appearance.

Emulsifying Agent—an ingredient added to an emulsion that prevents the small particles of the internal phase from fusing together and separating from the external phase.

Emulsion—a mixture of two liquids that do not normally mix. A liquid broken into small particles (the internal phase) is evenly distributed throughout the other liquid (the external or continuous phase).

Emulsion Base—an ointment base that is made up of water and oil. An emulsion base may be water-in-oil (W/O) where water is the internal phase and an oil-based ingredient is the external phase, or oil-in-water (O/W) where an oil-based ingredient is the internal phase and water is the external phase.

End-product Evaluation—the act of performing the final inspection before a product is allowed to leave the pharmacy. It includes an inspection for leaks, cloudiness, particulate matter, color, solution volume, container integrity, verification of compounding accuracy (ingredients and quantities), and sterility testing.

Enema—an aqueous solution introduced into the rectum to empty the bowel or treat diseases of the lower gastrointestinal tract.

Enteral—within, or by way of, the gastrointestinal tract. Enteral feeding relies on absorption of food from the gastrointestinal tract.

Enteric Coated Tablet—a tablet with a coating that protects it from stomach acid and protects the lining of the gastrointestinal tract from damage or irritation the drug may cause.

Epilepsy—a disorder characterized by sudden onset of brain dysfunction usually associated with some alteration of consciousness. The clinical manifestations may vary from generalized convulsions to momentary spells of impaired consciousness.

Essence—see Spirit.

Expectorant—an agent that increases secretions from the linings of the airways and facilitates their expulsion. Often used by patients with bronchitis, colds, or flu.

Extemporaneous Packaging—the repackaging of unit-dose containers of a medication to be used in a short period of time.

Extended-release Dosage Form—a medication dosage form that slowly and consistently releases a drug over an extended period of time. Such a dosage form may be an oral tablet or capsule but could be a topical patch, implant, or intramuscular injection.

External Phase—the liquid phase of an emulsion that contains small, evenly distributed particles of another liquid (internal phase). The external phase is also called the continuous phase.

Extract—a concentrated preparation of a drug that is two to six times as potent as the crude drug. This alcoholic or hydroalcoholic solution is prepared by soaking plant or animal tissue in a solvent, which withdraws the crude drug. The solvent then evaporates, leaving the active compound behind. It differs from a fluidextract or tincture only in its potency.

Extractive—a concentrated preparation of active components obtained from plant or animal tissue.

Extrapyramidal Symptoms—symptoms associated with Parkinson's disease and caused by some drugs (adverse effects) that include muscle spasms, restlessness, slowed muscle movement, tremor, rigidity, and abnormal posture. Abbreviated "eps".

Fee-for-service—a type of third-party reimbursement in which the pharmacy bills the third party based on the price of the drug dispensed or services rendered.

Fellowship—a 2- or 3-year postgraduate training program that allows pharmacy graduates to gain experience in medical research.

Fluidextract—an alcoholic or hydroalcoholic solution with a potency adjusted so that each milliliter of tincture contains the equivalent potency of 1000 mg of crude drug. A fluidextract is prepared by the extraction method. It differs from a tincture or extract only in its potency.

Formulary—a continually revised compilation of approved pharmaceuticals that reflects the judgment of the hospital, managed care, or third party staff involved in the formulary process.

Fungus—an organism that grows in irregular masses, without roots, stems, or leaves. Each organism may be one-celled or many-celled filaments and possesses branched structures. Fungi can cause infections.

Gargle—an aqueous solution used to treat conditions of the throat. The gargle is held in the throat as the patient gurgles air through the solution.

Gastroesophageal Reflux Disease (GERD)—clinical symptoms or tissue changes that result from backward movement of stomach (gastric) contents into the esophagus.

Gel—a thick, viscous suspension of undissolved drug in water. A gel is similar to a milk or magma but the suspended particle size is smaller.

Generic Name—a noun that indicates class or type of a drug product that has proven likeness to a proprietary (brand name) product.

Glaucoma—a disease of the eye characterized by increased pressure within the eyeball that produces defects in vision.

Glycerin—a sweet, oily fluid made from fats and oils.

Glycerite—a nonaqueous solution that employs glycerin, with or without water and/or alcohol, as its solvent and/or vehicle.

Good Manufacturing Practices (GMP)—guidelines that were established by the U.S. Food and Drug Administration in 1963 to represent standards of operation in manufacturing practice. They are the standards by which the pharmaceutical industry's manufacturing practices are gauged.

Granule—a medication dosage form that is made by wetting, drying, and grinding a powder into coarse pieces. Water is usually added before it is used. Granules are different from powders in that the particle size is larger and is usually more stable.

Hard Gelatin Capsule—a capsule that consists of two oblong casings filled with dry, powdered ingredients.

Heart Failure—a medical condition in which the heart fails to maintain the circulation of blood, resulting in congestion in the tissues. This is a mechanical failure—the heart fails as a pump.

Horizontal Laminar Airflow (LAF) Hood—special hood designed to blow highly filtered air horizontally across a work surface, creating an ideal environment for the preparation of non-hazardous sterile products. The hood is designed to reduce the potential for contaminating product prepared within the hood.

Hospital-acquired Infection—an infection in which the infecting organisms are introduced into the patient in the hospital, often by exposure of tissues during surgery or insertion of devices such as needles or catheters or from other patients. Hospital-acquired infections are often more difficult to treat than community-acquired infections.

Human Immunodeficiency Virus—the virus believed to cause AIDS (acquired immunodeficiency syndrome). Abbreviated HIV.

Hydroalcoholic Solution—a nonaqueous solution that employs a mixture of alcohol and water as its solvent and/or vehicle.

Hydrocarbon Base—see Oleaginous Base.

Hyperlipidemia—the presence of abnormally large amounts of lipids (fats) in the blood. Hyperlipidemia is a risk factor for coronary artery disease (e.g., atherosclerosis) and stroke.

Hypertension—high blood pressure.

Implant—a medication pump or device that is inserted into the body for a long period of time or permanently.

Incident Report—a description of the situation, which resulted in or had the potential to lead to an unusual or negative outcome. The report usually identifies the date, time and place of occurrence, people involved, and action taken.

Infection—the unusual multiplication of an organism within the body. As a result, the body's immune system takes action to eliminate the infecting organism.

Inflammation—cellular and tissue reaction that occurs in response to an injury or abnormal stimulation caused by a physical, chemical, or biologic agent. Includes the destruction or removal of injurious material and responses leading to repair and healing. Signs of inflammation are redness, heat, swelling, pain, and loss of function.

Inhalant—a solution or finely powdered drug delivered as a mist through the mouth into the respiratory tract.

Inhalation Route of Medication Administration—the route of medication administration that delivers medication into the lungs after inhalation through the mouth.

Interface—connection between two or more computer systems that enable data to be transferred. The interface can be uni-directional, where one system always sends data and the other system always receives data, or bi-directional, where data is sent back and forth between systems.

Intermittent Systems—IV drug delivery systems designed to administer medications at defined time intervals (e.g., every 4 hours or every 8 hours) rather than continuously.

Internal Phase—the liquid of an emulsion that is broken into small particles and is evenly distributed throughout the second liquid (the external or continuous phase).

Internet—a global interconnection of computer networks that allows people to access and route information all over the world.

Intraarterial Route of Medication Administration—the route of medication administration that introduces medication into an artery by injecting it through a needle placed directly in the artery.

Intraarticular Route of Medication Administration—the route of medication administration that introduces medication into a joint, such as a knee or elbow, by injecting it through a needle placed in the joint.

Intracardiac Route of Medication Administration—the route of medication administration that introduces medication into the muscle of the heart by injection through a needle placed directly in the heart.

Intradermal (ID) Route of Medication Administration—the route of medication administration that introduces medication into the top layer of the skin by injection through a needle placed in the top layers of the skin. An intradermal injection is not as deep as a subcutaneous injection.

Intramuscular (IM) Route of Medication Administration—the route of medication administration that introduces medication into a muscle by injection through a needle placed in a large muscle mass such as the upper arm, thigh, or buttock.

Intraperitoneal Route of Medication Administration—the route of medication administration that introduces medication into the peritoneal, or abdominal cavity, by injection through a needle placed in the peritoneal, or abdominal cavity. One method of dialysis, peritoneal dialysis, uses the intraperitoneal route to remove waste products from the blood of patients with kidney failure.

Intrapleural Route of Medication Administration—the route of medication administration that introduces medication into the sac surrounding the lungs, the pleura, by injection through a needle placed in the pleura.

Intrathecal Route of Medication Administration—the route of medication administration that introduces medication into the space around the spinal cord by injection through a needle placed in the spinal cord.

Intravenous (IV) Route of Medication Administration—the route of medication administration that introduces medication into the body through a needle placed directly in a vein.

Intraventricular Route of Medication Administration—the route of medication administration that introduces medication into the brain by injection through a needle into the brain's cavities, or ventricles.

Intravesicular Route of Medication Administration—the route of medication administration that introduces medication into the urinary bladder by injection through a needle.

Intravitreous Route of Medication Administration—the route of medication administration that introduces medication into the eye by direct injection.

Irrigating Solution—an aqueous solution used to wash or cleanse a part of the body.

Jelly—a semisolid viscous aqueous solution that contains a high proportion of water. May be used as a lubricant or vehicle.

Job Description—see Position Description.

Large Volume Parenteral (LVP)—any parenteral solution greater than 100 ml in volume.

Licensure—the process by which a government agency grants an individual permission to engage in a given occupation upon finding that the individual applicant has attained the minimal degree of competency necessary to ensure that the public health, safety, and welfare will be reasonably well protected.

Liniment—a medication dosage form applied to the skin with friction and rubbing. A liniment may be a solution, emulsion, or suspension.

Liquid Medication Dosage Form—a medication dosage form in which the medication is delivered as a fluid medium or vehicle (water, alcohol, glycerin, mineral oil). It may be intended for oral use or use in, or on, other parts of the body. Examples of liquid medication dosage forms include solutions, emulsions, and suspensions.

Local Area Network (LAN)—a group of computers linked together so that multiple users can access and share information.

Lotion—a suspension intended for external application.

Lozenge—a hard, disk-shaped, solid medication dosage form that contains medication in a sugar base. Also known as a troche or pastille.

Lumen—access port on a catheter through which solutions are administered to a patient.

Lyophilized Powder—powder that was derived by freeze-drying a solution. The powder is reconstituted prior to administering the drug to the patient.

Magmas and Milks—thick, viscous suspensions of undissolved drug in water, similar to a gel.

Mainframe Computers—large, expensive, powerful computers, designed to process large amounts of data that are shared by people in the work place.

Medical Record Number—a unique numerical patient identifier commonly used in the hospital setting.

Medication Administration Record (MAR)—the document used by health care professionals to record the time a medication was administered to a patient. The document is primarily completed by nurses and produced by the pharmacy or nursing staff.

Medication Error—defined by ASHP as "episodes in drug misadventuring that should be preventable through effective system controls involving pharmacists, physicians and other prescribers, nurses, risk management personnel, legal counsel, administrators, patients, and others in the organizational setting, as well as regulatory agencies and the pharmaceutical industry."

Medication Order—a written requested drug order for a medication from a licensed prescriber. The order becomes part of the patient's permanent medical record.

Medication Use System—the system in which drugs are prescribed, prepared, dispensed, administered to or taken by a patient, and drug therapy is monitored.

Microcomputers or Personal Computers (PC)—stand-alone systems that run software programs and manage data that is accessed from a larger source such as a mainframe. PCs have traditionally been used for word processing, spreadsheets, database management, desktop publishing, and telecommunication programs.

Mid-Level Practitioner—licensed professionals who perform their duties under the supervision of a physician and may have limited authority to prescribe medications according to predefined protocols or within certain other legal limitations. Examples include Nurse Practitioners and Physician's Assistants.

Minicomputers—smaller scaled mainframe computers commonly used by several people on local area networks (LAN) or, within small organizations or departments of a large organization.

Mnemonic—a short code used to identify a medication in a pharmacy computer system. For example, the mnemonic for acetaminophen 325 mg tablets might be "acet325t."

Modem—an electronic device that allows two computers to communicate using a telephone line. With a modem and the proper communication software, users can transfer data from one PC to another, share data with a PC, or connect to an on-line service to read an article or research a subject.

Molded Tablet—a tablet made from wet material placed and formed in a mold.

Monographs—(mono= single; graph= writing.) a writing about a single subject. In the context of this book, a monograph provides comprehensive information about a single drug or a group of drugs. Information typically provided in a monograph includes: drug actions, indications, contraindications, warnings, precautions, drug interactions, patient information, product availability, and administration and dosage.

Morbidity—a rate of incidence of a disease.

Mouthwash—an aqueous solution used to deodorize, refresh, or disinfect the mouth.

Mucilage—a thick, viscous aqueous solution of water containing the sticky components of vegetable matter.

Multidisciplinary Health Care Team—a team of health care personnel that may include pharmacists and technicians, nurses, physicians, and therapists working together with patients to provide medical treatment.

Myocardial Infarction—the death of heart tissue caused by a lack of oxygen, usually due to an occluded coronary artery.

Nasal Route of Medication Administration—the route of medication administration that delivers medication into the nostrils. Nasally administered medications are usually administered as sprays or drops.

Neuromuscular Blocking Agent—a drug that primarily interrupts the transmission of the nerve impulse at the junction of skeletal muscle and nerves, resulting in paralysis.

Neurotransmitter—any specific chemical agent that crosses the junction between two nerve cells to stimulate or inhibit an action.

Nonaqueous Solution—a solution that uses solvents with, or instead of water, as the vehicle. Commonly used nonaqueous solvents include alcohol, glycerin, and propylene glycol.

Nonprescription Medications—medications that can be purchased by the consumer without a prescription. Also called over-the-counter drugs (OTCs).

Oil-in-Water (O/W) Emulsion—an emulsion where small oil globules (the internal phase) are dispersed throughout water (the external phase).

Ointment—a semisolid medication dosage form intended for application to the skin or mucous membranes. Ointments are divided into categories according to their characteristics: oleaginous or hydrocarbon base, anhydrous or absorption base, emulsion base, or water-soluble base.

Oleaginous Base—an ointment base that is hydrophobic and does not wash off with water. It is occlusive and protective. Also known as a hydrocarbon base.

Ophthalmic—a term that means, pertaining to the eye.

Ophthalmic Route of Medication Administration—the route of medication administration that delivers medication into the eye. Ophthalmic medications may be formulated as solutions, suspensions, ointments, or gels.

Opportunistic Infection—an infection caused by an organism capable of causing disease only in a patient whose immune defenses are lowered by diseases (such as HIV) or drugs.

Oral (p.o.) Route of Medication Administration—the route of medication administration that introduces medication into the gastrointestinal tract through the mouth. Abbreviated p.o. (from the Latin *per os*—by mouth).

Osteoporosis—reduction in the quantity of bone or atrophy of skeletal tissue.

Otic Route of Medication Administration—the route of medication administration that delivers medication into the ear canal. Otic medications may be formulated as solutions or suspensions.

Over-The-Counter Drugs (OTCs)—medications that can be purchased by the consumer without a prescription. Also called nonprescription medications.

Parenteral Route of Medication Administration—any route of medication administration that introduces medication into the body by some means other than the gastrointestinal tract.

Parkinson's Disease—a neurological syndrome characterized by rhythmical muscle tremors, rigidity of movement, droopy posture, mask-like expression, and shuffling gait.

Pastille—see Lozenge.

Patient Compliance—the degree to which patients take their medication as prescribed.

Patient-controlled Analgesia (PCA)—a system of pain control using a device that injects a programmed amount of pain medication to a patient when he/she pushes a button. PCA systems are most often used to deliver medication intravenously and epidurally.

Patient Profile—a list of the prescriptions received by a patient and all corresponding prescription information (e.g., original date, refill dates, prescribing physician). The patient profile is used by pharmacists to evaluate a patient's drug therapy for appropriateness, drug interactions, allergy contraindications, efficacy, and patient compliance.

Peptic Ulcer Disease—a group of disorders involving erosion of the lining of the gastrointestinal tract by acid and pepsin. Duodenal and gastric ulcers are the most common types.

Percutaneous Route of Medication Administration—see Transdermal Route of Medication Administration.

Peripherally Inserted Central Venous (PICC) Catheters—catheters inserted through a vein in the arm and threaded so that the tip rests in the superior vena cava (heart).

Peritoneal Cavity—the abdominal cavity.

Pharmacy Department—the department of a hospital/place of business that is responsible for all aspects of drug use in the hospital from the time a drug is delivered to the hospital/place of business until after it has been administered to a patient. Pharmacy departments may be classified by function (administrative, clinical, distributive) and/or physical location (centralized, decentralized).

Pharmacy Practice Setting—the environment in which pharmacists work. Common examples of pharmacy practice settings include community, hospital (institutional), managed care, home care, hospice care (long-term care), and pharmaceutical industry.

Pharmacy Technician—a person who assists licensed pharmacists in pharmacy practice activities that do not require professional judgment.

Phlebitis—inflammation of the wall of a vein.

Policies and Procedures (P&P)—documents that provide guidance about the expectations of the hospital or business and pharmacy department on the behavior of the employees. General policies and procedures cover broad areas such as hiring requirements and employee benefits while pharmacy department policies and procedures cover areas specific to pharmacy.

Position Description—a document that defines functions and tasks for which an employee in a specific position is responsible. The authority of the position and other expectations such as dress code, work schedule, and physical requirements of the position may be included. A position description may also be referred to as a job description.

Postural Hypotension—a drop in blood pressure related to changes in position from lying or sitting to standing, often resulting in dizziness.

Pouch Package—a flexible package that is composed of two parts: a paper-foil laminate that is joined to another paper-foil laminate or to a clear cellophane-like material to form a small pouch. Pouch packages are used to hold medications.

Powder—a medication dosage form that may be used internally or externally. An *internal powder* is dissolved in water before ingestion. An *external powder* or *dusting powder* is a mixture of finely ground dry drugs and inactive ingredients that is sprinkled or dusted on the skin.

Prepackaging—see Batch Repackaging and Unit-of-use Package.

Prescription—an order, from a licensed prescriber, that may be presented at an ambulatory care pharmacy for the purpose of obtaining medications.

Preservatives—substances added to maintain sterility by killing or inhibiting the growth of bacteria or other organisms should the product inadvertently become contaminated.

Primary References—research articles published in journals (or "medical magazines").

Process Validation—testing that ensures that the steps used in sterile product preparation consistently yield sterile products of acceptable quality. It involves demonstrating proper technique by manipulating microbial growth media without exposing the media to bacteria, which is then used to measure the sterility of the test product.

Profession—an occupation or vocation that required advanced training in a liberal art or science. Pharmacy is a profession.

Psychoactive—possessing the ability to alter mood, anxiety, behavior, cognitive processes, or mental tension.

Psychosis—a mental disorder causing gross distortion of a person's emotional response and capacity to recognize reality, communicate, and relate to others.

Pyrogen—the by-products or remnants of bacteria that can cause severe reactions (e.g., fever and chills) in patients if injected in large enough amounts.

Quality Assurance—an ongoing, systematic process for monitoring, evaluating, and improving the quality of a service provided. Quality assurance activities are often used to identify problems and opportunities for improvement.

Reconstitute—adding a liquid to dissolve a powdered drug (e.g., lyophilized powder).

Rectal Route of Medication Administration—the route of medication administration where medications are inserted through the anus into the rectum. Rectal suppositories, enemas, and aerosol foams are administered via this route.

Registration—the process of making a list or being enrolled in an existing list. In an occupational setting, it may or may not be illegal to carry out a particular function without being registered.

Repackaging—the process of taking medication from one container and placing it into another container. Generally the original container is the manufacturer's bulk container.

Residency—a 1- or 2-year postgraduate training program where graduates from colleges of pharmacy gain additional clinical experience.

Rhinitis—inflammation of the nasal mucous membrane.

Route of Administration—the manner in which a drug is given (by mouth, injection, etc.) to a patient.

Route of Medication Administration—the manner in which a drug enters the body. A drug may be administered via any body orifice, through the skin, or artificially made opening.

Secondary References—indexing systems that provide a list of journal articles related to various topics. Secondary systems are used when new or very up-to-date information is required, or when no information can be located in tertiary references. Examples are Medline and International Pharmaceutical Abstracts (IPA)®.

Seizure—a convulsion; a violent spasm or series of jerkings of the face, trunk, or extremities.

Single-dose or Unit Dose Package—a package that contains one dose of the medication. This type of package could contain two tablets or two capsules of medication if that was the dose ordered.

Single-unit Package—a package that contains a single unit of medication. For example, one tablet, one syringe, one ampoule, one 2-ml volume of liquid, one 2-g mass of ointment, etc.

Small Volume Parenteral (SVP)—any parenteral solution 100 ml or less in volume.

Soft Gelatin Capsule—a soft, squeezable, elastic capsule filled with liquid, paste, or powdered medication.

Software—a set of programmed instructions that tells a computer what to do. A computer cannot do anything itself; it needs to know how to react to the input it gets from the user. Software provides that instruction.

Solid Medication Dosage Form—a medication dosage form in which the medication is delivered as a solid. It may be intended for oral use or use in other parts of the body. Examples of solid medication dosage forms include tablets, capsules, lozenges, ointments, suppositories, and creams.

Solution—an evenly distributed, homogeneous mixture of dissolved medication in a liquid vehicle where the molecules of a solid, liquid, or gaseous medication are equally distributed among the molecules of the liquid vehicle. A solution may be classified as aqueous, viscous aqueous, or nonaqueous.

Solvent—a liquid used to dissolve other substances (e.g., medication). Commonly used nonaqueous solvents include alcohol, glycerin, and propylene glycol.

Spend-down—a portion of prescription costs passed on to the patient by a third-party payer over a defined period of time. A spend-down requires a patient to spend a defined amount of out-of-pocket dollars on prescriptions within a year before the third party pays anything.

Spirit—a hydroalcoholic or alcoholic solution that contains volatile (easily evaporated) substances.

Spray—an aqueous solution delivered as a mist against the mucous membranes of the nose and throat.

Stat—an abbreviation of *statim*, which is Latin for immediately. Used by medical personnel to communicate an urgent need.

Status Epilepticus—a repeated seizure or a seizure prolonged for at least 30 minutes.

Sterile Compounding Area—a room for sterile product preparation that is functionally separate from nonsterile product preparation, and constructed to minimize particulate and microbial contamination. Usually has special procedures for cleanliness and disinfection, such as a dress code to minimize introduction of microorganisms or particulate matter; means of minimizing traffic flow; and procedures that also minimize the introduction of particulate matter.

Sterility—freedom from all living microorganisms and their spores.

Strip Package—a package that is formed by most automated oral solid repackaging machines. The package is so named because it comes off the machine in one continuous strip that is perforated between doses. Individual doses are removed by tearing the perforation.

Stroke—the result of an impaired blood supply to the brain caused by a blood clot or bleeding. Neurological symptoms (e.g., paralysis) are often caused by a stroke. The medical term is cerebrovascular accident.

Subcutaneous—a term that refers to tissue just beneath the skin.

Subcutaneous (SC, subQ, SQ) Route of Medication Administration—the route of medication administration that introduces medication beneath the skin by injection through a needle placed into the tissue immediately underneath the skin. Sometimes referred to as a hypodermic injection.

Sublingual Route of Medication Administration—the route of medication administration that introduces medication into the bloodstream through the underlining of the tongue.

Sublingual Tablet—a tablet that is placed under the tongue and quickly dissolved. The active drug is absorbed into the bloodstream through the underlining of the tongue.

Suspension—a mixture of finely divided particles of an undissolved solid distributed through a gas, liquid, or solid.

Syrup—a viscous aqueous solution that is a concentrated mixture of sugar and purified water. Syrups may contain flavoring agents or medication. A flavored syrup without a medication is known as a *nonmedicated syrup* and is intended for use as a vehicle for medications to be added later. A syrup that contains medication is known as a *medicated syrup*.

Tablet—a compacted solid medication dosage form.

Technician—a person skilled in the practical or mechanical aspects of a profession. A technician assists professionals in routine, day-to-day functions that do not require professional judgment.

Tertiary References—general references that present documented information in a condensed and compact format and may include a textbook, a CD-ROM system, or review articles.

Therapeutic Range—the concentration range of drug in the blood in which the drug is most effective and least toxic.

Tincture—an alcoholic or hydroalcoholic solution adjusted so that each milliliter of tincture contains the equivalent potency of 100 mg of crude drug. A tincture is prepared by the extraction method. It differs from a fluidextract or extract only in its potency.

Topical Route of Medication Administration—the route of medication administration that refers to the application of medication to the surface of the skin or mucous membranes. In most cases, topically administered medications are not intended to reach the bloodstream.

Total Parenteral Nutrition (TPN)—the intravenous administration of nutrients such as carbohydrates, fats, protein, electrolytes, trace elements, vitamins, and water needed to sustain life.

Trade Name—a proprietary (manufacturer specific) name given to a drug (it also called the brand name).

Transdermal Route of Medication Administration—the route of medication administration that delivers medication across the skin. Also known as the percutaneous route of medication administration.

Transdermal Patch—a medication formulation intended to deliver medication through the skin. The medicine is usually held to the skin by an adhesive patch and is absorbed over time via the transdermal route.

Troche—see Lozenge.

Unit-of-Use Packaging—a package that contains the necessary number of doses of medication for a specific period of treatment for a patient.

Vaginal Route of Medication Administration—the route of medication administration where medications are inserted into the vagina. Vaginal suppositories, tablets, creams, ointments, gels, and solutions are administered via this route.

Vaginal Tablet—a tablet that is inserted into the vagina.

Vehicle—the fluid or liquid medium that serves as a carrier or means of delivery for medication in a liquid medication dosage form. Common vehicles include water, alcohol, glycerin, and mineral oil.

Venipuncture—the puncture of a vein for any therapeutic purpose (e.g., blood draw, catheter insertion).

Venous Access Device—catheter that resides in a patient's vein through which medications or solutions are administered.

Venous Thrombosis—formation or presence of a blood clot within a vein.

Verbal Order—a prescription that is communicated orally by a prescriber (as opposed to a written order).

Vertical Laminar Airflow (LAF) Hood—special hood designed to blow highly filtered air vertically down onto a work surface, creating an ideal environment for the preparation of sterile products. Certain vertical LAF hoods are also designed to be biological safety cabinets, intended for use in preparation of cytotoxic or hazardous drugs.

Virus—a microorganism, usually much smaller than bacteria, which is incapable of growth or reproduction apart from living cells.

Viscous Aqueous Solution—a solution that employs purified water as its vehicle. It is usually sticky, thick, and sweet and is intended for oral ingestion.

Wash—a solution used to clean or bathe a body part (e.g., mouthwash, eyewash.)

Water-in-Oil (W/O) Emulsion—an emulsion where small water droplets (the internal phase) are dispersed throughout oil (the external phase).

Water-Soluble Base—a non-greasy, non-occlusive ointment base that is easily washed off with water. It does not contain any fat and usually does not contain any water.

Y-sites—name for injection ports on tubing sets that allow for administration of drugs or other solutions through the same tubing set. The injection port protrudes from the tubing and looks like a "Y."